PUBLIC HEALTH NUTRITION

Principles and Practice in Community and Global Health

EDITED BY

NATALIE STEIN, MS, MPH

Assistant Professor
Program in Public Health
Michigan State University
East Lansing, Michigan

JONES & BARTLETT
LEARNING

World Headquarters
Jones & Bartlett Learning
5 Wall Street
Burlington, MA 01803
978-443-5000
info@jblearning.com
www.jblearning.com

Jones & Bartlett Learning books and products are available through most bookstores and online booksellers. To contact Jones & Bartlett Learning directly, call 800-832-0034, fax 978-443-8000, or visit our website, www.jblearning.com.

Production Credits
Executive Publisher: William Brottmiller
Publisher: Michael Brown
Associate Editor: Chloe Falivene
Associate Production Editor: Rebekah Linga
Senior Marketing Manager: Sophie Fleck Teague
Manufacturing and Inventory Control Supervisor: Amy Bacus
Composition: Cenveo Publisher Services
Cover Design: Kristin E. Parker
Rights and Permissions Coordinator: Ashley Dos Santos
Cover Image: © iStockphoto/Thinkstock.
Printing and Binding: Edwards Brothers Malloy
Cover Printing: Edwards Brothers Malloy

Library of Congress Cataloging-in-Publication Data
Stein, Natalie, author.
 Public health nutrition : principles and practice in community and global health / Natalie Stein.
   p. ; cm.
 Includes bibliographical references and index.
 ISBN 978-1-4496-9204-9 (paperback)
 I. Title.
 [DNLM: 1. Nutritional Physiological Phenomena. 2. Malnutrition—prevention & control. 3. Public Health. 4. World Health. QU 145]
 RA441
 362.1—dc23
                          2013038790

6048
Printed in the United States of America
18 17 16 15 14   10 9 8 7 6 5 4 3 2 1

Contents

Preface

Nutrition is a global public health problem. Worldwide, one in eight individuals faces chronic hunger. Billions more suffer from micronutrient deficiencies, with consequences ranging from death, disability, and impaired growth and development, to reduced productivity and national economic development. Maternal and child health remains a leading global concern, largely because of malnutrition. More than half of deaths among infants and young children are related to malnutrition; 20% of maternal deaths are related to anemia. The impact of micronutrient deficiencies is also evident with vitamin A and iodine deficiencies, which are the leading causes of preventable blindness and cognitive impairment, respectively, worldwide.

Ironically, while many nations continue to struggle to provide enough food and nutrients to their populations, overnutrition is an increasing burden in nearly every part of the world. Low-, middle-, and high-income countries are experiencing increased rates of obesity, and over one-third of the world's adults are overweight. Obesity is a risk factor for chronic diseases such as cardiovascular disease, some cancers, diabetes, respiratory conditions, and osteoarthritis. Other nutritional factors, such as dietary fat composition, salt and sugar consumption, and consumption of vegetables, fruits, and whole grains, also affect risk for chronic diseases. Nearly two-thirds of the world's population lives in nations where chronic diseases kill more people than infectious diseases. Children are also at risk for obesity and chronic diseases.[1]

The field of public health nutrition is uniquely poised to meet these challenges. The international community increasingly recognizes the critical nature of nutrition in maintaining healthy populations and supporting national growth. International agencies, such as the World Health Organization (WHO) and other United Nations (UN) agencies and programs, and government agencies, such as the Department of Health and Human Services (DHHS) in the United States, include nutrition among their health priorities. Examples of public health nutrition programs include basic research, nutrition assistance, food aid, nutrition education, school meals, food fortification, supplementation, assessment, and surveillance. Public health strategies target populations and focus on prevention. Also at the core of public health are efforts to reduce the consequences of disparities, such as wealth. For example, in developing and industrialized nations alike, the poor are more likely to be food insecure and consume nutrient-poor diets.

This textbook uses the Millennium Development Goals (MDGs) (**Appendix 1**) and *Healthy People 2020* (HP 2020) objectives (**Appendix 2**) to provide an international and national context. Established in 2000 at the Millennium Summit of the United Nations, the MDGs are eight goals to reduce disparities in the world by the year 2015. Each goal is divided into more specific targets with benchmarks for progress.[2]

The DHHS publishes the U.S.-focused *Healthy People* objectives decennially based on the most pressing health problems in the nation, within the four overarching categories of general health status, health-related quality of life and well-being, determinants of health, and disparities. HP 2020 topics, such as Nutrition and Weight Status, Physical Activity, Early and Middle Childhood, and Heart Disease and Stroke, include multiple objectives to be reached by 2020. The *Healthy People* objectives also include consumer information, clinical strategies, and evidence-based resources for public health policy interventions.[3]

This book integrates the core competencies of public health professionals (**Appendix 3**). These competencies were revised in 2010 by the Council on Linkages between Academia and Public Health Practice, which represents universities, government agencies, and professional organizations relating to public health. The competencies are multidisciplinary skills that are referenced in this book to assist users in developing their confidence in public health settings.[4]

The first chapter places public health nutrition in a modern context through defining the field and introducing today's major issues. The next section lays the foundations for public health nutrition practice, including research methods, approaches to developing public health programs, and background on disparities and malnutrition worldwide. The next major part provides an overview of public health nutrition from birth through older adulthood. Obesity and chronic diseases are the focus of the book's next section. The final chapters look to the future, discussing the nutrition transition and strategies to absorb its impact in developing nations, changes in livelihoods, and nutritional status resulting from changes in land use, and the potential for telehealth to improve nutrition and health outcomes in communities worldwide.

Each chapter of the book begins with a case study that serves as an example of an application of one or more of the chapter's topics. Chapters provide an overview of the basic public health and nutrition concepts, and use multiple global examples to allow readers to see how public

health programs and theories can be applied and modified in specific situations at the community level.

The book surveys significant topics in public health nutrition and is intended for students and professionals with or without previous training in public health and/or nutrition. For these reasons, different chapters focus on various levels of public health infrastructure and public health venues, including research, government, international agencies, communities, and clinical settings. To further increase relevancy to a wide range of public health professionals, some chapters focus on the United States and other industrialized nations, while others emphasize developing nations.

There is reason to be hopeful. Through collaboration, the wise use of limited resources, and evidence-based solutions, leaders in public health can affect significant progress in health and nutrition in today's world. This book aims to help enable such efforts.

References

1 World Health Organization. (2013, March). *Fact sheet on obesity and overweight*. Fact Sheet No. 311. Retrieved from http://www.who.int/mediacentre/factsheets/fs311/en/index.html.

2 United Nations. (n.d.). *2015 Millennium Development Goals*. Retrieved from http://www.un.org/millenniumgoals.

3 U.S. Department of Health and Human Services, Healthypeople.gov website, http://www.healthypeople.gov/2020/default.aspx.

4 Public Health Foundation. (n.d.). *Core competencies for public health professionals*. Retrieved from http://www.phf.org/Pages/default.aspx.

Acknowledgments

Thank you to each contributing author for making this book possible. I am indebted to you for sharing your expertise and experience while continuing to fulfill your personal obligations of teaching, researching, and participating in public health nutrition programs. Because of your dedication, this is truly a global book written by experts from all areas of public health nutrition.

I also want to acknowledge the staff at Jones & Bartlett Learning for their roles in facilitating this book. Chloe Falivene, Rebekah Linga, Ashley Dos Santos, and Mike Brown, in particular, moved the project forward. In addition, many reviewers, who are anonymous to me, provided insightful suggestions to greatly improve this book.

I want to thank the Michigan State University Program in Public Health for its support. Dr. Mike Rip was always willing to answer my questions and give me advice. Librarian Abraham Wheeler enthusiastically suggested numerous valuable resources on various topics in this book.

I am very grateful to Mindy Liberman, a professional librarian with more than 30 years of experience, for her countless hours of assistance. She reliably prepared references, proofread the manuscript, and organized the figures and tables, all in her usual cheerful and professional way. Thank you, Mom!

My father, Robert Stein, has always been my greatest source of support and best friend, and my sister, Robin Stein, is the smartest, most humble, and most selfless person I know. Thank you, Dad and Robin, for encouraging me while helping me keep perspective. Dad, thank you also for proofreading this book! I dedicate this book to Dad, Mom, and Robin.

Contributors

Farzana Afroze, MBBS
Senior Clinical Fellow
Centre for Nutrition and Food
   Security
International Centre for Diarrhoeal
   Disease Research
Dhaka, Bangladesh

Tahmeed Ahmed, MBBS, PhD
Director and Senior Scientist
Centre for Nutrition and Food
   Security
International Centre for Diarrhoeal
   Disease Research
Professor of Public Health Nutrition
James P. Grant School of Public Health
BRAC University
Dhaka, Bangladesh

**Mohammed K. Ali, MBchB, MSc,
MBA**
Assistant Professor
Departments of Global Health and
   Epidemiology
Rollins School of Public Health
Emory University
Atlanta, Georgia

Richmond Aryeetey, PhD, MPH
Senior Lecturer
Department of Population, Family,
   and Reproductive Health
School of Public Health
University of Ghana
Legon, Accra, Ghana

Hasan Ashraf, MBBS, MCPS, MD
Senior Scientist
Centre for Nutrition and Food
   Security
International Centre for Diarrhoeal
   Disease Research
Dhaka, Bangladesh

Odilia I. Bermudez, PhD, MPH, LND
Associate Professor
Department of Public Health and
   Community Medicine
Tufts University School of Medicine
Boston, Massachusetts

**Mohammod Jobayer Chisti, MBBS,
MMed**
Scientist
International Centre for Diarrhoeal
   Disease Research
Dhaka, Bangladesh

Juliana F. W. Cohen, ScD, ScM
Research Fellow
Department of Nutrition
Harvard School of Public Health
Boston, Massachusetts

Matthew B. Cross, MA
Department of Health and Human
   Performance
University of Houston
Houston, Texas

Kirsten K. Davison, PhD
Associate Professor
Departments of Nutrition and Social
   and Behavioral Sciences
Harvard School of Public Health
Boston, Massachusetts

Jennifer Falbe, MPH, ScD
Doctoral Candidate
Departments of Nutrition and
   Epidemiology
Harvard School of Public Health
Boston, Massachusetts

**Abu Syed Golam Faruque, MBBS,
MPH**
Consultant

Centre for Nutrition and Food
   Security
International Centre for Diarrhoeal
   Disease Research
Dhaka, Bangladesh

P. Greg Gulick, JD, MHA, MBA
Assistant Professor
Program in Public Health
Michigan State University
East Lansing, Michigan

**Rukhsana Haider, MBBS, MSc,
IBCLC, PhD**
Chairperson
Training and Assistance for
   Health and Nutrition (TAHN)
   Foundation
Dhaka, Bangladesh

Allen M. Hallett, BS
Texas Obesity Research Center
Department of Health and Human
   Performance
University of Houston
Houston, Texas

**Md. Iqbal Hossain, MBBS, DCH,
PhD**
Senior Scientist
Centre for Nutrition and Food
   Security
International Centre for Diarrhoeal
   Disease Research
Adjunct Faculty
James P. Grant School of Public Health
BRAC University
Dhaka, Bangladesh

Md. Munirul Islam, MBBS, PhD
Scientist
Centre for Nutrition and Food
   Security

International Centre for Diarrhoeal
  Disease Research
Dhaka, Bangladesh

Melissa Johnson, PhD, MS
College of Agriculture, Environment,
  and Nutrition Sciences
Tuskegee University
Tuskegee, Alabama

Shweta Khandelwal, PhD, MSc
Research Scientist and Adjunct
  Assistant Professor
Public Health Foundation of India
New Delhi, India

Stephen Kodish, MS
Department of International Health
Johns Hopkins Bloomberg School of
  Public Health
Baltimore, Maryland

Sumon Kumar Das, MBBS
Assistant Scientist
Centre for Nutrition and Food
  Security
International Centre for Diarrhoeal
  Disease Research
Dhaka, Bangladesh
PhD Candidate
School of Population Health
The University of Queensland
Herston, Queensland, Australia

Amos Laar, PhD, MPH
Senior Lecturer
Department of Population, Family,
  and Reproductive Health
School of Public Health
University of Ghana
Legon, Accra, Ghana

Heather J. Leach, PhD
Postdoctoral Fellow
Faculty of Kinesiology
University of Calgary
Calgary, Alberta, Canada

Tracey A. Ledoux, PhD, RD
Assistant Professor

Department of Health and Human
  Performance
University of Houston
Houston, Texas

Rebecca E. Lee, PhD
Professor
College of Nursing and Health
  Innovation
Arizona State University
Phoenix, Arizona

Seung Hee Lee-Kwan, PhD, MS, LD
Program Coordinator
Department of International Health
Johns Hopkins Bloomberg School of
  Public Health
Baltimore, Maryland
Adjunct Assistant Professor
Department of Global Community
  Health and Behavioral Sciences
Tulane School of Public Health and
  Tropical Medicine
New Orleans, Louisiana

Hala Madanat, PhD
Associate Professor and Chair
Division of Health Promotion and
  Behavior Science
Graduate School of Public Health
San Diego State University
Deputy Director
San Diego Prevention Research Center
San Diego, California

Scherezade K. Mama, DrPH
Postdoctoral Fellow
Department of Health Disparities
  Research
The University of Texas M.D.
  Anderson Cancer Center
Houston, Texas

Grace S. Marquis, PhD, LLD (*hc*)
Associate Professor and Canadian
  Research Chair in Social and
  Environmental Aspects of
  Nutrition
School of Dietetics and Human
  Nutrition

McGill University
Montreal, Quebec, Canada

Iyas Masannat, RPh, MS
Adjunct Assistant Professor
San Diego State University
San Diego, California

Tabashir Z. Nobari, MPH
PhD Student
Department of Community Health
  Sciences
Fielding School of Public Health
University of California at Los Angeles
Los Angeles, California

Ralphenia D. Pace, PhD, RD, LD
Professor
Department of Food and Nutritional
  Sciences
Tuskegee University
Tuskegee, Alabama

Nathan H. Parker, MPH
Research Assistant
Texas Obesity Research Center
Department of Health and Human
  Performance
University of Houston
Houston, Texas

Tina G. Sanghvi, PhD
Country Programs Director
Alive & Thrive Initiative
Washington, DC

Aenor J. Sawyer, MD, MS
Assistant Clinical Professor
Department of Othropaedic Surgery
Director
UCSF Skeletal Health Service
Director
Pediatric Bone Health Consortium
University of California, San Francisco
San Francisco, California

Karen R. Siegel, MPH
Nutrition and Health Sciences, Laney
  Graduate School, and Hubert
  Department of Global Health

Emory University
Atlanta, Georgia

Erica G. Soltero, BA
Texas Obesity Research Center
Department of Health and Human
 Performance
University of Houston
Houston, Texas

Lyn M. Steffen, PhD, MPH, RD
Associate Professor
School of Public Health
Division of Epidemiology and
 Community Health
University of Minnesota
Minneapolis, Minnesota

Elizabeth Stites, PhD
Senior Researcher
Feinstein International Center
Tufts University
Somerville, Massachusetts

Emily Mitchard Turano, MS, MPH

Kirstin R. Vollrath, RD, LD
Department of Health and Human
 Performance
University of Houston
Houston, Texas

May C. Wang, MA, DrPH
Associate Professor
Department of Community Health
 Sciences
Fielding School of Public Health
University of California at Los Angeles
Los Angeles, California

**Heather Wasser, PhD, MPH, RD,
IBCLC**
Project Director
Center for Women's Health Research
University of North Carolina at
 Chapel Hill
Chapel Hill, North Carolina

Hope Weiler, RD, PhD
Associate Professor
School of Dietetics and Human
 Nutrition
McGill University
Montreal, Quebec, Canada

Pattanee Winichagoon, PhD
Associate Professor
Community/International Nutrition
Institute of Nutrition
Mahidol University
Salaya, Nakhon Pathom, Thailand

Suzanna A. Young, RD, MPH
Wellness Director (Retired)
North Carolina Department of Health
 and Human Services
Raleigh, North Carolina

Introduction to Public Health Nutrition

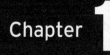
Introduction to Public Health Nutrition

Natalie Stein, MS, MPH

"Let food be thy medicine and medicine be thy food."—Hippocrates, 400 B.C.

Learning Objectives

- Define public health nutrition.
- Identify the role of public health nutrition in addressing the core functions of public health and the 10 essential public health services.
- Place public health nutrition in the context of global public health efforts.
- Recognize current and emerging global concerns in public health nutrition.
- Understand the roles of nutritionists and others who may be involved in public health nutrition efforts.

Case Studies: A Typical Monday in the Lives of Two Mothers

Case Study: Nicole, Los Angeles, California, United States

On this Monday morning in Los Angeles, California, 30-year-old Nicole wakes up at 5:00 a.m. to get ready for work. She lives with her 11-year-old son, John; her 3-year-old daughter, Paula; and her mother, Sarah, in a two-bedroom apartment. Nicole is a single mother.

Nicole leaves the apartment at 5:30 a.m. She rarely takes breakfast with her to work because she is in a rush and she knows that she can quickly get an inexpensive breakfast sandwich or burrito at any of the fast-food restaurants near her workplace, a courthouse in Los Angeles about

10 miles away from her mother's apartment. John participates in the national **School Breakfast Program (SBP)** and **National School Lunch Program (NSLP)**, and will eat a free breakfast at school, probably including cereal, a breakfast sandwich or burrito with cheese, egg, and sausage, or pancakes or waffles with sausage and syrup. After he leaves for school, Sarah will have fried eggs, with toast, and give her granddaughter cereal and whole milk. For lunch, the two of them usually have sandwiches with processed meat and American cheese, peanut butter and jelly sandwiches, or tortillas filled with ground beef and cheese. Sometimes they add some canned vegetables or potato chips. Sarah and Paula both enjoy oranges, bananas, and watermelon for snacks. Common options for John's school lunch include pasta with meat, turkey burgers, and sandwiches, served with a vegetable, a fruit, and reduced-fat milk.

Nicole does not have a car, so she walks a couple of blocks to the bus stop, catches the bus, and walks three blocks at the other end. She works as a cashier and dishwasher in a cafeteria in the basement of the courthouse from 6:30 a.m. to 3:30 p.m., Monday through Friday. She wishes that she could stay home with Paula as she did with John when he was little, but knows she can count on her mother to take good care of her. At work, Nicole gets free soft drinks and a $5 credit to use at the cafeteria for lunch. She usually gets the daily special, often a fried chicken sandwich or hamburger that comes with onion rings or French fries.

When she gets out of work, Nicole takes the bus back to her neighborhood. Because her neighborhood has a high crime rate, she is always grateful that her work hours allow her to get home before dark. On her walk home from the bus station, she buys a beef tamale from a local Mexican fast-food restaurant for her mother to take for dinner. Sarah leaves for her evening job as a custodian in a local elementary school, and Nicole gets to spend the evening with John and Paula. For dinner, Nicole makes macaroni and cheese from a box and serves it with frozen greens that she serves with butter.

After John finishes his homework and he and Paula go to bed, Nicole watches television to help her relax. She has a few cookies during the evening before going to bed at 10:30 p.m. Her mother will be home around 11:00 p.m. Sometimes Nicole thinks about going back to school, as she used to dream of, but she does not see how it can be possible when she and her mother are both working minimum-wage jobs to provide for John and Paula.

With a **body mass index (BMI)** of 31, Nicole is classified as obese. Since she has no health insurance and rarely visits a doctor, she does not know that her blood sugar levels are in the category of prediabetes. John is of normal weight, but Paula is already overweight. Sarah is also obese, and is on medications to control her high blood pressure.

Case Study: Buseje, Shire Highlands, Great Rift Valley, Malawi

On this same Monday morning, Buseje wakes up at dawn, 10,000 miles away from Nicole and Paula. She lives in a two-room thatched hut with her husband, her 8-year-old daughter, her 5-year-old son, and the 4-year-old boy who used to be their neighbor. Now, he is an orphan; the boy's mother died giving birth to him, and his father died from malaria last year. Buseje treats him like one of her own children, as is typical of how members of this community care for each other. He is about the same age as her second daughter would have been if she had not succumbed to malaria at the age of 2 years.

Millennium Development Goal 6: Combat HIV/AIDS, Malaria and Other Diseases. Target 6.C: Have halted by 2015 and begun to reverse the incidence of malaria and other major diseases

Reproduced from the United Nations. (n.d.). 2015 Millennium Development Goals. Retrieved from http://www.un.org/millenniumgoals/. Accessed August 13, 2013. This source is used for all Millennium Development Goals in this chapter.

Buseje makes breakfast for the family over the fire outside their home. They have a watery gruel, called *nsima*, made with corn meal. She gives the children and her husband some tea with sugar. She does all of the cooking over a fire in an adjacent room; only 9% of Malawi has electricity, and rates in rural areas range from 1–3% of households.[1] Her daughter joins the village schoolchildren as they pass by Buseje's hut on their walk to school. When there is too much work to be done at home, Buseje's daughter skips school. Although public school is free in Malawi, half of schoolchildren do not complete fourth grade.[2]

Millennium Development Goal 5: Improve Maternal Health. Target 5.A: Reduce by three-quarters the maternal mortality ratio

Buseje always puts the needs of her children and husband before her own needs. The warm, humid season in Malawi goes from November to April, and today, a day in October, marks the sixth month without rain. The family has been without much dietary diversity for weeks now. They still have plenty of corn and cassava, but not much else. Buseje suffers from iron-deficiency anemia, which makes her tired and susceptible to infections. Her children are already deficient not only in iron, but also in vitamin A. **Stunting** and **wasting** remain prevalent despite the nutrition rehabilitation units that are part of the World Food Programme's Country Program to fight malnutrition in Malawi.[3]

Millennium Development Goal 1: Eradicate Extreme Poverty and Hunger. Target 1.A: Halve, between 1990 and 2015, the proportion of people who suffer from hunger

During the day, Buseje watches the younger children. They feed the chickens, gather firewood, and then go to the market, where Buseje exchanges some fish for some fruit. After a lunch of more *nsima* and fruit, Buseje repairs a hole in the roof of their thatched-roof hut. This will help them stay dry during the coming rainy season. Buseje's daughter comes home from school, and her husband returns from the village, where he spent the day with the other men from the village. Buseje and her daughter serve *nsima*, some goat meat, and tea with sugar.

Discussion Questions

- Which nutritional concerns and associated health consequences do the women and their families face?
- What are the underlying causes of suboptimal diets and health for Nicole and Buseje?
- Which public health programs are available to assist the two women and their families?
- Which nutritional challenges do Nicole, Buseje, and their respective families face due to economic, racial/ethnic, geographic, gender, and other disparities?

Introduction

Adequate food and water are basic human needs. Sufficient energy (measured in calories), protein, fat, carbohydrates, water, vitamins, and minerals are necessary for preventing deficiencies, allowing proper growth, maintenance of body weight, and physiological function. Nutritional status is a significant determinant of health status. Malnutrition was, until recently, the main nutrition concern worldwide. Overnutrition, associated with obesity and chronic diseases, has now emerged as a significant and growing threat. Some regions simultaneously experience the presence and effects of undernutrition and overnutrition.

Each day consists of actions that affect dietary intake and nutritional status, but, as the above case studies illustrate, individual dietary behaviors vary greatly. Dietary patterns such as high consumption of added sugars, solid fats, and sodium, and low intakes of vegetables and whole grains put Nicole, and her family, at risk for obesity and chronic diseases that are prevalent in the United States and other industrialized nations. In contrast, Buseje's diet, frequently consisting of low energy intake and insufficient micronutrients due to poor dietary diversity, places her at risk for **underweight**, infections, and nutrient deficiency diseases. Each mother in the case studies could improve her nutrition status with healthier diet choices, but these choices are not always within an individual's capacity. Factors interfering with optimal nutrition may include the following:

- Inadequate knowledge about nutrient needs and how to meet them.
- High food cost or low personal income, making nutritious foods unaffordable.

- Lack of availability of nutritious foods for reasons such as lack of roads or means of transportation, seasonal unavailability, drought, natural disasters, war, and inability to store food.

Public health targets populations, with the objective of improving individuals' lives. Public health nutrition programs can lead to improvements in each of the mothers' diets and nutritional status, as well as better health, increased productivity, and higher quality of life.

- Nutrition education programs could help Nicole improve her choices for herself and her family. Improvements can include choosing more vegetables and whole grains, ordering lower-fat, lower-calorie menu items, and getting more physical activity. These changes could help her maintain a healthy weight, thus lowering the risk for obesity-related diseases.
- Nutrition assistance programs could provide healthy foods and information on how to use them. Interdisciplinary programs can help reduce crime rates and improve neighborhood sidewalks. Helpful policies could include a requirement for workplace cafeterias to sell low-cost healthy foods. These programs could help Nicole, her mother, and her daughter to eat better and exercise more.
- More widespread nutrition and community-based livelihood programs could lead to increased availability of nutritious foods in Malawi, while increased gender equality could lead to a greater contribution from Buseje's husband and a proportionate share of the nutritious foods for Buseje.

This chapter defines public health nutrition using an accepted definition of public health as a foundation, and expands on the basic concept. The chapter will also introduce some of the current primary nutrition-related concerns worldwide and the scope of public health programs in addressing them. Finally, identification of various careers pertinent to public health nutrition can engage readers from a variety of backgrounds in the book's content and assist them in planning their own careers.

What Is Public Health Nutrition?

Public health does not have a formal universal definition; rather, it is often described by its theories, roles, objectives, and/or approaches. Charles-Edward A. Winslow, an influential American bacteriologist, was an early and strong supporter of public health. His description from 1920 is still accurate today. According to Winslow, public health is:

> the science and the art of preventing disease, prolonging life, and promoting physical health and efficiency through organized community efforts of the sanitation of the environment, the control of community infections, the education of the individual in principles of personal hygiene, the organization of medical and nursing services for the early diagnosis and preventive treatment of disease, and the development of the social machinery which will ensure to every individual in the community a standard of living adequate for the maintenance of health.[4]

Reproduced from Winslow, C. E. A. (1920). The untilled field of public health. *Modern Medicine, 2*, 183.

No single, universally accepted definition of public health nutrition exists, but it can be described by adapting Winslow's portrayal of public health to the arena of nutrition. This will be done in the following sections.

"the science and the art..."

Science is objective, and art is subjective. This description of public health is just as appropriate for public health nutrition. Nutrition is the study of nutrient digestion, absorption, transportation, metabolism, and storage in the body and excretion from the body. This science recognizes six classes of nutrients: water, carbohydrates, fat, protein, vitamins, and minerals. The objective nutritional sciences, drawing on sciences such as biology, biochemistry, and immunology, describe nutrient metabolism and function, human requirements for energy and nutrients, and food sources of nutrients.

As much as possible, public health nutrition programs should be evidence-based, the product of gathering evidence through scientific studies and critical appraisal of that evidence.[5]

Nutritional epidemiology generates data on nutrition and health outcomes in populations through observational studies and experimental trials. Epidemiologists study population-wide patterns, such as prevalence and changes in patterns, and investigate possible causes. Biostatisticians use data to assess and identify widespread nutritional deficiencies or unhealthy eating patterns, draw conclusions about potential relationships between dietary intake and health outcomes, monitor nutrient status in populations, and design and evaluate interventions.

Public health nutrition is a combination of science and art. Existing scientific evidence regarding a specific nutritional issue is not always complete or consistent; even when it is, the healthiest course is not always taken. Returning to the second case study as an example, gender equality generally is associated with increased societal productivity and better nutrition and health; however, persistent disparities in gender roles continue to harm Malawian families like Buseje's. The art of public health nutrition may be necessary to understand and overcome political, logistical, and cultural barriers before science-based public health nutrition interventions can be successful.

"... of preventing disease, prolonging life, and promoting physical health and efficiency..."

While clinical healthcare in general and clinical nutrition in particular focus on treatment and rehabilitation, public health and, more specifically, public health nutrition emphasize disease prevention and promotion of well-being. More than half of the world's population is malnourished and currently experiencing or at risk for experiencing nutrition-related diseases. Consumption of adequate quantities of nutritious food reduces protein-energy malnutrition and nutrient deficiency diseases and infectious diseases. In contrast, overnutrition leads to obesity, which affects 500 million adults worldwide[6] and increases the risk of chronic diseases, such as type 2 diabetes, heart disease, and cancer, which are expected to threaten more than two-thirds of the world's population by 2020.[7] Public health nutrition focuses on healthy eating to prevent these diseases and minimize their effects.

The availability and accessibility of sufficient healthy foods, and encouragement of people to eat them, fall within the domain of public health nutrition.

"... through organized community efforts..."

Community-based approaches allow programs to reach large numbers of people. A pediatrician's recommendation that a child be provided with more foods high in calcium and vitamin D, for example, may result in that child's parents seeking more food sources. On a larger scale, a national policy requiring that fortified milk, a high-calcium food, contain vitamin D, together with a national school meal program that includes vitamin D–fortified milk, can result in improved calcium and vitamin D status for millions of schoolchildren.

A vitamin A supplementation program serves as an example of efforts that require careful organization as well as support by various community members to be successful. An intervention designed to reduce vitamin A deficiency among schoolchildren includes children who receive supplements, parents who encourage their children to take them, teachers who dispense the supplements, physicians to oversee local programs, public health educators to explain why the supplements are needed and how to take them, and government at various levels to regulate and administer the program.

> **Public Health Core Competency 4: Cultural Competency Skills 2: Recognizes the role of cultural, social, and behavioral factors in the accessibility, availability, acceptability, and delivery of public health services**
>
> Reproduced from Council on Linkages Between Academia and Public Health Practice. 2010 May. Core Competencies for Public Health Professionals. Washington, DC: Public Health Foundation. http://www.phf.org/resourcestools/Documents/Core_Competencies_for_Public_Health_Professionals_2010May.pdf. Accessed August 13, 2013. This source is used for all Public Health Core Competencies in this chapter.

> **Public Health Core Competency 5: Community Dimensions of Practice Skills 3: Identifies stakeholders**

"... of the sanitation of the environment, the control of community infections, the education of the individual in principles of personal hygiene..."

A premise of public health is that individuals and communities require wholesome environments to be healthy. Interventions can include regulations on pollutants, vaccinations, and education on—and facilities for—handwashing. More specific to nutrition are clean water for drinking and irrigation and clean soil for crops. Prevention of nutrient deficiencies, such as vitamin A and iron, can reduce the impact of infectious diseases, such as diarrheal diseases, which currently kill millions of children annually worldwide. Education on handwashing and other personal hygiene measures can reduce foodborne illness. A clean environment

and personal hygiene can mitigate millions of annual cases of food poisoning and illness due to contaminated water.[8,9,10]

"... the organization of medical and nursing services..."

Health care is basic to health. To effectively reach the public, rather than just a privileged minority, medical and nursing services must be organized into functional health-care systems. Along with care facilities and medical supplies, infrastructure required to deliver the 10 essential public health services includes "a capable and qualified workforce,"[11] which can be achieved with a greater number and consistency of education programs for health professionals, such as more dietetics programs. "Up-to-date data and information systems" may include laws requiring better records as well as use of the latest technology, such as mobile health applications for smartphones that allow patients to remotely interact with dietitians to manage diabetes through diet. "Public health agencies capable of assessing and responding to public health needs" require funding to operate, authority to respond to needs, and regulations outlining administration and duties.

> **Healthy People 2020: Objective PHI 4: Increase the proportion of 4-year colleges and universities that offer public health or related majors and/or minors**
> **Healthy People 2020: Objective PHI 8: (Developmental) Increase the proportion of Healthy People 2020 objectives that are tracked regularly at the national level**
>
> Reproduced from the U.S. Department of Health and Human Services. Healthypeople.gov. Retrieved from http://www.healthypeople.gov/2020/default.aspx. Last updated July 30, 2013. Accessed August 13, 2013.

"... for the early diagnosis and preventive treatment of disease..."

With its focus on prevention, public health can be thought of as "going upstream." Rather than intervening downstream, when people are already in need of treatment, public health attempts to intervene upstream, nearer to the source of health threats, to promote favorable and prevent poor health outcomes as much as possible. **Primary prevention** targets healthy individuals to prevent diseases and their risk factors. An example is the mandatory addition of thiamin (vitamin B1), riboflavin (vitamin B2), and niacin

"upstream effect"

(vitamin B3) to fortified grains in the United States to prevent deficiencies of these nutrients among healthy adults. **Secondary prevention**, which often includes screening to enable early detection of risk factors, targets individuals with risk factors to prevent the disease from developing. With objectives including reduced mortality from heart disease and better management and awareness of blood cholesterol levels by patients and health professionals, the National Cholesterol Education Program (NCEP) promotes regular screening for and rapid treatment of high cholesterol levels, a risk factor for heart disease.[12] **Tertiary prevention** aims to prevent or delay complications of a disease. Children with night blindness, an early sign of vitamin A deficiency, can be given vitamin A supplements to prevent progression to permanent blindness and/or death.

Early diagnosis and preventive treatment are also evident in surveillance programs. National surveys for surveillance include the National Health and Nutrition Examination Survey (NHANES) in the United States[13] and the China Health and Nutrition Survey (CHNS).[14] Such surveys can expose trends such as changes in nutritional status and their potential relationships with social patterns, policy changes, and economic patterns. The United Nations Administrative Committee on Coordination/Subcommittee on Nutrition identifies long-term program planning, timely warning (for example, early warning of famine conditions to allow for implementation of emergency food aid), and program management as additional purposes of nutrition surveillance.[15]

> **". . . and the development of the social machinery which will ensure to every individual in the community a standard of living adequate for the maintenance of health."**

Public health nutrition programs are cooperative social efforts. They can include government at national, state, and local levels; private sector entities; families or other target populations; community leaders, such as religious leaders and nonprofit organizations. A school-based community garden program, for example, might be targeted toward elementary school children in a low-income neighborhood. In addition to involving the children and their teachers, the project might involve parents, who could volunteer to help with the gardening; local stores, which could donate seeds and tools; media, which could publicize the program; and local council members, who could advocate for continued funding.

The infrastructure supporting medical services must not only exist but be accessible in order to be effective for the public. Supplementary nutrition programs increase the likelihood of low-income households receiving enough food. Referral programs, such as the Women, Infants, and Children (WIC) program in the United States, can assess nutritional status of participants and refer to needed medical services. Developing nations may struggle to provide their communities with food or nutrition education for reasons including remoteness, political turmoil, and lack of adequate foods.

Core Functions and Essential Public Health Services

The **core functions** of public health are **assessment**, **policy development**, and **assurance**. The Institute of Medicine has identified 10 essential public health services that fulfill these functions.[16]

Essential Public Health Services and Examples Within Assessment

1. Monitor health status to identify community health problems.
   Example: National surveys can assess diet intake and nutritional status measures to identify potential problems, such as obesity, nutrient deficiencies, and chronic disease prevalence.[17]

2. Diagnose and investigate health problems and health hazards in the community.
   Example: Ongoing surveys can identify alarming trends, such as increases in obesity rates or nutrient deficiencies, or widening disparities between different communities.

Essential Public Health Services and Examples Within Policy Development

3. Inform, educate, and empower people about health issues.
   Example: Messages regarding healthy food choices, such as encouragement to consume three high-calcium foods per day, delivered through media such as billboards, social media, and newspaper and television campaigns; in addition, healthcare providers can distribute similar messages via brochures provided by campaign leaders.

4. Mobilize community partnerships to identify and solve health problems.

   Example: Health fairs are collaborative opportunities. Employers and local businesses can sponsor the events, schools can host them, healthcare providers can provide screenings and information on health resources, dietitians can supply educational materials on healthy eating, and children and parents can participate in activities such as healthy cooking classes, gardening, and a fun walk.

5. Develop policies and plans that support individual and community health efforts.

   Example: To support a fortification program aimed at schoolchildren, the national government might require all schools to provide fortified foods in school meals in order to receive government reimbursement.

Essential Public Health Services and Examples Within Assurance

6. Enforce laws and regulations that protect health and ensure safety.

   Example: State and local health departments can regularly inspect[18] providers that administer public health programs, such as food retailers that participate in the Supplemental Nutrition Assistance Program to supply low-income households with food.

7. Link people to needed personal health services and ensure the provision of health care when otherwise unavailable.

   Example: Medicare, the U.S. federal health insurance program for adults over age 65 and individuals with disabilities, covers medical nutrition therapy for patients with diabetes whose doctors refer them, and diabetes management education and supplies for individuals with diabetes.[19]

8. Assure a competent public health and personal healthcare workforce.

   Example: Public health degree programs can include standardized objectives, such as the core competencies of public health.

9. Evaluate effectiveness, accessibility, and quality of personal and population-based health services.

   Example: Regular program evaluation, which may consider cost-effectiveness; outcomes such as dietary intake, blood sugar, or serum folate; or program reach, can allow programs to be improved, expanded, and/or modified.

10. Research for new insights and innovative solutions to health problems.

    Example: The Health Professionals Follow-up Study (HPFS)[20] and Nurses' Health Study,[21] led by Harvard School of Public Health with funding from the National Cancer Institute, include more than three decades' worth of data investigating diet–disease relationships. This information can be used to develop policies and public health recommendations.

Courtesy of NPHPS/CDC.

The Global Public Health Nutrition Landscape

International organizations, such as the World Health Organization (WHO) within the United Nations (UN), may coordinate emergency food aid and micronutrient supplement programs and work with communities and nations to implement successful programs.[22] National and state governments collect surveillance data, provide technical assistance as needed, evaluate programs, and develop and enforce policies, such as allotment of funds for nutrition assistance programs. Local entities, such as local health departments, schools, and food banks, are responsible for directly supplying health services, such as enrollment for nutrition assistance programs, provision of school meals, and referrals to healthcare providers. Nonprofit and volunteer organizations, university extension programs, workplaces, and hospitals are additional partners in improving the public's nutrition.

Traditionally, the major global nutrition concern was undernutrition. Hunger and protein deficiencies cause mortality, stunting, wasting, and underweight, and impair immune function. **Micronutrient** deficiencies also increase risk of mortality and infections, and specific vitamin and mineral deficiency diseases have their own consequences. Better nutrition knowledge and public health programs, such as surveillance, food fortification, and nutrition education, have greatly reduced or virtually eliminated certain deficiencies in many parts of the world; for example, **pellagra**, or deficiency of niacin (vitamin B3), is rare among healthy Americans due to grain fortification programs, and mandatory universal salt iodation can effectively eliminate endemic **goiter** due to iodine deficiency. However, hunger and protein and micronutrient deficiencies remain prevalent in developing nations. Deficiencies of iron, iodine, and vitamin A affect billions worldwide and can increase risk of death, blindness, infections, impaired cognitive and physical growth, and numerous other morbidities.[23] Various forms of undernutrition are familiar to Buseje, introduced in the second case study at the beginning of this chapter, and her community.

While continuing efforts to reduce undernutrition, global public health nutrition attention must increasingly be paid to overnutrition. Since 1980, obesity and overweight have doubled in prevalence worldwide, and 35% of adults are overweight or obese.[24] Obesity is not only a grave problem in wealthy nations; as developing nations experience the **nutrition transition**, they face the **dual burden of malnutrition**, or coexistence of obesity and undernutrition. Obesity increases the risk for numerous noncommunicable chronic diseases (NCDs), such as heart disease, diabetes, stroke, and osteoarthritis, and NCDs are now responsible for more than half of all deaths in the world.[25] Many of these deaths and diseases are preventable with improved diet, including weight control, and physical activity, which are WHO public health priorities.[26] Nicole and her family, introduced in the first case study at the beginning of this chapter, experience many of the nutritional and health concerns attributable to a Westernized diet and lifestyle.

Maternal and child nutrition is another area with increasing recognition of its significance. Maternal malnutrition can lead to poor pregnancy outcomes such as maternal perinatal death and **low birthweight (LBW)** or premature babies. Breastfed infants can develop nutrient deficiencies if maternal nutritional status is not adequate. Another way to improve infant health is by promoting **exclusive breastfeeding** and eventually the appropriate addition of **complementary foods** to the infant's diet. Public health nutrition, supplementary food, education, and policy programs can address these and other areas, such as nutrition for children in preschool and grade school. The WHO's Global Targets 2025 "to improve maternal, infant and young child nutrition" include reducing maternal anemia, reducing stunting and wasting, increasing exclusive breastfeeding, reducing LBW incidence, and avoiding an increase in childhood overweight.[27]

Careers in Public Health Nutrition

Whether the concern is obesity, chronic diseases, micronutrient deficiencies, suboptimal maternal and young children nutrition, chronic undernutrition, or acute malnutrition in emergency situations, public health nutrition relies on numerous professionals with diverse background and talents, and varying degrees of training specifically in public health and nutrition. The public health nutrition workforce carries out the essential functions of public health. People involved in any particular public health nutrition program depend on the community-specific factors such as needs, resources, culture, and history. They can work in clinics and hospitals, state and local health departments, government agencies, food manufacturers and health clubs in the private sector, schools, workplaces, faith-based and other community organizations, and research institutions.

Professionals specifically trained in nutrition or dietetics can work with any of the above institutions. Health educators can deliver messages to patients, employees, healthcare professionals, and students in hospitals, university extension programs, grade schools, and workshops. Sample topics include diet and exercise for diabetes management, weight loss and/or control, prenatal nutrient needs, and healthy cooking. Lactation consultants promote and facilitate breastfeeding through education and support. Specialists in specific life stages can assist with menu planning in schools, hospitals, and senior centers.

Because of the scope of nutrition problems, public health professionals both with and without much formal nutrition training are likely to be directly or tangentially involved in public health scenarios related to nutrition. Researchers design, conduct, and analyze data from scientific studies, and epidemiologists also examine surveillance data to identify potential areas of concern and the effects of public health programs.

Other experts may seem farther afield, but they are just as critical. Economists can guide cost-effective programs as well as make policy recommendations based on larger regional, national, and international interests. Land use and transportation experts, agriculturists, and urban planners help develop communities that make the best use of their food resources and have the roads and transportation available so that individuals can access food sources and so that food can be transported in and out of the region as needed. Environmentalists need consider implications for food production as they develop land use policies. Politicians and advocates influence policy decisions ranging from healthcare benefits, nutrition labeling requirements, and funding of research and other programs to requirements for school meals.

Conclusion

Poor nutrition is among the leading global causes of mortality and morbidity, with obesity, chronic and acute undernutrition, and nutrient deficiencies threatening more than half of the world's population. Nutritional status can be improved, but community-based, population-level efforts are required to have significant impact. Governments, nonprofit and community organizations, universities, and the private sector can effectively collaborate to develop programs with greater and more lasting impact than individuals' own efforts.

References

1 U.S. Department of State, Bureau of African Affairs. (2012, December 17). *U.S. relations with Malawi: Fact sheet*. Retrieved from http://www.state.gov/r/pa/ei/bgn/7231.htm

2 UNICEF. (n.d.). *Malawi: The situation of women and children*. Retrieved from http://www.unicef.org/malawi/children.html

3 World Food Programme. (n.d.). *Malawi*. Retrieved from http://www.wfp.org/countries/Malawi/Operations

4 Winslow, C. E. A. (1920). The untilled field of public health. *Modern Medicine, 2*, 183.

5 Partners in Information Access for the Public Health Workforce. (2013). *Public health information and data tutorial: References*. Retrieved from http://phpartners.org/tutorial/04-ebph/6-references/4.6.1.html

6 World Health Organization (WHO). (2013). *Media centre: Obesity and overweight*. Fact sheet 311. Retrieved from http://www.who.int/mediacentre/factsheets/fs311/en/index.html

7 Chopra, M., Galbraith, S., & Darnton-Hill, I. (2002). A global response to a global problem: The epidemic of overnutrition. *Bulletin of the World Health Organization, 80* (12), 952-58.

8 Fryczkowski, M. (1977). [Effect of the site of uretero-intestinal anastomosis on the magnitude of electrolyte disorders and acid-base equilibrium in patients following total cystectomy for neoplasms]. [Article in Polish]. *Polski Przeglad Chirurgiczny, 49*(10 A), 991-96. Retrieved from http://www.ncbi.nlm.nih.gov/pubmed/928238

9 World Health Organization (WHO). (2012). *Food safety: Initiative to estimate the global burden of foodborne diseases*. Retrieved from http://www.who.int/foodsafety/foodborne_disease/ferg/en/index.html

10 World Health Organization (WHO). (n.d.). *Food safety: Initiative to estimate the global burden of foodborne diseases. Information and publications*. Retrieved from http://www.who.int/foodsafety/foodborne_disease/ferg/en/index7.html

11 HealthyPeople.gov. (2013). *Public health infrastructure*. Retrieved from http://www.healthypeople.gov/2020/topicsobjectives2020/overview.aspx?topicid=35

12 National Institutes of Health, National Heart, Lung, and Blood Institute. (n.d.). *National Cholesterol Education Program: Program description*. Retrieved from http://www.nhlbi.nih.gov/about/ncep/ncep_pd.htm

13 Centers for Disease Control and Prevention (CDC). (2013). *National Health and Nutrition Examination Survey*. Retrieved from http://www.cdc.gov/nchs/nhanes.htm

14 University of North Carolina Population Center. (n.d.). *China Health and Nutrition Survey*. Retrieved from http://www.cpc.unc.edu/projects/china

15 Beaton, G., Kelly, A., Kevany, J., Martorell, R., & Mason, J. (1990). Table of contents. In *Appropriate uses of anthropometric indices in children*. Nutrition Policy Discussion Paper No. 7. ACC/SCN State-of-the-Art Series. Geneva: UN Administrative Committee on Coordination/Subcommittee on Nutrition. Retrieved from http://www.unsystem.org/scn/archives/npp07/begin.htm

16 Institute of Medicine (IOM), Committee on Assuring the Health of the Public in the 21st Century. (2003). *The future of the public's health in the 21st century*. Washington, DC: National Academies Press. Retrieved from http://books.nap.edu/openbook.php?record_id=10548&page=R2

17 National Statistical Coordination Board, Makati City, Philippines. Statistical Survey Review and Clearance System. (1998). *National nutrition survey: Philippines, 1998*. Retrieved from http://www.nscb.gov.ph/ssrcs/ssrcsDB_maintableviewP1.asp?key=21&psearch=

18 The local health department: Services and responsibilities: An Official Statement of the American Public Health Association Adopted November 1, 1950. (1951). *American Journal of Public Health and the Nation's Health, 41*(3), 302-7. doi:10.2105/AJPH.41.3.302. Retrieved from http://ajph.aphapublications.org/doi/abs/10.2105/AJPH.41.3.302

19 Medicare.gov. (n.d.). *Your Medicare coverage*. Retrieved from http://www.medicare.gov/coverage/nutrition-therapy-services.html

20 Harvard School of Public Health. (n.d.). *Health Professionals Follow-Up Study: About the study*. Retrieved from http://www.hsph.harvard.edu/hpfs/hpfs_about.htm

21 *The Nurses' Health Study*. (n.d.). Retrieved from http://www.channing.harvard.edu/nhs

22 UNICEF. (2003). *Nutrition: UNICEF in action*. Retrieved from http://www.unicef.org/nutrition/index_action.html

23 World Health Organization. (n.d.). *Nutrition: Micronutrients*. Retrieved from http://www.who.int/nutrition/topics/micronutrients/en/index.html

24 World Health Organization. (2013, March). *Fact sheet on obesity and overweight*. Fact sheet No. 311. Retrieved from http://www.who.int/mediacentre/factsheets/fs311/en/index.html

25 World Health Organization. (2007). *Working for health: An introduction to the World Health Organization*. Retrieved from http://www.who.int/about/brochure_en.pdf

26 World Health Organization. (n.d.). *Diet and physical activity: A public health priority*. Retrieved from http://www.who.int/dietphysicalactivity/en

27 World Health Organization. (n.d.). *Global targets 2025: To improve maternal, infant and young child nutrition*. Retrieved from http://www.who.int/nutrition/topics/nutrition_globaltargets2025/en/index.html

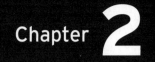
Nutritional Epidemiology: Application to Cardiovascular Disease

Lyn M. Steffen, PhD, MPH, RD
Natalie Stein, MS, MPH

"One should eat to live, not live to eat."–Benjamin Franklin

Learning Objectives

- Describe the major study designs in nutritional epidemiology.

- Explain implications of study design and population when addressing a study question using nutritional epidemiology studies.

- Describe common methods of diet assessment.

- Describe the factors that contribute to measurement error.

- Explain the significance of cardiovascular disease as a major public health problem and the role of nutritional epidemiology in addressing this problem.

- Describe relationships between dietary intake, including nutrients, foods, diet patterns, and cardiovascular disease.

Case Study: Using Nutritional Epidemiology to Study the Mediterranean Diet and Cardiovascular Disease

Cardiovascular disease (CVD) refers to any of the diseases affecting the heart and blood vessels. They include ischemic heart disease, coronary heart disease (CHD), peripheral artery disease, cerebrovascular disease, or stroke, and **hypertension**. Together, the CVDs are the leading cause of death worldwide, causing 30% of total deaths.[1] Despite their impact, the World Health Organization reports that the majority of CVD is preventable through behaviors such as avoiding tobacco, increasing physical activity, maintaining a healthy weight and eating a more nutritious diet.[2] Westernized diet patterns, characterized by high intakes of sugar, sodium, and saturated fat, are linked to increased risk of CVD. More prudent diet patterns, based on more nutritious, less processed foods, can lower the risk of CVD.

More accurately described as one of several similar dietary patterns than as a single specific diet, the Mediterranean diet is an example of a prudent diet. This type of diet is traditional in Mediterranean nations such as Italy, Greece, and Spain. Compared with Westernized diets, Mediterranean diets are generally higher in plant-based foods and fish, and lower in red meats, sweets, and saturated and trans fats. Monounsaturated fats from olive oil are the major fat source.

Investigation of Mediterranean Diets and CVD

Mediterranean-style diets are increasingly linked to reduced risk for CVD and improvements in risk factors, such as inflammation, high serum LDL cholesterol, and high blood pressure.[3] Many observational studies suggest the benefits of Mediterranean-style diets.[4] These studies provide important clues about the possible effects of a Mediterranean diet, but experimental trials are considered to be stronger sources of evidence than observational studies.

The PREDIMED Trial

The PREDIMED (Prevención con Dieta Mediterranea) was a groundbreaking multi-site clinical trial conducted in Spain from 2003 to 2008.[5] The 7,447 participants were 55 to 80 years old and had diabetes or at least three risk factors for heart disease. The control group was asked to follow a balanced diet falling within dietary guidelines for percentage of calories from fat, protein, and carbohydrates; the experimental groups were asked to follow a Mediterranean diet and provided with dietary counseling. Both experimental groups were provided either with nuts or with olive oil to supplement their diets. During the follow-up period of nearly five years, individuals in the Mediterranean diet groups experienced fewer cardiovascular events.

Clinical trials such as the PREDIMED trial can provide convincing evidence of links between diet and disease, but more research remains to be done to verify these results and resolve uncertainties. For example, monounsaturated fats are likely to be responsible for at least some of the cardiovascular benefits of a Mediterranean diet,[6] but current evidence is conflicting.[7]

Discussion Questions

- How does a Mediterranean diet differ from a typical Westernized diet? Which characteristics might contribute to its apparent cardioprotective effects?

- What is the role of nutritional epidemiology in combating significant public health nutrition concerns?

- Why can results from a clinical trial, such as the PREDIMED trial, be considered more convincing than results of observational studies? What further research is needed to provide more conclusive

evidence on the link between the Mediterranean diet and cardiovascular disease?

- How can appropriate studies be designed to answer specific research questions? What are the strengths and limitations of the major study designs used in nutritional epidemiology?

- How can results from research studies guide the development of public health nutrition policy?

Introduction

Cardiovascular disease is a major public health problem and is the leading cause of death in the United States and the world. Although the mortality rate of CVD has declined over the past 30 years, nearly one-third of adult deaths are from CVD. The high prevalence of hypertension is a significant reason; one in three adults has high blood pressure, which is a modifiable risk factor for CVD. Blood pressure increases with age, and currently 75% of older women and 65% of older men have high blood pressure. Slowing the progression of age-related increase in blood pressure in older adults and reducing blood pressure levels among younger individuals are examples of strategies to ultimately reduce CVD mortality.

Dietary intake influences blood pressure levels as well as risk for CVD. Healthy diet patterns lower the risk of developing CVD and its risk factors, such as high blood pressure, high total and LDL cholesterol, triglycerides, and **type 2 diabetes**.

Many associations between dietary intake and CVD are now widely accepted, but they were discovered and confirmed through scientific studies in the field of **nutritional epidemiology**. For example, a number of studies have led to broad acceptance that certain food types, including dairy products, fruit, whole grains, and nuts, are inversely related to the risk of **elevated blood pressure (EBP)** in young African American and Caucasian adults, and consumption of red and processed meat was positively related to higher blood pressure in younger and middle-aged populations. Using nutritional epidemiologic methods will facilitate the elucidation of diet–disease relationships.

Nutritional epidemiology is based on classic methods of epidemiology.[8,9] This chapter discusses research design components in nutritional epidemiology and the application of these concepts in the published literature. The chapter presents the most common types of epidemiologic studies, including experimental trials and observational studies.

Nutritional Epidemiology

Background

Public Health Core Competency 6: Basic Public Health Science Skills 4: Identifies the basic public health sciences (all fields)

Reproduced from Council on Linkages Between Academia and Public Health Practice. 2010 May. Core Competencies for Public Health Professionals. Washington, DC: Public Health Foundation. http://www.phf.org/resourcestools/Documents/Core_Competencies_for_Public_Health_Professionals_2010May.pdf. Accessed August 13, 2013. This source is used for all Public Health Core Competencies in this chapter.

Epidemiology is the study of the distribution and determinants of disease in human populations. The objective of an epidemiologic study is to answer a research question about the relation between an **exposure**, such as dietary intake, and an **outcome**, such as CVD, using an appropriate study design, population, and methods of data collection and analysis.

Epidemiologists use both experimental and observational study designs to investigate hypotheses about etiologic associations between exposures and an outcome. The research question determines the study design and selection criteria of study participants. **Table 2-1** matches a research question about sodium intake and blood pressure to the appropriate study design and population.

Experimental Studies

Experimental studies are designed to manipulate an exposure (sodium intake) to change an outcome (blood pressure) in specific populations. A **randomized clinical trial (RCT)** is the gold standard study design to determine **causality** between an exposure and an outcome. Many RCTs have examined the effectiveness of modified diets to change a clinical measure, such as weight, cholesterol, or blood pressure. Disadvantages include its short duration and expense.

Conducted from 1993 to 1997, the Dietary Approaches to Stop Hypertension (DASH) trial was a multicenter, randomized, outpatient feeding study designed to test the effectiveness of three different dietary patterns on lowering blood pressure among adults with high normal to high blood pressure over eight weeks.[10] The five clinical centers participating in this trial were Johns Hopkins University (Baltimore, Maryland), Duke University Medical Center (Durham, North Carolina), Kaiser Permanente (Portland, Oregon), Brigham and Women's Hospital (Boston, Massachusetts), and Pennington Biomedical Research Center (Baton Rouge, Louisiana).

Table 2-1 Research question matched to the study design and population

Research Question	Study Design	Study Population
Does decreasing dietary sodium lower the risk of developing high blood pressure?	Experimental	Selection is based on study inclusion criteria, including a diastolic blood pressure range between 80 and 85 mm Hg.
Observational Study Designs		
Do adults who have high blood pressure consume a diet higher in sodium than those without high blood pressure?	Cross-sectional	Select adults from a *defined population*. Selection is not based on blood pressure or diet criteria.
Did adults who had high blood pressure consume a diet higher in sodium than those without high blood pressure?	Case-control	Cases: Adults who have high blood pressure Controls: Adults without high blood pressure
Do those who typically consume a high-sodium diet have a higher incidence of high blood pressure than those who typically consume a diet lower in sodium over 15 years of follow-up?	Cohort	Adults who do not have high blood pressure at baseline and who also reported dietary intake at baseline and have both diet and blood pressure measures during follow-up

Over 8,800 adults were screened for eligibility. Eligibility criteria included age 22 years or older, systolic blood pressure less than 160 mm Hg, and diastolic blood pressure 80 to 95 mm Hg.[11] Exclusionary criteria included poorly controlled diabetes mellitus, hyperlipidemia, a cardiovascular event within the previous six months, chronic diseases that might interfere with participation, pregnancy or lactation, **body mass index (BMI)** over 35, the use of medications that affect blood pressure, unwillingness to stop taking vitamin and mineral supplements or antacids containing magnesium or calcium, renal insufficiency, and an alcoholic beverage intake of more than 14 drinks per week.[12] The final study population consisted of 459 Caucasian and African American healthy men and women average age 46 years with high normal blood pressure to mild hypertension at enrollment.

The two experimental diets were a diet pattern rich in fruit and vegetables and low in dairy products, and the DASH diet pattern, which is rich in low-fat dairy products, fruits, vegetables, and fish, and low in meat, sugar-sweetened beverages, saturated fats, and added sugars. Effects of these diets were compared with those of the control diet, or typical American diet. Adults who consumed the DASH diet had lower blood pressure after eight weeks than those who consumed the other two diets.[13]

Observational Studies

The most common observational study designs include (1) cross-sectional, (2) case-control, and (3) cohort.

Cross-Sectional Studies *prevalence*

The cross-sectional study is based on observing a group of individuals on a single occasion, or "snapshot" of time, to estimate the **prevalence** of a condition. In addition, the study findings may be used for hypothesis-generating. Surveillance studies, which are population surveys, use a cross-sectional study design, usually designed to determine the prevalence of a condition (high blood pressure) or a behavior (sodium consumption) in a **probability sample**. Cross-sectional studies cannot determine the sequence of events, or whether the exposure or outcome occurred first.

The **National Health and Nutrition Examination Study (NHANES)** is a surveillance study conducted annually and designed to monitor the health of the U.S. population. NHANES investigators select a probability sample of U.S. noninstitutionalized children and adults to participate in this survey. The survey combines interviews and physical examinations to gather data on the health of children and adults. Researchers can then use cross-sectional techniques to examine the data.

For example, Welch et al. studied the cross-sectional relation between added sugar intake and CVD risk factors in U.S. adolescents.[14] Using NHANES data collected from 1999 to 2004, investigators identified 2,157 adolescents eligible for this study and observed that over 21% of total daily energy intake came from added sugars. Further, added sugar intake was inversely related to **high-density lipoprotein (HDL) cholesterol** and positively related to **low-density lipoprotein (LDL) cholesterol** and **triglyceride** levels.

Case-Control Studies

In a case-control study, the exposure is compared between a group of study participants who have a disease or condition (cases) and another group who do not have the disease/condition (controls). Since cases are selected based on their case status, the case-control study is more efficient in studying a rare disease than using a cohort study design. Another benefit of case-control studies is that they can be conducted quickly, since the disease of interest has already developed by the time the study period begins.

A disadvantage of case-control studies is that they are more prone to **recall bias** and **selection bias** than other study designs. For example, in a case-control study examining the relation between coffee intake and pancreatic cancer, recall bias may occur when the cases inaccurately recall their dietary (coffee) intake prior to their diagnosis of disease. Further, selection bias can occur in a case-control study, when the selection of controls is related to the exposure-of-interest (coffee). For example, when the controls are recruited from a pool of patients with gastrointestinal (GI) conditions, these GI patient controls are not likely to drink coffee. Thus, the **measure of association** between the exposure (coffee consumption) and outcome (pancreatic cancer) will be over- or underestimated due to recall bias and/or selection bias. Another limitation of case-control studies is that the disease may influence the exposure rather than vice versa. For example, upon diagnosis of diabetes, saturated fat consumption may decrease as patients follow medical nutrition therapy recommendations. Finally, the measure of association between the exposure and outcome or odds ratio is an estimate of the relative risk, which is a measure of association in a cohort study.

One example of a population-based case-control study evaluated the relationship between alcohol intake and the risk of having a venous thromboembolism (VTE) event.[15]

Patients, or cases, attending one of six anticoagulation clinics in the Netherlands were asked to enroll in this study if they had had an incident or first VTE between March 1999 and September 2004. The control population included partners/spouses of patients and adults who were randomly selected from the same community as the cases. Cases (n = 4,423) and controls (n = 5,235) completed a standardized questionnaire about demographic characteristics, alcohol intake, and physical activity, and a blood sample was collected. The investigators found that alcohol consumption of two to four drinks per day compared with no alcohol was associated with a lower risk of VTE. However, lower fibrinogen levels in those who consumed alcohol may partly explain this association between alcohol intake and VTE.

Cohort Studies   *incidence*

The cohort study observes a group of participants over time, and can evaluate a range of effects related to one exposure. Unlike cross-sectional studies, which can measure only prevalence, cohort studies can estimate incidence of a disease or condition. Measurement of exposure is less likely to be affected by recall bias than in a case-control study because it occurs prior to development of the outcome. However, cohort studies are usually more expensive and time consuming than case-control studies.

As an example of a cohort study, a 15-year prospective cohort study examined the relationship between consumption of a plant-based diet and EBP among young African American and Caucasian adults.[16] The study population included young adult men and women enrolled in the Coronary Artery Risk Development in Young Adults (CARDIA) study. Exclusion criteria included reporting consumption of extreme caloric intakes at baseline and at exam 7 (less than 800 or more than 8,000 kcal/day for men and less than 600 or more than 6,000 kcal/day for women) (n = 119), lactating or pregnant at baseline (n = 54) or year 7 exam (n = 134), EBP (n = 443) or diabetes (n = 34) at baseline, or lack of fasting blood sample (n = 147). The remaining sample size was 4,304, consisting of 883 black men, 1,249 black women, 989 white men, and 1,183 white women. Standardized questionnaires were administered to obtain information about demographics, physical activity, smoking, and medical history. Trained staff measured blood pressure, weight, height, and waist circumference, and trained diet interviewers assessed dietary intake, using the CARDIA Diet History method, at baseline and at the year 7 exam. To assess the relation between plant-based food intake and EBP, investigators created food groups of meat, fish/seafood, dairy products, whole grains, refined grains, fruit, vegetables, legumes, and nuts. Individual food groups, including fruit, whole grains, nuts, and dairy, were inversely related to the risk of developing EBP over 15 years of follow-up, while meat intake was positively related to developing EBP.

Readers are referred to epidemiology textbooks for more details about epidemiologic methods and concepts.[17]

Data Collection Methods in Nutritional Epidemiology: Assessment of Dietary Intake

Part of designing a study is deciding which methods will be used. The following are common methods for assessing dietary intake.

24-Hour Diet Recall Interview Method

The objective of the **24-hour recall** is to obtain information about food and beverage intake during the previous 24 hours. It may be interviewer-administered in person or over the telephone. The multiple-pass interview is a standard 24-hour recall technique to (1) obtain a list of reported foods and beverages consumed, (2) review the list, (3) collect details about each food and beverage, and (4) review the details.[18] Dietary supplement use within the recall period, including use of antacids, may also be assessed. Food models, household measures, and pictures facilitate portion size estimation during in-person interviews, while for telephone interviews a two-dimensional booklet is mailed to participants prior to the telephone interview for use in estimating food and beverage amounts.[19]

In many cases, 24-hour dietary recalls can provide the least-biased dietary data.[20] In a **validation study** using **doubly-labeled water** to calculate **total energy expenditure**, energy intake estimated by the 24-hour recall was underreported by a relatively small 12–14% in men and 16–20% among women.[21] However, 24-hour recalls are expensive and impractical for large studies because multiple recalls per participant would be necessary to gather usual diet intake data, such as that required for predicting disease outcomes. The method can be useful for assessing the usual intake of populations.

Food Records

A **food record** or food diary is a detailed description of all foods and beverages consumed over a period of three to seven days. Staff sometimes train participants on food recording procedures; often, participants meet later with staff to review and document their records' accuracy. Then study staff can enter the data into a food and nutrient data entry system. Little difference is apparent between the quality of the food records from participants trained on techniques versus not trained.[22,23] This suggests that the use of undocumented food records is feasible for use in large cohort studies.

In validation studies, usual energy intake by seven-day food records has been underreported by 20% when compared with doubly-labeled water estimated energy expenditure in women.[24]

Direct Diet Data Entry and Analysis Systems

Available data entry and analysis systems for direct data entry of reported 24-hour recalls or food and beverage records or diaries include the Nutrition Data System for Research (NDSR; University of Minnesota Nutrition Coordinating Center), the Automated Self-Administered 24-hour recall (ASA24; National Cancer Institute), and the Food Intake Analysis System (University of Texas, Houston). NDSR and ASA24 use multiple-pass 24-hour recalls. These systems generally use the Food and Nutrient Databases produced by the U.S. Department of Agriculture (USDA); however, the NDSR system periodically supplements its nutrient and food database with food items and their nutrient values from food manufacturers. In addition, the NDSR has a Dietary Supplement Assessment Module (DSAM)[25] with a database of more than 2,000 dietary supplements and antacids. Direct data entry is more efficient and less costly than data entry of participants' completed paper forms by research staff. However, a disadvantage is the time gap when new foods become available in the marketplace and when the food and nutrient values are entered into the USDA food and nutrient database.

Each data entry and analysis system has advantages and disadvantages. Systems should be selected based on study objectives and budget constraints.

Food Frequency Questionnaires

The **food frequency questionnaire (FFQ)** consists of a structured list of food items. Participants indicate frequency of food intake, such as number of times per day, week, or month, and often the portion size, which is generally a standard serving size, such as one-half cup of vegetables, a slice of bread, or one cup of cereal. Serving sizes may also be estimated, using categories such as small,

medium, and large. An open-ended question is available to report any other food consumed that was not listed on the FFQ. The time period representing usual intake is often one month to a year.

The nutrient and food databases for FFQs typically use USDA Food and Nutrient Databases and can also include nutrition data reported by food manufacturers. However, the nutrients for each food on the FFQ food list are fixed; that is, the listed food item is generic as brand name information is not coded. In addition, food preparation is usually not taken into account. Data entry methods for FFQs may be direct entry by trained staff or by the participant, or electronic scanning of completed paper questionnaires.

The FFQ may be more economical to administer, since it can be self- or interviewer-administered. Nurses and health professionals have successfully completed self-administered questionnaires and mailed them back to the investigators.[26] An FFQ can also be used to screen for adherence to certain diet patterns. For example, in Spain, individuals who scored high on a Mediterranean Diet Adherence screener, a short FFQ, were categorized as adhering to a Mediterranean diet pattern.[27] The screener included 14 yes-no questions regarding frequency of consumption or use of various food types, such as fruits, vegetable, red meat and olive oil, and submissions with at least 7 "yes" responses indicated adherence. Other food frequency screeners might be used to identify individuals who meet dietary guidelines, or to divide individuals into percentiles.

A drawback of FFQs is that children, adolescents, and less-educated adults may require help completing the FFQ because of low literacy. Interviewer-administered FFQs are better for these populations. Another limitation is that FFQs rely on memory.

Validation studies show the FFQ to have substantial measurement error. One European study of more than 3,000 adults found that 33% of the study population underestimated usual energy intake from an FFQ compared with doubly-labeled water estimation of total energy expenditure.[28] In a recent study of U.S. adults, the self-reported FFQ energy intake compared with doubly-labeled water total energy expenditure underestimated energy intake by 31–36% in men and 34–38% in women. Self-reported protein intake was also underreported in both men and women compared with the gold standard urinary nitrogen biomarker.[29] Validation of the FFQs against multiple 24-hour recalls have yielded low to moderate correlations for nutrients and moderate correlations for reported food intake.[30,31]

Diet History

A **diet history (DH)** is a structured interview to gather data on usual dietary intake over a selected period of time, such as a month or year. Participants provide a list of food items, frequency of consumption, and portion size. Participants are also asked to report brand names or nutrient-modified food items, as well as additions to foods and beverages, such as sauces, condiments, butter, or margarine. Portion sizes are estimated by use of food models, household measures, or pictures. The DH may ask about food preparation and cooking fats, type or brand name of additions to foods at the table, and brand names of study foods-of-interest, such as ready-to-eat cereals with the information used to categorize the item as a whole or refined grain. Traditionally, the DH is followed by a 3-day food record or 24-hour recall interview; however, this component is sometimes omitted. Data entry may be direct or from a paper DH form.[32] The nutrient and food database for a DH uses the USDA Food and Nutrient Database and may also include food manufacturer nutrient values.

The DH method was developed by Bertha Burke in 1947[33,34] and later used in the Western Electric Study,[35] the CARDIA study,[36] and in several European studies.[37,38] In one study among children and adolescents, reported energy intake from a DH was overestimated compared with doubly-labeled water energy expenditure estimates.[39]

Measurement Error

Incorporating quality assurance (QA) and quality control (QC) activities into the study design can assure quality data and reduced **measurement error**, which occurs when random or systematic error is present (**Table 2-2**). QA activities before data collection consist of standardized study procedures and tools or instruments available to the diet interviewers as well as training and certification of the diet interviewers in study procedures prior to the start of data collection. QC activities during data collection consist of recording a proportion of the diet interviews to review interviewer performance, reviewing the data for irregularities, implementing automated software edits, and conducting analytic processing.

Table 2-2 Types of measurement error

Type of Error	Problem	Solution
Systematic error (bias) influences the validity of the measure		
Observer bias	When the interviewer is not accurate in measuring or reporting the participant's response	Implement quality control measures; retraining
Instrument bias	Inaccurate measurement due to a questionnaire or device that is not calibrated *(BodPod)*	Calibrate the instrument; pilot test the questionnaire
Subject or recall bias	A distortion in the subject's response; e.g., underreporting or overreporting dietary intake by certain groups	Neutral probing; review the questions and check the response
Random error is a wrong result occurring by chance that influences precision		
Observer variability	Possibly due to lack of training and certification	Training, certification
Instrument variability	Due to environmental factors (age of device, temperature, different assay lots, etc.)	Calibrate the device; buy the same device model across studies; regularly check the room temperature; order the same assay lot for all blood samples
Subject variability	Due to intrinsic variability of the individual, such as mood swings, illness, etc.	Reschedule the study exam; record the subject characteristic

Differential Reporting

A concern about the accuracy of self-reported dietary intake is the differential underreporting of food intake between groups, such as overweight versus normal-weight individuals. Differential reporting obscures associations between diet exposures and disease outcomes.[40,41] For example, diet–CHD relations were null before calibration, but the study found significant positive relations of calibrated-energy intake with CHD and inverse relations of percent energy from calibrated-protein intake with CHD risk in older, mostly white women.[42]

Objective biomarkers, such as doubly-labeled water, are accurate but expensive methods to calibrate and improve the accuracy of self-reported data. Another objective biomarker is urinary nitrogen to calibrate self-reported protein intake. Electrolytes help calibrate noncaloric sodium and potassium. Findings from the use of doubly-labeled water include decreasing energy expenditure with age and higher total energy expenditure among men than women for both whites[43] and African Americans.[44] Underreporting of energy expenditure is more likely among overweight or obese adults than normal weight,[45] younger versus older women and African Americans compared with whites.[46,47] Although energy and protein intakes may be calibrated, foods that have been underreported or omitted from the diet interview are still unknown; therefore, other nutrients may be misrepresented. Commonly underreported foods include cakes, pies, regular soft drinks, savory snacks, cheese, fat-type spreads, meats, and condiments, or items high in energy, sugar, sodium, and/or fat.[48,49]

Diet, Nutrition, and Cardiovascular Disease

HP 2020 Objectives

HDS-1 (Developmental): Increase overall cardiovascular health in the U.S. population

HDS-2: Reduce coronary heart disease deaths

HDS-3: Reduce stroke deaths

HDS-5: Reduce the proportion of persons in the population with hypertension

Reproduced from the U.S. Department of Health and Human Services. Healthypeople.gov. Retrieved from http://www.healthypeople.gov/2020/default.aspx. Last updated July 30, 2013. Accessed August 13, 2013.

Cardiovascular Disease Is a Public Health Problem

Public Health Core Competency 1: Analytical/ Assessment Skills 2: Describes the characteristics of a population-based health problem

Cardiovascular disease is the leading cause of death in the United States, while stroke follows in third place.[50] Ischemic heart disease is the top cause of death worldwide, along with stroke and other cerebrovascular diseases. Despite its impact, however, CVD is largely affected by modifiable risk factors, such as high blood pressure, high cholesterol, cigarette smoking, diabetes, poor diet, physical inactivity, obesity, and **metabolic syndrome**.[51] Epidemiological studies have exposed relationships between nutrients, food groups or diet patterns, and CVD.[52] This section highlights some of these studies.

Public Health Core Competency 1: Analytical/ Assessment Skills 1: Identifies the health status of populations and their related determinants of health and illness

Public Health Core Competency 6: Public Health Science Skills 5: Describes the scientific evidence related to a public health issue, concern, or intervention

Nutrient Intake and Hypertension

Higher sodium intake is related to higher blood pressure and risk for developing hypertension, but other nutrients may prevent high blood pressure. One cross-sectional study that assessed diet intake using four 24-hour recall in-person interviews found that dietary phosphorous, calcium, and magnesium were inversely associated with blood pressure among 4,680 men and women ages 40 to 59 from Japan, China, the United Kingdom, and the United States.[53] Calcium and magnesium were significantly correlated with phosphorus. A diet pattern rich in food sources of these nutrients, or dairy products, fruits and vegetables, and fish, is likely related to lower blood pressure. A meta-analysis of eight RCTs found substantially lower systolic blood pressure but smaller reductions in diastolic blood pressure with higher flavonoid intake; however, the optimal dose is still unknown.[54] A separate meta-analysis demonstrated marginally lower systolic and diastolic blood pressure with vitamin D supplementation among adults with hypertension,[55] although no effect of supplementation on blood pressure in individuals with normal blood pressure.

Food Groups and Hypertension

In the Atherosclerosis Risk in Communities (ARIC) study of middle-aged adults, higher consumption of low-fat milk, assessed by FFQ at baseline and six years later, was associated with smaller increases in blood pressure in whites but not in African Americans over nine years of follow-up.[56] In the same population, consumption of more full-fat or reduced-fat dairy products was associated with lower risk of developing high blood pressure.[57] In the CARDIA study, which included whites and African Americans aged 18–30 years at baseline, dietary intake was assessed with a diet history questionnaire at baseline and seven years later. Steffen et al. examined the relation between consumption from major food groups, defined as fruit, vegetables, legumes, nuts, meat, dairy, refined grains, whole grains; intakes; and the risk of developing EBP over 15 years of follow-up.[58] Greater intakes of plant foods and dairy products were associated with 31% and 15% lower risks, respectively, of developing EBP, while risk of EBP was increased by 50% with greater consumption of red and processed meat. In subgroup analysis of plant foods, whole-grain products, fruit, and nuts were each significantly and inversely related to EBP.

Investigations of Diet Patterns and CVD Risk Factors

As earlier described, DASH was a randomized clinical trial that demonstrated lower blood pressure among middle-aged adults with high normal or high blood pressure who were randomized to the DASH diet pattern compared with those randomized to the fruit and vegetable or control groups.[59] A different nutrient-rich diet pattern, the Mediterranean diet, was found to lower blood pressure, according to a meta-analysis of 14 clinical trials conducted in the United States, Europe, and Australia.[60] The diet is rich in fruit, vegetables, fish, nuts, and monounsaturated fat from olive oil. Multiple observational studies have demonstrated that healthy diet patterns, including the Mediterranean diet,[61] healthy diet score,[62] and a prudent diet pattern,[63] were related to lower risk of developing high blood pressure. In contrast, a cross-sectional study found higher blood pressure among Japanese adults who consumed a "Western" diet pattern, characterized by higher meat and lower vegetable intake.

Application of Research Findings to Public Health Policy

The DASH trial and other research studies have helped shape nutrition policies, including the Dietary Guidelines, to educate the general population in making changes in their eating habits. The 2010 Dietary Guidelines for Americans, for example, recommend choosing whole-grain products, reduced-fat dairy products, and a variety of protein foods, including lean meat, poultry, seafood, legumes, nuts and seeds, and increasing intake of fruit and vegetables.[64] However, despite consistent epidemiologic evidence relating greater red and processed meat consumption to higher risk of hypertension and other chronic diseases, these foods remain in the list of recommended foods.

Dietary Intake and CVD

The Seven Countries study, an **ecologic study** conducted in 1980 by Ancel Keys and colleagues, linked CHD incidence to greater intake of dietary saturated fat.[65] Based on this landmark study and other studies about dietary fat, subsequent versions of the U.S. Dietary Guidelines for Americans recommended consumption of a lower intake of total and saturated fat.[66] Since then, epidemiologic evidence has been accumulating regarding other diet–disease relationships.

Nutrient Intake and CVD

Few studies have shown a positive relation between total energy relative and risk of developing CHD, possibly due to underestimation of total energy intake due to underreporting of consumption of high-calorie snack foods, such as salty snacks, crackers, cake, cookies, pastries, candy, sugar-sweetened beverages, and alcohol.[67,68,69] Foods consumed at main meals tend to be more accurately reported than foods consumed between meals; thus the resulting micronutrient intake may be sufficiently accurate to predict diet–disease relations if it can be assumed that the majority of micronutrients are contributed by foods eaten at meals. Evidence reported from observational studies is inconsistent for the associations of the dietary antioxidants vitamin C and beta-carotene with CHD,[70] although a protective effect of the antioxidant vitamin E on CHD is consistent in observational studies. However, RCTs have not reproduced these results. Findings have been similarly inconsistent for supplemental vitamin C and beta-carotene.[71]

It appears that one supplemental antioxidant is not protective against CHD. However, numerous observational studies have reported significant and inverse associations of dietary **omega-3** fatty acids with CHD, congestive heart failure, and stroke.[72] In these studies, dietary intake was measured using 24-hour recall interviews, FFQ, or diet history questionnaires.

Food Groups and CVD

Numerous studies have examined the relation of single food groups relative to CVD. The evidence is consistent for whole-grain products and red and processed meat, but not for refined grains, dairy, or fruit and vegetable intakes. For example, in a prospective cohort study among over 15,000 white and African American middle-aged adults where dietary intake was assessed by FFQ, whole-grain products protected against the development of coronary artery disease (CAD) over 11 years of follow-up.[73] Fruit and vegetable intake was also protective only among African American adults. Refined grain products were not related to CAD in the whole group, and in subgroup analysis, refined grains were positively related to CAD in African Americans. It is not clear why these food groups were predictive in African Americans and not whites in the ARIC study.

Findings from a meta-analysis of 13 cohort studies with an average of 11 years of follow-up showed a 17% lower risk of CHD for adults consuming more than five servings of fruit and vegetables per day compared with those consuming less than three servings per day.[74] For red and processed meat, the risk of ischemic stroke increased by 13% with each 100g increase for red meat, and the risk increased by 11% for each 50g increase in processed meat intake according to a meta-analysis of five cohort studies.[75] Similar results have been reported for CHD in single studies using an FFQ to assess dietary intake. Finally, consumption of fish has been consistently related to lower CVD mortality, including fatal heart attack and sudden death.[76] Mechanisms that explain lower CVD with greater fish intake have been proposed.[77] In contrast, although the majority of evidence for whole grains and red and processed meats is consistent for CVD, the causal mechanisms have yet to be elucidated.

Diet Patterns and CVD

Numerous epidemiologic studies have examined the relations between diet patterns and risk of CVD. Diet patterns or scores have created **a priori** (based on an established concept) or generated **a posteriori** (data driven).[78,79] Data-driven-derived "prudent" diet patterns, a priori–derived healthy diet scores, the DASH diet pattern, and the Mediterranean diet pattern have been inversely related to mortality from all causes and CHD in several populations.[80,81,82,83,84] These diet patterns or scores have some common characteristics. The Mediterranean and DASH diet patterns are rich in fruits, vegetables, and nuts, while the Mediterranean diet pattern is rich in olive oil and the DASH diet pattern is higher in low-fat dairy products. A Norwegian healthy food score was rich in fruit, vegetables, and high-fat fish.[85] All three of these diet patterns were low in red and processed meat. In a Danish study, the prudent diet pattern, rich in fruits, vegetables, and whole-meal bread, was inversely related to all-cause and CVD mortality in men and women, after adjusting for relevant confounding factors; however, the Western diet, represented by greater meat, potatoes, white bread, and butter, was not significantly related to mortality.[86]

Conclusion

Although single nutrients, but not all, have been significantly related to CVD and its risk factors, such as high blood pressure, it is evident that combinations of nutrients and compounds in foods as well as the combination of foods in diet patterns work synergistically and, therefore, have greater health benefits or risks than individual nutrients or foods.[87] However, to understand the mechanisms underlying these relations, further nutrition research is warranted. Recent research in the field of nutritional metabolomics has focused on correlations between diet patterns and biomarkers.[88] These correlations may vary between individuals, with more pronounced differences between healthy individuals and those with heart disease, diabetes, and hypertension.[89,90,91] As nutritional epidemiology continues to provide new knowledge, public health nutritionists can work to improve diets through multilevel interventions.

References

1 World Health Organization. (2011). *The top 10 causes of death*. Fact Sheet No. 310. Retrieved from http://www.who.int/mediacentre/factsheets/fs310/en/index.html

2 World Health Organization. Media Center. (2011). *The top 10 causes of death*. Fact Sheet No. 310. Retrieved from http://www.who.int/mediacentre/factsheets/fs310/en/index.html

3 Willett, W. C. (2006). The Mediterranean diet: Science and practice. *Public Health Nutrition, 9*(1A), 105-10.

4 Estruch, R., Ros, E., Salas-Salvadó, J., Covas, M. I., Corella, D., Arós, F., . . . Martínez-González, M. A.; PREDIMED Study Investigators. (2013). Primary prevention of cardiovascular disease with a Mediterranean diet. *New England Journal of Medicine, 368*(14), 1279-90. doi:10.1056/NEJMoa1200303. Epub 2013 Feb 25.

5 Whayne, T. F., & Maulik, N. (2012). Nutrition and the healthy heart with an exercise boost. *Canadian Journal of Physiology and Pharmacology, 90,* 967-76.

6 Ruiz-Canela, M., & Martinez-Gonzalez, M. A. (2011). Olive oil in the primary prevention of cardiovascular disease. *Maturitas, 68*(3), 245-50. doi:10.1016/j.maturitas.2010.12.002

7 Degirolamo, C., & Rudel, L. L. (2010). Dietary monounsaturated fatty acids appear not to provide cardioprotection. *Current Atherosclerosis Reports, 12*(6), 391-96.

8 Margetts, B. M., & Nelson, M. (1997). *Design and concepts in nutritional epidemiology* (2nd ed.). New York, NY: Oxford University Press.

9 Willett, W. (2013). *Nutritional epidemiology* (3rd ed.) New York, NY: Oxford University Press.

10 Appel, L. J., Moore, T. J., Obarzanek, E., Vollmer, W. M., Svetkey, L. P., Sacks, F. M., . . . Harsha, D. W., for the DASH Collaborative Research Group. (1997). A clinical trial of the effects of dietary patterns on blood pressure. *New England Journal of Medicine, 336,* 1117-24.

11 Appel, L. J., Moore, T. J., Obarzanek, E., Vollmer, W. M., Svetkey, L. P., Sacks, F. M., . . . Harsha, D. W., for the DASH Collaborative Research Group. (1997). A clinical trial of the effects of dietary patterns on blood pressure. *New England Journal of Medicine, 336,* 1117-24.

12 Appel, L. J., Moore, T. J., Obarzanek, E., Vollmer, W. M., Svetkey, L. P., Sacks, F. M., . . . Harsha, D. W., for the DASH Collaborative Research Group (1997). A clinical trial of the effects of dietary patterns on blood pressure. *New England Journal of Medicine, 336,* 1117-24.

13 Appel, L. J., Moore, T. J., Obarzanek, E., Vollmer, W. M., Svetkey, L. P., Sacks, F. M., . . . Harsha, D. W., for the DASH Collaborative Research Group. (1997). A clinical trial of the effects of dietary patterns on blood pressure. *New England Journal of Medicine, 336,* 1117-24.

14 Welsh, J. A., Sharma, A., Cunningham, S. A., & Vos, M. B. (2011). Consumption of added sugars and indicators of cardiovascular disease risk among U.S. adolescents. *Circulation, 123,* 249-57. doi:10.1161/CIRCULATIONAHA.110.972166

15 Pomp, E. R., Rosendaal, F. R., & Doggen, C. J. (2008). Alcohol consumption is associated with a decreased risk of venous thrombosis. *Thrombosis and Haemostasis, 99,* 59-63.

16 Steffen, L. M., Kroenke, C. H., Yu, X., Pereira, M. A., Slattery, M. L., Van Horn, L., . . . Jacobs, D. R., Jr. (2005). Associations of plant food, dairy product, and meat intake with 15-y incidence of elevated blood pressure in young black and white adults: The Coronary Artery Risk Development in Young Adults (CARDIA) Study. Quiz 1363-4. *American Journal of Clinical Nutrition, 82*(6), 1169-77.

17 Rothman, K. J., Greenland, S., & Lash, T. L. (2008). *Modern epidemiology* (3rd ed.). Philadelphia, PA: Lippincott Williams & Wilkins.

18 Johnson, R. K., Driscoll, P., & Goran, M. I. (1996). Comparison of multiple-pass 24-hour recall estimates of energy intake with total energy expenditure determined by the doubly labeled water method in young children. *Journal of the American Dietetic Association, 96*(11), 1140-44.

19 Van Horn, L. V., Stumbo, P., Moag-Stahlberg, A., Obarzanek, E., Hartmuller, V. W., Farris, R. P., . . . Liu, K. (1993). The Dietary Intervention Study in Children (DISC): Dietary assessment methods for 8- to 10-year-olds. *Journal of the American Dietetic Association, 93*(12), 1396-1403.

20 Carroll, R. J., Midthune, D., Subar, A. F., Shumakovich, M., Freedman, L. S., Thompson, F. E., & Kipnis, V. (2012). Taking Advantage of the Strengths of 2 Different Dietary Assessment Instruments to Improve Intake Estimates for Nutritional Epidemiology. *Am J Epidemiol, 175*(4), 340-47.

21 Subar, A. F., Kipnis, V., Troiano, R. P., Midthune, D., Schoeller, D. A., Bingham, S., . . . Schatzkin, A. (2003). Using intake bio-markers to evaluate the extent of dietary misreporting in a large sample of adults: The OPEN Study. *American Journal of Epidemiology, 158*(1), 1-13.

22 Kolar, A. S., Patterson, R. E., White, E., Neuhouser, M. L., Frank, L. L., Standley, J., . . . Kristal, A. R. (2005). A practical method for collecting 3-day food records in a large cohort. *Epidemiology, 16*(4), 579-83.

23 Kwan, M. L., Kushi, L. H., Song, J., Timperi, A. W., Boynton, A. M., Johnson, K. M., . . . Kristal, A. R. (2010). A practical method for collecting food record data in a prospective cohort study of breast cancer survivors. *Journal of the American Dietetic Association, 172*(11), 1315-23.

24 Martin, L. J., Su, W., Jones, P. J., Lockwood, G. A., Tritchler, D. L., & Boyd, N. F. (1996). Comparison of energy intakes determined by food records and doubly labeled water in women participating in a dietary-intervention trial. *American Journal of Clinical Nutrition, 63*(4), 483-90.

25 Harnack, L., Stevens, M., Van Heel, N., Schakel, S., Dwyer, J. T., & Himes, J. (2008). A computer based approach for assessing dietary supplement use in conjunction with dietary recalls. *Journal of Food Composition and Analysis: An official publication of the United Nations University, International network of food data systems, 21*(Suppl. 1), S78-S82.

26 Barton, J., Bain, C., Hennekens, C. H., Rosner, B., Belanger, C., Roth, A., & Speizer, F. E. (1980). Characteristics of respondents and non-respondents to a mailed questionnaire. *American Journal of Public Health, 70,* 823-25.

27 Muñoz-Pareja, M., León-Muñoz, L. M., Guallar-Castillón, P., Graciani, A., López-García, E., Banegas, J. R., & Rodríguez-Artalejo, F. (2012). The diet of diabetic patients in Spain in 2008-2010: Accordance with the main dietary recommendations—A cross-sectional study. *PLoS One, 7*(6):e39454. doi:10.1371/journal.pone.0039454

28 Schoeller, D. A. (2002). Validation of habitual energy intake. *Public Health Nutrition, 5*(Suppl. 6A), 883-88. doi: http://dx.doi.org/10.1079/PHN2002378

29 Subar, A. F., Kipnis, V., Troiano, R. P., Midthune, D., Schoeller, D. A., Bingham, S., . . . Schatzkin, A. (2003). Using intake biomarkers to evaluate the extent of dietary misreporting in a large sample of adults: The OPEN Study. *American Journal of Epidemiology, 158*(1), 1-13.

30 Willett, W. C., Sampson, L., Stampfer, M. J., Rosner, B., Bain, C., Witschi, J., . . . & Speizer, F. E. (1985). Reproducibility and validity of a semiquantitative food frequency questionnaire. *American Journal of Epidemiology, 122*(1), 51-65.

31 Salvini, S., Hunter, D. J., Sampson, L., Stampfer, M. J., Colditz, G. A., Rosner, B., & Willett, W. C. (1989). Food-based validation of a dietary questionnaire: The effects of week-to-week variation in food consumption. *International Journal of Epidemiology, 18*(4), 858-67.

32 Rosner, B., Spiegelman, D., & Willett, W. C. (1990). Correction of logistic regression relative risk estimates and confidence intervals for measurement error: The case of multiple covariates measured with error. *American Journal of Epidemiology, 132*(4), 734-45.

33 Slattery, M. L., Murtaugh, M. A., Schumacher, M. C., Johnson, J., Edwards, S., Edwards, R., . . . Lanier, A. P. (2008). Development, implementation, and evaluation of a computerized self-administered diet history questionnaire for use in studies of American Indian and Alaskan Native people. *Journal of the American Dietetic Association, 108*(1), 101-9.

34 Burke, B. (1947). The dietary history as a tool in research. *Journal of the American Dietetic Association, 23*, 1041-46.

35 Shekelle, R. B., Shryock, A. M., Paul, O., Lepper, M., Stamler, J., Liu, S., & Raynor, W. J., Jr. (1981). Diet, serum cholesterol, and death from coronary heart disease. The Western Electric study. *New England Journal of Medicine, 304*(2), 65-70.

36 McDonald, A., Van Horn, L., Slattery, M., Hilner, J., Bragg, C., Caan, B., . . . Gernhofer, N. (1991). The CARDIA dietary history: Development, implementation, and evaluation. *Journal of the American Dietetic Association, 91*(9), 1104-12.

37 van Staveren, W. A., de Groot, L. C., & Haveman-Nies, A. (2002). The SENECA study: Potentials and problems in relating diet to survival over 10 years. *Public Health Nutrition, 5*(6A), 901-5.

38 deVries, J. H., deGroot, L. C., van Staveren, W. A. (2009). Dietary assessment in elderly people: Experiences gained from studies in the Netherlands. *European Journal of Clinical Nutrition, 63*(Suppl. 1), S69-74. doi:10.1038/ejcn.2008.68

39 Livingstone, M. B., & Black, A. E. (2003). Markers of the validity of reported energy intake. *Journal of Nutrition, 133*(Suppl. 3), 895S-920S.

40 Prentice, R. L., Shaw, P. A., Bingham, S. A., Beresford, S. A., Caan, B., Neuhouser, M. L., . . . Tinker, L. F. (2009). Biomarker-calibrated energy and protein consumption and increased cancer risk among postmenopausal women. *American Journal of Epidemiology, 169*(8), 977-89. doi:10.1093/aje/kwp008. Epub 2009 Mar 3.

41 Prentice, R. L., Huang, Y., Kuller, L. H., Tinker, L. F., Van Horn, L., Stefanick, M. L., . . . Johnson, K. C. (2011). Biomarker-calibrated energy and protein consumption and cardiovascular disease risk among postmenopausal women. *Epidemiology, 22*(2), 170-79. doi:10.1097/EDE.0b013e31820839bc

42 Prentice, R. L., Huang, Y., Kuller, L. H., Tinker, L. F., Van Horn, L., Stefanick, M. L., . . . Johnson, K. C. (2011). Biomarker-calibrated energy and protein consumption and cardiovascular disease risk among postmenopausal women. *Epidemiology, 22*(2), 170-79. doi:10.1097/EDE.0b013e31820839bc

43 Martin, L. J., Su, W., Jones, P. J., Lockwood, G. A., Tritchler, D. L., & Boyd, N. F. (1996). Comparison of energy intakes determined by food records and doubly labeled water in women participating in a dietary-intervention trial. *American Journal of Clinical Nutrition. 63*(4), 483-90.

44 Gannon, B., DiPietro, L., & Poehlman, E. T. (2000). Do African Americans have lower energy expenditure than Caucasians? *International Journal of Obesity and Related Metabolic Disorders, 24*(1), 4-13.

45 Heitman, B. L., & Lissner, L. (1995). Dietary underreporting by obese individuals: Is it specific or non-specific? *British Medical Journal, 311*(7011), 986-89.

46 Martin, L. J., Su, W., Jones, P. J., Lockwood, G. A., Tritchler, D. L., & Boyd, N. F. (1996). Comparison of energy intakes determined by food records and doubly labeled water in women participating in a dietary-intervention trial. *American Journal of Clinical Nutrition. 63*(4), 483-90.

47 Neuhouser, M. L., Tinker, L., Shaw, P. A., Schoeller, D., Bingham, S. A., Van Horn, L., . . . Prentice, R. L. (2008). Use of recovery biomarkers to calibrate nutrient consumption self-reports in the Women's Health Initiative. *American Journal of Epidemiology, 167*(10), 1247-59.

48 Livingstone, M. B., & Black, A. E. (2003). Markers of the validity of reported energy intake. *Journal of Nutrition, 133*(Suppl. 3), 895S-920S.

49 Poppitt, S. D., Swann, D., Black, A. E., & Prentice, A. M. (1998). Assessment of selective under-reporting of food intake by both obese and non-obese women in a metabolic facility. *International Journal of Obesity and Related Metabolic Disorders: Journal of the International Association for the Study of Obesity, 22*(4), 303-11.

50 Expert Panel on Detection, Evaluation, and Treatment of High Blood Cholesterol in Adults. (2001). Executive Summary of the Third Report of the National Cholesterol Education Program (NCEP) Expert Panel on Detection, Evaluation, and Treatment of High Blood Cholesterol in Adults (Adult Treatment Panel III). *JAMA, 285*(19), 2486-97. doi:10.1001/jama.285.19.2486

51 Steffen, L. M., Folsom, A. R., Cushman, M., Jacobs, D. R., Jr., & Rosamond, W. D. (2007). Greater fish, fruit, and vegetable intakes are related to lower incidence of venous thromboembolism: The Longitudinal Investigation of Thromboembolism Etiology. *Circulation, 115*(2), 188-95.

52 Roger, V. L., Go, A. S., Lloyd-Jones, D. M., Benjamin, E. J., Berry, J. D., Borden, W. B., . . . Turner, M. B. (2012). Heart disease and stroke statistics–2012 update: A report from the

American Heart Association statistics committee and stroke statistics subcommittee. *Circulation, 125*, e2–e220. doi:10.1161 /CIR.0b013e31823ac046

53 Elliott, P., Kesteloot, H., Appel, L. J., Dyer, A. R., Ueshima, H., Chan, Q., . . . Stamler, J., INTERMAP Cooperative Research Group. (2008). Dietary phosphorus and blood pressure: International study of macro- and micro-nutrients and blood pressure. *Hypertension, 51*(3), 669–75.

54 Hooper, L., Kroon, P. A., Rimm, E. B., Cohn, J. S., Harvey, I., Le Cornu, K. A., . . . Cassidy, A. (2008). Flavonoids, flavonoid-rich foods, and cardiovascular risk: A meta-analysis of randomized controlled trials. *American Journal of Clinical Nutrition, 88*(1), 38–50.

55 Witham, M. D., Nadir, M. A., & Struthers, A. D. (2009). Effect of vitamin D on blood pressure: A systematic review and meta-analysis. *Journal of Hypertension, 27*(10), 1948–54. doi:10.1097 /HJH.0b013e32832f075b

56 Alonso, A., Steffen, L. M., & Folsom, A. R. (2009). Dairy intake and changes in blood pressure over 9 years: The ARIC study. *European Journal of Clinical Nutrition, 63*(10), 1272–75. doi:10.1038/ejcn.2009.50. Epub 2009 Jun 17.

57 Steffen, L. M., unpublished data.

58 Steffen, L. M., Kroenke, C. H., Yu, X., Pereira, M. A., Slattery, M. L., Van Horn, L., . . . Jacobs, D. R., Jr. (2005). Associations of plant food, dairy product, and meat intake with 15-y incidence of elevated blood pressure in young black and white adults: The Coronary Artery Risk Development in Young Adults (CARDIA) Study. Quiz 1363-4. *American Journal of Clinical Nutrition, 82*(6), 1169–77.

59 Appel, L. J., Moore, T. J., Obarzanek, E., Vollmer, W. M., Svetkey, L. P., Sacks, F. M., . . . Harsha, D. W., for the DASH Collaborative Research Group. (1997). A clinical trial of the effects of dietary patterns on blood pressure. *New England Journal of Medicine, 336*, 1117–24.

60 Kastorini, C. M., Milionis, H. J., Esposito, K., Giugliano, D., Goudevenos, J. A., & Panagiotakos, D. B. (2011). The effect of Mediterranean diet on metabolic syndrome and its components: A meta-analysis of 50 studies and 534,906 individuals. *Journal of the American College of Cardiology, 57*(11), 1299–313. doi:10.1016/j.jacc.2010.09.073

61 Psaltopoulou, T., Naska, A., Orfanos, P., Trichopoulos, D., Mountokalakis, T., & Trichopoulou, A. (2004). Olive oil, the Mediterranean diet, and arterial blood pressure: The Greek European Prospective Investigation into Cancer and Nutrition (EPIC) study. *American Journal of Clinical Nutrition, 80*(4), 1012–18.

62 Steffen, L. M., Kroenke, C. H., Yu, X., Pereira, M. A., Slattery, M. L., Van Horn, L., . . . Jacobs, D. R., Jr. (2005). Associations of plant food, dairy product, and meat intake with 15-y incidence of elevated blood pressure in young black and white adults: The Coronary Artery Risk Development in Young Adults (CARDIA) Study. Quiz 1363-4. *American Journal of Clinical Nutrition, 82*(6), 1169–77.

63 Sadakane, A., Tsutsumi, A., Gotoh, T., Ishikawa, S., Ojima, T., Kario, K., . . . Kayaba K. (2008). Dietary patterns and levels of blood pressure and serum lipids in a Japanese population. *Journal of Epidemiology /Japan Epidemiological Association, 18*(2), 58–67.

64 United States Department of Agriculture and United States Department of Health and Human Services (USDA/HHS). (2011). 2010 dietary guidelines for Americans. Retrieved from http://www.cnpp.usda.gov/DietaryGuidelines.htm

65 Keys, A., Aravanis, C., Blackburn, H, Buzina, R., Djordjevic, B. S., Dontas, A. S., . . . Van Buchem, F. S. P. (1980). *Seven countries: A multivariate analysis of death and coronary heart disease.* Cambridge, MA: Harvard University Press.

66 United States Department of Agriculture and United States Department of Health and Human Services (USDA/HHS). (2011). 2010 Dietary guidelines for Americans. Retrieved from http://www.cnpp.usda.gov/DietaryGuidelines.htm

67 Livingstone, M. B., & Black, A. E. (2003). Markers of the validity of reported energy intake. *Journal of Nutrition, 133*(Suppl. 3), 895S–920S.

68 Prentice, R. L., Huang, Y., Kuller, L. H., Tinker, L. F., Van Horn, L., Stefanick, M. L., . . . Johnson, K. C. (2011). Biomarker-calibrated energy and protein consumption and cardiovascular disease risk among postmenopausal women. *Epidemiology, 22*(2), 170–79. doi:10.1097/EDE.0b013e31820839bc

69 Poppitt, S. D., Swann, D., Black, A. E., & Prentice, A. M. (1998). Assessment of selective under-reporting of food intake by both obese and non-obese women in a metabolic facility. *International Journal of Obesity and Related Metabolic Disorders: Journal of the International Association for the Study of Obesity, 22*(4), 303–11.

70 Honarbakhsh, S., & Schachter, M. (2009). Vitamins and cardiovascular disease. *British Journal of Nutrition, 101*(8), 1113–31. doi:10.1017/S000711450809123X. Epub 2008 Oct 1.

71 Honarbakhsh, S., & Schachter, M. (2009). Vitamins and cardiovascular disease. *British Journal of Nutrition, 101*(8), 1113–31. doi:10.1017/S000711450809123X. Epub 2008 Oct 1.

72 Mozaffarian, D., & Wu, J. H. (2011). Omega-3 fatty acids and cardiovascular disease: Effects on risk factors, molecular pathways, and clinical events. *Journal of the American College of Cardiology, 58*(20), 2047–67. doi:10.1016/j.jacc.2011.06.063

73 Steffen, L. M., Jacobs, D. R. Jr., Stevens, J., Shahar, E., Carithers, T., & Folsom, A. R. (2003). Associations of whole-grain, refined grain, and fruit and vegetable consumption with risk of all-cause mortality and incident coronary heart disease and ischemic stroke: The Atherosclerosis Risk in Communities (ARIC) Study. *American Journal of Clinical Nutrition, 78*(3), 383–90.

74 He, F. J., Nowson, C. A., Lucas, M., & MacGregor, G. A. (2007). Increased consumption of fruit and vegetables is related to reduced risk of coronary heart disease: Meta-analysis of cohort studies. *Journal of Human Hypertension, 21*(9), 717–28.

75 Chen, G. C., Lv, D. B., Pang, Z., & Liu, Q. F. (2013). Red and processed meat consumption and risk of stroke: A meta-analysis of prospective cohort studies. *European Journal of Clinical Nutrition, 67*(1), 91–95. doi:10.1038/ejcn.2012.180. Epub 2012 Nov 21.

76 Mozaffarian, D., & Wu, J. H. (2011). Omega-3 fatty acids and cardiovascular disease: Effects on risk factors, molecular pathways, and clinical events. *Journal of the American College of Cardiology, 58*(20), 2047-67. doi:10.1016/j.jacc.2011.06.063

77 Mozaffarian, D., & Wu, J. H. (2011). Omega-3 fatty acids and cardiovascular disease: Effects on risk factors, molecular pathways, and clinical events. *Journal of the American College of Cardiology, 58*(20), 2047-67. doi:10.1016/j.jacc.2011.06.063

78 Takata, Y., Shu, X. O., Gao, Y. T., Li, H., Zhang, X., Gao, J., . . . Zheng, W. (2013). Red meat and poultry intakes and risk of total and cause-specific mortality: Results from cohort studies of Chinese adults in Shanghai. *PLoS ONE 8*(2), e56963. doi:10.1371/journal.pone.0056963

79 Newby, P. K., & Tucker, K. L. (2004). Empirically derived eating patterns using factor or cluster analysis: A review. *Nutrition Reviews, 62*(5), 177-203.

80 Kant, A. K., & Graubard, B. I. (2005). A comparison of three dietary pattern indexes for predicting biomarkers of diet and disease. *Journal of the American College of Nutrition, 24*(4), 294-303.

81 Lockheart, M. S., Steffen, L. M., Rebnord, H. M., Fimreite, R. L., Ringstad, J., Thelle, D. S., . . . Jacobs, D. R., Jr. (2007). Dietary patterns, food groups and myocardial infarction: A case-control study. *British Journal of Nutrition, 98*(2), 380-87.

82 Trichopoulou, A., Costacou, T., Bamia, C., & Trichopoulos, D. (2003). Adherence to a Mediterranean diet and survival in a Greek population. *New England Journal of Medicine, 348*(26), 2599-2608.

83 Fung, T. T., Chiuve, S. E., McCullough, M. L., Rexrode, K. M., Logroscino, G., & Hu, F. B. (2008). Adherence to a DASH-style diet and risk of coronary heart disease and stroke in women. *Archives of Internal Medicine, 168*(7), 713-20. doi:10.1001/archinte.168.7.713

84 Estruch, R., Ros, E., Salas-Salvadó, J., Covas, M. I., Corella, D., Arós, F., . . . Martínez-González, M. A.; PREDIMED Study Investigators. (2013). Primary prevention of cardiovascular disease with a Mediterranean diet. *New England Journal of Medicine, 368*(14), 1279-90. doi:10.1056/NEJMoa1200303. Epub 2013 Feb 25.

85 Kant, A. K., & Graubard, B. I. (2005). A comparison of three dietary pattern indexes for predicting biomarkers of diet and disease. *Journal of the American College of Nutrition, 24*(4), 294-303.

86 Osler, M., Heitmann, B. L., Gerdes, L. U., Jørgensen, L. M., & Schroll, M. (2001). Dietary patterns and mortality in Danish men and women: A prospective observational study. *British Journal of Nutrition, 85*(2), 219-25.

87 Jacobs, D. R., Jr., & Steffen, L. M. (2003). Nutrients, foods, and dietary patterns as exposures in research: A framework for food synergy. *American Journal of Clinical Nutrition, 78*(3 Suppl.), 508S-513S.

88 O'Sullivan, A., Gibney, M. J., & Brennan, L. (2011). Dietary intake patterns are reflected in metabolomic profiles: Potential role in dietary assessment studies. *American Journal of Clinical Nutrition, 93*(2), 314-21. doi:10.3945/ajcn.110.000950. Epub 2010 Dec 22.

89 Wang, T. J., Larson, M. G., Vasan, R. S., Cheng, S., Rhee, E. P., McCabe, E., . . . Gerszten, R. E. (2011). Metabolite profiles and the risk of developing diabetes. *Nature Medicine, 17*(4), 448-53. doi:10.1038/nm.2307. Epub 2011 Mar 20.

90 Lewis, G. D., Asnani, A., & Gerszten, R. E. (2008). Application of metabolomics to cardiovascular biomarker and pathway discovery. *Journal of the American College of Cardiology, 52*(2), 117-23. doi:10.1016/j.jacc.2008.03.043

91 Holmes, E., Loo, R. L., Stamler, J., Bictash, M., Yap, I. K., Chan, Q., . . . Elliott, P. (2008). Human metabolic phenotype diversity and its association with diet and blood pressure. *Nature, 453*(7193), 396-400. doi:10.1038/nature06882. Epub 2008 Apr 20.

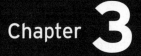

Chapter 3

Theories of Behavior Change and Their Application to Public Health Nutrition

Jennifer Falbe, MPH, ScD
Kirsten K. Davison, PhD

"He who loves practice without theory is like the sailor who boards ship without a rudder and compass and never knows where he may cast."–Leonardo da Vinci

Learning Objectives

- Define *health behavior* and provide examples related to nutrition.

- Describe the basic constructs of major theories and models of behavior change.

- Identify strengths and limitations of each theory and model described in this chapter.

- Identify similarities among constructs across the different theories and models.

- Describe how a theory or model can be used to inform the development of a nutrition intervention or program.

- Explain the process of selecting a theory or model when designing a program.

Case Study: Communities for Healthy Living

Once limited to children 4 years and older,[1] obesity is now epidemic in very young children. Today, 1 in 10 infants and 1 in 4 toddlers and preschool-aged children are overweight or obese.[2] The extreme public health burden of obesity results from its health consequences, such as high blood pressure, type 2 diabetes, polycystic ovary syndrome, sleep apnea,[3] and a lower life expectancy.[4] Low-income and ethnic minority families are most vulnerable to this burden, which perpetuates health disparities.[5,6] Elevated risk of obesity in vulnerable families can result from food

insecurity,[7] poor diet quality,[8] maternal stress,[9] low neighborhood safety,[10] higher density of fast-food restaurants, and limited access to fresh fruits and vegetables in low-income neighborhoods.[11]

The Communities for Healthy Living (CHL) program is a family-centered obesity-prevention intervention for children from low-income families. Based on theoretical models including the Family Ecological Model, Social Cognitive Theory, and Empowerment Theory, CHL was developed in collaboration with low-income parents using community-based participatory research. The intervention targeted parents' awareness and understanding of child weight status and of local resources for obesity prevention and treatment, parent self-efficacy to promote a healthy lifestyle in children, parenting practices linked with a healthy lifestyle, and skills valued by parents, including effective communication, conflict resolution, and advocacy. A pre-post cohort design was used to evaluate the CHL program.

Discussion Questions

- What motivated the development of CHL?
- How were multiple theories combined to inform the development and evaluation of CHL?
- How does CHL differ from traditional family interventions targeting childhood obesity?
- When attempting to improve a community's nutritional status and health outcomes, which health behaviors should be targeted for change, and how might an intervention change those behaviors? Where should the intervention take place, and how would each intervention component be used to change behavior?

Introduction

Where does the task of designing an intervention to improve health behaviors and health outcomes begin? Effective programs include multiple well-planned components. This chapter describes common theories and models of behavior change that can guide program development.

What Are Health Behaviors?

Gochman's[12,13] working definition of **health behaviors** is "those personal attributes such as beliefs, expectations, motives, values, perceptions, and other cognitive elements; personality characteristics, including affective and emotional states and traits; and overt behavior patterns, actions and habits that relate to health maintenance, to health restoration and to health improvement." Examples of individual overt health behaviors include regularly attending weight-loss sessions through a workplace wellness program, taking an iron supplement to treat anemia, exercising at least 2.5 hours per week, participating in health screenings, and drinking water instead of soda. Individual health behaviors to promote health can fall into the category of **preventive behaviors**, **illness behaviors**, or **sick-role behaviors**.[14,15]

Another definition extends beyond the individual to define *health behaviors* as "the actions, responses, or reactions of an individual, group, or system that prevent illness, promote health, and maintain quality of life."[16] Health behaviors exist at and are influenced by multiple levels, such as factors at the individual, interpersonal, institutional, community, and policy levels.

Behavioral Theories

Behavioral Theories and Models

Behavioral theories and models are those that provide a foundation for explaining why individuals behave the way that they do and how behavior can be changed.[17] For example, the Health Belief Model was developed primarily to explain behavior, while the stages of change of the Transtheoretical Model were developed to suggest how behavior can be changed.

Use of Theories in Research and Practice

Public Health Core Competency 2: Policy Development/ Program Planning Skills 6: Participates in program planning processes

Reproduced from Council on Linkages Between Academia and Public Health Practice. 2010 May. Core Competencies for Public Health Professionals. Washington, DC: Public Health Foundation. http://www.phf.org/resourcestools/Documents/Core_Competencies_for_Public_Health_Professionals_2010May.pdf. Accessed August 13, 2013. This source is used for all Public Health Core Competencies in this chapter.

For public health nutrition professionals, the primary function of theory is to inform the development, implementation, and evaluation of effective interventions and programs to change behavior and ultimately improve health. By mapping relationships among behavior change and hypothesized determinants of behavior change, and the factors that modify those relationships, theory can guide the choice of appropriate intervention strategies for specific populations and identify the variables that should be measured for evaluation.[18] Theoretical **constructs** are used to identify potential mediators between interventions and behavior change. Therefore, mediators specified in theories become the targets of theory-based interventions. For example, if using Social Cognitive Theory to develop an intervention to promote breastfeeding among new mothers, a key target of the intervention should be increasing a mother's *self-efficacy* to breastfeed.

Theories can reduce guessing and relying on intuition when planners and researchers are designing programs. They are not definitive recipes for programs, but, instead, are blueprints.[19] Selecting theories appropriate for specific purposes is discussed later in this chapter.

Some programs, such as those intended to investigate or change health behaviors, should be theory-based. Examples include the design and evaluation of a smart-phone application to increase physical activity and the development of a media campaign encouraging mothers to breastfeed. However, health behavior theories are not always applicable, such as when measuring distribution of health outcomes in a population (for example, the percentage of South Africans who are obese) or for examining the biological relationship between an exposure and outcome (for example, estimating the dose-response relationship between vitamin A intake and night vision).

Theory-based behavior change interventions appear to be more effective than those not based on theory.[20–22] The extent to which theory can be used falls along a continuum with the following categories:

1. informed by theory: a theoretical framework is specified but limitedly or not applied to study components;

2. applied theory: several constructs of a theoretical framework are applied to study components;

3. testing theory: measurement and testing of more than half the constructs of a framework or comparing two or more theories; or

4. building theory: developing new theories or revising existing ones using constructs specified, measured, and analyzed.[23]

This chapter includes examples that fall within each category along this continuum.

Early theories and models explaining behavior were focused on **intraindividual factors**, but more recent theories and models increasingly recognize the influence of interpersonal relationships and factors at the organizational, community, and policy levels. Multiple theoretical frameworks now address different levels of influence by explaining individual behavior as a function of one's social and physical environments. The theories and models presented in this chapter include both those with a focus on individual factors and those that go beyond the individual. These frameworks were selected because they are among those most commonly used in public health nutrition research and program development.

Health Belief Model

The Health Belief Model (HBM) is one of the earliest models used in public health (**Figure 3-1**). Developed in the 1950s by the U.S. Public Health Service to *explain* low participation in disease prevention and detection programs,

such as screening for tuberculosis,[24,25] it has since been applied to lifestyle behaviors requiring long-term change.

The HBM explains behavior as a function of the constructs in **Table 3-1**. The HBM also specifies **modifying factors** that can influence the nature and strength of the relationships between HBM constructs and behavior. Examples of modifying factors include age, gender, ethnicity, income, education, personality, peer pressure, and knowledge.

> *Healthy People 2020: Objective D-1: Reduce the annual number of new cases of diagnosed diabetes in the population*
>
> Reproduced from the U.S. Department of Health and Human Services. Healthypeople.gov. Retrieved from http://www.healthypeople.gov/2020/default.aspx. Last updated July 30, 2013. Accessed August 13, 2013.

Strengths and Limitations of HBM

The HBM is appealing due to its simplicity and parsimony. It can be particularly useful for designing programs focused on illness and sick-role behaviors among patient populations, such as obese or diabetic individuals, with heightened perceived severity and susceptibility. However, the

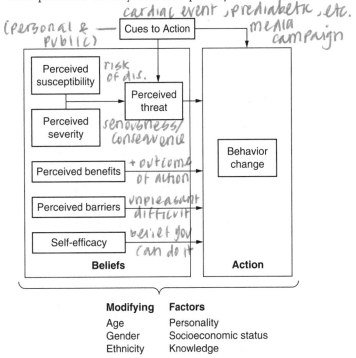

Figure 3-1 Health Belief Model

Data from Champion VL, Skinner CS. (2008). The Health Belief Model. In: Glanz K, Rimer BK, Viswanath K, eds. *Health behavior and health education: Theory, research, and practice* (pp. 49). San Francisco: Jossey-Bass.

Table 3-1 Main constructs of the Health Belief Model

Main Constructs	Description	Example
Perceived susceptibility	Perceived risk of contracting an illness or health condition.	Perceived risk of getting type 2 diabetes.
Perceived severity	Perceived seriousness of personal consequences of an illness. Together, perceived susceptibility and severity compose *perceived threat*.	Perception that consequences of type 2 diabetes are severe. Consequences can be either clinical (e.g., pain, amputation, kidney disease, blindness, or death from type 2 diabetes) or personal (e.g., ability to work, relationships with friends and family).
Perceived benefits	Perception of positive outcomes that will result from a particular action.	Perception that type 2 diabetes can be prevented by weight loss through diet and exercise. Also encompasses benefits unrelated to health, such as saving money by replacing soda with tap water as a primary beverage.
Perceived barriers	Perception of unpleasantness, difficulty, inconvenience, or other negative aspects of a behavior. A course of action is selected based on a person's cost-benefit analysis weighing perceived effectiveness of behaviors against perceived negative aspects of those behaviors.[26]	Perceptions that weight loss will be difficult and that exercise and diet change will be unpleasant and inconvenient.
Cues to action	Stories or events that trigger action.	Being diagnosed with prediabetes and experiencing symptoms such as fatigue. Environmental cues may include a media campaign on the consequences of uncontrolled blood sugar levels.
Self-efficacy	Belief that one can perform a specific behavior. Defined by Bandura as "the conviction that one can successfully execute the behavior required to produce the outcomes,"[27] self-efficacy was originally developed for Social Cognitive Theory and added to later versions of the HBM as suggested by Rosenstock and colleagues.[28]	Belief that one can adhere to a healthy diet and exercise routine to lose weight and prevent diabetes.

Data from: Rosenstock, I. M., Strecher, V. J., & Becker, M. H. (1988). Social Learning Theory and the Health Belief Model. *Health Education Quarterly 15*(2), 175-183 and Strecher, V. J., Champion, V. L., & Rosenstock, I. M. (1997). Handbook of Health Behavior Research I: Personal and Social Determinants. In D.S. Gochman (Ed.), (pp. 74). New York: Plenum Press.

HBM was originally developed to explain one-time behaviors and not necessarily long-term behavior change, such as consuming a more nutrient-dense diet, particularly among populations that do not generally feel threatened by long-term effects of poor diet, such as children and adolescents.[26]

Constructs of the HBM can predict behavior,[27] but relationships among its constructs are not yet well defined.[28]

Additionally, little research has been done to determine the utility of cues to action in changing behavior. Another limitation is its focus on individual and cognitive factors: the HBM does not directly address the social, cultural, and environmental factors that shape nutrition-related behaviors, and it has been suggested that inclusion of emotional components, such as fear, might improve the model's predictiveness.[29,30]

Applying Theory to Research and Practice: Health Belief Model

Application of the HBM to a Nutrition Education Worksite Intervention for University Staff

A university in the United States tested an HBM-based worksite nutrition education program to promote dietary behaviors that would reduce risk of cardiovascular disease (CVD) and cancer.[31] Employees were assigned to a control group or to attend eight one-hour educational sessions covering such topics as CVD and cancer, macronutrients, fruits and vegetables, physical activity, weight control, and meal planning. HBM constructs were integrated into lesson content. For example, *perceived severity* was addressed by teaching about health consequences of CVD and cancer, and *perceived benefits* were addressed by providing information on benefits of reducing saturated fat and increasing fruits and vegetables.

Outcome variables included five HBM constructs (*perceived susceptibility, perceived severity, perceived benefits, perceived barriers,* and *self-efficacy*), nutrition knowledge, and dietary intake. The intervention led to increased knowledge, more perceived benefits of healthy eating, and healthier dietary behaviors, such as consumption of fewer calories.

Using HBM to Develop an Intervention to Increase Whole Grain Consumption Among Older Americans

The "Whole Grains and Your Health" program was developed to increase voluntary consumption of whole-grain (WG) foods among people 59 years of age or older participating in government-funded congregate meals (that is, community meals) in senior centers in the state of Georgia.[32] Five lessons based on the following HBM constructs were delivered at senior centers.

- *Perceived susceptibility and severity:* Emphasizing common health conditions associated with low WG intake in seniors.

- *Perceived benefits:* Explaining potential for WGs to reduce disease risk.

- *Perceived barriers:* Providing information and correcting misinformation about WG labels.

- *Cues to action:* Providing "how-to" material (recipes and tips) on including WGs at meals.

- *Self-efficacy:* Teaching ways to identify, cook, and store WG foods.

Participants reported increases in consumption of whole-grain bread, whole-grain cereal, and whole-wheat crackers. A limitation of the HBM in this population is that it does not address environmental factors that affect behavior, such as availability of whole grains through congregate meals. Georgia law did not require congregate meals to include whole grains, and the intervention did not require centers to provide them either.

Theory of Reasoned Action and Theory of Planned Behavior

According to the Theory of Reasoned Action (TRA), *intention* to perform a behavior is the primary determinant of actually performing that behavior.[33] The two main constructs in the TRA that determine *intention* are **attitude** and **subjective norm** toward the behavior.[34] A person's

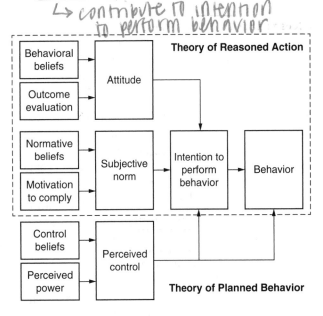

Figure 3-2 Theory of Reasoned Action and Theory of Planned Behavior

Data from Montaño, D. E., & Kasprzyk, D. (2008). Theory of Reasoned Action, Theory of Planned Behavior, and the Integrated Behavioral Model. In K. Glanz, B. K. Rimer, & K. Viswanath (Eds.), *Health behavior and health education: Theory, research, and practice* (pp. 67-96). San Francisco: Jossey-Bass; and Madden, T. J., Ellen, P. S, & Ajzen, I. (1992). A Comparison of the Theory of Planned Behavior and the Theory of Reasoned Action. *Personality and Social Psychology Bulletin, 18*(1), 3-9.

Table 3-2 Main constructs of the Theory of Reasoned Action and the Theory of Planned Behavior

Main Constructs	Description	Example
Attitude toward behavior	Positive or negative evaluation of the behavior in question, which is determined by beliefs about outcomes that may result from the behavior, weighted by the importance of those outcomes.	In regions of the world with a high prevalence of vitamin A deficiency, attitudes toward purchasing vitamin A-fortified cooking oil may be shaped by beliefs that consumption will prevent deficiency-related outcomes, the importance of those outcomes, and beliefs about the taste of fortified oil.
Subjective norm	Perceptions of social pressure to perform a behavior, which is shaped by one's beliefs that others think she or he should perform a behavior and motivation to comply with those others.	Also in settings of vitamin A deficiency, a pregnant woman's perception that family members, friends, or other important people want her to buy and use vitamin A-fortified cooking oil to prevent birth defects, night blindness, and impaired immunity that may result from vitamin A deficiency.
Perceived control (TPB)	Perceptions of how difficult or easy it is to perform a behavior, which is based on beliefs about the resources and opportunities one possesses to perform a behavior.	Perceptions of how difficult it is to obtain vitamin A-fortified cooking oil, which may be a function of beliefs about opportunities to shop for groceries, availability of the product, and ability to afford it.

Data from Ajzen, I. (1991). The Theory of Planned Behavior. *Organizational Behavior and Human Decision Processes, 50*, 179-211 and Ajzen, I., & Madden, T. J. (1986). Prediction of goal-directed behavior: Attitudes, intentions, and perceived behavioral control. *Journal of Experimental Social Psychology, 22*(5), 453-474.

intention to perform a behavior will be stronger if a person has a favorable *attitude* toward a behavior and believes that important people want him or her to perform that behavior. Other constructs are shown in **Table 3-2**.

Subjective norms may be more important for some behaviors, such as breastfeeding, while *attitudes* may play a larger role for other behaviors, such as using olive oil, which is high in monounsaturated fat, for cooking instead of butter, which is high in saturated fat.

The TRA is pertinent only to behaviors under **volitional control**.[35] External factors, such as inability to obtain out-of-season fresh vegetables, are not within an individual's volitional control.

To account for the variability in control individuals have over their actions, **perceived control** was added as another determinant of *intention* and behavior, and the revised model was named the Theory of Planned Behavior (TPB).[36,37] When the potential for volitional control is lacking, TPB states that higher *perceived control* predicts performance of a behavior.[38] As volitional control increases, the influence of *perceived control* decreases, leaving *intention* as the primary determinant of behavior.

According to the TPB, each of the main constructs is determined by two sets of factors. *Attitude* is determined by (1) behavioral beliefs, or beliefs about potential outcomes that may result from performing a behavior, and (2) outcome evaluation, or the value attached to results of a behavior. *Subjective norms* are shaped by (1) normative beliefs, or an individual's belief of whether other people think she or he should perform a behavior, and (2) one's motivation to comply with specific other people, which is affected by factors including individual personality traits, the other person's power to reward or punish the individual, how much an individual likes the other person, and the other person's perceived expertise.[39] *Perceived control* is determined by (1) control beliefs, or perceptions about factors, such as opportunities and skills, that can facilitate or impede performance of a behavior, and (2) perceived power, or perceptions about the power of each factor to facilitate or inhibit the behavior.

Strengths and Limitations of the TPB

The TPB is parsimonious, applicable to a wide range of behaviors, and clearly operationalized with guidelines on how to measure and analyze constructs and develop interventions based on the theory.[40] The theory better predicts physical activity and diet than disease detection, safer sex, and abstinence from substances,[41] but significant variation remains unaccounted for, suggesting that other variables not included in the TPB could enhance prediction. Compared with other theories, more focus has been placed on expanding the TPB, such as by incorporating variables related to emotion.[42]

The TRA and the TPB have been criticized as being too logical or rational, since individuals themselves do not always act rationally.[43,44] However, defenders note that these theories do not assume that beliefs are developed rationally or that they accurately reflect reality.[45,46] Rather, they assume that regardless of how biased beliefs may be, those beliefs result in *attitudes*, *subjective norms*, and *perceived control* consistent with those beliefs. Another limitation of the TRA and the TPB is that they are not applicable to behaviors over which there is no volitional control, such as ensuring nutrient intake during famine, or to habits that are so ingrained that they do not require *intention* or conscious reasoning. These theories may also be less applicable to youth, possibly due to the lack of control over diet or lack of reasoning around dietary behaviors in this group.[47]

Applying Theory to Research and Practice: Theory of Planned Behavior

Using the Theory of Planned Behavior to Develop The Infant Feeding Series (TIFS) Curriculum

The American Academy of Pediatrics (AAP) recommends introduction of solid foods no earlier than 4 to 6 months of age to reduce risk for health problems later in life.[48] Low-income mothers are less likely to meet AAP recommendations than higher-income mothers.[49] Therefore, the TIFS curriculum was developed for this population to promote appropriate transition to solids foods during infancy through education and behavior change.[50] A pilot study of TIFS among 16 African American and 15 Caucasian low-income mothers included six lessons delivered by paraprofessionals during home visits. The TPB guided the developers' understanding of the individual and contextual factors leading to early introduction of solid foods. The curriculum included the following determinants of TPB constructs:

- *Determinants of attitudes* included beliefs about feeding practices and consequences of early introduction

of solid foods. Relevant lessons aimed to increase knowledge of infant anatomy, cues, temperament, and indicators of readiness for solid foods.

- *Determinants of subjective norms* included a mother's beliefs about how family and healthcare providers think she should feed her infant and her motivation to comply. Lessons to enhance communication skills and increase the view of oneself as an information consumer were developed so mothers could communicate effectively with important others who may encourage early introduction of solid foods.

- *Determinants of perceived control* included perceptions of the presence or absence of resources, barriers, and the impact of each resource or barrier on feeding decisions. Lessons focused on alternatives to early feeding, such as nonfeeding methods for calming infants, and on normative sleep patterns.

After TIFS, mothers had greater knowledge about feeding practices, more accurately identified infant engagement cues, and had higher *self-efficacy* for adhering to AAP guidelines.[51] Nearly all women assessed six months after the intervention reported adhering to AAP guidelines. TIFS is currently being used in the Healthy Babies interventions—a community-based randomized trial of an in-home intervention.[52]

Evaluation of the TPB to Explain Dietary Behavior in Global Settings

In one study, investigators used a questionnaire to assess TPB constructs and fish consumption among a sample of 612 adults living in Vietnam.[53] In this study, the TPB was extended to include **descriptive norms**, or perceptions of whether others engage in a behavior. *Intention* to consume fish was associated with participants' positive evaluations about eating fish (*attitude*), perceptions that family and other important people want them to eat fish (*social norms*), perceptions of how often others eat fish (*descriptive norms*), and perceptions of how much control they have over eating fish (*perceived control*). Intentions and *perceived control* were associated with greater frequency of consumption.

A prospective study in Uganda investigated how well the TPB predicted *intention* and self-perceived consumption of sugars among adolescents,[54] who completed surveys at baseline and three months later. *Attitudes* and *perceived control* predicted intended sugar consumption at baseline, explaining 58% of the variance, and study conclusion, explaining 19% of variance. Baseline *intention* also predicted self-perceived sugar consumption three months later, supporting the validity of the TPB in predicting sugar consumption in this population. Results from these studies suggest that the TPB may be useful in designing interventions to increase fish intake among Vietnamese adults and reduce sugar intake among youth in Uganda.

Social Cognitive Theory

Social Cognitive Theory (SCT)[55,56] is among the most common theories used to design nutrition and physical activity interventions. **Reciprocal determinism**, or the idea that behavior is a function of the reciprocal and dynamic interactions between people and their environments, describes behavior. Environments affect individual actions, and individuals can change their environments to promote healthier behaviors. For example, residents in an urban community lacking access to produce may transform abandoned spaces into community gardens, thereby changing their neighborhood food environment. Key constructs of SCT focus on both personal and environmental characteristics that determine behavior (**Table 3-3**).

Principal Personal Constructs of SCT

Outcome expectations include physical outcomes, such as reduced risk of cancer, social outcomes, such as "my mother will be proud of me for eating my vegetables," or

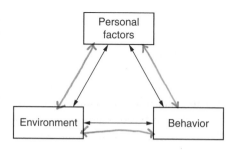

Figure 3-3 Social Cognitive Theory

Data from Bandura, A. (1986). *Social foundations of thought and action: A social cognitive theory.* Englewood Cliffs, NJ: Prentice-Hall.

self-evaluative outcomes, such as "I will feel better about myself by eating an apple instead of cake for dessert."

Self-efficacy is the foundation for motivation and action. The more difficult or complex a behavior, the more important *self-efficacy* is in performing that behavior.[57] Methods for increasing *self-efficacy* include enabling people to successfully perform behaviors in increasingly challenging situations, modeling of behaviors, improving people's emotional state before they attempt behavioral change, and providing verbal persuasion or encouragement to increase confidence in performing a behavior.[58]

Motivation alone is insufficient to change behavior, and SCT emphasizes the role of **self-regulation**, or self-control,

Table 3-3 Main constructs of Social Cognitive Theory

Main Constructs	Description	Example
Outcome expectations	Beliefs about the likelihood of potential physical, social, or self-evaluative outcomes of performing a behavior and the perceived value of those outcomes.	A pregnant woman's belief that prenatal vitamins will prevent birth defects.
Self-efficacy	Belief in one's ability to perform a specific action.	A mother's belief that she can exclusively breastfeed her infant for six months.
Self-regulation	Self-control, or ability to control one's behavior, which involves acquiring skills for self-management, identifying and monitoring behaviors, setting goals, evaluating performance in achieving goals, self-reward when goals are met, and problem solving when goals are not met.	Reducing intake of fast food by setting goals to limit intake, monitoring weekly intake, and self-reward when goals are met.
Observational learning	Learning by observing others perform a behavior and the consequences of those behaviors. Modeling (e.g., detailed demonstrations) of behaviors can be a useful educational strategy.	Learning how to prepare a healthy meal by watching detailed cooking demonstrations.

Data from Bandura, A. (1997). *Self-efficacy: The exercise of control.* New York, NY: W. H. Freeman.

in performing desired behaviors. Self-regulation requires short-term self-denial or hardship in anticipation of long-term benefits.[59] It depends not on "will power" but on acquisition of skills for self-management.[60] *Self-regulation* can be achieved through identification and monitoring of behaviors one wishes to change, setting achievable behavioral goals, evaluation of one's performance in achieving goals, rewarding oneself when goals are achieved, and problem solving and decision making when goals are not achieved.[61,62,63] Goal setting appears effective in interventions to change adults' dietary habits, but evidence for effectiveness among children and adolescents is lacking.[64,65]

Environmental Characteristics

The environment, both physical and social, is a key construct of SCT. Individuals' ability to exercise personal agency in their lives depends upon their environments and how modifiable these environments are.[66] Food availability, quality, and cost are aspects of the physical environment related to dietary behaviors. For example, in the home environment, a young child cannot drink sugar-sweetened beverages if family members do not bring these into the home. However, children can change their home environments by insisting their parents buy certain foods or beverages. They may also affect their parents' environments in other ways, such as by asking to go to a fast-food restaurant.[67] Likewise, a high school student may not eat vegetables during school lunch unless palatable options are included in school lunches. Safe and clean parks, sidewalks, and bicycle lanes contribute to physical activity–promoting neighborhood environments.

The social environment includes family, friends, peers, neighbors, co-workers, healthcare providers, and other individuals with whom people interact in their daily lives. Individuals can learn how to perform behaviors through **modeling**. For example, children may model healthy eating habits when they see child care providers eating the same healthy foods. Learning through personal experiences can be tedious, costly, and hazardous,[68] and **observational learning** can hasten the learning process and avoid personal consequences associated with trial and error. Technology and mass communications permit modeling to include media and no longer just models in immediate environments, such as one family, peers, co-workers, and classmates.[69] Individuals are more likely to emulate models who are similar to themselves,[70,71] an important consideration when designing interventions with modeling components.

Fictional media models have been used in entertainment education, and real media models have been featured in news stories. One example of entertainment education for observational learning was a television show with a side storyline on teen obesity, hypertension, and the 5 A Day campaign.[72] The show featured Elgin, an overweight African American teenager with poor eating habits and hypertension. Elgin was prescribed medication and counseled on diet and exercise, but was hospitalized after a cardiac event. When his doctor asks, "What do we learn from this?" Elgin responds, "5 A Day, exercise some, and find myself a job at a fruit and vegetable stand." An evaluation of the storyline showed positive effects on self-reported behaviors and modest impacts on knowledge, attitudes, and practices among viewers.[73]

Strengths and Limitations of SCT

SCT is a broad model that attempts to explain almost all human behaviors.[74] The concept of *self-efficacy*, which has also been incorporated into other frameworks, such as the HBM, has been validated extensively and found to be an important predictor of behavior. However, because of its breadth, SCT has not been tested as thoroughly as other theories have been.[75] The relationships among its constructs are not clearly specified, and it has often been used in a disordered manner by applying or testing only some constructs instead of the theory as a whole. Some SCT constructs may be differentially relevant to certain health conditions, behaviors, and populations. For instance, to address obesity, particularly among children, environmental factors may be more effective in changing diet and physical activity than attempts to influence *outcome expectations*, *self-efficacy*, or *self-regulation*. Additional testing of this theory using systematic experiments replicated over diverse behaviors and populations can help determine the relative importance of each construct for varying behaviors and populations.[76]

Applying Theory to Research and Practice: Social Cognitive Theory

Using Constructs of SCT to Reduce Television Viewing Among Preschool-Aged Children

Screen time is a risk factor for unhealthy weight gain in children. Growing evidence suggests that television viewing affects diet and weight through the influence of advertising.[77,78,79,80] Consequently, authorities including the

American Academy of Pediatrics, the Office of the Surgeon General, and the Commonwealth of Australia recommend limiting children's noneducational screen time to no more than two hours per day.[81,82,83]

A four–month pilot randomized controlled trial among 67 families in Seattle introduced an SCT-based behavior change intervention based on constructs with the following aims: (1) to reduce total amount of television watching among preschool-aged children and (2) to shift children's television exposure away from commercial content toward educational content to reduce exposure to advertising.[84] Each family was assigned a case manager who used in-person conferences, newsletters, email, and phone contact to motivate change in television viewing (intervention group) or child safety (control group). Communication with families addressed three SCT constructs by focusing on the following topics:

- Positive and negative effects of television on child health and development (*outcome expectations*);
- Encouraging mothers in building confidence to modify their child's television viewing (*self-efficacy*); and
- Strategies for modifying their child's television viewing (*volitional control*—a component of *self-regulation* akin to self-control).[85]

Children in the intervention group reduced total television viewing by 37 minutes/day and viewing of commercial content by 29 minutes/day. In the intervention group, parents improved *outcome expectations* compared with controls, but not *self-efficacy* or *volitional control*. Study authors concluded that this may be due to poor measurement of constructs or to the possibility that some other feature of the intervention not captured by the measured constructs was responsible for behavior change.

Using SCT to Inform a Qualitative Study of Mothers of Nutritionally At-Risk Children in Indonesia

A recent study used in-depth interviews to explore factors related to maternal *self-efficacy* in providing food for the home among low-income, urban mothers in the context of economic and nutritional transition in Indonesia.[86] In Indonesia, 11% of households contain both underweight and overweight individuals, with the prevalence being higher among urban residents.[87] Children are more likely to be underweight, while adults are more likely to be overweight.[88]

Researchers interviewed 19 mothers with a child enrolled in one of two elementary schools serving low-income

children in Jakarta. SCT constructs guided development of interview questions assessing food-related experience, parenting practices, management of income, social support, and the community setting. Results from coded interviews indicated high maternal *self-efficacy* to access and provide food for the family but low maternal *self-efficacy* in providing nutritious foods for children. Mothers believed that God and extended family would provide for them in times of economic need, but lacked nutrition knowledge and the confidence to choose appropriate meals for their children. Mothers also preferred ready-to-eat meals and meals requiring minimal preparation. This study suggests that this population would benefit from interventions designed to increase maternal knowledge and *self-efficacy* regarding healthy meal selection and preparation. *Self-efficacy* in selecting healthy meals could be increased by providing opportunities to develop sample menus and receive feedback on those menus. *Self-efficacy* cooking and preparing meals could be enhanced by participatory cooking demonstrations.

Transtheoretical Model and Change

The Transtheoretical Model (TTM) integrates multiple theories from psychotherapy.[89] Initially developed to explain how behavior change occurred through a series of stages that were predictive of successful smoking cessation,[90,91] the TTM has since been applied to a wide range of behaviors, including those related to obesity, eating disorders, and physical activity. According to the TTM, behavior change is a process that occurs in stages. For most health behaviors, such as eating a healthy diet, change is not a discrete event. Unlike other models, the TTM includes a temporal dimension appropriate for long-term behaviors, such that over time, an individual may make progress toward change or regress toward old behaviors through different stages. A major implication of the TTM is that there is no one-size-fits-all intervention that will be effective for everyone. Instead, interventions should be tailored to individuals based on their stages of change.

Stages of the Transtheoretical Model

The TTM posits that behavior change is a dynamic process that unfolds through six stages, although not always in a linear manner.[92,93] These **stages of change** are described in **Table 3-4**.

"Stages of Change"

Table 3-4 Main constructs of the Transtheoretical Model

Main Constructs (Stages of Change)	Description	Example
Precontemplation	No intention to change behavior in the near future, often defined as six months. Individuals may be unaware of the consequences of their behavior or be suppressing thoughts about change as a result of discouragement over past attempts and failures to change behavior.	No intention to replace sugar-sweetened beverages (SSBs) with low- or no-calorie drinks.
Contemplation *can be a long stage*	Considering or intending to change behavior in the near future, although this stage can last for a long time. People in this stage are more aware of the costs and benefits of taking action.	Considering giving up SSBs but weighing health benefits against the cost of giving up SSBs.
Preparation	Intends to change behavior very soon and has already taken steps toward change.	Plans to give up SSBs. Has done research on low-calorie alternatives and has purchased a refillable water bottle.
Action	Recent and overt changes in behavior, usually within the past six months. Generally, to be considered *"action"* in the TTM, changes in behavior should be substantial enough to reduce risk of disease—for example, choosing water instead of soft drinks every day and not just once a week.	Does not drink or purchase SSBs from the grocery store, cafeteria, or vending machine. Instead, purchases alternative drinks such as sparkling water.
Maintenance	Ongoing practice of behavior and engagement in efforts to prevent relapse. Has more confidence in ability to prevent relapse.	Maintains habits, in part by enlisting family to refrain from bringing SSBs into the home.
Termination *belief in one's ability to perform a certain action*	Complete self-efficacy and no temptation to return to old behaviors. This phase is not studied or used as widely as other stages, and there has been debate about whether one can ever truly reach termination, especially in the area of diet and exercise behaviors.	No further interest in SSBs; a genuine preference for water.
Decisional balance	Weighing of pros (benefits) and cons (costs) of behavior change.	Weighing pros (e.g., potential weight loss, increased insulin sensitivity, and financial savings) against the cons (e.g., reduced pleasure from giving up a favorite beverage and judgment from peers).
Self-efficacy	Confidence in one's ability to cope with high-risk situations without relapsing to unhealthy behaviors.	Confidence to resist drinking SSBs at a party when offered.
Temptation	Strength of urges to return to unhealthy behaviors.	Intense urge to purchase and drink SSBs when walking past a vending machine on a hot day.

Data from: Prochaska, J. O., Redding, C. A., & Evers, K. A. (2008). The Transtheoretical Model and Stages of Change. In K. Glanz, B. K. Rimer, & K. Viswanath (Eds.), *Health behavior and health education: Theory, research, and practice.* San Francisco: Jossey-Bass.

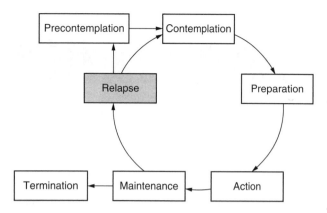

Figure 3-4 Stages of behavior change. This figure depicts how one might move through successive stages of change but does not show all possible arrows. Some individuals may not move through all stages, may not move through stages consecutively, and may return to a previous stage. For example, a person in action may return to precontemplation after repeated failures to maintain change.

Data from Prochaska, J. O., & DiClemente, C. C. (1982). Transtheoretical therapy: Toward a more integrative model of change. *Psychotherapy: Theory, Research & Practice, 19*(3), 276-288.

Processes of Change

Processes of change are activities that can be used by individuals to progress through stages of change. These processes can guide development of interventions or programs to change behavior. Processes with the strongest support from the literature are presented in **Table 3-5**.[94] Processes 1–4 may be more applicable to the earlier stages of *precontemplation, contemplation*, and *preparation*, and processes 5–9 to the later stages.[95]

Staging

Staging refers to determining a person's or group's stage of change to ensure that stage-matched interventions are delivered to the appropriate individuals or, conversely, that interventions are designed for the most common stages describing members of the target population. Staging of dietary behaviors is typically based on self-reported perceptions of behavior. At the community level, surveys or brief telephone interviews can be used. An example of a survey-based staging algorithm for fruit and vegetable intake is as follows:[96]

- The first question asks individuals how many servings per day of fruits and vegetables they usually consume.

Table 3-5 Processes of change

Processes of Change	Description
1. Consciousness raising	Increasing awareness of the causes, consequences, and remedies for particular behaviors through information, education, and personal feedback.
2. Dramatic relief	Experiencing negative emotions (e.g., fear and anxiety) about the risks of unhealthy behaviors, followed by anticipated relief if behavior is changed.
3. Self-reevaluation	Realizing that behaviors are an important aspect of one's identity.
4. Environmental reevaluation	Examining negative impacts of unhealthy behaviors on one's environment, including other people.
5. Self-liberation	Making a deep commitment to change.
6. Helping relationships	Enlisting the support of others to make and sustain changes in behavior.
7. Counterconditioning	Substituting unhealthy behaviors with healthier alternatives.
8. Reinforcement management	Increasing rewards for performing healthy behaviors and decreasing those for unhealthy behaviors.
9. Stimulus control	Adding cues to engage in healthy behavior and removing those for unhealthy behavior.
10. Social liberation	Realizing that social norms are changing to become supportive of desired behaviors.

Data from: Prochaska, J. O., Redding, C. A., & Evers, K. A. (2008). The Transtheoretical Model and Stages of Change. In K. Glanz, B. K. Rimer, & K. Viswanath (Eds.), *Health behavior and health education: Theory, research, and practice* (p. 99). San Francisco: Jossey-Bass.

- If less than two servings of fruit and less than three servings of vegetables are reported, the respondent is asked about intention to eat more fruits and vegetables in the next six months or 30 days. Those with no intention to eat more are classified in *precontemplation*. Those intending to eat more fruits and vegetables in the next six months or 30 days are classified in *contemplation* or *preparation*, respectively.

- Respondents initially reporting consumption of at least two servings per day of fruit or at least three servings per day of vegetables are asked whether they have been doing so for more than six months. Those who answer no are classified in *action*; those answering yes are classified in *maintenance*.

Another staging strategy involves asking people to rate whether their intake is very low, low, average, high, or very high and if intake has changed from one of these levels to another. This avoids the use of set cutoff points, such as five daily servings of fruits and vegetables, that may mask important changes, such as increasing intake from one to four servings of fruits and vegetables, that fall short of thresholds.

These staging methods both rely on perception of intake, which can be complicated by errors in reporting portion sizes and consumption of mixed dishes. Staging individuals for nutrient intake is more challenging.[97] In contrast, staging beverage intake can be easier since beverages are often consumed in standard containers, such as bottles or cans, and daily intake may be less variable.

Another method of staging includes using "actual" intake of foods or nutrients estimated from food frequency questionnaires (FFQs) or other dietary assessment methods, but this approach has limitations, such as the need to use a set cutoff point. In addition, using the dependent variable (nutrient intake) to also define the independent variable (stage) is problematic.[98]

Strengths and Limitations of the TTM

The TTM has intuitive appeal. Its assumption that people are at different stages of readiness to change is akin to the idea of "starting where people are," implying that tailored interventions appropriate for people's stages of change should be more effective than those using the same intervention for all people. The TTM specifies processes through which behavior change may occur, which can be used to identify types of intervention strategies most effective for

each stage or to deliver a sequence of interventions to move individuals through successive stages.

However, staging of certain dietary behaviors requires more clarity.[99] The TTM should be researched in a broader range of dietary behaviors to determine which stages are important and/or necessary, and which processes of change help people progress through stages for these particular behaviors.

Another concern about the TTM is that stages of change are often highly correlated with *intentions*, which brings to question whether measures of stages are actually measuring the construct of *intention*.[100] Lastly, durations that have commonly been specified for each stage (for example, the past six months for the *action* stage) may not be appropriate for all behaviors or populations. Overall, stage-based models have mixed utility.[101,102,103]

Applying Theory to Research and Practice: Transtheoretical Model

Computer-Based Intervention Tailored on TTM Stages and Processes of Change to Increase Fruit and Vegetable Intake Among African American Teens

One-fifth of African American youths consume five servings of fruits and vegetables a day.[104] Diet-related chronic diseases, including cardiovascular disease, cancer, and diabetes, disproportionately affect African Americans,[105] signifying a greater need for health promotion in this population. To increase fruit and vegetable intake among urban African American youth, a computer-based program was developed and delivered through youth services agencies. Previous research had found that the target population was mostly in *contemplation* or *preparation* (63%), followed by *precontemplation* (20%), and *action* or *maintenance* (17%) stages for fruit and vegetable intake.[106] Therefore, the program was designed to address these stages.[107] Youth in the intervention programs participated in four 30-minute CD-ROM sessions. Session 1 classified participants into their current stages, and sessions 2 to 4 were tailored to participants' stage by incorporating processes of change:

- *Precontemplation*: Included processes of consciousness raising, dramatic relief, and environmental reevaluation to enhance awareness of low intake of fruits and vegetables. For example, to raise consciousness, participants completed an assessment that provided personalized feedback about their usual daily servings.

- *Contemplation-preparation:* Included processes of self-reevaluation and self-liberation to increase confidence in ability to increase fruit and vegetable intake, resolve ambivalence, and facilitate a plan to change diet. A self-liberation strategy involved daily goal setting and development of a one-week menu and action plan.

- *Action-maintenance:* Included processes of reinforcement management, helping relationships, counterconditioning, and stimulus control to sustain recommended intake of fruit and vegetables. An example of a helping relationship strategy was to encourage youths to team up with another person to develop a "buddy contract" to identify strategies for supporting each other.

Youths completing the computer-based program had higher perceived pros of increasing fruit and vegetable consumption and higher consumption compared with the control group. They also progressed to the later stages of change and maintained the recommended intake of fruits and vegetables. Changes observed in this study were measured in the short term. Future studies using this approach should determine if dietary changes are sustained. As youths spend increasing amounts of time with computers and smartphones, tailored interventions delivered through electronic media may be both cost effective and appealing to them.

Effect of an Intervention to Change Dietary Behaviors for Diabetes Prevention Among Norwegian-Pakistani Women

Public Health Core Competency 4: Cultural Competency Skills 1: Incorporates strategies for interacting with persons from diverse backgrounds

Pakistanis compose the largest ethnic minority in Norway, and are at higher risk for type 2 diabetes than other Norwegian groups. InnvaDiab was a targeted intervention that included group sessions, individual counseling, and exercise group sessions. One hundred and ninety-eight women living in Norway who were either born in Pakistan or born in Norway with two Pakistani parents were randomized to the intervention or control group.[108] Through six group sessions over seven months, participants were encouraged to reduce sugar and refined carbohydrates; change to more complex carbohydrates; change cooking fat to rapeseed (canola) oil; eat more fatty fish, vegetables, and legumes; and consume fruit in small amounts. To examine the impact of the intervention on stages of change for these dietary behaviors, one question was asked about each behavior. Response options corresponded to each stage (for example, "I have not changed my behavior for the past six months, but I am considering doing so" [*contemplation*] and "during the past six months, I have changed my behavior" [*action*]).

At follow-up, the intervention group exhibited significant shifts from pre-*action* into *action* stages for changing type of fat, reducing sugar, and reducing white flour. Compared with the control group, the intervention group was more likely to be in *action* stages for reducing intake of sugar and white flour, changing type of fat, and increasing intake of vegetables and legumes. The odds of being in action or maintenance stages for sugar, white flour, and type of fat at follow-up increased with session attendance,[109] and changes in reported intake of sugar-rich drinks and rapeseed oil were significantly greater in the intervention group than in the control group.

In this example, investigators examined shifts in stages of change as an indicator of intervention effectiveness. However, they did not indicate that the intervention itself was based on any particular theoretical framework or that it was specifically designed to alter stage of change.

Ecological Models

Ecological models are the final set of models to be reviewed in this chapter. Authorities including the World Health Organization (WHO),[110] the Centers for Disease Control and Prevention (CDC),[111] the White House Task Force on Childhood Obesity,[112] and the Institute of Medicine (IOM)[113,114] identify policy and environmental interventions as among the most promising strategies for achieving population improvements in diet, physical activity, and obesity. A weakness of theories and models primarily concerned with individual cognitive processes is their limited capacity to guide environmental, community, and policy interventions. In contrast, ecological models (EMs) or social ecological models (SEMs) explain human behavior based on dynamic interactions between people and environments[115,116] and the multiple levels of influence over behavior,[117,118] which may include individual, interpersonal, organizational, environmental, community, and policy levels.

Table 3-6 Parent-centered Family Ecological Model

Proximal Factors	Broader contexts
• Family size, ethnicity, and structure	• Parent job demands
• Family health	• Child characteristics
• Parent modeling of nutrition and activity behaviors	• School policies
• Parent nutrition knowledge	• Media and food advertising
• Availability of healthy foods at home	• Nutrition labeling
	• The built environment

Data from: Davison, K. K., & Campbell, K. J. (2005). Opportunities to prevent obesity in children within families: An ecological approach. In D. Crawford & R. Jeffery (Eds.), *Obesity Prevention and Public Health*. Oxford: Oxford University Press.

helpful/effective ↓ for children

Levels of the Ecological Model

individual

Intrapersonal factors include an individual's characteristics, such as genetics, age, income, education, knowledge, attitudes, behavior, self-concept, and skills. As an example, the Planet Health curriculum addresses intrapersonal factors by increasing knowledge and skill building in the areas of diet, activity, and screen time among sixth to eighth graders by increasing knowledge and skill building in these areas. Lessons were designed to fit within existing school curricula and reinforce skills in other subjects as well, such as language arts and math. In a school-based **randomized controlled trial**, the two-year intervention reduced obesity among girls and reduced time spent watching television among both girls and boys.[119]

Interpersonal factors include social networks and support systems, such as the family, the work group, and friendship networks. The Pediatric Overweight Prevention through Parent Training program targeted interpersonal factors to reduce unhealthy weight gain among 2- to 4-year-old Latino children.[120] In a randomized controlled pilot study of the program, parents attended seven weekly educational classes designed to increase knowledge about the Dietary Guidelines, teach families behavior modification strategies and strategies to increase children's vegetable and fruit preferences, and to identify and address barriers to healthy lifestyles. At one year, body mass index (BMI) z-scores of children in the intervention group decreased compared with those of children in the control group.[121]

Institutional factors encompass social institutions such as worksites, schools, child care centers, churches, and neighborhood organizations. Interventions in these settings can be effective because of access to many individuals in confined settings where they spend much of their time. Interventions at this level include wellness policies, improving on-site food options, providing exercise facilities, and organizing walking groups for social support. To assist workplaces in developing obesity prevention programs, the CDC maintains the website "LEAN Works!"[122] The site has interactive tools and resources to help design evidence-based programs.

Community factors are relationships among organizations, institutions, and informal networks within defined boundaries. Community coalitions and partnerships can increase coordination to influence local and state food policies, community awareness of health problems and their causes, and coordination of resources. Coalitions can include non-profit organizations, schools, churches, employers, local government agencies, healthcare organizations, media, and private citizens. Community factors also include a community's built and social environment, such as the density of fast-food restaurants and presence of bicycle lanes.

Policy and society factors include policies at local, state, and national levels, industry activities, and mass media. Policies, such as food safety laws and local and state regulations of trans fats in restaurants, can affect the nature of the food supply. The ban on sales of sugary drinks exceeding 16 ounces in New York City restaurants, proposed in 2012 and met with ongoing resistance by 2013, is a policy that can affect behaviors.[123] Policies can also incentivize behaviors. For example, the **Women, Infants, and Children (WIC)** food package incentivizes breastfeeding by providing fully breastfeeding women greater amounts of food, including a higher dollar value for fruits and vegetables.[124] Agricultural subsidies may indirectly affect behaviors through their impact on food prices.

Vanaspati, a common butter substitute in India, provides an illustration of industry's effects on people's diets. The trans fat content of commercially prepared vanaspati can be up to 65% of total fatty acids.[125] Media can also influence health behaviors for better and for worse. Accurate news coverage, public service announcements, and authoritative websites on diet and physical activity can support healthy behaviors. In contrast, advertising of unhealthy products, misinformation on websites and news stories, and modeling of unhealthy behaviors in television shows can have detrimental impacts on health behaviors.

Culture includes those shared perceptions, beliefs, values, norms, customs, and behaviors of a group that are passed on to others, especially children,[126] and it affects dietary choices. For example, white rice, a source of refined carbohydrates, is a mainstay of many modern Asian diets, while brown rice and other whole grains are rarely consumed.[127] However, high consumption of refined carbohydrates is associated with increased risk of type 2 diabetes,[128,129] and high intake of whole grains is associated with lower risk.[130,131,132] Cultural barriers to acceptance of brown rice among Chinese adults have been identified as perceptions of unpalatable taste and low quality. **Acculturation** also affects diet. Mexican Americans with greater acculturation to the United States have lower intakes of fruits, beans, and whole-fat milk and higher intake of sugar-sweetened beverages and whole grains.[133,134,135]

EMs are consistent with the trend in public health toward increasing recognition of the role of external factors in individual health behavior. Interventions focused on changing characteristics of individuals have dominated many nutritional interventions, but these strategies may not work unless environments are supportive. Likewise, environmental strategies, such as increasing availability of fruits, vegetables, and whole grains in corner stores, may not work in absence of education and attention to psychological factors. Sallis and colleagues have proposed four core principles of EMs of health behavior:[136]

1. The multiple influences on specific health behaviors include factors at the intrapersonal, interpersonal, organizational, community, and public policy levels.

2. Influences on behaviors interact across these different levels.

3. Ecological models should be behavior-specific, identifying the most relevant potential influences at each level.

4. Multilevel interventions should be most effective in changing behavior.

EMs should be tailored for specific behaviors and contexts, and sample EMs are presented below.

Model of Community Nutrition Environments

This conceptual model was developed to study four types of nutrition environments and the environmental variables that exist in these settings: the community nutrition environment (location and type of food venues or outlets), organizational nutrition environment (workplace, school, home, and other environments), consumer nutrition environment (availability, price, promotion, placement, and nutrition information of healthy and unhealthy foods), and information environment (media and marketing).[137] This model proposes that within each environment, policy variables, including public and industry policy, affect environmental variables, which then affect consumption directly or indirectly.

Family Ecological Model

EMs aim to explain variations in the behavior of individuals, who are at the center of EMs. However, EMs go beyond

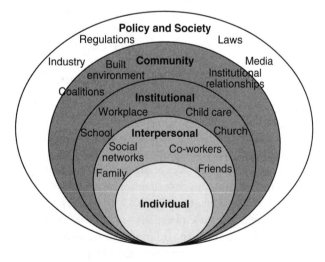

Figure 3-5   Ecological Model

Data from Bronfenbrenner, U. (1977). Toward an experimental ecology of human development. *American Psychologist, 32*(7), 513-531 and McLeroy, K. R., Bibeau, D., Steckler, A., & Glanz, K. (1988). An ecological perspective on health promotion programs. *Health Education Quarterly, 15*(4), 351-377.

explaining individual behaviors. For example, the EM was recently reconceptualized as the Family Ecological Model (FEM), which postulates that parenting specific to children's food, physical activity, and screen-related behaviors is shaped by factors proximal to families (for example, child characteristics, family history and structure, and family health) in combination with the broader contexts. Broader contexts can encompass parent job characteristics and demands, school policies, community food and activity resources, and neighborhood social capital. The FEM recognizes that effective family-centered interventions require understanding of contexts in which families are embedded.

Applying Theory to Research and Practice: FEM

The FEM was recently applied in a family-centered program to prevent obesity in preschool-aged children enrolled in Head Start, a federal program to promote school readiness among children from low-income households. In a small city in upstate New York, a **community-based participatory research (CBPR)** approach guided the overall process of intervention development and implementation.[138] Participants were children ages 2 to 5 years enrolled in Head Start and their parents or guardians.

A community advisory board (CAB) composed predominantly of parents of Head Start children was established. An early objective of the CAB was to conduct a community assessment to learn more about family lives, program outcomes valued by Head Start families, and family and community resources that could foster sustainability.

Researchers provided CAB members with the FEM to frame discussions around possible constructs to include in the community assessment. CAB members were asked to reflect on the FEM as they discussed how factors in their social, cultural, economic, and physical environments affected their obesity-related parenting behaviors, or those specific to children's diet and physical activity behaviors. These informal discussions led to the creation of an extensive list of factors that parents believed affected their parenting cognitions and behaviors specific to healthy lifestyles.[139] These factors were subsequently measured in the community assessment using a combination of **qualitative** and **quantitative** measures.[140]

From Assessment to Intervention

Results from the community assessment were reviewed with the CAB through a series of data workshops, which

enabled parents to provide their interpretation of the data.[141] Results were also shared with Head Start families at a town hall meeting and with Head Start staff and leadership and the broader community through a community forum to solicit further input on the interpretation of the data and the themes emerging. The data and interpretative feedback were used to refine the FEM[142] and identify priorities for the subsequent family-centered intervention—the Communities for Healthy Living (CHL) program.

The four key elements of the resulting CHL program (**Table 3-7**) were: (1) a health communication campaign to increase parents' awareness of childhood obesity and dispel myths around children's weight, (2) revisions to health letters sent home to Head Start families communicating the results of their child's body mass index assessments, (3) informal nutritional counseling sessions that were integrated into Head Start family outreach activities, and (4) a parent-led program to promote social networking and advocacy, communication, media literacy, and conflict resolution skills—all of which were identified in the community assessment as key outcomes of interest to parents.

Program Evaluation

A pre-post cohort design was used to evaluate the CHL program.[143] Because three of the four intervention components were integrated into preexisting Head Start activities, all families were at least minimally exposed to the intervention, and 154 families participated in its evaluation. Improvements in children's BMI z-score, light physical activity, and television viewing time were noted.[144] Improvements were also observed in parents' resource empowerment (that is, the ability to determine the resources needed to promote child health and to access such resources) and food, physical activity, and screen-related parenting practices.

Strengths and Limitations of EMs

EMs provide frameworks for intervening at multiple levels of influence. Intervening at the organizational, community, and policy levels affects more people, including those who had no intention of changing behaviors and those who are socially and economically vulnerable and unlikely to otherwise be reached by health promotion programs. Furthermore, interventions that create supportive environments and policies help to sustain behavior change over the long term. CHL, for example, initiated changes in organizational practices, through health letters sent home, and

Table 3-7 Components of the Communities for Healthy Living program

Intervention Component	Description	Intervention Principles
Health Communication Campaign	Posters were displayed in all Head Start centers for three to four weeks each. Quotes from the community assessment focus groups (e.g., "It's just baby fat, he'll grow out of it") were used as a basis of the campaign. Research negating each quote was highlighted.	Increase parents' awareness and recognition of their child's weight status. Dispel myths about children's weight status (e.g., he's just big for his age, my child is active so she can't be overweight, juice is good for my child).
Revised Body Mass Index (BMI) letters	Health letters sent to families with results from their child's height and weight measurements were revised to improve the accessibility of information for parents.	Increase parent awareness and understanding of child weight status. Increase parent awareness of local resources for obesity prevention and treatment.
Family nutrition counseling	Informal nutrition counseling sessions were integrated into Head Start family engagement activities. Local nutrition graduate students attended Head Start family events, provided samples of healthy foods, and answered questions parents had regarding their child's and their own nutrition and weight status.	Foster parent social networking. Promote parent resource empowerment. Increase parent nutrition knowledge.
Parents Connect for Healthy Living Program	Six weekly two-hour sessions implemented in each center. All sessions addressed skills that parents were most interested in gaining, incorporated materials/examples around healthy living, and included workshops by local organizations (e.g., media literacy training led by local public broadcasting station). Sessions were led by trained parent leaders in conjunction with an experienced group moderator.	Sessions included materials/examples specific to healthy living and addressed the following: • Resource identification and utilization • Effective communication • Conflict resolution • Media literacy • Professionalism

Modified from Davison, K. K., Jurkowski, J. M., Li, K., Kranz, S., & Lawson, H. A. (2013). A childhood obesity intervention developed by families for families: results from a pilot study. *International Journal of Behavioral Nutrition and Physical Activity, 10,* 3.

community capacity to support a healthy body weight in children, by linking Head Start families with nutrition students from a local college. These supported long-term ability of parents to promote healthy body weights in their children.

A limitation of EMs is their lack of clarity around which levels of influence are most important for different behaviors and how variables interact across levels. EM-based interventions demand time, labor, and resources. They require developing and delivering interventions, collecting and/or developing measures of influence at multiple levels, and sophisticated statistical approaches.[145] Changing environments may take many years to achieve, exceeding

grant timelines and making evaluation difficult. Since these changes often require legislation and regulation, building relationships with policy makers and advocates can be efficacious.[146] Since EMs generally lack inclusion of cognitive variables, combining them with other models may be effective in designing multilevel interventions that address the intrapersonal level. In the case of the CHL intervention, SCT and empowerment theory[147] were used in conjunction with FEM to specify anticipated cognitive mechanisms of change. Consistent with these models, increases in parents' *self-efficacy* to promote a healthy lifestyle and perceived resource empowerment, or knowing which resources are needed and how to acquire such resources, were linked to improvements in diet, physical activity, and screen-related parenting practices and children's behavioral and weight-related outcomes.

How Is Theory Tested?

A theory is tested to determine how its constructs are related and if those constructs—separately and in total—predict behavior in the manner specified by the theory. Theories can be tested alone or against one another. The majority of research testing theory comes from **observational studies**. Most of these studies are **cross-sectional**, thus preventing ability to determine the direction of causation. **Longitudinal/prospective** observational studies can investigate how cognitive constructs are associated with future performance of a behavior. However, they are still prone to bias due to unmeasured confounding by previous performance of a behavior[148] and other variables. Randomized controlled trials and other experimental designs are less prone to these biases.[149] The most critical question theory testing should seek to answer is "whether changes in particular theory-based constructs lead to changes in health behavior."[150] Noar and Mehrotra have proposed the multi-methodological theory-testing (MMTT) framework for testing health behavior theory that, in addition to including observational studies, also includes randomized lab and field experiments, mediation analysis of theory-based interventions, and meta-analysis to test theory.[151] While some experimental studies explicitly aim to test theory (for example, by translating one or more theories into intervention conditions and testing those conditions against one another), others use theory to develop intervention components aimed at changing constructs hypothesized to induce behavior change. The latter designs should still be used to test theory by including valid and reliable measures of theoretical constructs and conducting a mediation analysis. A recent review of dietary behavior change interventions among youth[152] found that interventions were generally unsuccessful in changing mediators (that is, theoretical constructs), but *self-efficacy* and *outcome expectations* were most consistently associated with changes in diet. *Outcome expectations* was the only construct identified as a mediator in multiple interventions.

Public Health Core Competency 1: Analytical/ Assessment Skills 4: Uses methods and instruments for collecting valid and reliable quantitative and qualitative data

---

How to Select Theory

Currently, no single theory or model is universally superior. This is partly due to the need for further research, and also due to the need to select a theory based on the particular circumstances. A review found only 19 published articles with empirical comparisons of theories, and only a fraction included diet-related interventions.[153] Similarly, a systematic review of research on health behavior and health promotion in 10 major peer-reviewed journals from 2000 to 2005 found that only five articles focused on testing theory.[154] Until more complete data are available, practitioners and researchers should consider each model in the context of the target population (for example, high school students in urban Mexico or mothers of young children in Malawi), health problem (for example, obesity or severe malnourishment), desired behavior (for example, replacing soda with water or feeding one's child protein-rich foods), and setting (for example, school, home, or worksite). They should also review the literature to select behaviors causally and strongly related to the outcome of interest and to review empirical evidence that constructs outlined in a specific theory predict these behaviors in populations similar to the target group.

Theory selection can proceed by working backward from a logic model of the problem.[155] A logic model is a planning tool that requires program planners to specify a framework's components, such as inputs (resources that go into a program), outputs (program activities and population reached), and outcomes (changes resulting from program outputs).[156] The PRECEDE-PROCEED model[157] provides a structure for applying theories for planning and evaluating interventions and programs.[158] After theory selection, researchers should determine and clearly specify how to use the theory. This may include specifying the components of an intervention based on theory, the specific constructs used to inform those components, methods and procedures to change mediators, instruments used to measure constructs, and validity and reliability of those instruments.

Conclusion

This chapter describes widely used theories and models of behavior change and provides examples of each theory's application to public health nutrition. Theories of health behavior guide the development of programs by specifying which behavioral determinants (for example, cognitive and/or environmental constructs) to target and how to measure outcomes. However, most theories and models do not specify the procedures for *changing* mediators identified by theories. Interventions have often "used intuitively reasonable procedures," but future research should focus on developing and testing specific procedures for altering mediating variables among various populations.[159,160]

In addition, theories should continue to be tested to determine their abilities to explain nutritional behaviors among different populations. Since existing theories generally explain no more than 30% of the variance in diet and physical activity behaviors,[161,162] inclusion of new constructs may improve prediction. Combining theories to include cognitive and environmental factors can also help.[163]

References

1 Ogden, C. L., Troiano, R. P., Briefel, R. R., Kuczmarski, R. J., Flegal, K. M., & Johnson, C. L. (1997). Prevalence of overweight among preschool children in the United States, 1971 through 1994. *Pediatrics, 99*(4), E1.

2 Ogden, C. L., Carroll, M. D., & Flegal, K. M. (2008). High body mass index for age among U.S. children and adolescents, 2003-2006. *Journal of the American Medical Association, 299*(20), 2401-5.

3 Daniels, S. R. (2006). The consequences of childhood overweight and obesity. *Future of Children, 16*(1), 47-67.

4 Olshansky, S. J., Passaro, D. J., Hershow, R. C., Layden, J., Carnes, B. A., Brody, J., . . . Ludwig, D. S. (2005). A potential decline in life expectancy in the United States in the 21st century. *New England Journal of Medicine, 352*(11), 1138-45.

5 Anderson, S. E., & Whitaker, R. C. (2009). Prevalence of obesity among U.S. preschool children in different racial and ethnic groups. *Archives of Pediatrics and Adolescent Medicine, 163*(4), 344-48.

6 Wang, Y., & Beydoun, M. A. (2007). The obesity epidemic in the United States–gender, age, socioeconomic, racial/ethnic, and geographic characteristics: A systematic review and meta-regression analysis. *Epidemiologic Reviews, 29*, 6-28.

7 Gundersen, C., Lohman, B. J., Garasky, S., Stewart, S., & Eisenmann, J. (2008). Food security, maternal stressors, and overweight among low-income US children: Results from the National Health and Nutrition Examination Survey (1999-2002). *Pediatrics, 122*(3), e529-540.

8 Leung, C. W., Ding, E. L., Catalano, P. J., Villamor, E., Rimm, E. B., & Willett, W. C. (2012). Dietary intake and dietary quality of low-income adults in the Supplemental Nutrition Assistance Program. *American Journal of Clinical Nutrition, 96*(5), 977-88.

9 Gundersen, C., Lohman, B. J., Garasky, S., Stewart, S., & Eisenmann, J. (2008). Food security, maternal stressors, and overweight among low-income U.S. children: Results from the National Health and Nutrition Examination Survey (1999-2002). *Pediatrics, 122*(3), e529-540.

10 Burdette, H. L., Wadden, T. A., & Whitaker, R. C. (2006). Neighborhood safety, collective efficacy, and obesity in women with young children. *Obesity (Silver Spring), 14*(3), 518-25.

11 Larson, N. I., Story, M. T., & Nelson, M. C. (2009). Neighborhood environments: Disparities in access to healthy foods in the U.S. *American Journal of Preventive Medicine, 36*(1), 74-81.

12 Gochman, D. S. (1988). Health behavior: Plural persepctives. In D. S. Gochman (Ed.), *Health behavior: Emerging research perspectives* (pp. 3-17). New York: Plenum Press.

13 Gochman, D. S. (1982). Labels, systems and motives: Some perspectives for future research. *Health Education Quarterly, 9*, 167-74.

14 Kasl, S. V., & Cobb, S. (1966). Health behavior, illness behavior, and sick role behavior. I. Health and illness behavior. *Archives of Environmental Health, 12*(2), 246-66.

15 Kasl, S. V., & Cobb, S. (1966). Health behavior, illness behavior, and sick-role behavior. II. Sick-role behavior. *Archives of Environmental Health, 12*(4), 531-41.

16 Salazar, L. F., Crosby, R. A., & DiClemente, R. J. (2013). Health behavior in the context of the "new" public health. In R. J. DiClemente, L. F. Salazar, & R. A. Crosby (Eds.), *Health behavior theory for public health principles, foundations and applications*. Burlington, MA: Jones & Bartlett Learning.

17 Kerlinger, F. N. (1986). *Foundations of behavioral research* (3rd ed.). New York: Holt, Rinehart & Winston.

18 Glanz, K., Rimer, B. K., & Viswanath, K. (2008). The scope of health behavior and health education. In K. Glanz, B. K. Rimer, & K. Viswanath (Eds.), *Health behavior and health education: Theory, research, and practice* (4th ed.). San Francisco, CA: Jossey-Bass.

19 Lytle, L. A. (2005). Nutrition education, behavioral theories, and the scientific method: Another viewpoint. *Journal of Nutrition Education and Behavior, 37*(2), 90-93.

20 Ammerman, A. S., Lindquist, C. H., Lohr, K. N., & Hersey, J. (2002). The efficacy of behavioral interventions to modify dietary fat and fruit and vegetable intake: A review of the evidence. *Preventive Medicine, 35*(1), 25-41.

21 Noar, S. M., Benac, C. N., & Harris, M. S. (2007). Does tailoring matter? Meta-analytic review of tailored print health behavior change interventions. *Psychological Bulletin, 133*(4), 673-93.

22 Legler, J., Meissner, H. I., Coyne, C., Breen, N., Chollette, V., & Rimer, B. K. (2002). The effectiveness of interventions to promote mammography among women with historically lower rates of screening. *Cancer Epidemiology, Biomarkers and Prevention, 11*(1), 59-71.

23 Painter, J. E., Borba, C. P., Hynes, M., Mays, D., & Glanz, K. (2008). The use of theory in health behavior research from 2000 to 2005: A systematic review. *Annals of Behavioral Medicine, 35*(3), 358-62.

24 Rosenstock, I. M. (1966). Why people use health services. *Milbank Memorial Fund Quarterly, 44*, 94-124.

25 Hochbaum, G. M. (1958). *Public participation in medical screening programs: A socio-psychological study.* PHS Publication No. 572. Washington, DC: Public Health Service, Division of Special Health Services.

26 Baranowski, T., Cullen, K. W., Nicklas, T., Thompson, D., & Baranowski, J. (2003). Are current health behavioral change models helpful in guiding prevention of weight gain efforts? *Obesity Research, 11*(Suppl.), 23S-43S.

27 Janz, N. K., & Becker, M. H. (1984). The Health Belief Model: A decade later. *Health Education & Behavior, 11*(1), 1-47.

28 Champion, V. L., & Skinner, C. S. (2008). The Health Belief Model. In K. Glanz, B. K. Rimer, & K. Viswanath (Eds.), *Health behavior and health education: Theory, research, and practice.* San Francisco, CA: Jossey-Bass.

29 Champion, V. L., & Skinner, C. S. (2008). The Health Belief Model. In K. Glanz, B. K. Rimer, & K. Viswanath (Eds.), *Health behavior and health education: Theory, research, and practice.* San Francisco, CA: Jossey-Bass.

30 Champion, V. L., Skinner, C. Sugg, Menon, U., Rawl, S., Giesler, R. B., Monahan, P., & Daggy, J. (2004). A breast cancer fear scale: Psychometric development. *Journal of Health Psychology, 9*(6), 753-62.

31 Abood, D. A., Black, D. R., & Feral, D. (2003). Nutrition education worksite intervention for university staff: Application of the Health Belief Model. *Journal of Nutrition Education and Behavior 35*(5), 260-67.

32 Ellis, J., Johnson, M. A., Fischer, J. G., & Hargrove, J. L. (2005). Nutrition and health education intervention for whole grain foods in the Georgia Older Americans Nutrition Program. *Journal of Nutrition for the Elderly, 24*(3), 67-83.

33 Fishbein, M., & Ajzen, I. (1975). *Belief, attitude, intention and behavior: An introduction to theory and research.* Reading, MA: Addison-Wesley.

34 Ajzen, I. (1991). The Theory of Planned Behavior. *Organizational Behavior and Human Decision Processes, 50*, 179-211.

35 Ajzen, I. (1991). The Theory of Planned Behavior. *Organizational Behavior and Human Decision Processes, 50*, 179-211.

36 Fishbein, M., & Ajzen, I. (1975). *Belief, attitude, intention and behavior: An introduction to theory and research.* Reading, MA: Addison-Wesley.

37 Ajzen, I., & Madden, T. J. (1986). Prediction of goal-directed behavior: Attitudes, intentions, and perceived behavioral control. *Journal of Experimental Social Psychology, 22*(5), 453-74.

38 Madden, T. J., Scholder, E. P., & Ajzen, I. (1992). A Comparison of the Theory of Planned Behavior and the Theory of Reasoned Action. *Personality and Social Psychology Bulletin, 18*(1), 3-9.

39 Ajzen, I. (1991). The Theory of Planned Behavior. *Organizational Behavior and Human Decision Processes, 50*, 179-211.

40 McEachan, R. R. C., Conner, M., Taylor, N. J., & Lawton, R. J. (2011). Prospective prediction of health-related behaviours with the Theory of Planned Behaviour: A meta-analysis. *Health Psychology Review, 5*(2), 97-144.

41 McEachan, R. R. C., Conner, M., Taylor, N. J., & Lawton, R. J. (2011). Prospective prediction of health-related behaviours with the Theory of Planned Behaviour: A meta-analysis. *Health Psychology Review, 5*(2), 97-144.

42 Baranowski, T., Cullen, K. W., Nicklas, T., Thompson, D., & Baranowski, J. (2003). Are current health behavioral change models helpful in guiding prevention of weight gain efforts? *Obesity Research, 11*(Suppl.), 23S-43S.

43 Allen, C. T., Machleit, K. A., Schultz Kleine, S., & Notani, A. S. (2005). A place for emotion in attitude models. *Journal of Business Research, 58*(4), 494-99.

44 Armitage, C. J., Conner, M., & Norman, P. (1999). Differential effects of mood on information processing: Evidence from the theories of reasoned action and planned behaviour. *European Journal of Social Psychology, 29*(4), 419-33.

45 Fishbein, M. (2008). A reasoned action approach to health promotion. *Medical Decision Making, 28*(6), 834-44.

46 Ajzen, I. (2011). The theory of planned behaviour: Reactions and reflections. *Psychology & Health, 26*(9), 1113-27.

47 McEachan, R. R. C., Conner, M., Taylor, N. J., & Lawton, R. J. (2011). Prospective prediction of health-related behaviours with the Theory of Planned Behaviour: A meta-analysis. *Health Psychology Review, 5*(2), 97-144.

48 American Academy of Pediatrics. (2009). *Pediatric nutrition handbook* (6th ed.). Elk Grove Village, IL: American Academy of Pediatrics.

49 Hendricks, K., Briefel, R., Novak, T., & Ziegler, P. (2006). Maternal and child characteristics associated with infant and toddler feeding practices. *Journal of the American Dietetic Association, 106*(1, Suppl.), 135-48.

50 Brophy-Herb, H., Silk, K., Horodynski, M., Mercer, L., & Olson, B. (2009). Key theoretical frameworks for intervention: Understanding and promoting behavior change in parent-infant feeding dhoices in a low-income population. *Journal of Primary Prevention, 30*(2), 191-208.

51 Brophy-Herb, H., Silk, K., Horodynski, M., Mercer, L., & Olson, B. (2009). Key theoretical frameworks for intervention: Understanding and promoting behavior change in parent-infant feeding dhoices in a low-income population. *Journal of Primary Prevention, 30*(2), 191-208.

52 Horodynski, M. A., Olson, B., Baker, S., Brophy-Herb, H., Auld, G., Van Egeren, L., . . . Singleterry, L. (2011). Healthy babies through infant-centered feeding protocol: An intervention targeting early childhood obesity in vulnerable populations. *BMC Public Health, 11*, 868.

53 Tuu, H. H., Olsen, S. O., Thao, D. T., & Anh, N. T. (2008). The role of norms in explaining attitudes, intention and consumption of a common food (fish) in Vietnam. *Appetite, 51*(3), 546-51.

54 Astrom, A. N. (2004). Validity of cognitive predictors of adolescent sugar snack consumption. *American Journal of Health Behavior, 28*(2), 112-21.

55 Bandura, A. (1986). *Social foundations of thought and action: A social cognitive theory*. Englewood Cliffs, NJ: Prentice-Hall.

56 Bandura, A. (1977). *Social learning theory*. Englewood Cliffs, NJ: Prentice Hall.

57 Bandura, A. (1997). *Self-efficacy: The exercise of control*. New York: W. H. Freeman.

58 Bandura, A. (1997). *Self-efficacy: The exercise of control*. New York: W. H. Freeman.

59 Bandura, A. (1997). *Self-efficacy: The exercise of control*. New York: W. H. Freeman.

60 Bandura, A. (1997). Self-efficacy: The exercise of control. New York, NY: W. H. Freeman.

61 Baranowski, T., Cullen, K. W., Nicklas, T., Thompson, D., & Baranowski, J. (2003). Are current health behavioral change models helpful in guiding prevention of weight gain efforts? *Obesity Research, 11*(Suppl.), 23S-43S.

62 Bandura, A. (1997). *Self-efficacy: The exercise of control*. New York: W. H. Freeman.

63 McAlister, A. L., Perry, C. L., & Parcel, G. S. (2008). How individuals, environments, and health behaviors interact: Social Cognitive Theory. In K. Glanz, B. K. Rimer, & K. Viswanath (Eds.), *Health behavior and health education: Theory, research, and Practice* (4th ed.). San Francisco, CA: Jossey-Bass.

64 Cullen, K. W., Baranowski, T., & Smith, S. P. (2001). Using goal setting as a strategy for dietary behavior change. *Journal of the American Dietetic Association, 101*(5), 562-66.

65 Shilts, M. K., Horowitz, M., & Townsend, M. S. (2004). Goal setting as a strategy for dietary and physical activity behavior change: A review of the literature. *American Journal of Health Promotion, 19*(2), 81-93.

66 Bandura, A. (1997). *Self-efficacy: The exercise of control*. New York: W. H. Freeman.

67 Baranowski, T. (1997). Families and health sctions. In D. S. Gochman (Ed.), *Handbook of health behavior research I: Personal and social determinants*. New York: Plenum Press.

68 Wood, R., & Bandura, A. (1989). Social Cognitive Theory of Organizational Management. *Academy of Management Review, 14*(3), 361-84.

69 Bandura, A. (2001). Social Cognitive Theory of Mass Communication. *Media Psychology, 3*(3), 265-99.

70 Bandura, A. (2001). Social Cognitive Theory of Mass Communication. *Media Psychology, 3*(3), 265-99.

71 Schunk, D. H. (1987). Peer models and children's behavioral change. *Review of Educational Research, 57*(2), 149-74.

72 Valente, T. W., Murphy, S., Huang, G., Gusek, J., Greene, J., & Beck, V. (2007). Evaluating a minor storyline on *ER* about teen obesity, hypertension, and 5 A Day. *Journal of Health Communication, 12*(6), 551-66.

73 Valente, T. W., Murphy, S., Huang, G., Gusek, J., Greene, J., & Beck, V. (2007). Evaluating a minor storyline on *ER* about teen obesity, hypertension, and 5 A Day. *Journal of Health Communication, 12*(6), 551-66.

74 Bandura, A. (1986). *Social foundations of thought and action: A social cognitive theory*. Englewood Cliffs, NJ: Prentice-Hall.

75 Tuu, H. H., Olsen, S. O., Thao, D. T., & Anh, N. T. (2008). The role of norms in explaining attitudes, intention and consumption of a common food (fish) in Vietnam. *Appetite, 51*(3), 546-51.

76 McAlister, A. L., Perry, C. L., & Parcel, G. S. (2008). How individuals, environments, and health behaviors interact: Social Cognitive Theory. In K. Glanz, B. K. Rimer, & K. Viswanath (Eds.), *Health behavior and health education: Theory, research, and Practice* (4th ed.). San Francisco, CA: Jossey-Bass.

77 Gortmaker, S. L. (2008). Innovations to reduce television and computertime and obesity in childhood. *Archives of Pediatric and Adolescent Medicine, 162*(3), 283-84.

78 Pearson, N., & Biddle, S. J. (2011). Sedentary behavior and dietary intake in children, adolescents, and adults: A systematic review. *American Journal of Preventive Medicine, 41*(2), 178-88.

79 Harris, J. L., Bargh, J. A., & Brownell, K. D. (2009). Priming effects of television food advertising on eating behavior. *Health Psychology, 28*(4), 404-13.

80 Halford, J. C., Boyland, E. J., Hughes, G. M., Stacey, L., McKean, S., & Dovey, T. M. (2008). Beyond-brand effect of television food advertisements on food choice in children: The effects of weight status. *Public Health Nutrition, 11*(9), 897-904.

81 Strasburger, V. C. (2011). Children, adolescents, obesity, and the media. *Pediatrics, 128*(1), 201-8.

82 Commonwealth of Australian Government, Department of Health and Ageing. (2004). *Australia's physical activity recommendations for 5-12 year olds*. Retrieved from http://www .health.gov.au/internet/main/publishing.nsf/Content/9D7D393 564FA0C42CA256F970014A5D4/$File/kids_phys.pdf

83 Office of the Surgeon General. (2007). *The Surgeon General's call to action to prevent and decrease overweight and obesity*. Retrieved from http://www.surgeongeneral.gov/topics /obesity/calltoaction/fact_adolescents.htm

84 Zimmerman, F. J., Ortiz, S. E., Christakis, D. A., & Elkun, D. (2012). The value of social-cognitive theory to reducing preschool TV viewing: A pilot randomized trial. *Preventive Medicine, 54*(3-4), 212-18.

85 Zimmerman, B. J. (2000). Attaining self regulation: A social cognitive perspective. In M. Boekaerts, P. R. Pintrich, & M. Zeidner (Eds.), *Handbook of self-regulation*. San Diego, CA: Academic Press.

86 Kolopaking, R., Bardosono, S., & Fahmida, U. (2011). Maternal self-efficacy in the home food environment: A qualitative study among low-income mothers of nutritionally at-risk children in an urban area of Jakarta, Indonesia. *Journal of Nutrition Education and Behavior, 43*(3), 180-88.

87 Doak, C. M., Adair, L. S., Bentley, M., Monteiro, C., & Popkin, B. M. (2005). The dual burden household and the nutrition transition paradox. *International Journal of Obesity, 29*(1), 129-36.

88 Doak, C. M., Adair, L. S., Bentley, M., Monteiro, C., & Popkin, B. M. (2005). The dual burden household and the nutrition transition paradox. *International Journal of Obesity, 29*(1), 129-36.

89 Prochaska, J. M., & DiClemente, C. C. (1984). *The transtheoretical approach: Crossing traditional boundaries of change.* Homewood, IL: Dow Jones/Irwin.

90 Prochaska, J. O., & DiClemente, C. C. (1983). Stages and processes of self-change of smoking: toward an integrative model of change. *Journal of Consulting and Clinical Psychology, 51*(3), 390-95.

91 DiClemente, C. C., & Prochaska, J. O. (1982). Self-change and therapy change of smoking behavior: A comparison of processes of change in cessation and maintenance. *Addictive Behaviors, 7*(2), 133-42.

92 Prochaska, J. O., Redding, C. A., & Evers, K. A. (2008). The Transtheoretical Model and stages of change. In K. Glanz, B. K. Rimer, & K. Viswanath (Eds.), *Health behavior and health education: Theory, research, and practice.* San Francisco, CA: Jossey-Bass.

93 Prochaska, J. O., Velicer, W. F., Rossi, J. S., Goldstein, M. G., Marcus, B. H., Rakowski, W., . . . Rossi, S. R. (1994). Stages of change and decisional balance for 12 problem behaviors. *Health Psychology, 13*(1), 39-46.

94 Prochaska, J. O., Redding, C. A., & Evers, K. A. (2008). The Transtheoretical Model and stages of change. In K. Glanz, B. K. Rimer, & K. Viswanath (Eds.), *Health behavior and health education: Theory, research, and practice.* San Francisco, CA: Jossey-Bass.

95 Prochaska, J. O., DiClemente, C. C., & Norcross, J. C. (1992). In search of how people change: Applications to addictive behaviors. *American Psychologist, 47*(9), 1102-14.

96 Ma, J., Betts, N. M., Horacek, T., Georgiou, C., & White, A. (2003). Assessing stages of change for fruit and vegetable intake in young adults: A combination of traditional staging algorithms and food-frequency questionnaires. *Health Education Research, 18*(2), 224-36.

97 Baranowski, T., Cullen, K. W., & Baranowski, J. (1999). Psychosocial correlates of dietary intake: Advancing dietary intervention. *Annual Review of Nutrition, 19*(1), 17.

98 Kristal, A. R., Glanz, K., Curry, S. J., & Patterson, R. E. (1999). How can stages of change be best used in dietary interventions? *Journal of the American Dietetic Association, 99*(6), 679-84.

99 Baranowski, T., Cullen, K. W., Nicklas, T., Thompson, D., & Baranowski, J. (2003). Are current health behavioral change models helpful in guiding prevention of weight gain efforts? *Obesity Research, 11*(Suppl.), 23S-43S.

100 Brewer, N. T., & Rimer, B. K. (2008). Perspectives on health behavior theories that focus on individuals. In K. Glanz, B. K. Rimer, & K. Viswanath (Eds.), *Health behavior and health education: Theory, research, and practice.* San Francisco, CA: Jossey-Bass.

101 Bridle, C., Riemsma, R. P., Pattenden, J., Sowden, A. J., Mather, L., Watt, I. S., & Walker, A. (2005). Systematic review of the effectiveness of health behavior interventions based on the Transtheoretical Model. *Psychology & Health, 20*(3), 283-301.

102 Spencer, L., Wharton, C., Moyle, S., & Adams, T. (2007). The Transtheoretical Model as applied to dietary behaviour and outcomes. *Nutrition Research Review, 20*(1), 46-73.

103 Horwath, C. C., Nigg, C. R., Motl, R. W., Wong, K. T., & Dishman, R. K. (2010). Investigating fruit and vegetable consumption using the Transtheoretical Model. *American Journal of Health Promotion, 24*(5), 324-33.

104 Krebs-Smith, S., Cook, D., Subar, A. F., Cleveland, L., Friday, J., & Kahle, L. L. (1996). Fruit and vegetable intakes of children and adolescents in the United States. *Archives of Pediatrics & Adolescent Medicine, 150*(1), 81-86.

105 U.S. Department of Health and Human Services, Office of Minority Health. (2007). *Minority health disparities at a glance.* HHS Fact Sheet. Retrieved from http://minorityhealth.hhs.gov/templates/content.aspx?ID=2139

106 Di Noia, J., Schinke, S. P., Prochaska, J. O., & Contento, I. R. (2006). Application of the Transtheoretical Model to fruit and vegetable consumption among economically disadvantaged African-American adolescents: Preliminary findings. *American Journal of Health Promotion, 20*(5), 342-48.

107 Di Noia, J., Contento, I. R., & Prochaska, J. O. (2008). Computer-mediated intervention tailored on Transtheoretical Model stages and processes of change increases fruit and vegetable consumption among urban African-American adolescents. *American Journal of Health Promotion, 22*(5), 336-41.

108 Johansen, K. S., Bjørge, B., Telle Hjellset, V., Holmboe-Ottesen, G., Råberg, M., & Wandel, M. (2010). Changes in food habits and motivation for healthy eating among Pakistani women living in Norway: Results from the InnvaDiab-DEPLAN study. *Public Health Nutrition, 13*(6), 858-67.

109 Raberg Kjollesdal, M. K., Hjellset, V. T., Bjorge, B., Holmboe-Ottesen, G., & Wandel, M. (2011). Intention to change dietary habits, and weight loss among Norwegian-Pakistani women participating in a culturally adapted intervention. *Journal of Immigrant and Minority Health, 13*(6), 1150-58.

110 World Health Organization. (2010). *Global recommendations on physical activity for health.* Retrieved from http://www.who.int/dietphysicalactivity/factsheet_recommendations/en

111 Koplan, J. P., & Dietz, W. H. (1999). Caloric imbalance and public health policy. *Journal of the American Medical Association, 282*(16), 1579-81.

112 White House Task Force on Childhood Obesity. (2010). *Solving the problem of childhood obesity within a generation.* Retrieved from http://www.letsmove.gov/pdf/TaskForce_on_Childhood_Obesity_May2010_FullReport.pdf

113 Committee on an Evidence Framework for Obesity Prevention Decision Making, Food and Nutrition Board of the Institute of Medicine. (2010). *Bridging the evidence gap in obesity prevention: A framework to inform decision making.* Washington, DC: The National Academies Press. Retrieved from http://books.nap.edu/openbook.php?record_id=12847

114 Committee on Health and Behavior: Research, Practice, and Policy, Board on Neuroscience and Behavioral Health, and the Institute of Medicine. (2001). *Health and behavior: The interplay of biological, behavioral, and societal influences.* Washington, DC: National Academies Press. Retrieved from http://www.nap.edu/openbook.php?record_id=9838

115 Stokols, D. (1992). Establishing and maintaining healthy environments: Toward a social ecology of health promotion. *American Psychologist, 47*(1), 6-22.

116 Sallis, J. F., Owen, N., & Fisher, E. B. (2008). Ecological models of health behavior. In K. Glanz, B. K. Rimer, & K. Viswanath (Eds.), *Health behavior and health education: Theory, research, and practice*. San Francisco, CA: Jossey-Bass.

117 Bronfenbrenner, U. (1979). *The ecology of human development*. Cambridge, MA: Harvard University Press.

118 McLeroy, K. R., Bibeau, D., Steckler, A., & Glanz, K. (1988). An ecological perspective on health promotion programs. *Health Education Quarterly, 15*(4), 351-77.

119 Gortmaker, S. L., Peterson, K., Wiecha, J., Sobol, A. M., Dixit, S., Fox, M. K., & Laird, N. (1999). Reducing obesity via a school-based interdisciplinary intervention among youth: Planet Health. *Archives of Pediatrics and Adolescent Medicine, 153*(4), 409-18.

120 Slusser, W., Frankel, F., Robison, K., Fischer, H., Cumberland, W. G., & Neumann, C. (2012). Pediatric overweight prevention through a parent training program for 2-4 year old Latino children. *Childhood Obesity, 8*(1), 52-59.

121 Slusser, W., Frankel, F., Robison, K., Fischer, H., Cumberland, W. G., & Neumann, C. (2012). Pediatric overweight prevention through a parent training program for 2-4 year old Latino children. *Childhood Obesity, 8*(1), 52-59.

122 Centers for Disease Control and Prevention. (2011). *CDC's LEAN Works! A workplace obesity prevention program*. Retrieved from http://www.cdc.gov/leanworks/index.html

123 Department of Health and Mental Hygiene Board of Health. (2012). *Notice of Adoption of an Amendment (§81.53) to Article 81 of the New York City Health Code*. Retrieved from http://www.nyc.gov/html/doh/downloads/pdf/notice/2012/notice-adoption-amend-article81.pdf

124 U.S. Department of Agriculture Food & Nutrition Services. (2012, February 17). *Questions and answers about the WIC food packages*. Retrieved from http://www.fns.usda.gov/wic/benefitsandservices/foodpkgquestions.HTM

125 L'Abbe, M. R., Stender, S., Skeaff, C. M., Ghafoorunissa, & Tavella, M. (2009). Approaches to removing trans fats from the food supply in industrialized and developing countries. *European Journal of Clinical Nutrition, 63*(S2), S50-67.

126 Altman, I., & Chemers, M. M. (1984). Some definitions: Culture, environment, and psychological processes. In *Culture and Environment*. New York: Cambridge University Press.

127 Zhang, G., Malik, V. S., Pan, A., Kumar, S., Holmes, M. D., Spiegelman, D., . . . Hu, F. B. (2010). Substituting brown rice for white rice to lower diabetes risk: A focus-group study in Chinese adults. *Journal of the American Dietetic Association, 110*(8), 1216-21.

128 Hu, F. B., Manson, J. E., Stampfer, M. J., Colditz, G., Liu, S., Solomon, C. G., & Willett, W. C. (2001). Diet, lifestyle, and the risk of type 2 diabetes mellitus in women. *New England Journal of Medicine, 345*(11), 790-97.

129 Villegas, R., Liu, S., Gao, Y. T., Yang, G., Li, H., Zheng, W., & Shu, X. O. (2007). Prospective study of dietary carbohydrates, glycemic index, glycemic load, and incidence of type 2 diabetes mellitus in middle-aged Chinese women. *Archives of Internal Medicine, 167*(21), 2310-16.

130 de Munter, J. S., Hu, F. B., Spiegelman, D., Franz, M., & van Dam, R. M. (2007). Whole grain, bran, and germ intake and risk of type 2 diabetes: A prospective cohort study and systematic review. *PLoS Medicine, 4*(8), e261.

131 Fung, T. T., Hu, F. B., Pereira, M. A., Liu, S., Stampfer, M. J., Colditz, G. A., & Willett, W. C. (2002). Whole-grain intake and the risk of type 2 diabetes: A prospective study in men. *American Journal of Clinical Nutrition, 76*(3), 535-40.

132 McKeown, N. M., Meigs, J. B., Liu, S., Wilson, P. W., & Jacques, P. F. (2002). Whole-grain intake is favorably associated with metabolic risk factors for type 2 diabetes and cardiovascular disease in the Framingham Offspring Study. *American Journal of Clinical Nutrition, 76*(2), 390-98.

133 Batis, C., Hernandez-Barrera, L., Barquera, S., Rivera, J. A., & Popkin, B. M. (2011). Food acculturation drives dietary differences among Mexicans, Mexican Americans, and Non-Hispanic Whites. *Journal of Nutrition, 141*(10), 1898-1906.

134 Ayala, G. X., Baquero, B., & Klinger, S. (2008). A systematic review of the relationship between acculturation and diet among Latinos in the United States: Implications for future research. *Journal of the American Dietetic Association, 108*(8), 1330-44.

135 Liu, J. H., Chu, Y. H., Frongillo, E. A., & Probst, J. C. (2012). Generation and acculturation status are associated with dietary intake and body weight in Mexican American adolescents. *Journal of Nutrition, 142*(2), 298-305.

136 Sallis, J. F., Owen, N., & Fisher, E. B. (2008). Ecological models of health behavior. In K. Glanz, B. K. Rimer, & K. Viswanath (Eds.), *Health behavior and health education: Theory, research, and practice*. San Francisco, CA: Jossey-Bass.

137 Glanz, K., Sallis, J. F., Saelens, B. E., & Frank, L. D. (2005). Healthy nutrition environments: Concepts and measures. *American Journal of Health Promotion, 19*(5), 330-33.

138 Jurkowski, J. M., Green Mills, L. L., Lawson, H. A., Bovenzi, M. C., Quartimon, R., & Davison, K. K. (2013). Engaging low-income parents in childhood obesity prevention from start to finish: A case study. *Journal of Community Health, 38*(1), 1-11.

139 Davison, K. K., Jurkowski, J. M., & Lawson, H. A. (2013). Reframing family-centered obesity prevention using the Family Ecological Model. *Public Health Nutrition, 16*(10), 1861-69.

140 Davison, K. K., Jurkowski, J. M., & Lawson, H. A. (2013). Reframing family-centered obesity prevention using the Family Ecological Model. *Public Health Nutrition, 16*(10), 1861-69.

141 Davison, K. K., Jurkowski, J. M., Li, K., Kranz, S., & Lawson, H. A. (2013). A childhood obesity intervention developed by families for families: Results from a pilot study. *International Journal of Behavioral Nutrition and Physical Activity, 10*, 3.

142 Davison, K. K., Jurkowski, J. M., Li, K., Kranz, S., & Lawson, H. A. (2013). A childhood obesity intervention developed by families

for families: Results from a pilot study. *International Journal of Behavioral Nutrition and Physical Activity, 10*, 3.

143 Davison, K. K., Jurkowski, J. M., & Lawson, H. A. (2013). Reframing family-centered obesity prevention using the Family Ecological Model. *Public Health Nutrition, 16*(10), 1861-69.

144 Davison, K. K., Jurkowski, J. M., Li, K., Kranz, S., & Lawson, H. A. (2013). A childhood obesity intervention developed by families for families: Results from a pilot study. *International Journal of Behavioral Nutrition and Physical Activity, 10*, 3.

145 Sallis, J. F., Owen, N., & Fisher, E. B. (2008). Ecological models of health behavior. In K. Glanz, B. K. Rimer, & K. Viswanath (Eds.), *Health behavior and health education: Theory, research, and practice*. San Francisco, CA: Jossey-Bass.

146 Sallis, J. F., Owen, N., & Fisher, E. B. (2008). Ecological models of health behavior. In K. Glanz, B. K. Rimer, & K. Viswanath (Eds.), *Health behavior and health education: Theory, research, and practice*. San Francisco, CA: Jossey-Bass.

147 Israel, B. A., Checkoway, B., Schulz, A., & Zimmerman, M. (1994). Health education and community empowerment: conceptualizing and measuring perceptions of individual, organizational, and community control. *Health Education Quarterly, 21*(2), 149-70.

148 Weinstein, N. D. (2007). Misleading tests of health behavior theories. *Annals of Behavioral Medicine, 33*(1), 1-10.

149 Weinstein, N. D. (2007). Misleading tests of health behavior theories. *Annals of Behavioral Medicine, 33*(1), 1-10.

150 Noar, S. M., & Mehrotra, P. (2011). Toward a new methodological paradigm for testing theories of health behavior and health behavior change. *Patient Education and Counseling, 82*(3), 468-74.

151 Noar, S. M., & Mehrotra, P. (2011). Toward a new methodological paradigm for testing theories of health behavior and health behavior change. *Patient Education and Counseling, 82*(3), 468-74.

152 Cerin, E., Barnett, A., & Baranowski, T. (2009). Testing theories of dietary behavior change in youth using the mediating variable model with intervention programs. *Journal of Nutrition Education and Behavior, 41*(5), 309-18.

153 Noar, S. M., & Zimmerman, R. S. (2005). Health Behavior Theory and cumulative knowledge regarding health behaviors: are we moving in the right direction? *Health Education Research, 20*(3), 275-90.

154 Painter, J. E., Borba, C. P., Hynes, M., Mays, D., & Glanz, K. (2008). The use of theory in health behavior research from 2000 to 2005: A systematic review. *Annals of Behavioral Medicine, 35*(3), 358-62.

155 Green, L. W., & Kreuter, M. W. (2005). *Health program planning: An educational and ecological approach* (4th ed.). New York: McGraw-Hill.

156 Medeiros, L. C., Butkus, S. N., Chipman, H., Cox, R. H., Jones, L., & Little, D. (2005). A logic model framework for community nutrition education. *Journal of Nutrition Education and Behavior, 37*(4), 197-202.

157 Green, L. W., & Kreuter, M. W. (2005). *Health program planning: An educational and ecological approach* (4th ed.). New York: McGraw-Hill.

158 Gielen, A. C., McDonald, E. M., Gary, T. L., & Bone, L. R. (2008). Using the PRECEDE-PROCEED model to apply health behavior theories. In K. Glanz, B. K. Rimer, & K. Viswanath (Eds.), *Health behavior and health education: Theory, research, and practice*. San Francisco, CA: Jossey-Bass.

159 Medeiros, L. C., Butkus, S. N., Chipman, H., Cox, R. H., Jones, L., & Little, D. (2005). A logic model framework for community nutrition education. *Journal of Nutrition Education and Behavior, 37*(4), 197-202.

160 Abraham, C., & Michie, S. (2008). A taxonomy of behavior change techniques used in interventions. *Health Psychology, 27*(3), 379-87.

161 McEachan, R. R. C., Conner, M., Taylor, N. J., & Lawton, R. J. (2011). Prospective prediction of health-related behaviours with the Theory of Planned Behaviour: A meta-analysis. *Health Psychology Review, 5*(2), 97-144.

162 Baranowski, T., Cullen, K. W., & Baranowski, J. (1999). Psychosocial correlates of dietary intake: Advancing dietary intervention. *Annual Review of Nutrition, 19*(1), 17.

163 Jeffery, R. W. (2004). How can Health Behavior Theory be made more useful for intervention research? *International Journal of Behavioral Nutrition and Physical Activity, 1*(1), 10.

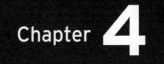
The Food Environment and Prepared Foods

Seung Hee Lee-Kwan, PhD, MS, LD
Natalie Stein, MS, MPH

"We can make a commitment to promote vegetables and fruits and whole grains on every part of every menu. We can make portion sizes smaller and emphasize quality over quantity. And we can help create a culture—imagine this—where our kids ask for healthy options instead of resisting them."—Michelle Obama

First Lady of the U. S., Remarks to the Congressional Black Caucus Conference September 16, 2010

Learning Objectives

- Define the food environment.

- Associate the food environment with socioeconomic status, nutritional status, and health outcomes.

- Discuss the relationship between prepared food consumption and obesity and explain several factors affecting the relationship.

- Describe disparities in prepared food consumption and health outcomes based on culture, race/ethnicity, and socioeconomic status.

- Discuss the role of the food environment in individual food choices.

- Explain how to assess the community food environment.

- Recognize point-of-purchase, price manipulation, and menu labeling as public health approaches to improve the food environment.

- Recognize the need to consider cultural diversity when planning interventions.

Case Study: Baltimore Healthy Carry-Outs

The city of Baltimore has a prevalence of obesity of 35% compared with the U.S. national prevalence of 26.3%,[1] and significant socioeconomic and racial disparities related to food access.[2,3] Forty-six percent of predominantly African American neighborhoods have low healthy food availability, compared with only 4% of predominantly white neighborhoods. Sixty-eight percent of white neighborhoods and only 19% of African American neighborhoods have high availability of healthy foods.[4] Many residents lack cars and are limited in their abilities to purchase foods from outside the neighborhood.[5]

Providing 75% of prepared foods in low-income neighborhoods in Baltimore,[6] **carry-outs** are similar to franchised fast-food restaurants, but have no or limited seating and parking, and often offer few or no healthy choices.[7]

Prepared food consumption is a public health concern in the United States, and predominantly African American neighborhoods in Baltimore are particularly affected.[8]

On average, low-income African American adults in Baltimore spend $288 per month on prepared foods and only $274 per month at supermarkets,[9] and more than half of daily energy intake comes from prepared food sources such as fried chicken, submarine sandwiches, and soda.[10] Daily energy intake is 200 calories above the national average.[11] Low-income, urban African American adults reported eating at local carry-out restaurants more than three times per week on average. At each carry-out visit, they spent an average of $10.[12] Although the number of carry-outs is up to 10 times higher than the number of fast-food restaurants in low-income areas, few studies have focused on the impact of these venues on health and obesity of low-income populations.[13] Carry-outs remain potentially effective but untapped targets for public health nutrition interventions to promote healthy eating and prevent obesity.

The Baltimore Healthy Carry-outs (BHC) intervention was developed, using formative research, to improve the prepared food environment of low-income African Americans. Point-of-purchase (POP) strategies included menu board revision (**Figure 4-1**), menu labeling, and price reduction. A seven-month trial was conducted in four intervention and four comparison (control) carry-outs (**Figure 4-2**). The

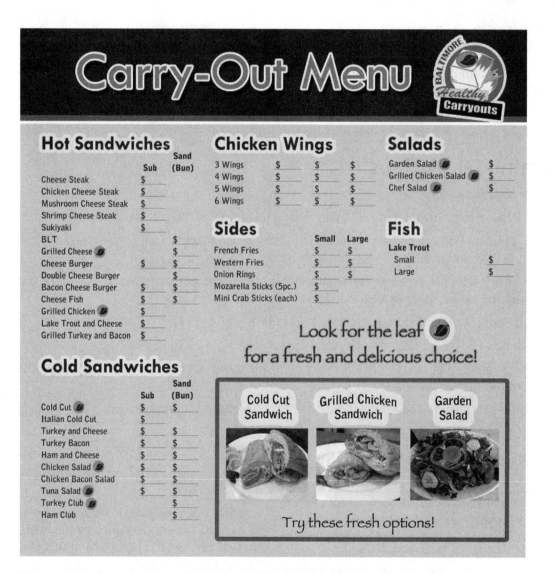

Figure 4-1 Sample menu from the Baltimore Healthy Carry-out intervention

Reproduced from Lee-Kwan, S. H., Goedkoop, S., Young, R., Batorsky, B., Hoffman, V., Jeffries, J., Hamouda, M., & Gittelsohn, J. (2013). Development and implementation of the Baltimore healthy carry-outs feasibility trial: process evaluation results. *BMC Public Health, 13*, 638.

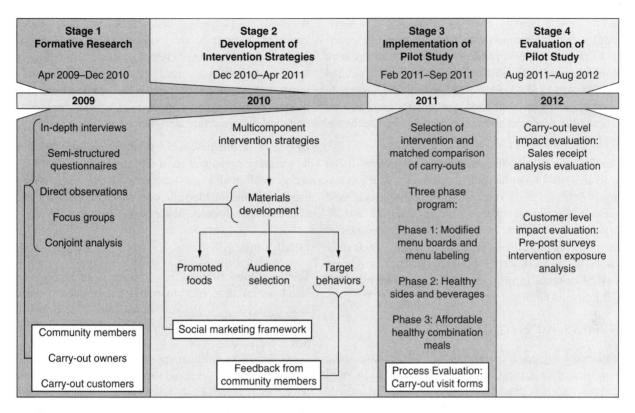

Figure 4-2 Baltimore Healthy Carry-outs timeline

Reproduced from Lee, S. H. (2012). Changing the food environment in Baltimore City: Impact of an intervention to improve carry-outs in low-income neighborhoods. Doctoral dissertation. Johns Hopkins University.

BHC trial included three phases: (1) Improve menu boards and labeling to promote healthier items; (2) Promote healthy sides and beverages and introduce new items; and (3) Introduce healthier combo meals and change food preparation methods. Participant carry-outs increased healthy food sales and total revenue, and their customers purchased healthier foods. The study confirms the potential for future programs to focus on carry-outs.

Discussion Questions

- Which characteristics place the BHC target population as an at-risk community for poor nutrition?
- Why is high consumption of carry-out food associated with poor nutrition and unfavorable health consequences?
- What features of BHC made it an example of a successful public health intervention?
- How might lessons learned from BHC be applied in other communities?

Introduction

Profound changes in the **food environment** and in individual nutrition have taken place in the United States in the past few decades.[14] The food environment consists of environmental and structural factors that affect food choice.[15] Available foods consist of two elements: (1) foods that can be purchased for home consumption, and (2) **prepared foods (PFs)**,[16] interchangeably called foods away from home (FAFH).[17] Food availability, accessibility, and affordability are also part of the food environment. The food environment has received recent attention as an important determinant of individual eating behaviors. Largely modifiable, the food environment is a likely target of nutrition interventions for health promotion.

Food Deserts and Food Swamps in the United States

The word "desert" evokes an image of a dry vast land where access to necessary resources is limited, and "**food deserts**" are areas where residents have inadequate access to nutritious foods.[18,19] Cummins describes food deserts as "populated urban areas where residents do not have access to an affordable and healthy diet."[20] The 2008 Farm Bill defined it as "an area in the United States with limited access to affordable and nutritious food, particularly such an area composed of predominantly lower income neighborhoods and communities."[21]

A food desert has no single operational definition. It can be an area within a radius of a quarter-mile, in urban settings,[22] or 10 miles, in rural areas.[23] "Lack of access" and measure of access are not standardized either. Some studies define food deserts as areas without supermarkets,[24] while others allow one or more such stores in their definitions of "food deserts."[25,26] Nearly all studies rely on physical distance from healthy foods, although variable, to define food deserts.

Urban vs. Rural Food Deserts

While most research focuses on urban food environments, their rural counterparts are equally influential. In rural food deserts where the population is less dense, the average distance to the supermarket is greater than in urban areas. To account for differences in distance and lifestyle, the U.S. Department of Agriculture (USDA) includes a "drivable" distance measure for rural areas and uses a **"walkability"** measure for urban areas in assessment of food deserts.[27]

Another transportation-related distinction between urban and rural communities is method of transportation; urban areas tend to have more thorough public transportation systems, and rural residents rely more on personal transportation to access food outlets. Still, living closer to a supermarket is associated with higher fruit and vegetable consumption in rural residents.[28]

Rural communities may have only a few or a limited variety of stores. Greater proportions of small grocery stores and convenience stores compared with full-service supermarkets are associated with lower availability and/or selection of nutrient-dense foods, such as skim milk, fruits, vegetables, and bread.[29] Rural communities tend to be less reliant on formal food and nutrition assistance systems and more likely to obtain food through gardening, hunting, and food exchange systems.[30] These sources can be seasonal and unreliable.

In contrast, urban areas have robust food environments, including supermarkets, convenience stores, coffee shops, fast-food and full-service restaurants, and street vendors. However, disparities are evident within a large city. Supermarkets have largely relocated to suburbs with more space for parking lots.[31] Inner-city neighborhoods are left to rely instead on corner stores, which tend to have a limited variety of foods for higher prices.[32,33] Fast-food restaurants and carry-outs are abundant.[34]

Despite these differences, the food environment has similar effects in urban and rural settings. Individuals without access to affordable and healthy foods are more likely to experience malnutrition and poorer health outcomes, such as obesity and chronic diseases.

Food Swamps

The term "**food swamps**" has emerged as an alternative to "food deserts" in an effort to more accurately describe areas lacking access to healthy foods. Food swamps are areas that suffer from overnutrition resulting from energy-dense foods, often offered by small stores and fast-food restaurants.[35] As an illustrate of the utility of the concept of food swamps compared with deserts, the prevalence of obesity is more closely linked to the presence of many fast-food outlets with unhealthy offerings than to a lack of supermarkets that carry healthy foods.[36] For example, in New Orleans, Louisiana, one study found that fast-food restaurant density was independently correlated with median household income and percentage of African American residents, and predominantly African American neighborhoods had 60% more fast-food restaurants per square mile than in predominantly white neighborhoods.[37] Similarly, in Los Angeles, California, restaurants located in predominantly African American and low-income neighborhoods were less likely to offer healthier options.[38]

Prepared Foods and the Food Environment

In addition to foods purchased for home preparation, the built food environment also consists of PFs. In 2012, Americans spent nearly half of their food dollars eating out,[39,40] an increase of 18% from 1977 to 1978.[41] The number of fast-food restaurant locations has doubled since the 1970s. These trends parallel increases in obesity.[42]

Foods away from home (FAFH) include "full meals and single ready-to-eat items" from restaurants and grocery stores. Fast-food restaurants and carry-outs are the main sources of FAFH.[43] Common PFs include fried chicken, burgers, submarine sandwiches, pizza, French fries, and soda. Burritos and tacos are common at Mexican restaurants, pizza and pasta dishes are prevalent in Italian eateries, and dishes based on white rice are integral to Asian restaurants.

Disparities in the Food Environment and Diet Intake

Food deserts are not ubiquitous in industrialized nations, but **socioeconomic status (SES)** is a consistent determinant of diet intake. Lower SES is associated with poorer diet in industrialized nations, including in North America, Europe, Asia, and Australia.

Lower SES Associated with Poorer Diet

Individuals with lower incomes tend to have higher intakes of refined grains, potatoes, fatty meats, sweets, sugar-sweetened beverages, and whole milk.[44,45,46,47] **Saturated fat**, **sodium**, and added sugar consumption is also higher. Furthermore, nutrient intake can be lower because of their relatively high cost. Iron, dietary fiber, vitamin C, and **beta-carotene** intakes are often lower among low-income individuals. These nutrients are associated with fruits and vegetables and whole and fortified grains. Seafood, a source of **omega-three fatty acids**, is consumed less frequently among lower-income populations.[48] Lower nutrient intake and high-calorie food consumption is also observed among low-income rural children.[49]

Relationship Between the Food Environment, Diet, and Health

The food environment is a source of health disparities, and living in neighborhoods with poor food environments is associated with poorer diet and health. Studies using **market-basket** approaches and geographic surveys demonstrate the influence of the food environment on diet.[50] Residents of food deserts depend on small stores that offer limited and/or expensive healthy foods, while energy-dense foods are less expensive.[51,52]

Obesity and some diet-related health conditions will be discussed later in the chapter. Additional consequences of poor nutrition and a poor food environment include decreased work productivity among adults[53] and poorer academic performance[54] and behavior in children.[55] These effects in turn can perpetuate a cycle of poverty that continues to include poor nutrition and health outcomes.

Obesity and the Food Environment

After smoking and tobacco use, obesity and overweight are the leading actual causes of preventable death in the United States.[56] Although the prevalence of obesity may have plateaued, more than two-thirds of Americans are overweight and obese.[57,58] The prevalence of obesity in the United States has more than doubled from 15% in 1976–80.[59] Obesity is a risk factor for many chronic health conditions, including cardiovascular disease (CVD), type 2 diabetes mellitus (T2D), obstructive sleep apnea, osteoarthritis, hypertension, and some cancers.[60,61,62] In 2008, an estimated $146 billion of U.S. adult medical expenditures were attributed to obesity.[63] Compared with normal-weight individuals, obese individuals spend on average 30% more, or $1,429 annually, in medical expenses.[64]

Causes of obesity include genetic makeup and factors that affect diet and exercise behaviors. These include culture, socioeconomic status, and food availability. The food environment is a major factor in obesity. A lower ratio of nearby fast-food restaurants and convenience stores to supermarkets and grocery stores is associated with lower risk of obesity.[65] Low nutrient-dense, high energy-dense foods are cheaper per calorie than healthier counterparts, making them more affordable on limited budgets.[66]

> *Public Health Core Competency 4: Cultural Competency Skills 1: Incorporates strategies for interacting with persons from diverse backgrounds*
>
> Reproduced from Council on Linkages Between Academia and Public Health Practice. 2010 May. Core Competencies for Public Health Professionals. Washington, DC: Public Health Foundation. http://www.phf.org/resourcestools/Documents/Core_Competencies_for_Public_Health_Professionals_2010May.pdf. Accessed August 13, 2013. This source is used for all Public Health Core Competencies in this chapter.

Foods Away from Home and Obesity

An obesogenic environment can be defined by its prevalence of FAFH or PF, whose consumption is linked to obesity. Fast-food outlet and restaurant prevalence is correlated with prevalence of obesity,[67,68,69] and a higher number of fast-food restaurants per capita is associated with faster body mass index (BMI) gain in children.[70] Among adults, fast-food restaurant density and a higher ratio of fast-food to full-service restaurants is associated with higher BMI, risk of obesity, and weight gain.[71,72,73,74] Americans who eat at least one fast-food meal per week are more likely to be obese than those who eat out less often.[75]

The increase in away-from-home foods since 1977–78 parallels the increase in obesity rates in the United States.[76] Possible explanations for this relationship include larger portions, higher calorie density of PF,[77] and more frequent eating occasions. Each meal eaten away from home is associated with consumption of an additional 134 calories.[78] Many of the top sources of calories (**Table 4-1**) in the average American diet are fat, sugar, and refined carbohydrates, and are common PF options.[79]

Another factor contributing to obesity is increased portion sizes at restaurants and in processed foods and beverages.[80,81] Large portions encourage people to consume more calories.[82,83,84] Since the 1970s, standard soft drink servings have increased by 49 calories, French fries by 68 calories, and hamburgers by 97 calories.[85] This equates to an increase of 200 calories in a standard order of a hamburger with fries and a beverage. A 200-calorie daily increase in consumption correlates with a 21-pound weight gain over the course of one year.

Disparities in PF Availability and Obesity

Links between PF availability and racial differences in obesity,[86] neighborhood characteristics such as median household income, presence of food outlets,[87,88,89] and lower-quality diets, often defined using the Healthy Eating Index (HEI), are complex.[90] Higher proportions of PFs have been found in predominantly African American neighborhoods, as compared with white neighborhoods in the various locations in the United States.[91,92,93,94] Racial differences are seen in rural settings as well. In a rural Texas community, non-whites had a higher risk of obesity and higher frequency of fast-food consumption when more fast-food outlets were accessible, while this effect was not seen among whites.[95]

Characteristics of Obesogenic Environments and SES

Low-income neighborhoods are often obesogenic[96] environments because of fewer resources, such as grocery stores and places to exercise, and problems such as crime and traffic that interfere with healthy eating and physical activity.[97] Lack of healthy food sources within walking distance is associated with obesity incidence.[98] Investigating disparities in the food environment disparities can help understand obesity disparities in different race, ethnic, and socioeconomic groups and vulnerable populations such as children and the elderly.

For instance, children are heavily influenced by the neighborhood food environment. Living in close proximity (defined as 400 meters) to food retail stores is associated with obesity.[99]

Table 4-1 Selected top sources of calories in the typical American diet that are commonly eaten as foods away from home or prepared foods

Food Category	Includes
1. Grain-based desserts	Cakes, cookies, pies, doughnuts, pastries
3. Chicken and chicken mixed dishes	Fried and baked chicken strips, patties and wings, chicken sandwiches, and chicken stir-fries
4. Soda/energy/sports drinks	Sweetened sodas, waters, energy drinks
5. Pizza	Cheese pizza and pizza with toppings
7. Pasta and pasta dishes	Macaroni and cheese, pasta with sauce, filled pasta
8. Mexican dishes	Tortillas, burritos, tacos, quesadillas, nachos
9. Beef and beef mixed dishes	Steak, meatloaf, beef with noodles
10. Dairy desserts	Ice cream, milkshakes, frozen yogurt
12. Burgers	Hamburgers, cheeseburgers
17. Fried potatoes	French fries, hash browns
21. Rice and rice mixed dishes	White rice, fried rice

Data from U.S. Department of Agriculture, U.S. Department of Health and Human Services. (2010). *Dietary Guidelines for Americans 2010*. Washington, DC: U.S. Government Printing Office. http://www.health.gov/dietaryguidelines/dga2010/DietaryGuidelines2010.pdf. Accessed September 4, 2013.

The Neighborhood Impact on Kids study described relationships between SES, an obesogenic environment, and childhood obesity in selected regions of San Diego, California, and King's County, Washington. A better nutrition environment was characterized by nearby supermarkets and fewer fast-food outlets. The physical activity categorization was based on **walkability**, or proximity of food retail outlets, and **playability**, or proximity and number of parks in the area. Children living in better nutrition and physical activity environments were less likely to be obese, although slightly more likely to be overweight.[100] Lower income was associated with poorer nutrition and physical activity environments.

Demographics and Disparities in Obesity

Disparities in obesity prevalence among minority populations are present in the United States. The obesity rates of non-Hispanic blacks and Hispanics are 49.5% and 40.4%, respectively, compared with 34.3% in non-Hispanic whites.[101] Approximately 60% of non-Hispanic black women are obese, compared with only 41.4% of Hispanic women and 32.2% of non-Hispanic white women.[102] Non-Hispanic blacks have a mean BMI of 28.6, followed by Hispanics, non-Hispanic whites, and non-Hispanic Asians, with averages of 27.7, 26.9, and 24.0, respectively.[103]

Racial and Geographic Disparities in Obesity

Racial disparities in obesity prevalence are often linked to disparities in the food environment. In the United States, racial minorities are more likely to have risk factors for obesity, such as being impoverished[104] and living in high-density metropolitan areas.[105,106] Among women, low income and less education are additional risk factors for obesity.[107]

The concept of **block groups** exists in non-Hispanic black and Hispanic communities. More than 60% of non-Hispanic blacks and Hispanics live in segregated neighborhoods, defined as non-Hispanic blacks and Hispanics, respectively, making up at least 25% of residents. These communities have higher obesity rates. Non-Hispanic white and non-Hispanic Asian men living in Hispanic block groups are also more likely to be obese. In contrast, communities with a high rate of non-Hispanic Asians are less likely to be obese, as are non-Hispanics and non-Hispanic blacks living in these block groups. The Coronary Artery Risk Development in Young Adults study, **Project CARDIA**, followed 3,031 young adults, aged 18 to 30 years at baseline, for 15 years starting in 1985 or 1986. Blacks frequented fast-food restaurants more

often than whites and were most likely to be obese, implicating a role of the food environment.[108] Further data show that in communities in the United States consisting of at least 35% African Americans and 35% whites with similar education and income, health status is similar between whites and African Americans.[109] These findings, along with findings that being nonwhite is associated with poorer health in urban but not rural settings,[110] are evidence for the role of determinants of obesity aside from race.

Socioeconomic Disparities and Obesity

Many studies have linked SES and obesity. For example, individuals with lower education and income are more likely to be obese.[111,112] SES is also associated with short-term weight gain, as individuals with the lowest SES were 30% more likely to gain weight during a yearlong prospective study than those classified as highest SES.[113] Longitudinal studies have also associated weight gain with living in a lower-SES neighborhood.[114,115]

Gender, Income, and Obesity

The association between SES and obesity has gender differences. Women, but not men, with lower education and income are more likely to be obese than their counterparts.[116,117] One study found that women whose properties had the lowest values were 3.4 times more likely to be obese than those whose properties had the highest values.[118] Again, the relationship was not significant for men. A study conducted in Canada found that while women who lived in a disadvantaged neighborhood had higher BMI scores than those who lived in affluent areas, men in wealthy areas had higher BMI scores than those in poor areas.[119]

Conclusion

Public health interventions must target environmental, social, and cultural factors[120,121] to reduce disparities in obesity and other determinants of health. This chapter next discusses relationships between the food environment and diet and health. Then, it discusses strategies to improve the food environment.

Chronic Diseases and the Food Environment

Chronic diseases are the leading causes of death in the United States, with cardiovascular disease, cancer, stroke, and diabetes being the first, second, fourth, and seventh leading causes of death, respectively. Their causes and risk factors are largely modifiable, and include poor nutrition and obesity. Diets high in high-sodium, high-fat, and high-sugar foods, such as many fast foods and other PFs, are risk factors for chronic diseases.

Diabetes and Prepared Foods

Diabetes mellitus, or DM, is a condition in which an individual's blood sugar levels are uncontrolled.[122] Nearly 8% of Americans, and nearly one-quarter of adults over 60, have diabetes. The seventh-leading direct cause of death in the United States, DM is a secondary cause of many more mortalities. Risk factors for **type 2 diabetes mellitus** include obesity, lack of physical activity, older age, and belonging to certain minority groups, including African American, American Indian, Hispanic/Latino, and Asian American. Type 2 DM is largely considered preventable by maintaining a healthy weight, achieving recommended levels of physical activity, and choosing a healthy diet. These same behaviors can improve diabetes management and prevent or delay diabetes-related complications, such as kidney disease, blindness, heart disease, and infections.

PF Consumption and Incidence of Diabetes

Patterns associated with higher intake of PF foods and increased risk for type 2 diabetes mellitus include greater consumption of saturated fat[123] and added sugars,[124] and lower consumption of whole grains,[125] dietary fiber, and vegetables. The 2010 Dietary Guidelines for Americans suggest that individuals with diabetes limit sodium intake to 1,500 mg per day, compared with 2,300 milligrams per day for healthy adults, but PFs are often high in sodium.[126]

Consistent with expectations, one prospective study confirmed a relationship between consumption of fast food and diabetes incidence. In the study, African American women were 29–68% more likely to develop diabetes if they consumed at least two servings per week of fried chicken, Chinese food, or burgers than women who did not consume these foods, although no relationship was seen between diabetes and eating pizza, Mexican fast food, or fried fish.[127] The observed relationship might be related to higher rates of obesity among women who consumed more fried chicken, pizza, and burgers. Other studies have confirmed associations between fast-food consumption and diabetes development among Latino and non-Latino women in urban areas[128] and Mexican Americans in rural Texas.[129] Increased fast-food consumption and similar patterns, such as eating more fried chicken, are associated with diabetes among

American Indians.[130] Western-style fast-food consumption is associated with diabetes risk not only in the United States and other Western nations, but also in Asia.[131]

PF Consumption and Risk Factors for Diabetes

Increased consumption of PFs has been directly linked to three primary risk factors of diabetes mellitus: high fasting blood glucose, weight gain, and insulin resistance.[132,133,134] The CARDIA study found that more frequent fast-food restaurant use at both baseline and follow-up led to 4.5 kg (10 pounds) greater weight gain and two-fold greater increase in insulin resistance.[135] Weight gain and obesity appear to be **mediators** of the association between PF and diabetes.

↑Energy dense prepared foods → ↑Energy consumption → Weight gain → Obesity → Diabetes

Cardiovascular Diseases and Prepared Foods

Heart disease, or **cardiovascular disease**, is the leading cause of death in the United States[136] and the world.[137] **Dyslipidemia** obesity and diabetes mellitus are risk factors for heart disease. Consumption of PFs may be linked to increased incidence of heart disease or risk factors for CVD.

Prepared Foods and Hypertension

Hypertension, or HTN, affects about one-third of Americans, and nearly one-third of American adults are prehypertensive, or at risk for high blood pressure.[138] HTN is a risk factor for strokes and heart attacks. The World Health Organization lists hypertension as the top risk factor for mortality worldwide.[139] Lifestyle choices to lower HTN risk include maintaining a healthy body weight, getting adequate physical activity, and following a sodium-controlled, high-nutrient diet, such as the Dietary Approaches to Stop Hypertension, or DASH, eating pattern.

Prepared and restaurant foods contribute the majority of sodium in the American diet. Chicken and beef dishes, pizza, pasta, cold cuts, condiments, Mexican-style fast foods, burgers, and rice dishes are common fast foods and are among the top sources of sodium in the typical American diet.[140] The link between PF consumption and high blood pressure has been confirmed in a variety of adult and children populations in the United States and the world.[141,142,143] Further suggesting a negative impact of PF, availability of nearby supermarkets is associated with lower blood pressure.[144] Lower intake of fast foods is associated with diets more consistent with DASH

> ### Factors to Consider in the Food Environment Research
>
> Literature related to obesity and the built food environment has received increased attention because individuals' eating behavior is highly affected by the environment. Many studies have examined the association between the **built food environment** in the form of foods purchased for home consumption and diet quality and obesity. For example, the availability of supermarkets in neighborhoods was positively associated with diet quality[145,146] and inversely associated with obesity prevalence.[147] However, more recent studies using longitudinal data have shown no direct association between presence of supermarkets and BMI and/or diet quality.[148,149]
>
> Drewnowski et al. found that supermarkets, when sorted by price, were inversely associated with BMI, suggesting a possible mediating effect of price on the relationship between supermarkets and obesity.[150] In addition, Gustafson et al. found that availability of transportation was an **effect modifier** when assessing supermarket density and fruit and vegetable consumption; in other words, having access to transportation reduces the obesogenic effect of lack of supermarkets nearby.[151] Additionally, validation of food outlet databases, such as Dunn & Bradshaw, has been an issue. This difficulty may be due to rapidly changing food landscapes and out-of-date databases unable to make temporal relationships.[152] Therefore, associations between built food environments and obesity must take into account important confounders such as price and transportation.

recommendations, including lower intake of saturated fat and sodium, and higher intake of fruits, vegetables, low-fat dairy products, and whole grains.

Prepared Foods and Dyslipidemia

Dyslipidemia refers to abnormal blood lipid levels.[153] One-sixth of Americans have high total cholesterol, and one-third have high LDL cholesterol. Dyslipidemia is associated with obesity, physical inactivity, and a poor diet.[154] **Saturated fat** raises total and LDL cholesterol levels; **trans fats** raise LDL cholesterol and lower HDL cholesterol levels.

PFs are likely to have negative consequences for blood lipid levels. Many foods commonly eaten as prepared foods or foods away from home are among the top sources of saturated fat in the typical American diet. Examples include pizza, dairy desserts (such as ice cream), chicken and beef dishes, pasta dishes, Mexican-style fast food, and fried potatoes. Trans fats may be in fried foods, such as French fries and doughnuts, and processed snack foods, such as crackers, snack cakes, and cookies.

Assessing the Food Environment

Risk factors such as low-income neighborhood, lack of transportation, high proportion of ethnic minorities, and a poor food environment can alert public health workers to the likelihood of suboptimal health outcomes in the community. Assessing the food environment allows public health nutritionists to evaluate the likelihood of poor nutrition and impaired health. Food environment assessments may describe types and numbers of available food sources in a community, the foods they offer, and their prices. Researchers have developed and used several different methods for assessing the food environment depending on the specific situation and desired information. Results of the assessment can be used to identify potential targets and approaches for intervention, advocate for political support, and/or evaluate current interventions.

Community Assessment: Nutrition Environment Assessment Tool (NEAT)

The Nutrition Environment Assessment Tool (NEAT) assesses a community's environment and policies related to promoting and supporting healthy eating and the provision of access to healthy foods within the workplace, community, and school settings. Communities in Michigan may use the online tool to identify their food environments' strengths and weaknesses. The assessment can lead to ideas on ways to improve the nutritional environment.[155]

Site-Specific Food Environment Assessment

Site-specific food environment assessments look at the food environment within a specific location, such as a restaurant, supermarket, or school. They might investigate factors such as food item variety, availability of specific foods, marketing, and cost. Multiple tools are available.

Nutrition Environmental Measurement Survey—Stores (NEMS-S)

The Nutrition Environmental Measurement Survey— Stores (NEMS-S) is a structured survey to measure store nutrition environments. It assesses availability and pricing of foods within 11 categories: milk, fresh fruits and vegetables, ground beef, hot dogs, frozen dinners, baked goods, beverages (soda/juice), whole-grain bread, baked chips, and cereal. A higher NEMS score indicates availability of healthier choices, lower prices, and better quality of foods.

The NEMS-S can evaluate community food environments and identify barriers, such as unavailability of skim milk, to healthy eating behaviors.[156,157,158] Higher income neighborhoods are associated with a higher score.[159,160] Supermarkets have higher availability and lower price of healthy foods, such as fresh fruits, vegetables, and low-fat milk, than grocery stores.[161,162]

Nutrition Environmental Measurement Survey—Restaurant (NEMS-R)

The NEMS-R assesses eight types of indicators: low-fat, low-calorie, healthy main dish options; availability of fruits and vegetables without added sauce; whole-grain bread and baked chips; beverages; children's menus; signage and promotions; facilitators and barriers to healthy eating; and pricing and accessibility. Similar to NEMS-S, NEMS-R is used to collect baseline data on food environment, characterize healthy food availability, and evaluate nutritional information in restaurants and fast-food outlets.

A study using NEMS-R found that nonfranchised PF sources have fewer healthy choices than fast-food outlets.[163] A NEMS-R in a children's hospital setting found a prevalence of less healthy items despite the presence of healthy food items, and nutritional information and signage promoting healthy eating are underused.[164] The NEMS-R indicated that sit-down restaurants offered more healthy food items than food trucks on a college campus.[165] Like NEMS-S, NEMS-R utilizes widespread research, initiatives, and interventions.

The BHC program used a modified version of a NEMS-R that was a one-page checklist focused primarily on health-promoting foods at prepared food sources. The 10-minute survey allowed assessment of a large number of prepared food sources in Baltimore City and facilitated data collection in the face of store owners' resistance to detailed surveying.[166]

Assessment of Food Deserts

The USDA defines a food desert as a *low-income census tract* with *low access* to a supermarket. The poverty rate is at least 20% , and at least 500 people or 33% of the population live at least one mile from a supermarket or large grocery store, or 10 miles in rural areas. Food deserts are mapped on the USDA's Food Desert Locator, which can be a good resource for public health professionals who are investigating the possible implementation of interventions.

The Healthy Food Financing Initiative (HFFI) is part of First Lady Michelle Obama's Let's Move program.[167] Its objective is to work with grocery stores, corner stores, and other small food retailers to increase healthy food offerings in low-income communities. It focuses on food deserts as identified using the USDA's definition.

Assessing Diet Quality

Predictors of disparities in the food environment are similarly linked to disparities in diet quality, and include socioeconomic status, including income and level of education,[168] degree of acculturation of ethnic minorities,[169,170] and proximity and density of fast-food outlets.[171] Low income is associated with poorer diet quality characteristics, such as lower intake of vegetables and whole grains, and higher intake of sodium.[172]

Diet Quality Assessment

To be practical for public health applications on a population level, a diet quality assessment method needs to be rapid, inexpensive, and quantifiable. The **Healthy Eating Index (HEI)** is a common psychometric measure of diet quality developed by the USDA in 1995 and revised in 2006; the HEI-2005 is based on the 2005 Dietary Guidelines for Americans.[173] The HEI awards points for diet variety and for limiting intake of saturated fat, sodium, and calories from solid fats, alcoholic beverages, and added sugars (**Table 4-2**). A perfect score is 100 points.

Improving the Food Environment and Dietary Intake

Given the significance of the food environment in diet and health status, effective programs to improve the food environment are a priority in public health nutrition.

Table 4-2 Components of the Healthy Eating Index-2005*

Component	Maximum Points	Criteria
Total fruit (including 100% juice)	5	≥ 0.8 cup equivalent per 1,000 calories
Whole fruit (not juice)	5	≥ 0.4 cup equivalent per 1,000 calories
Total vegetables	5	≥ 1.1 cup equivalent per 1,000 calories
Dark green and orange vegetables and legumes	5	≥ 0.4 cup equivalent per 1,000 calories
Total grains	5	≥ 3 oz. equivalent per 1,000 calories
Whole grains	5	≥ 1.5 oz. equivalent per 1,000 calories
Milk[a]	10	≥ 1.3 cup equivalent per 1,000 calories
Meat and beans	10	≥ 2.5 oz. equivalent per 1,000 calories
Oils[b]	10	≥ 12 grams per 1,000 calories
Saturated fat[d]	10	≤ 7% of energy[c]
Sodium[d]	10	≤ 0.7 gram per 1,000 calories[c]
Calories from solid fats, alcoholic beverages, and added sugars (SOFAS)	20	≤ 20% of energy

*A diet meeting the listed requirements would receive a score of 100, which is the highest possible HEI-2005 score.

[a]Legumes count as vegetables after Meat and Beans requirement is met.

[b]Includes all milk products, including fluid milk, yogurt and cheese, and soy beverages.

[c]Include nonhydrogenated vegetable oils and oils in fish, nuts, and seeds.

[d]Saturated fat and sodium get a score of 8 for intake levels reflecting the 2005 Dietary Guidelines: ≤ 10% of energy from saturated fat and ≤ 1.1 grams of sodium per 1,000 calories.

Modified from the Center for Nutrition Policy and Promotion, USDA. (2008). *Healthy Eating Index-2005*. Retrieved from http://www.cnpp.usda.gov/Publications/HEI/healthyeatingindex2005factsheet.pdf. Accessed September 4, 2013.

Elements of Successful Interventions

Development and implementation of successful interventions requires: (1) **formative research**, (2) **process evaluation**, and (3) **impact evaluation**. Formative research helps researchers identify and understand the target population's characteristics, or interests, behaviors, and needs, that influence decisions and actions.[174,175] Methods include interviews, observations, and focus groups. Process evaluation assesses whether the intervention was implemented as planned. The intervention's delivery may be altered by controllable or uncontrollable factors, such as when a rainstorm and broken roof forced the week-long closure of a carry-out during the BHC intervention. Process evaluation in BHC included assessment of poster and menu board placement, and counting the number of healthy menu items at each carry-out. Impact evaluation measures success of the intervention. In BHC, sales of healthy food items and behavior changes of customers were measured to assess its impact (**Figure 4-3**).

Examples of Previous Interventions

Many successful interventions have been in hospital, college, and worksite cafeterias,[176] likely because they are contained environments in which customers use the cafeterias repeatedly and have high exposure to intervention materials. Limited environmental interventions have been conducted in "real-world"[177,178] prepared food sources such as restaurants, department-store food service areas,[179] and fast-food restaurants.[180] These studies were conducted in primarily white and affluent neighborhoods, in which residents may react differently to health-promoting advertisements and intervention strategies as compared with low-income ethnic neighborhoods.

Despite the difficulty of conducting environmental interventions targeted to the general population in noncontained environments, the importance is recognized. The Dietary Guidelines Advisory Committee suggests the need for improved, easy-to-understand labels listing energy content and portion size for restaurant meals.[181]

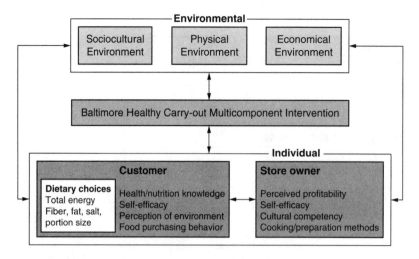

Figure 4-3 Baltimore Healthy Carry-out conceptual framework

Reproduced from Lee, S. H. (2012). Changing the food environment in Baltimore City: Impact of an intervention to improve carry-outs in low-income neighborhoods. Doctoral dissertation. Johns Hopkins University.

Multiple studies have investigated the providing of nutrition information through health messages, menu labeling, and promotions in PF sources. Menu labeling of low-fat/low-cholesterol entrées at a steakhouse led to significant increases in sales of all labeled menu entrées.[182] In seven department-store cafeterias, labeling on low-fat items on menu boards resulted in significant sales increases.[183] A fast-food restaurant found that visual messages promoting low-fat salads increased sales of side salads, but not entrée salads.[184] Most of these studies, however, had weak study designs with small sample sizes or lacked comparison sites. Moreover, all of these interventions were conducted in affluent white neighborhoods, and have not been tested in low-income urban areas.

In a low-income area of Montreal, "Coeur en santé St. Henri" was an intervention focused on offering healthy menu options.[185] Self-administered questionnaires investigated frequency of ordering healthy options and customer reactions to the intervention. Store-level impact was not measured, but 20% of customers had heard about the intervention prior to their current visit, and intentions to eat healthier improved. Also, regular customers were more likely than those who visited less than once per week to order healthy options,[186] suggesting that environmental interventions of this kind can be more effective in reaching low-income subgroups who are more difficult to reach with traditional education strategies. One limitation of this study is that it did not consider the storeowner's perspective.

Such perspectives are crucial because storeowners can tailor their merchandise to meet community needs and preferences and therefore mediate access to healthy foods.[187] Successful store-based interventions required understanding of storeowner motivation and which intervention strategies are feasible.[188,189]

Steps to a Healthier Salinas

The Steps to a Healthier Salinas program was a multifaceted five-year plan to reduce obesity and diabetes rates among Mexican Americans in Salinas, California. The taqueria-based portion of the program was a successful PF source intervention in low-income areas, and it included both restaurant owners and customers.[190] In Salinas, taquerias, with standard options including burritos and tacos, were more concentrated in low-income neighborhoods. They were less likely than fast-food chains to provide nutrition information.

The intervention included nutrition education and social marketing components. A health department educator and nutritionists developed materials describing healthier methods of food preparation and suggestions for increasing servings of fruits and vegetables and reducing fat content. Social marketing occurred as owners highlighted the healthier options. Many owners modified their recipes to make them healthier and offered more healthy foods. Also, taqueria owners began to see themselves as having roles in their community's health. The program's success led to developing a nutrition toolkit for future interventions. The toolkit has educational materials for taqueria owners and customers, case studies of participants, and outreach information.

Its cultural relevance helped make the taqueria-based portion of the Steps to a Healthier Salinas intervention successful. The more traditional Mexican dishes were found to be healthier than Americanized versions, and taqueria owners tended to be Latinos serving Latino communities. Other settings may need modified approaches. Many urban carry-outs in cities such as New York, Baltimore, and Washington, D.C., have Korean American owners serving African American communities.[191,192] Community-specific interventions are necessary to motivate owners because owners' changes in food preparation practices would not be affecting their own race/ethnicity groups.

In BHC, primary customers were African Americans. Owners, mainly Korean immigrants, reported limited English proficiency as a barrier to serving healthy foods in carry-outs. The BHC team considered cultural barriers when designing the intervention by, for example, promoting new healthy combo meals in posters so that the owners would not have to verbally promote those items.

> *Public Health Core Competency 4: Cultural Competency Skills 2: Recognizes the role of cultural, social, and behavioral factors in the accessibility, availability, acceptability, and delivery of public health services*

Multiple Policy Changes in New York City

Recent policies in New York City that aim to reduce obesity by improving the PF environment include mandatory calorie counts on menus and a ban on added trans fats in restaurants and other PF outlets. In 2012, the city proposed a ban on the sale of sugar-sweetened beverages larger than 16 ounces in PF establishments.[193]

Mandatory Posting of Calorie Counts on Menus

Beginning in 2008, calorie counts on menus were required in New York City.[194] A cross-sectional survey conducted nine months later found that the average energy content of meals was not different than the average energy content of meals purchased before policy implementation, and only 15% of customers used the point-of-purchase information. However, those who did consumed 106 fewer calories per meal.

A similar cross-sectional survey among low-income consumers found that nearly 56% noticed the menu labeling, and those who saw it consumed 100 fewer calories.[195] However, overall, purchasing behaviors did not change significantly.[196] While supportive of the regulation, low-income residents were doubtful that caloric labeling would change purchasing behaviors, since factors such as poverty and hunger greatly affect food ordering decisions.[197] Furthermore, menus displayed total calories in the order, regardless of whether a single order was intended to contain multiple servings.[198] In addition, low-income individuals may order foods that cost less per calorie to increase the meal's perceived value.[199] Different approaches to menu labeling may therefore be more appropriate in low-income neighborhoods.

Trans Fat Ban

Reducing trans fats consumption can potentially lower the risk of heart disease by lowering **LDL cholesterol** and raising **HDL cholesterol** levels. In an effort to improve cholesterol levels and reduce the risk of heart disease in New York City, the Board of Health approved a ban on trans fats in all prepared food establishments.[200] Only foods still in the manufacturer's original packaging may contain 0.5 grams or more of trans fats per serving. Trans fat consumption decreased by an average of 2.4 grams per purchase with the ban,[201] while saturated fat increased by a relatively inconsequential 0.5 grams per purchase.

Price Manipulations

A price manipulation is a policy designed to influence consumption of products or services by making them artificially more or less expensive. Artificial raising or lowering costs or profits for producers or consumers can occur through taxes on foods to be discouraged and subsidies, leading to lower costs, for foods to be encouraged. Examples include federal agricultural subsidies to encourage growth of specific crops, and snack taxes levied on high-fat, high-calorie, and/or high-sugar snack foods, such as candy bars.

Food Cost and Obesity

Some research suggests that increased prevalence of obesity may be due to increased consumption of soda and chips with artificially low prices due to government subsidies for corn and soy.[202,203] Nutrient-dense foods, such as fruits, vegetables, whole grains, and fat-free dairy products, cost far more per calorie than high-sugar, high-fat foods, which, in the United States, often contain corn syrup, a refined sugar, and soybean oil. If healthy food prices were comparable, consumers could theoretically be more likely to purchase those foods. Therefore, researchers must consider the mediating effect of food pricing when investigating the relationship between the availability of foods and consumption.[204]

Examples of Price Manipulations to Improve the Food Environment

Methods of manipulating prices include providing discount coupons, lowering healthy food prices, and increasing unhealthy food prices. Steps to a Healthier Salinas disseminated 10% discount coupons in newspapers and at taquerias. The TrEAT Yourself Well program[205] conducted in the greater San Diego area implemented an intervention to promote healthy eating in fine dining, Mexican, upscale pizza, and "40s-style diner" restaurants. The intervention provided discount cards for healthy menu items, as well as waitstaff incentives of $1 per healthy item they sell. Sales of healthy items increased by nearly 5%.

One study at a delicatessen restaurant in Connecticut compared health message only, price reduction only, and health message with price reduction interventions.[206] Price reductions involved 20–30% discounts on low-fat items. The combination of health message and price reduction led to increased sales of target food items, with most of the increase due to the price reduction. Interestingly, the authors suggest that health message interventions can have paradoxical effects if foods labeled as healthy are assumed to taste worse than other foods.

In another study of price manipulations, education promoting low-fat snacks and price reductions of healthy snacks in vending machines of 10%, 25%, or 50% led to increases in sales of 9%, 39%, or 93%, respectively.[207] Due to the increase in sales, the price reduction did not affect the profit per machine, although the burden of restocking the vending machine more frequently due to an increase in sales could discourage price reductions.

Price Manipulations Targeted Toward Store Owners: Baltimore Healthy Stores

A form of price manipulation targeting store owners is to help with initial stocking, as in the Baltimore Healthy

Stores intervention trials in 16 corner stores and supermarkets in East and West Baltimore.[208] Investigators providing shelf labels, posters, fliers, taste tests, and educational sessions to promote healthy foods, such as cooking spray and low-fat products. Participating store owners received a $25 gift card to purchase promoted products. Sales of selected promoted foods increased after the intervention, suggesting the potential of incentives for storeowners in helping initiate interventions.[209]

Voluntary Healthy Restaurant Programs

North Carolina's Winner's Circle Healthy Dining Program was among the first statewide community-based interventions to work with various food venues, such as local health departments, cooperative extension services, and schools, to establish unified nutrition criteria and develop an icon to promote healthy foods.[210] The program was implemented in 65 out of 100 counties in North Carolina. Participants included 75 restaurants, more than 400 McDonald's restaurants, and all 2,400 public K–12 schools in the state. At each location, menu and recipe analysis allowed identification of healthy choices, which were marked with a promotional icon. The majority of participating restaurants and all schools increased the quantity of healthy items once they had their menus analyzed.

In Massachusetts, Shape Up Somerville (SUS) was a community-based participatory program to reduce obesity by increasing access to healthy foods and physical activity opportunities.[211] In the part of SUS targeting family restaurants, goals included increasing the availability of half-size portions, offering more fruits and vegetables, and providing low-fat milk or water as beverage options. The program was voluntary, and approximately 12% of restaurants that were recruited achieved criteria for SUS approval. However, in six months only half of these restaurants remained compliant.

In Howard County, Maryland, the Healthy Howard Healthy Restaurant program is a voluntary initiative to promote healthier menu options. Menu analysis was conducted to identify healthy entrées meeting certain nutrition criteria.[212] Meals could be designated as healthy if they contained less than 750 calories, including less than 30% of calories from fat and less than 10% of calories from saturated fat, a lean protein source, and fruits and vegetables. As of January 2012, the Healthy Howard program was implemented in 96 out of 870 restaurants in the county, suggesting moderate reach.

Operated by local health departments, Winner's Circle, SUS, and Healthy Howard exemplify programs with potentially large impacts. However, the voluntary nature of these programs may have contributed to their relatively low reach. Restaurant owners may view the interventions as a burden or devoid of benefit for their business.[213] Another limitation is that these programs did not all measure impact on consumer choices.

Implementation of BHC

Evaluation of BHC included measurement of sales data as well as associations between customers' exposure level to the intervention materials and purchasing behavior. Trained data collectors visited carry-outs weekly to retrieve sales receipts (**Figure 4-4**) during the 4-week baseline period and 28-week intervention period. Carry-out owners

received $25 gift cards each week for collecting the receipts. Sales receipts contained detailed information about entrées, side dishes, and beverages purchased, both in person and over the phone, and cost of each item.

To evaluate customer-level impact, consumers took three post-intervention surveys at each of the eight carry-outs in BHC (**Figure 4-5**). The Customer Impact Questionnaire (CIQ) reported height and weight and examined consumer behaviors, such as frequency of visits to carry-outs, to other restaurants and to the particular carry-out, and amount spent on each food purchase. Also used were the National Cancer Institute Percent energy from fat (NCI Pfat) screener and the Intervention Exposure Assessment (IEA) to assess intervention-specific knowledge and purchasing behaviors, with questions such as "Have you seen this poster [photo provided]?" and "Have you purchased

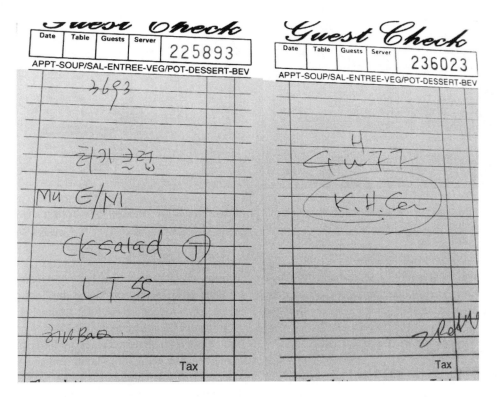

Figure 4-4 A photo of two hand written guest checks. Examples of hand-written menu orders (Left: "3693" indicates the last 4 digits of the customer's phone number, Turkey club, mustard, everything without mayonnaise, Chicken Salad sandwich, toasted, lettuce, tomatoes, seasoned salt, honey barbeque sauce. Right: Four wings and French fries, fry hard (fried until crispy), ketchup, hot sauce and seasoned salt)

Reproduced from Lee, S. H. (2012). Changing the food environment in Baltimore City: Impact of an intervention to improve carry-outs in low-income neighborhoods. Doctoral dissertation. Johns Hopkins University.

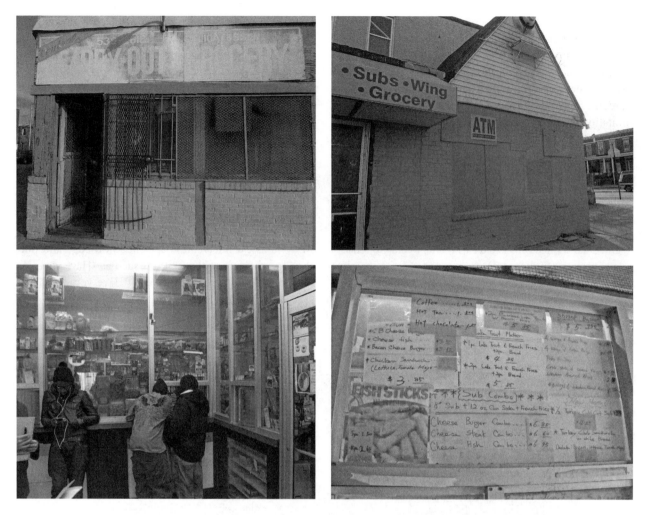

Figure 4-5 Two exterior photos of carry-outs and two interior photos of carry-outs

Reproduced from Lee, S. H. (2012). Changing the food environment in Baltimore City: Impact of an intervention to improve carry-outs in low-income neighborhoods. Doctoral dissertation. Johns Hopkins University.

watermelon at this carry-out?" These assessments allowed measurement of the level of intervention exposure among customers and association with purchases of healthy foods.

Evaluation and Future Directions for BHC

Process evaluation in BHC assessed intervention reach, dose received, and fidelity using sales receipts, carry-out visit evaluation, and intervention exposure assessment. On average, the intervention carry-outs reached 36.8% more customers during the intervention relative to baseline. The menu boards and labels were seen by 100.0% and 84.2% of individuals, respectively. Promoted entrée availability and revised menu and poster presence all had high fidelity and feasibility.

Impact evaluation at the carry-out level utilized sales receipts from seven carry-outs and found an increase in healthy food sales and total revenues in the intervention group. Customer-level impact evaluation found that intervention customers were more likely to purchase promoted healthy items, and a dose-response relationship was observed between intervention exposure and amount of healthy food purchased. In the intervention group, the turkey club sandwich, fruit cup, cooked greens, side salad, and baked chips had increased odds of being purchased among customers when coupled with the BHC intervention.

Future programs to improve the food environment should be evidence-based, feasible to implement, and culturally acceptable for prolonged sustainability. Moreover, collaborating with local health departments and incorporating certification to provide incentives for food stores can improve reach and implementation.

Role of Culture in Food Environment Interventions

While public health programs should be based on past experiences and fundamental concepts, each also needs to consider factors particular to its situation. These include available funding and other resources, community and government support, and cultural factors. Interventions to improve the food environment must include culturally appropriate training programs, materials in the appropriate language(s), and accepted foods.

Staff and Others Involved in Implementation

Since half of carry-out owners participating in BHC were first-generation Korean Americans, Korean-speaking study coordinators and staff were essential. Moreover, to ensure positive interaction between study staff and carry-out owners, cultural sensitivity training was conducted with all study staff. The training session covered Korean core cultural values, basic Korean greetings, and Korean manners.

Select Foods That Are Culturally Acceptable

The availability of low-cost, affordable foods does no good if people won't eat them. Offered foods and recipes must be culturally acceptable. Among a variety of healthy foods promoted in BHC, some appeared more "culturally acceptable" to carry-out owners and customers based on increased sales at intervention carry-outs. For instance, fruit cups were preferred to bananas, baked chips to pretzels, and turkey sandwiches to grilled cheese sandwiches. Including culturally acceptable foods early in the intervention can motivate carry-out owners to participate.

Use Culturally Appropriate Intervention Strategies

In BHC, researchers incorporated community feedback into the design of intervention materials such as posters and menu labels. Suggestions included: (1) using specific colors, such as orange and purple, which reflect the colors of professional sports teams in Baltimore, (2) avoiding the word "health," which invokes "bland" and "disgusting," and instead using "fresh" to evoke positive associations, and (3) creating gender-specific messages for posters, such as focusing on weight loss for females and increasing energy for males.

Collaboration with Local Food Policy Initiatives and Government Involvement

Collaborating with local food policy initiatives allows programs to use existing materials and infrastructure for programs. Government involvement not only increases the chances of gaining funds and supportive policies in the future, but can also increase program credibility and therefore participation.

From the beginning, the BHC project shared progress and findings with the Baltimore Food Policy Initiative and Department of Planning. This partnership allowed policy briefs to be generated when communicating with policy makers about the need to disseminate such carry-out interventions. Moreover, the collaboration was crucial to demonstrate the cost-effectiveness, short- and long-term success, and potential sustainability of the BHC intervention.

With strong leadership from the initiatives and support from the Baltimore mayor's office, BHC strategies were implemented in 100 carry-outs in six public food markets in Baltimore.[214] The initiative, called Get Fresh Public Markets, targets four areas: (1) Healthy carry-outs, (2) customer demand, (3) local farmer day stalls, and (4) a healthy food and fitness strategy. BHC directly addresses goals 1 and 4. By 2012, 36 carry-outs in three public markets had received some or all of the intervention components, and by 2015, all carry-outs in all public markets are scheduled to participate.

Healthy Carry-Out Certification

A certification program increases the prestige of offering healthier foods, thus encouraging food vendors to improve their selections. Certification also helps guide consumers so that they can choose healthier foods without much effort or background knowledge.

Healthy carry-out certification in Baltimore is a citywide standard for identifying prepared food sources that provide and promote healthy food options. To be certified, sites must offer more than two choices each of healthy side dishes, healthy beverages, and healthy entrées. Future certification could make use of BHC intervention strategies, such as menu analysis to identify more-healthy food options and menu labeling for items that qualify as "healthy." The Department of Health currently conducts Food Service

Facility Inspection Reports two to three times annually. Including questions to assess healthy carry-out certification compliance could promote healthier food offerings.

Conclusion

The food environment includes characteristics such as proximity to restaurants and stores, food prices, and availability of healthy foods. Inadequate access to affordable and healthy foods can lead to poor individual food choices and health problems, such as obesity, heart disease, and cardiovascular diseases. Certain groups, such as low-income individuals, minorities, and inner-city dwellers, are disproportionately exposed to poor food environments.

Foods prepared away from home, such as in restaurants and carry-outs, are often high in calories, fat, sugar, and sodium. Carry-out foods compose a significant portion of the diet within some disadvantaged communities, and public health interventions to improve foods offered at carry-outs can potentially greatly impact the public's health (**Figure 4-6**). Possible approaches include menu labeling, price manipulations, and education for consumers and restaurant owners. As discovered from various programs, successful interventions are culturally appropriate and include means for evaluation.

Baltimore Healthy Carry-Outs:
Changing the prepared food environment
Policy Brief #7 (June 17, 2011)

INTERVENTION STRATEGIES

Interventions must consider strategies that are culturally acceptable for both the owners and the customers.
- Promote healthy foods that are culturally acceptable and desirable.
- Promote and advertise healthy foods in store to increase customer demand.
- Provide incentives for the owners to reduce the economic burden on serving healthy foods

The Baltimore Healthy Carryout project is a pilot trial of a multi-component intervention in prepared food sources in low-income urban neighborhoods, which specifically targets both carry-out owners and customers in Baltimore City. The BHC project has a quasi-experimental study design including 8 carry-outs, located in East and West Baltimore. Four carry-outs will receive 6 months pilot intervention consisting of 3 phases (2 months per phase) with the focus of changing the food environment through point-of-purchase promotions, and four carry-outs will serve as comparison.

THREE PHASES OF THE INTERVENTION

Phase 1: Physical Environment and Menu Labeling Modifications
- *Menus:* Replace current menus with new menu by identifying healthier foods that are currently offered, including pictures of healthy items. The menus are in large format and also available in paper format for customers to take with them.
- *Leaf Logo:* The green leaf logo is used to identify a healthy choice signifying "fresh is best". The logo is used consistently in all promoted choices.
- *Visual Posters:* A variety of small posters are used to promote healthy eating and advertise healthier foods.

Urban carryout owners were enthusiastic and cooperative about implementing new menus, which highlighted healthy options. The menu continues to be sustainable and highly regarded.

Modified menu boards and posters were highly acceptable due to the perceived minimal burden on the carry-out owners and the perceived aesthetic improvement.

Sales of highlighted healthy items in carry-outs continue to increase.

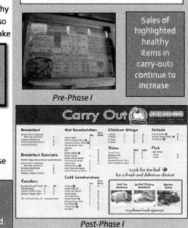

Pre-Phase I

Post-Phase I

Figure 4-6   An example of a BHC policy brief

Reproduced from Lee, S. H. (2012). Changing the food environment in Baltimore City: Impact of an intervention to improve carry-outs in low-income neighborhoods. Doctoral dissertation. Johns Hopkins University.

References

1 Baltimore City Health Department. (2008, July 23). *Fact sheet: Overweight and Obesity in Baltimore City, 1997-2007.* Fact Sheet, 1(1). Retrieved from http://www.baltimorehealth .org/info/2008_07_22.ObesityFactSheet.pdf

2 Franco, M., Diez Roux, A. V., Glass, T. A., Caballero, B., & Brancati, F. L. (2008). Neighborhood characteristics and availability of healthy foods in Baltimore. *American Journal of Preventive Medicine, 35*(6), 561-67.

3 Gittelsohn, J., Franceschini, M., Rasooly, I., Ries, A., Ho, L., Santos, V., Jennings, S., et al. (2007). Understanding the food environment in a low-income urban settings: Implications for food store interventions. *Journal of Hunger and Environmental Nutrition, 2*(2/3), 33-50.

4 Franco, M., Diez Roux, A. V., Glass, T. A., Caballero, B., & Brancati, F. L. (2008). Neighborhood characteristics and availability of healthy foods in Baltimore. *American Journal of Preventive Medicine, 35*(6), 561-67.

5 Antin, T. M., & Hora, M. T. (2005). Distance and beyond: Variables influencing conceptions of food store accessibility in Baltimore, Maryland. *Practicing Anthropology, 27*(2), 15-17.

6 Lee, S. H., Rowan, M., Powell, L. M., Newman, S., Klassen, A. C., Frick, K. D., et al. (2010). Characteristics of prepared food sources in low-income neighborhoods of Baltimore City. *Ecology of Food and Nutrition, 49*(6), 409-30.

7 Lee, S. H., Rowan, M., Powell, L. M., Newman, S., Klassen, A. C., Frick, K. D., et al. (2010). Characteristics of prepared food sources in low-income neighborhoods of Baltimore City. *Ecology of Food and Nutrition, 49*(6), 409-30.

8 Noormohamed, A., Lee, S. H., Batorsky, B., Jackson, A., Newman, S., & Gittelsohn, J. (2012). Factors influencing ordering practices at Baltimore City carryouts: Qualitative research to inform an obesity prevention intervention. *Ecology of Food and Nutrition, 51*(6), 481-91.

9 Palmer, A., Haering, S., Smith, J., & McKenzie, S. (2007). *Understanding and addressing food security in southwest Baltimore.* Retrieved from Johns Hopkins Center for a Livable Future website, http://www.jhsph.edu/bin/o/u /OROSWreport2009-1-1.pdf

10 Gittelsohn, J., & Sharma, S. (2009). Physical, consumer, and social aspects of measuring the food environment among diverse low-income populations. *American Journal of Preventive Medicine, 36*(4 Suppl.), S161-65.

11 Sharma, S., Cao, X., Arcan, C., Mattingly, M., Jennings, S., Song, H. J., & Gittelsohn, J. (2009). Assessment of dietary intake in an inner-city African American population and development of a quantitative food frequency questionnaire to highlight foods and nutrients for a nutritional invention. *International Journal of Food Sciences and Nutrition, 60*(Suppl. 5), 155-67.

12 Lee, S. H., Hoffman, V., Bleich, S. N., & Gittelsohn, J. (2012). Frequency of visiting and food dollars spent at carry-outs among low-income, urban African-American adults. *Journal of Hunger & Environmental Nutrition, 7,* 459-67.

13 Lee, S. H., Rowan, M., Powell, L. M., Newman, S., Klassen, A. C., Frick, K. D., et al. (2010). Characteristics of prepared food sources in low-income neighborhoods of Baltimore City. *Ecology of Food and Nutrition, 49*(6), 409-30.

14 Krishnan, S., Coogan, P. F., Boggs, D. A., Rosenberg, L., & Palmer, J. R. (2010). Consumption of restaurant foods and incidence of type 2 diabetes in African American women. *American Journal of Clinical Nutrition, 91*(2), 465.

15 Darmon, N., & Drewnowski, A. (2008). Does social class predict diet quality? *American Journal of Clinical Nutrition, 87,* 1107-17.

16 Cummins, S., & Macintyre, S. (2002). "Food deserts": Evidence and assumption in health policy making. *British Medical Journal, 325*(7361), 436.

17 Todd, J., Mancino, L., & Lin, B-H. (2010). *The impact of food away from home on adult diet quality.* USDA Economic Research Report No. (ERR-90). Washington, DC: U.S. Government Printing Office.

18 Reisig, V., & Hobbiss, A. (2000). Food deserts and how to tackle them: A study of one city's approach. *Health Education Journal, 59*(2), 137-49.

19 Ver Ploeg, M., Breneman, V., Farrigan, T., et al. (2009, June). Access to affordable and nutritious food—measuring and understanding food deserts and their consequences: Report to Congress. Administrative Publication No. (AP-036). Retrieved from http://www.ers.usda.gov/publications/ap-administrative-publication/ap-036.aspx

20 Cummins, S., & Macintyre, S. (2002). "Food deserts": Evidence and assumption in health policy making. *British Medical Journal, 325*(7361), 436.

21 United States Department of Agriculture. Agricultural Marketing Service. (n.d.). *What is the definition of a food desert?* Retrieved from http://apps.ams.usda.gov/fooddeserts /FAQ.aspx#definition

22 Gordon-Larsen, P., Nelson, M. C., Page, P., & Popkin, B. M. (2006). Inequality in the built environment underlies key health disparities in physical activity and obesity. *Pediatrics, 117*(2), 417-24.

23 Hubley, T. A. (2011). Assessing the proximity of healthy food options and food deserts in a rural area of Maine. *Applied Geography, 31,* 1224-31.

24 Blanchard, T., & Lyson, T. (2006). *Access to low cost groceries in nonmetropolitan counties: Large retailers and the creation of food deserts.* Paper presented at the Measuring Rural Diversity Conference, Washington, DC. Retrieved from http://srdc.msstate.edu/trainings/presentations_archive /2002/2002_blanchard.pdf

25 Guy, C., Clarke, G., & Eyre, H. (2004). Food retail change and the growth of food deserts: A case study of Cardiff. *International Journal of Retail and Distribution Management, 32,* 72-88.

26 Morton, L. W., & Blanchard, T. C. (2007) Starved for access: Life in rural America's food deserts. *Rural Realities, 1*(4), 20-29.

27 Ver Ploeg, M., Breneman, V., Farrigan, T., Hamrick, K., Hopkins, D., Kaufman, P., et al. (2009). *Access to affordable and nutritious food: Measuring and understanding food deserts and their consequences: Report to Congress. Appendix C. Methods, supporting tables, and maps for national-level analysis of supermarket access.* Retrieved from http://www.ers.usda.gov/media/242642/ap036l_1_.pdf

28 Dean, W. R., & Sharkey, J. R. (2011). Rural and urban differences in the associations between characteristics of the community food environment and fruit and vegetable intake. *Journal of Nutrition Education and Behavior, 43*(6), 426-33.

29 McGee, B. B., Johnson, G. S., Yadrick, M. K., Richardson, V., Simpson, P. M., Gossett, J. M., . . . Bogle, M.L. (2011). Food shopping perceptions, behaviors and ability to purchase healthful food items in the lower Mississippi delta. *Journal of Nutrition Education and Behavior, 43*(5), 339-48.

30 Smith, C., & Miller, H. (2011). Accessing the food systems in urban and rural Minnesotan communities. *Journal of Nutrition Education and Behavior, 43*(6), 492-504.

31 Policylink. (n.d.). *Grocery store development.* Retrieved from http://www.policylink.org/site/c.lkIXLbMNJrE/b.7962289/k.8730/Grocery_Store_Development/apps/nl/newsletter2.asp

32 McGee, B. B., Johnson, G. S., Yadrick, M. K., Richardson, V., Simpson, P. M., Gossett, J. M., . . . Bogle, M. L. (2011). Food shopping perceptions, behaviors and ability to purchase healthful food items in the lower Mississippi delta. *Journal of Nutrition Education and Behavior, 43*(5), 339-48.

33 Steward, H., & Dong, D. (2012, June 5). Fresh vegetables and salty snacks cost more in urban locales. *Amber Waves.* Retrieved from USDA Economic Research Service website, http://www.ers.usda.gov/amber-waves/2012-june/fresh-vegetables.aspx#.UkMxlhXD8y8

34 Gittelsohn, J., & Sharma, S. (2009). Physical, consumer, and social aspects of measuring the food environment among diverse low-income populations. *American Journal of Preventive Medicine, 36*(4 Suppl.), S161-65.

35 Rose, D., Bodor, J. N., Swalm, C. M., Rice, J. C., Farley, T. A., & Hutchinson, P. L. (2009). *Deserts in New Orleans? Illustrations of urban food access and implications for policy.* Paper prepared for University of Michigan National Poverty Center and USDA Economic Research Service Review. Retrieved from http://www.npc.umich.edu/news/events/food-access/rose_et_al.pdf

36 Woodham, C. (2009). Food desert or food swamp? An in-depth exploration of neighbourhood food environments in Eastern Porirua and Whitby. In University of Otago, *Public Health.* Dunedin, New Zealand: Wellington.

37 Block, J. P., Scribner, R. A., & DeSalvo, K. B. (2004). Fast food, race/ethnicity, and income: A geographic analysis. *American Journal of Preventive Medicine, 27*(3), 211-17.

38 Lewis, L. B., Sloane, D. C., Nascimento, L. M., Diamant, A. L., Guinyard, J. J., Yancey, A. K., et al. (2005). African Americans' access to healthy food options in south Los Angeles restaurants. *American Journal of Public Health, 95*(4), 668-73.

39 U.S. Department of Agriculture. (2011). *ERS/USDA Briefing Room: Food CPI and Expenditures: Table 10.* Retrieved from http://www.ers.usda.gov/briefing/cpifoodandexpenditures/data/Expenditures_tables/table10.htm

40 Guthrie, J. F., Lin, B. H., & Frazao, E. (2002). Role of food prepared away from home in the american diet, 1977-78 versus 1994-96: Changes and consequences. *Journal of Nutrition Education and Behavior, 34*(3), 140-50.

41 U.S. Department of Agriculture. (2003). Profiling food consumption in America. Ch. 2 in *Agriculture fact book, 2001-2002.* Washington, DC: U.S. Government Printing Office.

42 U.S. Department of Agriculture, U.S. Department of Health and Human Services. (2010). *Dietary guidelines for Americans 2010.* Washington, DC: U.S. Government Printing Office.

43 U.S. Department of Agriculture. (2011). *ERS/USDA Briefing Room: Food CPI and Expenditures: Table 15.* Retrieved from http://www.ers.usda.gov/Briefing/CPIFoodAndExpenditures/Data/Expenditures_tables/table15.htm

44 Darmon, N., & Drewnowski, A. (2008). Does social class predict diet quality? *American Journal of Clinical Nutrition, 87,* 1107-17.

45 Rolland-Cachera, M. F., & Bellisle, F. (1986). No correlation between adiposity and food intake: Why are working class children fatter? *American Journal of Clinical Nutrition, 44,* 779-87.

46 Xie B., Gilliland, F. D., Li, Y. F.,& Rockett, H. R. (2003). Effects of ethnicity, family income, and education on dietary intake among adolescents. *Preventive Medicine, 36,* 30-40.

47 Oh, S. Y., & Hong, M. J. (2003). Food insecurity is associated with dietary intake and body size of Korean children from low-income families in urban areas. *European Journal of Clinical Nutrition, 57,* 1598-1604.

48 Hulshof, K. F. A. M., Brussaard, J. H., Kruizinga, A. G., Telman, J., & Lowik, M. R. H. (2003). Socio-economic status, dietary intake and 10 y trends: The Dutch National Food Consumption Survey. *European Journal of Clinical Nutrition, 57,* 128-37.

49 Sharkey, J. R., Nalty, C., Johnson, J. M., & Dean, W. R. (2012). Children's low food security is associated with increased dietary intakes in energy, fat, and added sugar among Mexican-American children (6-11y) in Texas border colonias. *BMC Pediatrics, 12,* 16.

50 Beaulac, J., Kristjansson, E., & Cummins, S. (2009). A systematic review of food deserts, 1996-2007. *Preventing Chronic Diseases, 6*(3), A105.

51 Economic Research Service. (2009) *Access to affordable and nutritious food: Measuring and understanding food deserts and their consequences. Report to Congress.* Washington, DC: U.S. Department of Agriculture. Retrieved from http://www.ers.usda.gov/Publications/AP/AP036/AP036.pdf

52 Cummins, S., & Macintyre, S. (2002). "Food deserts": Evidence and assumption in health policy making. *British Medical Journal, 325*(7361), 436.

53 Thomas, D., & Strauss, J. (1997). Health and wages: Evidence on men and women in urban Brazil. *Journal of Econometrics, 77*(1), 159-85.

54 Kleinman, R. E., Hall, S., Green, H., Korzec-Ramirez, D., Patton, K., Pagano, M. E., & Murphy, J. M. (2002). Diet, breakfast and academic performance in children. *Annals of Nutrition & Metabolism, 42*(Suppl. 1), 24-30.

55 Walter, T., De Andraca, I., Chadud, P., & Perales C. G. (1989). Iron deficiency anemia: Adverse effects on infant psychomotor development. *Pediatrics, 84*(1), 7.

56 Gostin, L. O. (2007). Law as a tool to facilitate healthier lifestyles and prevent obesity. *JAMA, 297*(1), 87-90.

57 Flegal, K. M., Carroll, M. D., Ogden, C. L., & Curtin, L. R. (2010). Prevalence and trends in obesity among US adults, 1998-2008. *JAMA, 303*(3), 235-41.

58 Wang, Y., & Beydoun, M. A. (2007). The obesity epidemic in the United States—gender, age, socioeconomic, racial/ethnic, and geographic characteristics: A systematic review and meta-regression analysis. *Epidemiologic Reviews, 29*, 6-28.

59 Centers for Disease Control and Prevention. (2009). *Prevalence of overweight, obesity and extreme obesity among adults: United States, trends 1960-62 through 2005-2006.* NCHS Health e-stat. Retrieved from http://www.cdc.gov/nchs/data/hestat/overweight/overweight_adult.htm

60 Maryland Department of Health & Mental Hygiene Family Health Administration, Family Health Administration, Center for Preventive Health Services. (2005, May). *Burden of overweight and obesity in Maryland.* Retrieved from http://www.kentonthemove.org/pdf/burden.pdf

61 Kopelman, P. G. (2000). Obesity as a medical problem. *Nature, 404*(6778), 635-43.

62 National Institutes of Health & National Heart, Lung, and Blood Institute. (1998). *Clinical guidelines on the identification, evaluation, and treatment of overweight and obesity in adults: The evidence report.* Retrieved from http://www.nhlbi.nih.gov/guidelines/obesity/ob_gdlns.pdf

63 Finkelstein, E. A., Trogdon, J. G., Cohen, J. W., & Dietz, W. (2009). Annual medical spending attributable to obesity: Payer-and service-specific estimates. *Health Affairs, 28*(5), w822-w831.

64 Withrow, D., & Alter, D. (2011). The economic burden of obesity worldwide: A systematic review of the direct costs of obesity. *Obesity Reviews, 12*(2), 131-41.

65 Spence, J. M., Cutumisu, N., Edwards, J., Raine, K. D., & Smoyer-Tomic, K. (2009). Relation between local food environments and obesity among adults. *BMC Public Health, 9*, 192.

66 Drewnowski, A. (2004). Obesity and the food environment: Dietary energy and diet costs. *American Journal of Preventive Medicine, 27*, 154-62.

67 Chou, S. Y., Grossman, M., & Saffer, H. (2004). An economic analysis of adult obesity: Results from the behavioral risk factor surveillance system. *Journal of Health Economics, 23*(3), 565-87.

68 Maddock, J. (2004). The relationship between obesity and the prevalence of fast food restaurants: State-level analysis. *American Journal of Health Promotion: AJHP, 19*(2), 137-43.

69 McCrory, M. A., Fuss, P. J., Hays, N. P., Vinken, A. G., Greenberg, A. S., & Roberts, S. B. (1999). Overeating in America: Association between restaurant food consumption and body fatness in healthy adult men and women ages 19 to 80. *Obesity Research, 7*(6), 564-71.

70 Sturm, R., & Datar, A. (2005). Body mass index in elementary school children, metropolitan area food prices and food outlet density. *Public Health, 119*(12), 1059-68.

71 Mehta, N. K., & Chang, V. W. (2008). Weight status and restaurant availability: A multilevel analysis. *American Journal of Preventive Medicine, 34*(2), 127.

72 Beydoun, M. A., Powell, L. M., & Wang, Y. (2009). Reduced away-from-home food expenditure and better nutrition knowledge and belief can improve quality of dietary intake among US adults. *Public Health Nutrition, 12*(3), 369-81.

73 Duffey, K. J., Gordon-Larsen, P., Jacobs, D. R., Jr., Williams, O. D., & Popkin, B. M. (2007). Differential associations of fast food and restaurant food consumption with 3-y change in body mass index: The Coronary Artery Risk Development in Young Adults study. *American Journal of Clinical Nutrition, 85*(1), 201-8.

74 Tucker, K. L., Maras, J., Champagne, C., Connell, C., Goolsby, S., Weber, J., et al. (2007). A regional food-frequency questionnaire for the U.S. Mississippi Delta. *Public Health Nutrition, 8*(1), 87-96.

75 U.S. Department of Agriculture, U.S. Department of Health and Human Services. (2010). *Dietary guidelines for Americans 2010.* Washington, DC: U.S. Government Printing Office.

76 Lin, B. H., Guthrie, J., & Frazao, E. (1999). Nutrient contribution of food away from home. In Frazao, F. (ed.), *America's eating habits: Changes and consequences* (pp. 213-42). Washington, DC: U.S. Government Printing Office.

77 Lee, S. H., Rowan, M. T., Newman, S., Anderson, J., Suratkar, S. R., Klassen, A. C., et al. (2010). Description of prepared foods around recreation centers in low income neighborhoods in Baltimore City [Abstract]. *FASEB Journal, 24*(1), 744.7.

78 Morrison, R., Mancino, L., & Variyam, J. (2011, March 11). Will calorie labeling in restaurants make a difference? *Amber Waves. 7*(2). Retrieved from USDA Economic Research Service website, http://www.ers.usda.gov/amber-waves/2011-march/will-calorie-labeling.aspx

79 U.S. Department of Agriculture, U.S. Department of Health and Human Services. (2010). *Dietary Guidelines for Americans 2010.* Washington, DC: U.S. Government Printing Office.

80 Bowman, S. A., Gortmaker, S. L., Ebbeling, C. B., Pereira, M. A., & Ludwig, D. S. (2004). Effects of fast-food consumption on energy intake and diet quality among children in a national household survey. *Pediatrics, 113*(1), 112-18.

81 Guthrie, J. F., Lin, B. H., & Frazao, E. (2002). Role of food prepared away from home in the American diet, 1977-78 versus 1994-96: Changes and consequences. *Journal of Nutrition Education and Behavior, 34*(3), 140-50.

82 Diliberti, N., Bordi, P. L., Conklin, M. T., Roe, L. S., & Rolls, B. J. (2004). Increased portion size leads to increased energy intake in a restaurant meal. *Obesity Research, 12*(3), 562-68.

83 Rolls, B. J., Morris, E. L., & Roe, L. S. (2002). Portion size of food affects energy intake in normal-weight and overweight men and women. *American Journal of Clinical Nutrition, 76*(6), 1207-13.

84 Wansink, B., & Cheney, M. M. (2005). Super bowls: Serving bowl size and food consumption. *JAMA, 293*(14), 1727.

85 Young, L. R., & Nestle, M. (2007). Portion sizes and obesity: Responses of fast-food companies. *Journal of Public Health Policy, 28*(2), 238-48.

86 Lovasi, G. S., Hutson, M. A., Guerra, M., & Neckerman, K. M. (2009). Built environments and obesity in disadvantaged populations. *Epidemiologic Reviews, 31*, 7-20.

87 Franco, M., Diez-Roux, A. V., Nettleton, J. A., Lazo, M., Brancati, F., Caballero, B., et al. (2009). Availability of healthy foods and dietary patterns: The multi-ethnic study of atherosclerosis. *American Journal of Clinical Nutrition, 89*(3), 897-904.

88 Galvez, M. P., Morland, K., Raines, C., Kobil, J., Siskind, J., Godbold, J., et al. (2008). Race and food store availability in an inner-city neighbourhood. *Public Health Nutrition, 11*(6), 624-31.

89 Powell, L. M., Slater, S., Mirtcheva, D., Bao, Y., & Chaloupka, F. J. (2007). Food store availability and neighborhood characteristics in the united states. *Preventive Medicine, 44*(3), 189-95.

90 Moore, L. V., Diez Roux, A. V., Nettleton, J. A., Jacobs, D. R., & Franco, M. (2009). Fast-food consumption, diet quality, and neighborhood exposure to fast food: The multi-ethnic study of atherosclerosis. *American Journal of Epidemiology, 170*(1), 29-36.

91 Franco, M., Diez-Roux, A. V., Nettleton, J. A., Lazo, M., Brancati, F., Caballero, B., et al. (2009). Availability of healthy foods and dietary patterns: The multi-ethnic study of atherosclerosis. *American Journal of Clinical Nutrition, 89*(3), 897-904.

92 Galvez, M. P., Morland, K., Raines, C., Kobil, J., Siskind, J., Godbold, J., et al. (2008). Race and food store availability in an inner-city neighbourhood. *Public Health Nutrition, 11*(6), 624-31.

93 Lovasi, G. S., Hutson, M. A., Guerra, M., & Neckerman, K. M. (2009). Built environments and obesity in disadvantaged populations. *Epidemiologic Reviews, 31*, 7-20.

94 Powell, L. M., Slater, S., Mirtcheva, D., Bao, Y., & Chaloupka, F. J. (2007). Food store availability and neighborhood characteristics in the united states. *Preventive Medicine, 44*(3), 189-95.

95 Dunn, R. A., Sharkey, J. R., & Horel, S. (2012). The effect of fast food availability on fast-food consumption and obesity among rural residents: An analysis by race/ethnicity. *Economics and Human Biology, 10*(1), 1-13.

96 Hill, J. O., & Peters, J. C. (1998). Environmental contributions to the obesity epidemic. *Science, 280*(5368), 1371.

97 Lovasi, G. S., Hutson, M. A., Guerra, M., & Neckerman, K. M. (2009). Built environments and obesity in disadvantaged populations. *Epidemiology Reviews, 31*, 7-20.

98 Auchincloss, A. H., Mujahid, M. S., Shen, M., Michos, E. D., Whitt-Glover, M. C., Diez Roux, A. V. (2012). Neighborhood health-promoting resources and obesity risk (the Multi-Ethnic Study of Atherosclerosis). *Obesity (Silver Spring)*. doi:10.1038/oby.2012.91 [Epub ahead of print]

99 Leung, C. W., Gregorich, S. E., Laraia, B. A., Kushi, L. H., & Yen, I. H. (2010). Measuring the neighborhood environment: Associations with young girls' energy intake and expenditure in a cross-sectional study. *International Journal of Behavioral Nutrition and Physical Activity, 7*, 52.

100 Frank, L. D., Saelens, B. E., Chapman, J., Sallis, J. F., Kerr, J., Glanz, K., . . . Cain, K. L. (2012). Objective assessment of obesogenic environments in youth: Geographic information system methods and spatial findings from the Neighborhood Impact on Kids Study. *American Journal of Preventive Medicine, 42*, e47-e55.

101 Flegal, K. M., Carroll, M. D., Kit, B. K., Ogden, C. L. (2012). Prevalence of obesity and trends in the distribution of body mass index. *JAMA, 307*(5), 491-97.

102 Flegal, K. M., Carroll, M. D., Kit, B. K., Ogden, C. L. (2012). Prevalence of obesity and trends in the distribution of body mass index. *JAMA, 307*(5), 491-97.

103 Kirby, J. B., Liang, L., Chen, H. J., & Wang, Y. (2012). Race, place, and obesity: The complex relationships among community racial/ethnic composition, individual race/ethnicity, and obesity in the United States. *American Journal of Public Health, 102*(8), 1572-1578.

104 U.S. Census Bureau. (2010). *Table 697. Income, poverty and health insurance coverage in the United States, 2009. Current Population Reports, P60-238, and Historical Tables-Table F-05*. Retrieved from http://www.census.gov/compendia/statab/cats/income_expenditures_poverty_wealth.html

105 U.S. Census Bureau. (2012). *Statistical of the United States: 2012. Table 23. Metropolitan statistical areas with more than 750,000 persons in 2010—Population by race and Hispanic or Latino origin: 2010* (p. 31). Retrieved from http://www.census.gov/compendia/statab/2012/tables/12s0023.pdf

106 Lopez, R. (2004, September). Urban sprawl and risk for being overweight or obese. *American Journal of Public Health, 94*(9), 1574-79.

107 Centers for Disease Control and Prevention. (2010, December). *Obesity and socioeconomic status in adults: United States, 2005-2008*. NCHS Data Brief No. 50. Retrieved from http://www.cdc.gov/nchs/data/databriefs/db50.pdf

108 Pereira, M. A., Kartashov, A. I., Ebbeling, C. B., Van Horn, L., Slattery, M. L., Jacobs, D. R., Jr., et al. (2005). Fast-food habits, weight gain, and insulin resistance (the CARDIA study): 15-year prospective analysis. *Lancet, 365*(9453), 36-42.

109 Laveist, T., Pollack, K., Thorpe, R., Fesahazion, R., & Gaskin, D. (2011). Place, not race: Disparities dissipate in southwest Baltimore when blacks and whites live under similar conditions. *Health Affairs, 30*, 1880-87.

110 Sharkey, J. R., Johnson, C. M., & Dean, W. R. (2011). Relationship of household food insecurity to health-related quality of life

in a large sample of urban and rural women. *Women Health, 51*(5), 442-60.

111 Loucks, E. B., Rehkopf, D. H., Thurston, R. C., & Kawachi, I. (2007). Socioeconomic disparities in metabolic syndrome differ by gender: Evidence from NHANES III. *Annals of Epidemiology, 17*(1), 19-26.

112 Wang, Y., & Chen, X. (2011). How much of racial/ethnic disparities in dietary intake, exercise, and weight status can be explained by nutrition- and health-related psychosocial factors and socioeconomic status among US adults? *Journal of American Dietetic Association, 111*(12), 1904-11.

113 Purslow, L. R., Wareham, N. J., Forouhi, N., Brunner, E. J., Luben, R. N., Welch, A. A., Khaw, K. T., Bingham, S. A., & Sandhu, M. S. (2008). Socioeconomic position and risk of short-term weight gain: Prospective study of 14,619 middle-aged men and women. *BMC Public Health, 9*(8), 112.

114 Stafford, M., Brunner, E. J., Head, J., & Ross, N. A. (2010). Deprivation and the development of obesity a multilevel longitudinal study in England. *American Journal of Preventive Medicine, 39*(2), 130-39.

115 Coogan, P. F., White, L. F., Evans, S. R., Adler, T. J., Hathaway, K. M., Palmer, J. R., & Rosenberg, L. (2011). Longitudinal assessment of urban form and weight gain in African American women. *American Journal of Preventive Medicine, 40*(4), 411-48.

116 McLaren, L. (2007). Socioeconomic status and obesity. *Epidemiologic Reviews, 29*(10), 29-48.

117 Coogan, P. E., Wise, L. A., Cozier, Y. C., Palmer, J. R., Rosenberg, L. (2012). Lifecourse educational status in relation to weight gain in African American women. *Ethnic Disparities, 22*(2), 198-206.

118 Rehm, C. D., Moudon, A. V., Hurvitz, P. M., & Drewnowski, A. (1982). Residential property values are associated with obesity among women in King County, WA, USA. *Social Science and Medicine, 75*(3), 491-95.

119 Matheson, F. I., Moineddin, R., Glazier, R. H. (2008). The weight of place: A multilevel analysis of gender, neighborhood material deprivation and body mass index among Canadian adults. *Social Science & Medicine, 66*, 675-90.

120 Neff, R. A., Palmer, A. M., McKenzie, S. E., & Lawrence, R. S. (2009). Food systems and public health disparities. *Journal of Hunger & Environmental Nutrition, 4*(3), 282-314.

121 Wang, Y., & Zhang, Q. (2006). Are American children and adolescents of low socioeconomic status at increased risk of obesity? Changes in the association between overweight and family income between 1971 and 2002. *American Journal of Clinical Nutrition, 84*(4), 707-16.

122 National Diabetes Information Clearinghouse (NDIC). (2012). *Diabetes overview*. NIH Publication No. 09-3873. Retrieved from National Institute of Diabetes and Digestive and Kidney Diseases, National Institutes of Health website, http://diabetes.niddk.nih.gov/dm/pubs/overview/index.aspx

123 Savil, P. (2012). Identifying patients at risk of type 2 diabetes. *Practitioner, 256*(1753), 25-27.

124 Fitch, C., Keim, K. S., Academy of Nutrition and Dietetics. (2012). Position of the Academy of Nutrition and Dietetics: Use of nutritive and nonnutritive sweeteners. *Journal of the Academy of Nutrition and Dietetics, 112*(5), 739-58.

125 U.S. Department of Agriculture, U.S. Department of Health and Human Services. (2010). *Dietary guidelines for Americans 2010*. Washington, DC: U.S. Government Printing Office.

126 U.S. Department of Agriculture, U.S. Department of Health and Human Services. (2010). *Dietary guidelines for Americans 2010*. Washington, DC: U.S. Government Printing Office.

127 Krishnan, S., Coogan, P. F., Boggs, D. A., Rosenberg, L., & Palmer, J. R. Consumption of restaurant foods and incidence of type 2 diabetes in African American women. *American Journal of Clinical Nutrition, 91*(2), 465-71.

128 O'Brien, M. J., Davey, A., Alos, V. A., & Whitaker, R. C. (2013). Diabetes-related behaviors in Latinas and non-Latinas in California. *Diabetes Care, 36*(2), 355-61.

129 Heuman, A. N., Scholl, J. C., & Wilkinson, K. (2013). Rural Hispanic populations at risk in developing diabetes: Sociocultural and familial challenges in promoting a healthy diet. *Health Communication, 28*(3), 260-74.

130 Archer, S. L., Greenlund, K. J., Valdez, R., Casper, M. L., Rith-Najarian, S., & Croft, J. B. (2004). *Public Health Nutrition, 7*(8), 1025-32.

131 Odegaard, A. O., Koh, W. P., Yuan, J. M., Gross, M. D., & Pereira, M. A. (2012). Western-style fast food intake and cardiometabolic risk in an eastern country. *Circulation, 126*(2), 182-88.

132 Ludwig, D. S., Majzoub, J. A., Al-Zahrani, A., Dallal, G. E., Blanco, I., & Roberts, S. B. (1999). High glycemic index foods, overeating, and obesity. *Pediatrics, 103*(3), E26.

133 Pereira, M. A., Kartashov, A. I., Ebbeling, C. B., Van Horn, L., Slattery, M. L., Jacobs, D. R., Jr., et al. (2005). Fast-food habits, weight gain, and insulin resistance (the CARDIA study): 15-year prospective analysis. *Lancet, 365*(9453), 36-42.

134 Salmeron, J., Manson, J. E., Stampfer, M. J., Colditz, G. A., Wing, A. L., & Willett, W. C. (1997). Dietary fiber, glycemic load, and risk of non-insulin-dependent diabetes mellitus in women. *JAMA, 277*(6), 472-77.

135 Pereira, M. A., Kartashov, A. I., Ebbeling, C. B., Van Horn, L., Slattery, M. L., Jacobs, D. R., Jr., et al. (2005). Fast-food habits, weight gain, and insulin resistance (the CARDIA study): 15-year prospective analysis. *Lancet, 365*(9453), 36-42.

136 Centers for Disease Control and Prevention. (2012). *Heart disease*. Retrieved from http://www.cdc.gov/heartdisease/

137 World Health Organization. (2011). *The top 10 causes of death*. Retrieved from http://www.who.int/mediacentre/factsheets/fs310/en/index.html

138 Centers for Disease Control and Prevention. (2012). *High blood pressure fact sheet*. Retrieved from http://www.cdc.gov/DHDSP/data_statistics/fact_sheets/fs_bloodpressure.htm

139 World Health Organization. (2009). *Global health risks: Mortality and burden of disease attributable to selected major*

risks. Retrieved from http://www.who.int/healthinfo/global_burden_disease/GlobalHealthRisks_report_full.pdf

140 U.S. Department of Agriculture, U.S. Department of Health and Human Services. (2010). *Dietary guidelines for Americans 2010*. Washington, DC: U.S. Government Printing Office.

141 Liu, J., Hickson, D. A., Musani, S. K., Talegawkar, S. A., Carithers, T. C., Tucker, K. L., Fox, C. S., & Taylor, H. A. (2012). Dietary patterns, abdominal visceral adipose tissue and cardiometabolic risk factors in African-Americans: The Jackson Heart Study. *Obesity (Silver Spring)*.

142 Naja, F., Nasreddine, L., Itani, L., Adra, N., Sibai, A. M., & Hwalla, N. (2011). Association between dietary patterns and the risk of metabolic syndrome among Lebanese adults. *European Journal of Nutrition, 52*(1), 97-105.

143 Kollias, A., Skliros, E., Stergiou, G. S., Leotsakkos, N., Saridi, M., & Garifallos, D. (2011). Obesity and associated cardiovascular risk factors among schoolchildren in Greece: A cross-sectional study and review of the literature. *Journal of Pediatric Endocrinology and Metabolism, 24*(11-12), 929-38.

144 Dubowitz, T., Ghosh-Dastidar, M., Eibner, C., Slaughter, M. E., Fernandes, M., Whitsel, E. A., Bird, C. E., . . . Escarce, J. J. (2012). The Women's Health Initiative: The food environment, neighborhood socioeconomic status, BMI and blood pressure. *Obesity (Silver Spring), 20*(4), 862-71.

145 Franco, M., Diez-Roux, A. V., Nettleton, J. A., Lazo, M., Brancati, F., Caballero, B., et al. (2009). Availability of healthy foods and dietary patterns: The multi-ethnic study of atherosclerosis. *American Journal of Clinical Nutrition, 89*(3), 897-904.

146 Laraia, B. A., Siega-Riz, A. M., Kaufman, J. S., & Jones, S. J. (2004). Proximity of supermarkets in positively associated with diet quality index for pregnancy. *Preventive Medicine, 39*(5), 869-75.

147 Morland, K., Wing, S., & Diez Roux, A. (2006). Supermarkets, other food stores, and obesity: The atherosclerosis risk in communities study. *American Journal of Preventive Medicine, 30*(4), 333-39.

148 Boone-Heinonen, J., Gordon-Larsen, P., Kiefe, C. I., Shikany, J. M., Lewis, C. E., & Popkin, B. M. (2011). Fast food restaurants and food stores: Longitudinal associations with diet in young to middle-aged adults: The CARDIA study. *Archives of Internal Medicine, 171*(13), 1162-70.

149 Drewnowski, A., Aggarwal, A., Hurvitz, P. M., Monsivais, P., & Moudon, A. V. (2012). Obesity and supermarket access: Proximity or price? *American Journal of Public Health, 102*(8), e74-e80.

150 Drewnowski, A., Aggarwal, A., Hurvitz, P. M., Monsivais, P., & Moudon, A. V. (2012). Obesity and supermarket access: Proximity or price? *American Journal of Public Health, 102*(8), e74-e80.

151 Gustafson, A. A., Sharkey, J., Samuel-Hodge, C. D., Jones-Smith, J., Folds M. C., Cai, J., Ammerman, A. S. (2011). Perceived and objective measures of the food store environment and the association with weight and diet among low-income women in North Carolina. *Public Health Nutrition, 14*(6), 1032-38.

152 Liese, A. D., Colabianchi, N., Lamichhane, A. P., Barnes, T. L., Hibbert, J. D., Porter, D. E., Nichols, M. D., et al. (2010). Validation of 3 food outlet databases: Completeness and geospatial accuracy in rural and urban food environments. *American Journal of Epidemiology, 172*(11), 1324-33.

153 Miller, M. (2009). Dyslipidemia and cardiovascular risk: The importance of early prevention. *QJM, 102*(9), 657-67.

154 Centers for Disease Control and Prevention. (2012). *Cholesterol*. Retrieved from http://www.cdc.gov/cholesterol/index.htm

155 *Welcome to the online home of the Nutrition Environment Assessment Tool (NEAT)*. (n.d.). Retrieved from the Promoting Healthy Eating website, http://mihealthtools.org/neat/default.asp

156 Eisenmann, J. C., Gunderson, C., Lohman, B. J., Garasky, S., & Stewart, S. D. (2011). Is food insecurity related to overweight and obesity in children and adolescents? *Obesity Reviews, 12*(5), e73-83.

157 Moore, L. V., Diez Roux, A. V., & Franco, M. (2012). Measuring availability of healthy foods: agreement between directly measured and self-reported data. *American Journal of Epidemiology, 175*(10), 1341-47.

158 Gartin, M. (2012). Food deserts and nutritional risk in Paraguay. *American Journal of Human Biology, 24*(3), 296-301.

159 Andreyeva, T., Blumenthal, D. M., Schwartz, M. B., Long, M. W., & Brownell, K. D. (2008). Availability and prices of foods across stores and neighborhoods: The case of New Haven. *Health Affairs (Millwood), 27*(5), 1381-88.

160 Krukowski, R. A., West, D. S., Harvey-Berino, J., & Prewitt, E. T. (2010). Neigborhood impact on healthy food availability and pricing in food stores. *Journal of Community Health, 35*(3), 315-20.

161 Leone, A. F., Rigby, S., Betterley, C., Park, S., Kurtz, H., Johnson, M. A., & Lee, J. S. (2011). Store type and demographic influence on the availability and price of healthful foods, Leon County, Florida, 2008. *Preventing Chronic Diseases, 8*(6), A140.

162 Liese, A. D., Weis, K. E., Pluto, D., Smith, E., & Lawson, A. (2007). Food store types, availability, and cost of foods in a rural environment. *Journal of the American Dietetic Association, 107*(11), 1916-23.

163 Lee, S. H., Rowan, M. T., Newman, S., Anderson, J., Suratkar, S. R., Klassen, A. C., et al. (2010). Description of prepared foods around recreation centers in low income neighborhoods in Baltimore City [Abstract]. *FASEB Journal, 24*, 744.7.

164 Lesser, L. I., Hunnes, D. E., Reyes, P., Arab, L., Ryan, G. W., Brook, R. H., Cohen, D. A. (2012). Assessment of food offerings and marketing strategies in the food-service venues at California children's hospitals. *Academic Pediatrics, 12*(1), 62-67.

165 Erdman, M. B., Horacek, T., Phillips, B., Guo, W., Colby, S., . . . Greene, G. (2010). Assessment of the food and eating environment on college campus using a modified version of the Nutrition Environment Measures Survey for Restaurants (NEMS-R). *Journal of the American Dietetic Association, 110*(9), A24.

166 Lee, S. H., Rowan, M. T., Newman, S., Anderson, J., Suratkar, S. R., Klassen, A. C., et al. (2010). Description of prepared foods around recreation centers in low income neighborhoods in Baltimore City [Abstract]. *FASEB Journal, 24*, 744.7.

167 U.S. Department of Agriculture. (2012). *Food desert locator.* Retrieved from http://www.ers.usda.gov/data-products/food-desert-locator/about-the-locator.aspx

168 Darmon, N., & Drewnoski, A. (2008). Does social class predict diet quality? *American Journal of Clinical Nutrition, 87,* 1107-17.

169 Shin, C. N., & Lach, H. (2011). Nutritional issues of Korean Americans. *Clinical Nursing Research, 29*(2), 162-80.

170 Novotny, R., Chen, C., Williams, A. E., Albright, C. L., Nigg, C. R., Oshiro, C. E., Stevens, V. J. (2012). U.S. acculturation is associated with health behaviors and obesity, but not their change, with a hotel-based intervention among Asian-Pacific Islanders. *Journal of Academy of Nutrition and Dietetics, 112*(5), 649-56.

171 He, M., Tucker, P., Irwin, J. D., Gilliland, J., Larsen, K., & Hess, P. (2012). Obesogenic neighborhoods: The impact of neighborhood restaurants and convenience stores on adolescents' food consumption behaviors. *Public Health Nutrition, 15*(12), 2331-39.

172 U.S. Department of Agriculture, Center for Nutrition Policy and Promotion. (2008). *Diet quality of low-income and higher-income Americans in 2003-2004 as measured by the Healthy Eating Index-2005.* Nutrition Insight 42. Retrieved from http://www.cnpp.usda.gov/Publications/NutritionInsights/Insight42.pdf

173 U.S. Department of Agriculture, Center for Nutrition Policy and Promotion. (2008). *Healthy Eating Index-2005.* Retrieved from http://www.cnpp.usda.gov/Publications/HEI/healthyeating-index2005factsheet.pdf

174 Cortes, L. M., Gittelsohn, J., Alfred, J., & Palafox, N. A. (2001). Formative research to inform intervention development for diabetes prevention in the Republic of the Marshall Islands. *Health Education & Behavior, 28*(6), 696-715.

175 Strolla, L. O., Gans, K. M., & Risica, P. M. (2006). Using qualitative and quantitative formative research to develop tailored nutrition intervention materials for a diverse low-income audience. *Health Education Research, 21*(4), 465.

176 Seymour, J. D., Yaroch, A. L., Serdula, M., Blanck, H. M., & Khan, L. K. (2004). Impact of nutrition environmental interventions on point-of-purchase behavior in adults: A review. *Preventive Medicine, 39*(Suppl. 2), S108-36.

177 Albright, C. L., Flora, J. A., & Fortmann, S. P. (1990). Restaurant menu labeling: Impact of nutrition information on entree sales and patron attitudes. *Health Education & Behavior, 17*(2), 157.

178 Horgen, K. B., & Brownell, K. D. (2002). Comparison of price change and health message interventions in promoting healthy food choices. *Health Psychology, 21*(5), 505-12.

179 Eldridge, A. L., Snyder, M., Faus, N., & Kotz, K. (1997). Development and evaluation of a labeling program for low-fat foods in a discount department store foodservice area. *Journal of Nutrition Education, 29,* 159-61.

180 Wagner, J., & Winett, R. (1988). Prompting one low-fat, high-fiber selection in a fast-food restaurant. *Journal of Applied Behavior Analysis, 21*(2), 179.

181 Dietary Guidelines Advisory Committee. (2010). *Report of the Dietary Guidelines Advisory Committee on the Dietary Guidelines for Americans, 2010.* Retrieved from http://www.cnpp.usda.gov/DGAs2010-DGACReport.htm

182 Albright, C. L., Flora, J. A., & Fortmann, S. P. (1990). Restaurant menu labeling: Impact of nutrition information on entree sales and patron attitudes. *Health Education & Behavior, 17*(2), 157.

183 Eldridge, A. L., Snyder, M., Faus, N., & Kotz, K. (1997). Development and evaluation of a labeling program for low-fat foods in a discount department store foodservice area. *Journal of Nutrition Education, 29,* 159-61.

184 Wagner, J., & Winett, R. (1988). Prompting one low-fat, high-fiber selection in a fast-food restaurant. *Journal of Applied Behavior Analysis, 21*(2), 179.

185 Richard, L., O'Loughlin, J., Masson, P., & Devost, S. (1999). Healthy menu intervention in restaurants in low-income neighbourhoods: A field experience. *Journal of Nutrition Education, 31*(1), 54-59.

186 Richard, L., O'Loughlin, J., Masson, P., & Devost, S. (1999). Healthy menu intervention in restaurants in low-income neighbourhoods: A field experience. *Journal of Nutrition Education, 31*(1), 54-59.

187 Flournoy, R., & Treuhaft, S. (2005). *Healthy food, healthy communities: Improving access and opportunities through food retailing.* Oakland, CA: Policy Link.

188 Gittelsohn, J., Suratkar, S., Song, H. J., Sacher, S., Rajan, R., Rasooly, I. R., et al. (2010). Process evaluation of Baltimore healthy stores: A pilot health intervention program with supermarkets and corner stores in Baltimore city. *Health Promotion Practice, 11*(5), 723.

189 Song, H. J., Gittelsohn, J., Kim, M. Y., Suratkar, S., Sharma, S., & Anliker, J. (2010). Korean American storeowners' perceived barriers and motivators for implementing a corner store-based program. *Health Promotion Practice, 12*(3), 472-82.

190 Hanni, K. D., Garcia, E., Ellemberg, C., & Winkleby, M. (2009). Targeting the taqueria: Implementing healthy food options at Mexican American restaurants. *Health Promotion Practice. 10*(2 Suppl.), 91S-99S.

191 Min, P. G. (1996). *Caught in the middle: Korean communities in New York and Los Angeles.* Berkeley, CA: University of California Press.

192 Bailey, B. (2000). Communicative behavior and conflict between African-American customers and Korean immigrant retailers in Los Angeles. *Discourse and Society, 11*(1), 86-109.

193 Choi, R. B. (2012). *Notice of Public Hearing.* New York City Department of Health and Mental Hygiene. Retrieved from http://www.nyc.gov/html/doh/downloads/pdf/notice/2012/amend-food-establishments.pdf

194 Dumanovsky, T., Huang, C. Y., Nonas, C. A., Matte, T. D., Bassett, M. T., & Silver, L. D. (2011). Changes in energy content of lunchtime purchases from fast food restaurants after introduction of calorie labeling: Cross sectional customer surveys. *BMJ, 343,* d4464.

195 Dumanovsky, T., Huang, C. Y., Nonas, C. A., Matte, T. D., & Bassett, M. T., & Silver, L. D. (2011). Changes in energy content of lunchtime purchases from fast food restaurants after introduction of calorie labeling: Cross sectional customer surveys. *BMJ, 343*, d4464.

196 Elbel, B., Kersh, R., Brescoll, V. L., & Dixon, L. B. (2009). Calorie labeling and food choices: A first look at the effects on low-income people in New York City. *Health Affairs, 28*(6), w1110–w1121.

197 Gordon, C., & Hayes, R. (2012). Counting calories: Resident perspectives on calorie labeling in New York City. *Journal of Nutrition Education and Behavior, 44*(5), 454–58.

198 Cohn, E., Larson, E., Araujo, C., Sawyer, V., & Williams, O. (2012). Calorie postings in chain restaurants in a low-income urban neighborhood: Measuring practical utility and policy compliance. *Journal of Urban Health, 89*(4), 587–97.

199 Loewenstein, G. (2011). Confronting reality: Pitfalls of calorie posting. *American Journal of Clinical Nutrition, 93*(4), 679–80.

200 New York City Department of Health and Mental Hygiene. (n.d.). *Healthy heart: Avoid trans fat.* Retrieved from http://www.nyc.gov/html/doh/html/cardio/cardio-transfat.shtml

201 Angell, S. Y., Cobb, L. K., Curtis, C. J., Konty, K. J., & Silver, L. D. (2012). Change in trans fatty acid content of fast-food purchases associated with New York City's restaurant regulation: a pre-post study. *Annals of Internal Medicine, 157*(2), 81–86.

202 Andreyeva, T., Long, M. W., & Brownell, K. D. (2010). The impact of food prices on consumption: a systematic review of research on the price elasticity of demand for food. *American Journal of Public Health, 100*(2), 216–22.

203 Story, M., Kaphingst, K. M., Robinson-O'Brien, R., & Glanz, K. (2010). Creating healthy food and eating environments: Policy and environmental approaches. *Annual Reviews in Public Health, 29*, 253–72.

204 Drewnowski, A. (2012). The economics of food choice behavior: Why poverty and obesity are linked. *Nestle Nutrition Institution Workshop Series, 73*, 95–112.

205 Acharya, R. N., Patterson, P. M., Hill, E. P., Schmitz, T. G., & Bohm, E. (2006). An evaluation of the "TrEAT Yourself Well" restaurant nutrition campaign. *Health Education Behavior, 33*(3), 309–24.

206 Horgen, K. B., & Brownell, K. D. (2002). Comparison of price change and health message interventions in promoting healthy food choices. *Health Psychology, 21*(5), 505–12.

207 French, S. A., Story, M., Fulkerson, J. A., & Gerlach, A. F. (2003). Food environment in secondary schools: A la carte, vending machines, and food policies and practices. *American Journal of Public Health, 93*(7), 1161–67.

208 Gittelsohn, J., Suratkar, S., Song, H.-J., Sacher, S., Rajan, R., Rasooly, I. R., . . . Anliker, J. A. (2010). Process evaluation of Baltimore Healthy Stores: a pilot health intervention program with supermarkets and corner stores in Baltimore City. *Health Promotion Practice, 11*(5), 723–32.

209 Song, H.-J., Gittelsohn, J., Kim, M., Suratkar, S., Sharma, S., & Anliker, J. (2011). Korean American storeowners' perceived barriers and motivators for implementing a corner store-based program. *Health Promotion Practice, 12*(3), 472–82.

210 Molloy, M. (2002). Practice notes: Strategies in health education. Winner's Circle Healthy Dining program. *Health Education & Behavior, 29*, 406–8.

211 Economos, C. D., Folta, S. C., Goldberg, J., Hudson, D., Collins, J., Baker, Z., Lawson, E., & Nelson, M. (2009). A community-based restaurant initiative to increase availability of healthy menu options in Somerville, Massachusetts: Shape Up Somerville. *Preventing Chronic Disease, 6*(3), A102.

212 Healthy Howard. (2012). *Look for certified Healthy Restaurants.* Retrieved from http://www.healthyhowardmd.org/healthy-howard/healthy-restaurants

213 Gittelsohn, J., Lee, S. H., & Batorsky, B. (Under Review). A systematic review of community-based prepared food source interventions. *American Journal of Preventive Medicine.*

214 Freishtat, H. (2012). *Baltimore Food Policy Initiative/ Public Markets/ Get Fresh Lexington. Baltimore City Government.* Retrieved from baltimorecity.gov/Government/AgenciesDepartments/Planning/BaltimoreFoodPolicyInitiative/PublicMarkets/GetFreshLexington.aspx.

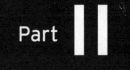

Global and Community Aspects of Undernutrition

Chapter 5

Public Health Nutrition Inequalities: The Global Context

Odilia I. Bermudez, PhD, MPH, LND

"A meaningful path out of poverty requires a strong economy that produces jobs and good wages; a government that can provide schools, hospitals, roads, and energy; and healthy, well-nourished children who are the future human capital that will fuel economic growth."

Courtesy of the World Bank. http://www.worldbank.org/mdgs/poverty_hunger.html

Learning Objectives

- Define health and nutrition inequalities.
- List social determinants that increase the risk of malnutrition in children and adults in developing countries.
- Identify major nutrition problems affecting the world population.
- Discuss public health efforts to alleviate health and nutrition inequalities.
- Identify characteristics of nutrition inequalities in low- and medium-income countries

Case Study: Malnutrition in Guatemala

Guatemala is a Central American nation with a diverse population of 14 million in 2013.[1] As a developing nation, Guatemala is experiencing the **nutrition transition** and **double burden of malnutrition**. One study in Guatemala examined malnutrition and its correlates.[2] Using data from the Guatemalan Living Standards Measurement Survey (LSMS), researchers determined that the prevalence of underweight children under 5 was 47%, 42% of mothers were overweight, and 17% of households had a stunted child and overweight mother (SCOM). Lower income was associated with underweight children, while higher income was more closely associated with overweight mothers.

Poor nutrition was more likely in rural areas, in households with lower maternal education, and among indigenous populations.

The prevalence of undernutrition is higher in Guatemala than in some Central American nations, such as Costa Rica, despite common historical and social development. For example, by 2009, the prevalence of chronic malnutrition (stunting) was estimated at 6% and 13% for Costa Rica and Guatemala, respectively, while the prevalence of underweight was 1% in Costa Rica and 48% in Guatemala **(Table 5-1)**. Furthermore, the prevalence of SCOM in Guatemala is the highest in Latin America.[3] Guatemalans, whose diets depend on sugars, beans, and maize, also experience anemia, regional iodine deficiencies, and

Table 5-1 Socioeconomic indicators for Costa Rica and Guatemala, 2009-2011

Indicator	Costa Rica	Guatemala
Total population, 2010	4,659,000	14,389,000
% of population urbanized, 2010	64	49
Adult literacy rate (%), 2005-2010	96	74
Life expectancy at birth (years), 2010	79	71
Maternal mortality (× 100,000 live births)	21	130
Infant mortality rate (× 1,000 live births)	15 (1990), 9 (2010)	56 (1990), 25 (2010)
Under-5 mortality (× 1,000 live births)	17 (1990), 10 (2010)	78 (1990), 32 (2010)
Improved sanitation (% households)	95 (urban), 96 (rural)	89 (urban), 81 (rural)

Data from UNICEF. (2013). *Information by country and region.* Retrieved March 4, 2013, from URL: http://www.unicef.org/infobycountry/latinamerica.html

vitamin A deficiency.[4] Although less severe than in Guatemala, nutrition concerns in Costa Rica include nutritional anemias, overweight in children and adults, hunger, and vitamin A deficiency.[5]

This chapter introduces malnutrition and its causes in Latin America and the world. It addresses the causes and consequences of malnutrition on a population level. The chapter describes the role of public health nutrition in improving global health, and the increasing focus on overnutrition.

Discussion Questions

- Which social determinants affect nutritional status and contribute to the dual burden of malnutrition in Guatemala?

- Why is assessment essential to improving nutritional status?

- Describe the major nutritional concerns in Guatemala.

- Which public health approaches might contribute to the observed disparities in nutritional status in various countries in Latin America despite commonalities in culture and history?

Introduction

Public health nutrition embraces those actions, activities, strategies, and interventions directed at the alleviation of nutritional imbalances, **food insecurity**, poverty, and nutrition-related health problems that affect population groups. The growing global focus of public health nutrition results from **globalization**, with patterns such as an increase in migration, globalization of the food supply, and better communication and information through technology.

Consequently, public health nutrition practitioners must be knowledgeable about global nutrition problems and responses from the international community when searching for strategies to alleviate those problems. In summary, public health nutrition reaches global proportions when those strategies and activities are directed to or involve the global community. This chapter presents an overview of the main nutrition and food security concerns in the global community and addresses social **determinants** modulating those nutrition problems.

To promote nutrition and **food security** globally, public health nutrition practitioners gain or reinforce core competencies that have been developed by the Association of Schools of Public Health (ASPH) as their master of public health (MPH) Core Competency Model.[6] The interdisciplinary/cross-cutting competencies in the model are especially relevant when working with diverse populations. Sociocultural norms, concepts about food systems, and the influence of traditional medicine, including the assigned value to specific food and food ingredients, are essential components of the lifestyles of populations in nations at any level of development. Examples of interdisciplinary/cross-cutting competencies are outlined in **Box 5-1**.

Concept of Global Public Health Nutrition

According to the World Health Organization (WHO), "Health is a state of complete physical, mental and social well-being and not merely the absence of sickness or disease."[7] This is an overarching concept applicable to both individuals and population groups across the lifespan, the health-disease continuum, and the stages of the **epidemiological transition**. Public health nutrition focuses

Box 5-1 Interdisciplinary/cross-cutting competencies required for MPH professionals, including those working across global boundaries

Competencies	Examples of Sub-competencies
Diversity and Culture	Describe the roles of history, power, privilege, and structural inequality in producing health disparities.
	Use the basic concepts and skills involved in culturally appropriate community engagement and empowerment with diverse communities.
	Develop public health programs and strategies responsive to the diverse cultural values and traditions of the communities being served.
Leadership	Describe alternative strategies for collaboration and partnership among organizations, focused on public health goals.
	Apply social justice and human rights principles when addressing community needs.
	Develop strategies to motivate others for collaborative problem solving, decision making, and evaluation.
Public Health Biology	Explain the role of biology in the ecological model of population-based health.
	Explain how genetics and genomics affect disease processes and public health policy and practice.
	Apply evidence-based biological and molecular concepts to inform public health laws, policies, and regulations.
Professionalism	Apply basic principles of ethical analysis (e.g., the Public Health Code of Ethics, human rights framework, and other moral theories) to issues of public health practice and policy.
	Apply evidence-based principles and the scientific knowledge base to critical evaluation and decision making in public health.
	Apply the core functions of assessment, policy development, and assurance in the analysis of public health problems and their solutions.
Program Planning	Describe how social, behavioral, environmental, and biological factors contribute to specific individual and community health outcomes.
	Differentiate among goals, measurable objectives, related activities, and expected outcomes for a public health program.
	Differentiate between qualitative and quantitative evaluation methods in relation to their strengths, limitations, and appropriate uses, and emphases on reliability and validity.
Systems Thinking	Explain how the contexts of gender, race, poverty, history, migration, and culture are important in the design of interventions within public health systems.
	Analyze the effects of political, social, and economic policies on public health systems at the local, state, national, and international levels.
	Analyze the impact of global trends and interdependencies on public health–related problems and systems.

Data from the Association of Schools of Public Health. (2012). *MPH Core Competency Model*. http://www.asph.org/publication/MPH_Core_Competency_Model/index.html. Accessed September 4, 2013.

Box 5-2 Key descriptors of public health nutrition

- Applies public health principles
- Is population-based
- Has global dimensions*
- Focuses on food and nutrition systems
- Focuses on health and nutrition promotion
- Promotes primary prevention
- Focuses on wellness maintenance
- Draws from many disciplines*
- Focuses on education
- Focuses on economic factors
- Promotes environmental behavior change

*Global-related descriptor added by the author

Data from Hughes, R. (2003). Definitions for public health nutrition: a developing consensus. *Pub Hlth Nutr*, Sep;6(6), 615-20.

Box 5-3 Examples of social determinants of nutrition and food security

- Availability of healthy and nutritious food from locally produced or purchased products
- Availability of healthy and nutritious food at local markets and stores
- Adequate education level of the population, including nutritional education
- Access and utilization of health services
- Access to job opportunities
- Availability of adequate living conditions, including proper sanitation conditions
- Exposure to a healthy environment
- Access to communication and information technology
- Adequate social support and social interactions
- Opportunities for participation in community organization and development

---

on health protection, disease prevention, and well-being in population groups. Global public health nutrition gives priority to those most affected by malnutrition, food insecurity, poverty, and social vulnerability. Some of the key descriptors that need to be present in a definition of public health nutrition were identified and reported by Hughes,[8] and used for the list of descriptors of Global Public Health Nutrition as seen in **Box 5-2**.

Social Determinants of Malnutrition and Food Insecurity

Social determinants of food and nutrition security are those conditions that affect the ability of societies and individuals to prevent **malnutrition** and food insecurity and promote health. Those social determinants include the conditions in which people are born, grow, live, work, and age (**Box 5-3**). The health, education, agriculture, housing, and environmental sectors impact social determinants, which are constantly modified by political, social, and economic forces.[9]

When the social determinants of nutrition and food security are unfavorable, food systems are limited or constrained, leading to poorer nutritional status with problems such as overnutrition, nutrient deficiencies, hunger,

nutrition-related chronic diseases, and food insecurity. Because these situations are widespread in developing nations, global public health must focus on the socioeconomic and cultural determinants of poor nutrition and health, with emphasis on the poorest, most neglected, and most vulnerable groups. The dimensions and complexities of the current public health nutrition problems and their social determinants demand the coordinated efforts of the global community of practitioners, scientists, and other stakeholders in setting the global public health nutrition agenda.

Nutrition and Food Inequalities

Inequalities in nutrition status or in food security exist in the presence of unfair or discriminatory differences between populations or members of a particular ethnic or racial group. Those differences are the manifestation of the unequal distribution of resources or of environmental, social, and economic conditions that influence the risk of those groups to becoming sick, malnourished, food insecure, poor, and with limited productivity.

Disparities affecting children under 5 years of age are more concerning because of their far-reaching consequences. Malnourishment impairs children's capacities to grow

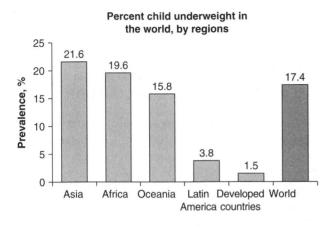

Figure 5-1 Child underweight (%) among children under 5 y, in the world and by regions

Data from the WHO. (2013). Global InfoBase: Global Comparable Estimates and Maps. Retrieved July 8, 2011, from URL: https://apps.who.int/infobase/

and develop normally, and interferes with their ability to become fully productive members of their countries. The United Nations Standing Committee on Nutrition (UNSCN) reported that, by the year 2007, the overall prevalence of child underweight was present in about 17% of the global population of children under 5 years of age;[10] however, a wide gap existed by region (**Figure 5-1**). The prevalence in Asian and African nations was 22% and 20%, respectively, as compared with 1.5% for developed countries. Among the most prevalent nutrient deficiencies is deficiency of vitamin A, whose essential roles include promoting vision and a healthy immune system. The worldwide prevalence of **hypovitaminosis A** is 30%, with a large difference between 40% for South Central Asia and Central and West Africa and 10% in South and Central America.[11]

Major Global Public Health Nutrition Problems Affecting the World Population

In a position paper, the Academy of Nutrition and Dietetics recognized the universal right to "safe, nutritious and culturally appropriate food" and identified global "nutrition insecurities" (**Figure 5-2**).[12] Inadequate sanitation is the most significant nutrition insecurity worldwide, affecting 36% of the population. Stunting and underweight in children under 5 years of age each affect 2–3% of the global population, and cause 25% and 16% of stunting and underweight, respectively, in children under 5.[13]

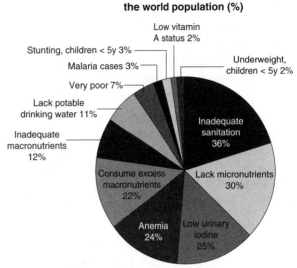

Figure 5-2 Proportion of the world's population, or 7 billion people, affected by nutrition insecurity problems

Data from: Nordin, S. M., Boyle, M., & Kemmer, T. M. (2013). Position of the Academy of Nutrition and Dietetics: Nutrition security in developing nations: Sustainable food, water, and health. *Journal of the Academy of Nutrition and Dietetics, 113*(4), 581-595.

Undernutrition is directly related to poverty, hunger, and infectious diseases among children under 5 years of age, and more so among those under 2 years. The Mother and Child Nutrition Initiative notes that "malnutrition kills 4 million children every year . . . one child every 4 seconds."[14] This is in comparison to a total of 10 million annual child deaths, with the vast majority in developing nations.[15] Mortality of children under 5 (U5MR) is affected by nutritional status and by sanitation conditions. Additional factors that modify U5MR are in **Box 5-4**.

> **Box 5-4** Factors affecting mortality in children under 5
>
> - Nutritional status and the health knowledge of mothers
> - Level of immunization and oral rehydration therapy
> - Availability of maternal and child health services (including prenatal care)
> - Income and food availability in the family
> - Availability of safe drinking water and basic sanitation
> - Overall safety of the child's environment

Infant mortality, which is often used as an overall indicator of a nation's health status, is affected by the nutritional status of both mother and child. Infant mortality is lower in the presence of higher quality of life, higher maternal education, improved perinatal care, better control of communicable diseases, and better nutrition interventions with emphasis on breastfeeding-related interventions.[16]

Inadequate quality and quantity of food continue to cause hunger, food insecurity, and nutrient deficiencies and their health consequences in billions of people. Simultaneously, shifts in the food supply and dietary patterns have led to increases in nutrition-related noncommunicable diseases, including obesity, type 2 diabetes, and cardiovascular disease. This section addresses those two categories of nutritional concerns.

About Malnutrition Problems Associated with Food Deprivation

Neglected and poor populations are often affected with specific nutritional diseases associated with low dietary intakes of specific micronutrients (**Box 5-5**), leading to "**hidden hunger**." Conditions such as hunger, iodine deficiency, iron-deficiency anemia, folate deficiency, and vitamin A deficiency are significant in the world. For example, hypovitaminosis A, while rare in industrialized nations, affects

Box 5-5 Major nutrition problems associated with lack of specific nutrients

Health Condition/ Disease	Nutrient Deficiency	Affected Groups
Hunger	Temporal or prolonged absence of food, creating severe food insecurity. Hunger exists when dietary energy (calorie) intake is inadequate for sustaining life and regular activities.	Poor, uneducated populations are at higher risk for hunger. Though present worldwide, hunger is most prevalent in certain regions of Southeast Asia and Africa.
Undernutrition	Lack of healthy, sufficient, and varied foods	Mother and child groups are most affected. Poverty, lack of healthy food, inadequate health care, and frequent illnesses are also risk factors for undernutrition.
Iron-deficiency anemia	Iron	Iron deficiency is the most common nutrient deficiency worldwide, affecting young children and women of childbearing age most.
Hypovitaminosis A	Vitamin A	Highly prevalent in the developing world, children with higher risk for deficiency are those with measles, respiratory infections, diarrhea, and other severe infectious diseases. Lack of vitamin A is the main cause of blindness in developing nations.
Neural tube defects	Folate	Babies born to women with low folate levels due to inadequate intake from food and supplements have higher risks of neural tube defects, such as spina bifida. Folic acid supplementation during pregnancy can reduce the prevalence of neural tube defects.
Goiter	Iodine	Iodine deficiency is likely in populations using non-iodized salt and/or living in regions where agricultural land is depleted of iodine. Goiter is more prevalent in adolescents, particularly girls.

about 5 million preschool-aged children and increases the risk of blindness and death due to infectious diseases.

Public Health Core Competency 1: Analytical/Assessment Skills 1: Identifies the health status of populations and their related determinants of health and illness

Reproduced from Council on Linkages Between Academia and Public Health Practice. 2010 May. Core Competencies for Public Health Professionals. Washington, DC: Public Health Foundation. http://www .phf.org/resourcestools/Documents/Core_Competencies_for_Public _Health_Professionals_2010May.pdf. Accessed August 13, 2013. This source is used for all Public Health Core Competencies in this chapter.

The Nutrition Transition and Its Effects on Diet

Globalization of the food supply and technological advances in information and communications have produced dramatic changes in the **food environment** and in behaviors related to nutrition and health. The result is an escalation of rates of nutritional origin diseases such as obesity and noncommunicable diseases, particularly diabetes, cardiovascular disease, and certain forms of cancer. The study of these diseases and their determinants is an active field in global public health nutrition.

The global **nutrition transition** has been characterized by adverse changes in populations' eating habits. Traditional diets were mostly plant-based and included high **nutrient-dense** foods, such as cereals, vegetables, and fruits.[17,18] More processed, less nutritious foods have frequently replaced these healthier choices (**Box 5-6**). This has led to the rise of nutrition-related chronic diseases.

These dietary changes have been accompanied by dramatic reduction in physical activity levels, with the adoption of sedentary lifestyles rather than more active traditional lifestyles. Factors associated with those changes in physical activity patterns include increased access to public or private transportation, **urbanization**, and the associated reduction in occupational physical activity, mechanization, and several determinants of personal and structural environments in which the new Central American societies operate.

The Worldwide Obesity Epidemic

While the prevalence of overweight and obesity is increasing worldwide, developing nations often must contend with the **double burden of malnutrition**, in which childhood undernutrition and adult overweight or obesity coexist in the same household.[19,20] Tobacco use, high blood pressure, and overweight and obesity are the three main risk factors for premature deaths and disability in the developed world.[21] The consequences of obesity in the developing world are also concerning for national governments and international organizations. Adult obesity is more common in the world than childhood undernutrition.[22] In 2002, about 200 million children were overweight or obese, plus more than a billion adults were either overweight or obese.[23] At that time, 20 nations worldwide had an average **body mass index** (BMI) greater than or equal to 30 among their female adult populations (**Figure 5-3**).

Box 5-6 Modern diets compared to traditional diets

Traditional Diets	Modern Diets
• High nutritional quality	• Low nutritional quality
• Adequate in energy intakes and nutrient density	• High energy intake and low nutrient density
• Low in commercially processed foods	• High in commercially processed foods
• High in whole grains and cereals	• High in grains and refined grains
• High consumption of fruits and vegetables	• Low consumption of fruits and vegetables
• Consumption of fresh fruit and juices	• High consumption of sweetened soft drinks
• Low consumption of salt and high-sodium products	• High consumption of salt and high-sodium products
• Low intake of saturated fats and oils	• High intake of saturated fats and oils
• No use of trans fatty acids	• High intake of trans fatty acids

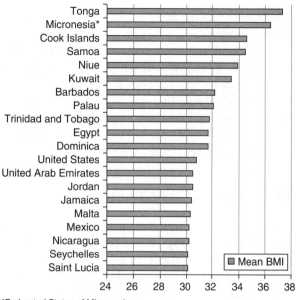

Countries with the highest mean BMI among their women populations

*Federated States of Micronesia

Figure 5-3　Countries with an average BMI > 30.0 in their female populations > 30 years

Data from the WHO. (2013). Global InfoBase: Global Comparable Estimates and Maps. Retrieved July 8, 2011, from URL: https://apps.who.int/infobase/

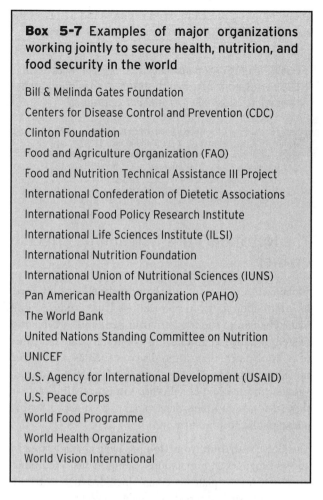

Box 5-7 Examples of major organizations working jointly to secure health, nutrition, and food security in the world

Bill & Melinda Gates Foundation

Centers for Disease Control and Prevention (CDC)

Clinton Foundation

Food and Agriculture Organization (FAO)

Food and Nutrition Technical Assistance III Project

International Confederation of Dietetic Associations

International Food Policy Research Institute

International Life Sciences Institute (ILSI)

International Nutrition Foundation

International Union of Nutritional Sciences (IUNS)

Pan American Health Organization (PAHO)

The World Bank

United Nations Standing Committee on Nutrition

UNICEF

U.S. Agency for International Development (USAID)

U.S. Peace Corps

World Food Programme

World Health Organization

World Vision International

Major Organizations and Initiatives Working to Improve Nutrition and Food Security in the World

The severity and magnitude of the nutrition and food security problems affecting the world population demands joint efforts and resources to work in coordination and with common goals. Several international organizations, initiatives, and programs are currently working on correcting the global public health nutrition inequalities present in the world (**Box 5-7**).

The Millennium Development Goals

All United Nations (UN) members have agreed to work toward achieving eight goals, known as the Millennium Development Goals (MDG), by 2015.[24] The MDGs are the product of the 2000 Millennium Summit at the UN world headquarters in New York. World leaders promised to combat poverty, hunger, illiteracy, gender discrimination, childhood death, maternal death, diseases, and environmental degradation and to develop global partnerships (**Box 5-8**).

Other Major Global Food and Nutrition Initiatives

Increased life expectancy in most nations is evidence of the improved public health status of the global community; however, solutions and new strategies are still needed to address the significant nutrition-related problems that remain. International and regional organizations and nongovernmental organizations have traditionally focused on long-existing problems such as infectious diseases, hunger, micronutrient deficiencies, and infant mortality. Structural changes in the population and the epidemiological and nutrition transitions are linked to emergent new health and nutrition problems, including adult and childhood obesity, type 2 diabetes, cardiovascular disease, and age-related diseases.

Box 5-8 Selected targets and progress reports of the Millennium Development Goals

MDGs	Targets	Progress Report
Goal 1: Eradicate extreme poverty and hunger	1.C: Halve, between 1990 and 2015, the proportion of people who suffer from hunger.	- Some progress, but one in five children under 5 years is underweight. - Rural children are more likely to be underweight.
Goal 2: Achieve universal primary education	2.A: Ensure that, by 2015, children everywhere, boys and girls alike, will be able to complete a full course of primary schooling.	- In developing nations, enrollment in primary education went from 82% in 1999 to 90% in 2010. - Demand for secondary education is growing.
Goal 3: Promote gender equality and empower women	3.A: Eliminate gender disparity in primary and secondary education, preferably by 2005, and in all levels of education no later than 2015.	- The world achieved gender parity in primary and secondary education, but still some regions are behind. - "Violence against women continues to undermine efforts to reach all goals."
Goal 4: Reduce child mortality (under-5 mortality rate/U5MR)	4.A: Reduce U5MR by two-thirds between 1990 and 2015.	- Child mortality is declining. - Increasing proportion of child deaths are in sub-Saharan Africa. - Children born into poverty are almost twice as likely to die before the age of 5 as those from wealthier families.
Goal 4: Reduce child mortality (U5MR)	4.A: Reduce U5MR by two-thirds between 1990 and 2015.	- Childhood mortality is declining. - An increasing proportion of child deaths is in sub-Saharan Africa. - Children born into poverty are almost twice as likely to die before the age of 5 as those from wealthier families.
Goal 5: Improve maternal health	5.A: Reduce by three-quarters the maternal mortality ratio (MMR).	- Since 1990, MMR declined by 47%. - MMR in developing regions is still 15 times higher than in industrialized regions.
Goal 6: Combat HIV/AIDS, malaria, and other diseases	6.A: Have halted by 2015 and begun to reverse the spread of HIV/AIDS.	- More people than ever are living with HIV due to fewer AIDS-related deaths and the continued large number of new infections. - Comprehensive knowledge of HIV transmission remains low among young people, along with condom use.
Goal 7: Ensure environmental sustainability	7.C: Halve, by 2015, the proportion of the population without sustainable access to safe drinking water and basic sanitation.	- Target of halving the proportion of people without access to improved sources of water was met in 2010. - Access to improved sanitation facilities in developing nations increased from 36% in 1990 to 56% in 2010. - 2.5 billion individuals in developing countries still lack access to improved sanitation facilities.
Goal 8: Develop a global partnership for development	8.B: Address the special needs of least developed countries.	- Debt relief initiatives have reduced the external debt of heavily indebted poor countries. - Twenty developing countries remain at high risk of debt distress.

Reproduced from the United Nations. (n.d.). 2015 Millennium Development Goals. Retrieved from http://www.un.org/millenniumgoals/. Accessed August 13, 2013. This source is used for all Millennium Development Goals in this chapter.

Box 5-9 Examples of other major global food and nutrition initiatives

Organization	Initiatives	Description
UN Standing Committee on Nutrition (UNSCN), U.S. Government, over 20 other countries, and over 100 agencies and organizations	Scaling Up Nutrition (SUN)	Focuses on the critical 1,000-day window between conception and a child's second birthday. Supports national efforts to improve diets, pregnancy nutrition. and breastfeeding.
World Food Programme (WFP)	Global Response to High Food Prices: The Comprehensive Framework for Action	Establishes mechanisms to increase the availability of adequate food products for the maternal and child group and for other vulnerable groups.
U.S. Government	Feed the Future	A global hunger and food security initiative focused on agricultural growth with the goal of promoting health and reducing poverty.
World Health Organization (WHO)	Global Strategy on Diet, Physical Activity and Health	Issues recommendations for countries, organizations, global partners focused on the promotion of healthy diets and regular physical activity for the prevention of noncommunicable diseases.

International organizations and national governments from several countries are engaged in addressing these problems (**Box 5-9**).

Conclusion

Major accomplishments of public health and nutrition programs include reductions in infection and malnutrition in children under 5 years of age and a slower rate of progression of unprecedented pandemics like obesity, type 2 diabetes, and hypertension that are highly prevalent across the world. However, undernutrition and overnutrition persist, and demonstrate gross inequalities, often linked to disparities in social determinants. Continued and improved public health support is necessary to address malnutrition and inequalities, and public health nutrition professionals have important roles in and opportunities to contribute to the correction of those inequalities.

References

1 Information retrieved from https://www.cia.gov/library/publications/the-world-factbook/geos/gt.html

2 Lee, J., Houser, R. F., Must, A., Palma de Fulladolsa, P., & Bermudez, O. I. (2012). Socioeconomic disparities and the familial coexistence of child stunting and maternal overweight in Guatemala. *Economics and Human Biology, 10,* 232-41.

3 Lee, J., Houser, R. F., Must, A., Palma de Fulladolsa, P., & Bermudez, O. I. (2012). Socioeconomic disparities and the familial coexistence of child stunting and maternal overweight in Guatemala. *Economics and Human Biology, 10,* 232-41.

4 Food and Agricultural Organization. (n.d.). *Nutrition country profiles: Guatemala.* Retrieved from http://www.fao.org/ag/agn/nutrition/gtm_en.stm

5 Chen, L. T., & Jimenez, L. A. E. S. (1999). FAO: Perfiles nutricionales por paises: Costa Rica. Retrieved from the Food and Agricultural Organization website, ftp://ftp.fao.org/ag/agn/nutrition/ncp/crimap.pdf

6 Association of Schools of Public Health. (2012). *MPH Core Competency Model.* Retrieved from http://www.asph.org/document.cfm?page=851

7 World Health Organization. (n.d.). *WHO definition of health*. Retrieved from http://www.who.int/about/definition/en/print.html

8 Hughes, R. (2003). Definitions for public health nutrition: A developing consensus. *Public Health Nutrition, 6*(6), 615-20.

9 World Health Organization, Commission on Social Determinants of Health. (2008). *Closing the gap in a generation: Health equity through action on the social determinants of health*. Geneva: World Health Organization. Retrieved from http://www.who.int/social_determinants/thecommission/finalreport/en/index.html

10 United Nations Standing Committee on Nutrition. (2010). *Sixth report on the world nutrition situation* (p. 47). Geneva: UNSCN.

11 United Nations Standing Committee on Nutrition. (2010). *Sixth report on the world nutrition situation* (p. 48). Geneva: UNSCN.

12 Nordin, S. M., Boyle, M., & Kemmer, T. M., for the Academy of Nutrition and Dietetics. (2013). Position of the Academy of Nutrition and Dietetics: Nutrition security in developing nations: Sustainable food, water, and health. *Journal of the Academy of Nutrition and Dietetics, 113*(4), 581-95.

13 Nordin, S. M., Boyle, M., & Kemmer, T. M., for the Academy of Nutrition and Dietetics. (2013). Position of the Academy of Nutrition and Dietetics: Nutrition security in developing nations: Sustainable food, water, and health. *Journal of the Academy of Nutrition and Dietetics, 113*(4), 584.

14 Mother and Child Nutrition Initiative. (2013). Malnutrition. Retrieved from http://motherchildnutrition.org/index.html#.UWMgdf7D-Cg

15 UNICEF. (2008). Child survival. In *State of the world's children 2008* (p. 2). New York: UNICEF. Retrieved from http://www.unicef.org/sowc08/docs/sowc08.pdf

16 UNICEF. (2008). Child survival. In *State of the world's children 2008* (pp. 1-3). New York: UNICEF. Retrieved from http://www.unicef.org/sowc08/docs/sowc08.pdf

17 Bermudez, O., & Tucker, K. L. (2003). Trends in dietary patterns of Latin American populations. *Cadernos de Saúde Pública. 19*(Suppl. 1), S87-S99.

18 Bermudez, O. I. , Hernandez, L. M., Mazariegos, M., & Solomons, N. S. (2008). Secular trends in food patterns of Guatemalan consumers: New foods for old. *Food and Nutrition Bulletin, 29*(4), 278-87.

19 Lee, J., Houser, R. F., Must, A., Fulladolsa, P. P., & Bermudez, O. I. (2012). Socioeconomic disparities and the familial coexistence of child stunting and maternal overweight in Guatemala. *Economics and Human Biology, 10*(3): 232-41. doi:10.1016/j.ehb.2011.08.002

20 Lee, J., Houser, R. F., Must, A., de Fulladolsa, P. P., & Bermudez, O. I. (2010). Disentangling nutritional factors and household characteristics related to child stunting and maternal overweight in Guatemala. *Economics and Human Biology, 8*(2), 188-96.

21 World Health Organization. (2006). *Global health risks: Mortality and burden of disease attributable to selected major risks*. Retrieved from http://www.who.int/healthinfo/global_burden_disease/GlobalHealthRisks_report_full.pdf

22 International Association for the Study of Obesity. (2010). *Obesity: Understanding and challenging the global epidemic*. Retrieved from http://www.iaso.org/site_media/uploads/IASO_Summary_ Report_2009.pdf

23 International Obesity Taskforce. (2011). *The global epidemic*. Retrieved from http://www.iaso.org/iotf/obesity/obesitytheglobalepidemic

24 UN Millennium Development Goals. (n.d.). Retrieved from http://www.un.org/millenniumgoals

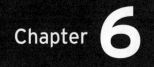

Chapter 6

Formative Research Approaches to Develop Undernutrition Interventions

Stephen Kodish, MS

"Human beings are quite simple. The apparent complexity of our behavior over time is largely a reflection of the complexity of the environment in which we find ourselves."–Herbert Simon

Learning Objectives

- Describe the global burden of undernutrition and current strategies to address it.
- Highlight the Millennium Development Goals (MDGs) relating to maternal and child undernutrition.
- Define formative research and highlight its value in public health nutrition programs to address undernutrition.
- Describe the complexities and considerations that surround the introduction of specialized food commodities.
- Consider the appropriateness of using specialized food commodities when addressing undernutrition.
- Provide an overview of research methods that are appropriate for nutrition-formative research and important to program design.

Case Study: Lessons Learned from a Nutrition Intervention at Kakuma Refugee Camp, Kenya

Kakuma Refugee Camp is near the border town of Lochichokio in the Turkana District of northwest Kenya, 30 miles from South Sudan. It was established in August 1992 for refugees fleeing the Sudanese civil war and decades of civil strife in eastern and central Africa. With refugees from Somalia, Sudan, and Ethiopia, and to a lesser extent from the Congo, Uganda, Rwanda, Eritrea, Namibia, and Zimbabwe,[1] Kakuma is a complex setting with numerous health challenges.

Although refugee populations receive food aid during emergencies and other protracted situations, malnutrition and related health problems remain widespread in refugee camps due to inadequate intake and nutrient deficiencies. Malnutrition impacts children especially because of their dependency on adults and their susceptibility to disease.[2] Malnutrition rates in refugee situations of sub-Saharan Africa are among the highest in the world.[3]

At Kakuma, prevalence of iron-deficiency **anemia** (IDA) in 2007 was 86% in children under 5 years, 80% among adolescent girls, and 41% among women of reproductive age.[4] Consequences of IDA include increased risk of maternal and child mortality as well as impaired cognitive function and physical growth and development among children.[5] Vitamin A deficiency is common among malnourished individuals, and consequences can include anemia, increased mortality risk, and xerophthalmia, which is the leading cause of blindness in children throughout the world.[6] Various strategies have been employed in refugee camps to ameliorate these health burdens **(Figure 6-1)**.

Dietary Diversification

Dietary diversification is a pragmatically difficult strategy in remote, arid locations such as Kakuma. Nevertheless, diversification of food and access to local markets are essential to the provision of **micronutrients** to vulnerable populations.[7] Local fresh foods provide refugees or internally displaced persons (IDP) with carotene, iron, vitamin C, thiamin, trace elements, and phytonutrients.[8] Remote locations like Kakuma, unreliable local markets, and high food costs are challenges to dietary diversification. In Kakuma, which has 70,000 inhabitants, purchasing sufficient quantities of food for general distribution is too expensive. A project using this strategy in Somalia in 1989 was too expensive and logistically difficult; it was discontinued not long after it started.[9]

Food Fortification

Supplementary feeding programs that provide fortified cereal–legume blends can be more feasible. Foods in such programs can be precooked to minimize micronutrient losses during preparation. Other benefits are that the nutrients are in one source, and that the fortified commodity can be stored as a contingency stock and mobilized when needed. In 1998, Oxfam/United Nations High Commissioner for Refugees (UNHCR) found no major problems with either the use or acceptability of blended foods at the household level,[10] although some technical and operational issues regarding quality control, acceptance of such products, and timely supply of locally produced food products have emerged since. For these reasons, food fortification has been criticized as a short-term strategy.

Fortification of cereals is a convenient way of preventing deficiency diseases, but it reduces shelf life of food and requires monitoring of quality control.[11] Micronutrient losses can occur during storage, transport, and preparation. Multiple nations, however, especially in Latin America and Asia, employ successful food fortification programs.[12,13]

Despite fortified foods distribution as part of the food ration at Kakuma, IDA rates among refugees there remained high in 2008,[14] prompting a **micronutrient powder (MNP)** program.

Nutrition Intervention in Kakuma Refugee Camp

The MNPs distributed at Kakuma were one-gram sachets to be added to meals just before eating. The sachets were formulated to be particularly beneficial for young children and pregnant and lactating women. MNPs, as part of **home food fortification**, are generally inexpensive to produce and are lightweight for commodity transportation and distribution.[15] Home fortification with MNP allows children aged 6 to 59 months to get two recommended nutrient intakes (RNIs) per week, which is the World Health Organization/UNICEF/World Food Programme recommendation for emergency settings where fortified foods are distributed, as at Kakuma.[16] There, corn-soy blend plus (CSB+), or fortified corn soy, was offered with the normal food ration. Packets of MixMe™—the MNP brand used in the initiative—had been distributed at no cost since 2008 by the United Nations World Food Programme (WFP), as part of its partnership with DSM Nutritional Products. The entire camp population received once-a-day MNP sachets through bimonthly distribution linked to normal food aid distribution.

Uptake of MNP at the distribution points was 99% at program launch in January 2009, but dropped 10% each month before reaching a low of 30% within seven months. Intensified communication activities led to a plateau between 40% and 48%, but again fell to 30% by year's end.[17] Initially, such low uptake was surprising given that the product was provided free and was intended to address IDA, which program staff considered an important health concern.

A subsequent qualitative assessment unveiled the complexities associated with improving the nutritional status of a population utilizing a specialized food commodity. The low uptake can largely be explained proximally by confusion and distrust among the beneficiary population related to the foreign food product. These feelings resulted from interrelated distal and proximal factors.[18] A fundamental determinant of low MNP acceptability was a very limited **formative research** phase. Behavior change communication and social marketing efforts did not have a foundation from which an acceptable and appropriate behavior-change intervention could be informed by and developed specifically for the target population. The result was a lack of impact on nutritional status of the targeted beneficiaries.[19]

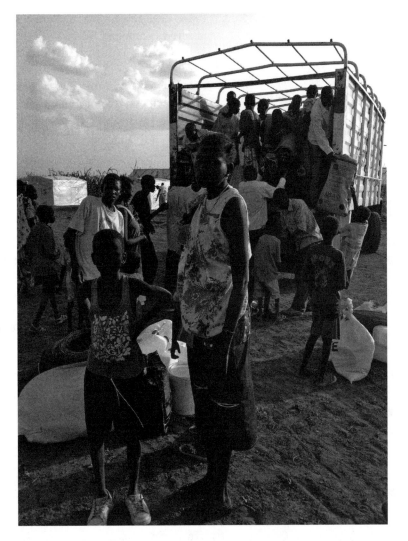

Figure 6-1 Kakuma Refugee Camp in Kenya

Courtesy of EC/ECHO Anna Chudolinska.

Discussion Questions

- Why are refugee populations at such high risk for malnutrition?
- What are the most common nutritional concerns among refugee populations, and what are their consequences?
- Which public health nutrition strategies can reduce the burden of malnutrition among vulnerable populations?
- Based on the experience at Kakuma Refugee Camp, what considerations should be made when introducing specialized food commodities as part of nutrition programming?

Introduction

Many lessons related to nutrition programming were learned from the complexities and challenges faced by the MNP program at Kakuma Refugee Camp. Consequently, stakeholders around the globe increasingly view detailed, multistage formative research and careful product introduction as essential to successful behavior-change interventions that use specialized food commodities to improve the nutritional status of vulnerable populations. This chapter explores the global burden of undernutrition and the role of formative research in developing programs to address undernutrition.

The Global Burden of Undernutrition

Poverty and food insecurity go hand in hand. Together, they restrict availability of and access to nutritious diets, which include **complete protein**, adequate micronutrient content and bioavailability, essential fatty acids, and low antinutrient content.[20] Low-quality diets lead to substantial burdens of preventable nutrition-related morbidity and mortality globally.

Undernutrition in Under-5 Children

Maternal and child undernutrition remains commonplace in low-income and middle-income countries. It is the underlying cause of 3.5 million deaths and blamed for 35% of the disease burden in children under age 5 and 11% of total global disability-adjusted life years (DALYs). Globally, among children under 5, the number of deaths and DALYs ascribed to chronic malnutrition (low height-for-age), severe acute malnutrition (low weight-for-height), and intrauterine growth restriction compose the largest percentage of any risk factor in this age group.[21] Regionally, in sub-Saharan Africa and south-central Asia, 178 million children under 5 are **stunted**, and an additional 55 million are **wasted**. Of this group, 19 million have severe wasting or severe acute malnutrition (SAM).[22]

Multilevel Approaches to Reduce Malnutrition

With short- and long-term population-level consequences, the burden of undernutrition results from synergy among basic, underlying, and immediate factors (**Figure 6-2**).[23] Accordingly, the international community employs numerous intervention strategies at various levels. Global nutrition efforts have significant political willpower and influence due to the **Millennium Development Goals**

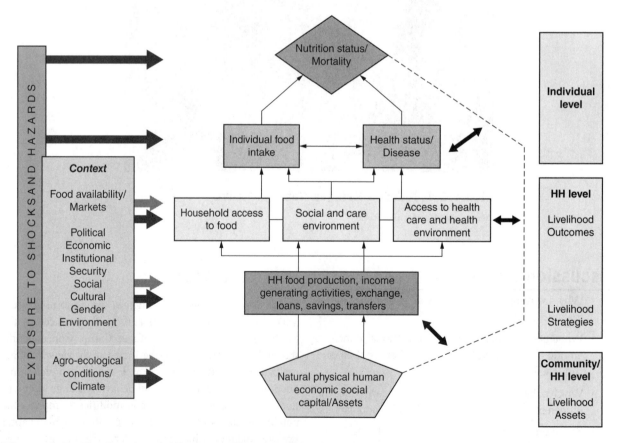

Figure 6-2 Food and nutrition security conceptual framework

Reproduced from the World Food Programme. *Emergency Food Security Assessment Handbook*, Second Edition. http://home.wfp.org/stellent/groups/public/documents /manual_guide_proced/wfp203246.pdf. Accessed September 6, 2013.

(MDGs), set to expire in 2015. Addressing undernutrition is necessary for nations to achieve the MDGs.

> *Millennium Development Goal 1: Eradicate Extreme Poverty and Hunger. Target 1. A: Halve, between 1990 and 2015, the proportion of people who suffer from hunger*
>
> Reproduced from the United Nations. (n.d.). 2015 Millennium Development Goals. Retrieved from http://www.un.org/millenniumgoals/. Accessed August 13, 2013. This source is used for all Millennium Development Goals in this chapter.

> *Millennium Development Goal 4: Reduce Child Mortality. Target 4. A: Reduce by two-thirds, between 1990 and 2015, the under-five mortality rate*

> *Millennium Development Goal 5: Improve Maternal Health Target 5. A: Reduce by three-quarters, between 1990 and 2015, the maternal mortality ratio*

> *Millennium Development Goal 6: Combat HIV/AIDS, Malaria and Other Diseases. Target 6. A: Have halted by 2015 and begun to reverse the spread of HIV/AIDS*

Economic Inequity

Some argue that addressing upstream factors, near the base of the United Nations Children's Emergency Fund (UNICEF) conceptual framework (Figure 6-2), could significantly reduce undernutrition, and thus should be the priority.[24] For example, in most countries, twice as many poor children as wealthier children suffer from chronic malnutrition. However, reversing systemic problems that have resulted from neo-liberal economic policies can be difficult or impossible.[25]

Behavior Change

Behavior-change interventions may have the potential to address maternal and child undernutrition.[26] Major reductions in undernutrition can be made more immediately through programmatic health and nutrition interventions[27] that address factors more proximal to nutritional status/mortality in the framework. These include dietary intake or health status. Behavior-change interventions could improve acute and chronic malnutrition among populations by reducing rates of stunting, micronutrient deficiencies, and child deaths.[28]

Examples of behavior-change interventions to address maternal and child undernutrition include variations of strategies to promote **exclusive breastfeeding, complementary feeding**, provision of food supplements, micronutrient interventions, supportive nutrition strategies (such as voucher systems), and large-scale nutrition programs.

Critical Window of Opportunity

Stunting is challenging or impossible to reverse after 36 months of age. Attention therefore must be on nutrition interventions during pregnancy and through 36 months.[29] Conception to 24 months is a critical "window of opportunity" to improve a child's health status.[30,31] The window represents the peak incidence of growth faltering, micronutrient deficiencies, and infectious diseases in low-income countries.[32] After 24 months, undernutrition can cause irreversible damage for future development toward adulthood.[33] Beyond 36 months, interventions might not reduce stunting, and can even have detrimental effects due to the association between rapid weight gain later in childhood and adverse long-term outcomes.[34] While there is currently no panacea to solve the global problem of undernutrition, scientific evidence is mounting to support interventions to effectively reduce stunting among other forms of undernutrition between conception and 24 months.

Global Efforts to Address Undernutrition

Since the early 1960s, the WFP and its partners, such as UNICEF, have provided food aid in emergency situations, including those resulting from droughts, floods, and famines. One of the seven guiding principles of WFP is to offer "a general food basket based on providing 2,100 kcal per person per day."[35] This addresses Article 25 of the Universal Declaration of Human Rights: "Everyone has the right to a standard of living adequate for the health and well-being of himself and of his family, including food."[36] However, evidence is mounting that simply providing more energy, or calories, from increased quantity of food cannot solve global chronic undernutrition.

In the mid-1980s, vitamin A, iron, and zinc were among the micronutrients identified as being "growth-limiting" and necessary for fighting infections.[37,38] The international nutrition community's focus shifted from diet quantity to diet quality. Although inadequate energy intake persists in many settings, suboptimal intakes of several micronutrients are more widespread and may be present despite adequate energy.[39] Multiple strategies have been enacted by United Nations bodies, academics, and nongovernmental organizations to address chronic undernutrition.

Micronutrient Fortification Programs

A strategy used in high-, medium-, and low-income countries is the fortification of staple foods with important micronutrients such as vitamin A, iodine, and zinc. This approach can address micronutrient deficiencies in the general population, but it is suboptimal among young children, particularly those 6 to 23 months of age, who rely solely on breastmilk and complementary foods. This age group consumes too little of fortified staple foods to obtain adequate amounts of each essential nutrient.[40] "Home fortification" addresses this challenge by making possible the provision of appropriate amounts of micronutrients without major changes in dietary practices. The strategy involves fortification of a staple food in the home by the primary caretaker after cooking.

Available home fortification products include spreads, such as Nutributter® and Plumpy'Nut™; crushable tablets, such as Foodlet; and MNPs, such as Sprinkles, Vitashakti, and MixMe™.[41] MNPs and lipid-based nutrient supplements (LNS) are two commonly used supplements for home fortification. While MNPs have the benefits of being low cost and easy to use, they provide only micronutrients.[42] In contrast, LNS also provide energy, thereby increasing the energy density as well as the micronutrient content of complementary foods.[43]

These food commodities are most often introduced as part of the programs of the WFP and other food assistance agencies. Supplementary feeding programs provide extra food and food commodities, usually in addition to general food rations, to specific vulnerable groups, typically pregnant and lactating women (PLW) and children under 5. Blanket programs supply all individuals within a population's vulnerable groups, while programs in less severe conditions can target undernourished children or mothers.[44]

Specialized Food Commodities

Available supplementary food products for children 6 to 23 months include fortified blended foods (FBF), complementary food supplements, ready-to-use supplementary foods (RUSF), and MNPs (**Table 6-1**). The appropriate choice of

Table 6-1 Specialized food commodities used by the World Food Programme (WFP)

Type of Food	Description
Fortified blended foods (FBF)	These foods have been developed for treating moderate malnutrition and developed with the assumption that they provide most of the child's energy intake along with breastmilk and a local, unfortified staple food. A FBF, such as corn-soy blend + + (CSB++): milk powder, soy bean oil, sugar, is added to a local staple food, such as corn or wheat. This can be used for blanket feeding of children 0-23 months because it provides approximately 70% of total energy intake.
Complementary food supplements	These are concentrated forms of high-quality nutrients that may come in powder or paste form and are used to complement or enhance a meal. Examples include lipid-based nutrient supplements (LNS), and they have provided the best results on linear growth among children 6-23 months.
Ready-to-use supplementary foods (RUSF)	RUF products include lipid-based pastes and are used for the treatment of SAM or MAM where cooking is not possible. They are used to replace a meal. Many products are peanut-based and fortified with micronutrients and either milk powder or whey protein and are primarily commercially produced. One example is Supplementary Plumpy™. RUF products do not require preparation, and they are formulated specifically to meet the nutritional needs of young children.
Micronutrient powders (MNP)	MNP is used for home fortification of foods and designed to cover the daily requirements of important vitamins and minerals. These may be used among children if the population has sufficient macronutrients, including animal protein from the regular diet, but lacks micronutrients. MNP is also used among PLW wherein the micronutrient gap tends to be most crucial.

Data from World Food Programme. (2013). Special nutrition products. Available at http://www.wfp.org/nutrition/special-nutritional-products. Accessed September 6, 2013.

product depends not only on nutritional appropriateness, but also on cost effectiveness and context.

Criticisms of Specialized Food Commodities

Despite context-specific differences, sweeping criticisms have arisen over the use of specialized food commodities. Energy and nutrients in the form of food are necessary but insufficient to address global childhood undernutrition, as highlighted by the UNICEF framework (Figure 6-2). Some critics argue that these products are unaffordable; they undermine other, more proven strategies; they medicalize and commercialize the prevention of undernutrition; and they are unrealistic solutions.[45] Furthermore, they argue, specialized food commodities are at best short-term solutions. At worst, they are damaging to other national and local work by distracting from more sustainable and proven maternal and child health policies and programs, such as breastfeeding initiatives.[46,47]

Results of research on the effectiveness of specialized food commodities as part of supplementary feeding programs are mixed.[48] Compared with standard fortified food blends, specialized food products can further improve nutritional status among children with acute malnutrition.[49] However, making comparisons between studies and various contexts is difficult. Formulations and quantities of specialized food products vary between studies. Also, the context-specific impact of such interventions depends on factors such as the initial prevalence of undernutrition, the degree of household food insecurity, the energy density of traditional complementary foods, and the availability of micronutrient-rich local foods.[50]

The Future of Specialized Food Commodity Programs

Despite controversy, specialized food commodity programs and evaluations of them continue. Questions remain regarding which specific food commodities are most appropriate in particular settings and the extent of their roles. According to Dewey and Adu-Afarwuah, "Complementary feeding interventions, by themselves, cannot change the underlying conditions of poverty and poor sanitation that contribute to child malnutrition. They need to be implemented in conjunction with a larger strategy that includes improved water and sanitation, better health care and adequate housing."[51] When introduced as part of multifaceted approaches, specialized food commodity programs can help reduce childhood morbidity and malnutrition.[52]

The novelty of supplemental foods to most targeted populations and local WFP staff and related agencies creates challenges related to programmatic feasibility of the various product options for different groups.[53] Careful and strategic product introduction can maximize acceptability and appropriate consumption. The effectiveness of a supplementary feeding program utilizing specialized food commodities to positively impact nutritional status hinges, in large, on product acceptability, consistent uptake, and appropriate usage.[54]

Key Considerations in Behavior Change with Specialized Food Commodities

Caretakers have the onus of regularly fortifying the complementary foods of their children aged 6 to 23 months. Home fortification programs therefore require caretaker behavior change to be effective.

Acceptability of Specialized Food Commodities

Data regarding population acceptability of specialized food commodities are limited and mixed. MNP programs in response to natural disasters in Indonesia and Haiti had high acceptability and compliance among beneficiaries;[55,56] similar programs in refugee camps in Bangladesh and Nepal also resulted in favorable acceptance.[57,58] However, at Kakuma Refugee Camp in Kenya, an MNP within a blanket supplementary feeding program had low acceptance and no impact on nutritional status, measured by hemoglobin levels, of children under 5 and PLW.[59]

Public Health Core Competency 4: Cultural Competency Skills 2: Recognizes the role of cultural, social, and behavioral factors in the accessibility, availability, acceptability, and delivery of public health services

Reproduced from Council on Linkages Between Academia and Public Health Practice. 2010 May. Core Competencies for Public Health Professionals. Washington, DC: Public Health Foundation. http://www.phf.org/resourcestools/Documents/Core_Competencies_for_Public_Health_Professionals_2010May.pdf. Accessed August 13, 2013. This source is used for all Public Health Core Competencies in this chapter.

LNS products can be considered acceptable if over 50% of a given dose is consumed, as seen among rural Malawians 8 to 12 months old in a two-week, home-use trial,[60] as well as in a two-week pilot trial to test the acceptability of LNS among Ghanaian infants and PLW,[61] and in Burkina Faso in a two-week trial providing zinc-fortified LNS to children aged 9 to 12 months and PLW. The product was highly accepted based on feeding observations and data from focus groups and interviews.[62] A similar acceptability study of LNS and MNP among PLW and infants and young children (IYC) in Bangladesh included a test feeding, a two-week home use trial, and feedback via focus group discussions.[63] All supplements (LNS for PLW; LNS for IYC; MNP for IYC) were acceptable to beneficiaries, based on amount of the test meal consumed and feedback in focus group discussions. Short home-feeding trials to determine acceptability have been the norm for testing acceptability of specialized food products, but more data are needed to ensure acceptability in long-term interventions.

As described earlier in the chapter, uptake of MNP, used as the indicator of acceptability at Kakuma Refugee Camp, fell from 99% to 30% in the first six months of a 17-month program.[64] So, while more data about food commodity acceptability are being made available, they should be interpreted carefully, especially if conducted over shorter periods of time than may be indicative of sustained acceptance.

Sharing of Specialized Food Products

Acceptability is just one barrier to the intended beneficiary receiving and consuming the specialized food product. Another is **misallocation**, or the inappropriate sharing of these food products among household and community members at the expense of the intended beneficiary.

To date, limited research examines how and why misallocation occurs, and how to reduce it. In-depth interview data from Uganda illustrate that sharing of RUSF rations is common and attributable to cultural values.[65] Unpublished WFP data from an LNS project in Somalia suggest evidence of sharing among children under 5 years.[66] Direct observations in Malawi found sharing of corn-soy blend and LNS 15% and 5% of the time, respectively, but no effect of the sharing on children's weight-for-age z scores.[67] In Tanzania, mothers reported that only leftover processed soy- and rice-based complementary food products that were not eaten by the intended child beneficiary were shared among household members.[68] From focus groups in Bangladesh, sharing is higher when supplements are intended for children rather than for PLW, yet it is still uncommon overall.[69] Limitations to this information include lack of primary caretakers' presence during all children's meals, resulting in inaccurate caregiver observations of what was being eaten[70] or shared. More accurate methods to capture and understand food product sharing practices are needed.

Importance of Formative Research in Nutrition Interventions

Formative research both enhances specialized food commodity acceptability and helps in the understanding of potential food commodity sharing practices. Nutrition programs providing humanitarian aid often do little or no formative work to understand the local context.[71] Formative research can help public health practitioners who are often cultural outsiders, lacking familiarity with the context and dynamics of target communities. Also, the provided products are typically novel to those populations. Kodish and colleagues found that at the front end of a specialized food commodity project, detailed, multistage formative research over multiple months is crucial for program success.[72] Moreover, culturally appropriate communication and promotion strategies and product packaging must be developed and pretested during this formative phase.

Need for Adequate Formative Research

This work provides critical information and is the keystone of an effective social marketing framework to be used to promote specialized food commodities during a nutrition program so that intended beneficiaries have access to and are able to appropriately utilize a product. Failure to employ formative research can lead to programmatic challenges, from sharing of the commodity among household (intra-household) and community members (inter-household), potentially limiting impact on targeted individuals, to commodity rejection by a target population.[73]

> *Public Health Core Competency 2: Policy Development/ Program Planning Skills 6: Participates in program planning processes*

Experts have made recommendations for organizations considering the implementation of a home fortification program using a specialized food commodity that is novel to the target population.[74] First, packaging must be "culturally appropriate and clear and self-explanatory with regard to content, target group, and methods and frequency of use." Next, social marketing, WHO's Information,

Education and Communication (IEC) materials, and training for product distributors are needed. Finally, to increase acceptance rates, caretakers must receive clear instructions on product use at the time of distribution. These suggestions demand significant labor and planning.

Formative research is now widely acknowledged, both in international nutrition specifically and public health at large, as the keystone to the development of evidence-based interventions for maternal and child health.[75,76,77,78] This is particularly true in specialized food commodity programs, where the acceptability and appropriate consumption of a food product hinge on the product's well-planned introduction.

Consider the 17-month intervention in Kakuma Refugee Camp, which saw distribution of 14.4 million sachets of MNP but no effect on anemia rates. Sachets cost $360,000 in addition to costs of shipping, distribution, personnel, and social marketing costs. Kodish and colleagues found that a main reason why this project fell short of its intended impact was the brevity of the three-week, superficial formative research period, lacking in thoroughness and methodological rigor.[79] More recent projects have been integrating longer formative research periods (three months in Kenya in an MNP project;[80] five months in Niger in an MNP and LNS project)[81] in order to develop culturally appropriate interventions, based on the understanding that collecting ethnographic information is necessary in order to understand the target population and to develop effective social marketing strategies.

Requirements for Successful Formative Research

Public health nutrition interventions are more likely to be successful when based on multiphase formative research plans that are community-led, use mixed methods, and are iterative in nature. This has been shown in nutrition projects among vulnerable populations in the Native American communities of North America, the Pacific Islander population of the Pacific, and the First Nations population in the Canadian north.[82,83,84] Due in part to variations in opportunities and constraints among different populations, no internationally agreed-upon approach to conduct high-quality formative research exists. However, the international health community has embraced it as an invaluable tool in intervention development.

Public Health Core Competency 5: Community Dimension of Practice Skills 2: Demonstrates the capacity to work in community-based participatory research efforts

Household Food Allocation and Food Sharing Practices

Formative research can help intervention staff understand local intra-household dynamics, such as household food allocation, cash income control, and decision-making patterns, which are culture-specific.[85] In rural Nepal, for example, shared plate eating is related to various negative caring practices and is a predictor of **xerophthalmia** status in children.[86] Conversely, separate research in Nepal found shared plate eating to be associated with more and different foods being offered to young children.[87] Because food sharing from a single bowl or plate is common in low-income settings, including sub-Saharan Africa,[88,89] understanding food sharing dynamics can help identify their potential influence on children's nutritional status and on implications for developing specialized food product interventions.

Understanding the existing patterns of intra-household allocation of food is a prerequisite for determining the effectiveness of specialized food commodity programs.[90] Household food allocation is part of a more comprehensive household system with four components: food selection, food preparation, food serving, and related food allocation patterns.[91] Inter-household food distribution, in contrast, is a social aspect of the larger food environment, and in low-income settings largely includes foods shared with extended family or community members outside of the immediate household.[92] Both intra- and inter-household food sharing must be understood to develop nutrition programs that channel specialized food commodities toward specific beneficiaries using a social marketing framework.

Successful maternal and child health intervention strategies, including supplementary feeding programs, require adaptation to make them local, community-based, and context-specific.[93] Meeting beneficiaries' needs most effectively and appropriately is a priority for nutrition programs, which serve the most vulnerable populations at times of greatest need.

Informing Social Marketing Strategy

Formative research can help development of a social marketing framework as a program base. Drawing upon ideas generated from decades of private-sector salesmanship, a social marketing framework is now central to many behavior change public health programs globally. In contrast to conventional information-heavy, educational approaches, community-based social marketing can more effectively lead to sustainable behavior change.[94] According to Kotler and Zaltman, "Social marketing is the design, implementation, and control of programs calculated to influence the acceptability of social ideas and involving considerations of product planning, pricing, communication, distribution, and marketing research."[95] This framework is not a theory, but rather a model that draws from such fields as psychology, sociology, anthropology, and communications to help public health practitioners understand how to positively influence people's behavior.[96]

Characteristics of Social Marketing

Approaches to social marketing can vary, but commonalities are evident across various descriptions.[97] First, social marketing is not about coercion or enforcement but voluntary behavior change. Second, change is sought through an exchange: a clear benefit to the beneficiary should be present if change is to occur.[98] Third, marketing techniques should use concepts such as audience segmentation and targeting.[99,100,101] Fourth, distinct from other forms of marketing, the goal of social marketing should be to improve individual welfare and society, and not to benefit the organization specifically.[102] This framework also often includes strategic planning, in-depth formative research, audience and channel analysis, tailoring of communication strategies according to the needs and desires of the audience, and multilevel evaluation and consumer feedback,[103] with four tenets central to its strategy: product, price, place, and promotion.

Social marketing should be a key aspect of behavior-change nutrition programming that involves specialized food commodities. A strong behavior change communication strategy with appropriate messaging, known as a social marketing approach, is essential to increase demand and promote the proper utilization of such food products.[104,105] This approach has been recently used with specialized food commodity programs in China,[106] Kenya,[107] and Zimbabwe.[108] In Zimbabwe, formative research was successfully conducted to develop culturally appropriate messages that addressed the barriers to complementary feeding with and without an LNS. Using formative research to develop an understanding of intra- and inter-household dynamics can help promote many aspects of health that contribute to phases 1 and 2 of a social marketing strategy (**Figure 6-3**).[109] These dynamics are a key aspect of food utilization—one of the three pillars of food security—and may be important to understand as part of social marketing efforts.

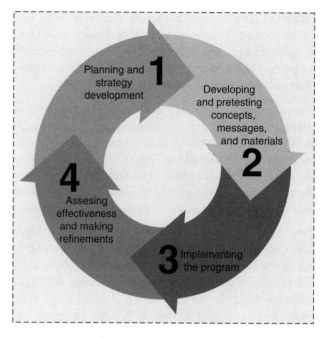

Figure 6-3 Social marketing cycle

Modified from NCI. (2005). Theory at a glance: A guide for health promotion practice. Washington, DC: U.S. Department of Health and Human Services. NIH Publication No. 05-3896. http://www.cancer.gov/cancertopics/cancerlibrary/theory.pdf. Accessed August 9, 2013.

Formative Research Methods to Engage Communities

Both qualitative and quantitative methods are available to formative researchers who aim to develop nutrition interventions with input from community members. Contracting a team of medical anthropologists to conduct in-depth ethnographic work that clarifies each social and cultural determinant of nutrition health community-wide is unrealistic due to labor and time requirements, and it rarely permits cross-cultural comparative work.

Alternatively, Rapid Assessment Procedures (RAP) can capture similar information more quickly, acting as compromises between deep, open-ended anthropological work and "quick-and-dirty" program assessment, which usually has very specific, predefined objectives. It is a field guide for using anthropological research techniques to gather community perspectives on health behaviors.[110] Qualitative and quantitative techniques include in-depth interviews, direct observations, community workshops, focus group discussions, free lists, and pile sorts, just to name a few. Methods used depend on the goals of the nutrition program, and can include community workshops, in-depth interviews, direct observations, focus group discussions, and systematic interviewing methods.

Community Workshops

Community participation in the planning, implementation, and evaluation of community-based interventions has been considered an effective strategy for implementing successful public health programs.[111] These workshops involve generation of new ideas as well as reviews of intervention materials developed by local artists that community members vote on to determine preferred intervention strategies and social marketing. Community workshops can actively engage the community, to identify intervention priority areas and to develop culturally salient messages as part of nutrition intervention formative research.[112]

Currently, in Ntchisi, Malawi, and Cabo Delgado, Mozambique, WFP efforts to develop culturally appropriate nutrition intervention trials with an LNS for children 6 to 23 months include community workshops. Community members help brainstorm and prioritize activities, strategies, and messages that will ultimately be the foundation of the intervention's behavior change communication strategy.

In-Depth Interviews

In-depth interviews are another data collection method that gives the community a voice in nutrition program design. Though based on a clear plan, they also display minimum control over participants' responses. This subjective assessment allows participants to express themselves in their own terms and at their own paces, so researchers can gather information and build rapport.[113] Interviewees may include caretakers, community leaders, community health workers, and other key stakeholders who are integral to program development.

Caretaker and Community Leader Interviews

Caretakers can be defined as male and female caretakers who play a role in the care of young children and household decision making that influences child growth;[114] they may be mothers, fathers, or grandmothers. Caretakers may be recruited as a single group, but their data may be stratified by type of caretaker during analysis should divergent

themes emerge. Community leaders to be interviewed can include religious leaders, elected officials, elders, and other individuals who play leadership roles in the communities and can speak as key informants about their communities at large. Interviews with these individuals build rapport and provide access to the community and sampling guidance. They can also be conducted in order to collect contextual information about community history, illnesses, meal preparation, eating/feeding behavior, food sharing, and suggestions for the development of a nutrition program based on previous programs that have been implemented in the community in question.

Structure of In-Depth Interviews

In-depth interviews can be unstructured, semi-structured, or structured.[115] The advantage of semi-structured interviews is their balance of data gathered for program design and room for participants to express themselves in their own words. These interviews usually begin with discussions of relatively nonthreatening, general constructs aimed at assessing the cultural perceptions and practices of the caretakers regarding their feeding and livelihood practices.[116] They are based on an interview guide, but the interviewer has discretion over whether and which probes are followed for deeper information.[117] Interviewers often aim to collect information about illnesses, meal preparation, and feeding/eating practices. More specific questions and probes attempt to elucidate the context and determinants related to the nutritional behavior of interest.

Direct Observations

Since nutrition practitioners are rarely trained in anthropological research methods, direct observations are not routine in nutrition programming. However, they can be valuable to formative research by increasing understanding of factors that influence food utilization at the household and community levels. For example, data from direct observations can help researchers gain an understanding of the food environment, including food availability, access, and utilization. They can also elucidate household feeding and food preparation behaviors, including the identification of key times during the day when home fortification with specialized food commodities may be most appropriate for an intended beneficiary to ensure high compliance or acceptability. At Kakuma Refugee Camp, for example, direct observations revealed that Royco®, a food flavoring additive, was commonly added to dishes during food preparation in the Somali communities—a practice similar to home fortification with micronutrient powder and one that social marketing efforts could have piggybacked had this finding been made available from formative work.

Direct observations can often address some household food-related behaviors that other methods cannot.[118] To avoid altering of food consumption patterns, households are not usually notified in advance that their meal will be observed.[119] On observation forms, research team members record descriptions of meal preparation and feeding/eating events as they occur. After observations, researchers expand upon these descriptions by writing field notes, or written accounts that provide the core data for ethnographic analysis.[120] These semi-structured field notes should be selective in what they include, since they inevitably are meant to answer specific research questions of interest. Notes written by the research team should have a strong descriptive thrust, providing accounts of people, scenes, and dialogues related to the context around food behaviors.[121]

Focus Group Discussions

Focus groups are effective qualitative research tools for identifying social norms and building consensus not only in public health, but also in marketing research.[122] Focus group discussions can be employed to build consensus around specific strategies for promoting a specialized food commodity during a nutrition intervention, as well as around key messages and media for promotion of key nutritional behaviors or products. They can also be used to identify social norms related to causes, perceptions, and practices of beneficiaries regarding nutrition-related behavior.

Methodologically, focus groups should include 6 to 10 homogenous caretakers who perceive themselves to be similar in gender, age, and social class.[123] Sessions should last no more than two hours each. The total number of groups should depend on how soon **data saturation** is reached; with homogenous groups of individuals allowing more free-flowing conversations, three to five groups is typically sufficient. During a focus group discussion, a funnel approach is used. It begins with a less structured approach, with questions that emphasize free discussion, and progresses to a more structured discussion of specific questions related to norms or social marketing materials themselves as stimulus aids. These general guidelines are flexible and should be adaptable to the specific situation.

Systematic Interviewing Methods: Free Lists and Pile Sorts

Less common but just as useful are **systematic interviewing methods**, which allow for **cultural domain analysis** during formative research. Used more often for ethnographic research in anthropology, systematic interviewing methods, especially free lists and pile sorts, have great utility in formative research.

Free Lists

Free listing is a simple listing activity of items within a cultural domain.[124] Eliciting free lists of local foods and nutritional illnesses can allow for an understanding of the foods available in a community and the foods most salient to community members. These types of questions allow researchers to determine how salient particular foods, illnesses, and preventative measures are within a community. The goal is to understand how a population interprets and understands the content of these domains in order to develop culturally appropriate messages that resonate with the target audience as part of a social marketing strategy to best promote key behaviors or food commodities. Determining the items that make up a "foods" domain, for example, would require identification of the full range of foods in a community, which would later allow an illustration of the relative importance that community members ascribe to those foods[125] and provide the basis for a model to explain factors related to a behavior of interest among community members. The same activity can be done for illnesses and preventative measures for a chosen nutritional illness of interest, or whatever else is deemed to be important to community members based on data collected from in-depth interviews.

Pile Sorts

After conducting free lists, pile sorts can be conducted with community members in order to define local food concepts. The free lists conducted with community members will reveal various lists that define cultural domains of local foods, illnesses, and preventive measures of a nutritional illness. Based on a cutoff, the most salient items will be chosen from these free lists in order to be included in the pile sorts. Then, pile sorting exercises can be conducted to assess the degree to which these issues mentioned in free lists are perceived to cluster together. These exercises are intended to collect data on the perceived interrelationships among different issues in relation to perceived similarities.[126,127] Caretakers are provided a stack of cards, with words or phrases written on them in local languages. If possible, pictures or photos will be provided in lieu of words for caretakers without literacy. The participants are then asked to sort those cards into piles, putting items that are similar together in a pile. Inquiries are then made to informants to explain why items appear in one pile or another to gather the "why" and "how" behind the data. Weller and Romney explain that pile sort data tend to be sparse, requiring 20 or more participants to obtain stable results.[128] They suggest using samples between 30 and 40 for reliable data. The pile sorting task has been used extensively in ethnographic research, is easy to use, and can facilitate useful data through conversation about ways to sort cards.[129] Visual Anthropac computer software[130] can be used in the analysis of both free list and pile sort data.

These mixed methods that can be implemented as part of a RAP approach give beneficiaries a voice in the way that they would prefer to receive food assistance as opposed to the way that we public health practitioners assume they would prefer. Doing so offers the best chance to have sustainable, effective, and impactful nutrition interventions.

Conclusion

Conducting formative research can increase the likelihood of interventions being successful. In recent years, the international nutrition community has made great efforts to develop evidence-based interventions derived at least partially from formative research. The era of top-down interventions is nearing its end, as evidenced by the many other areas of public health that have also turned to community-led behavior-change interventions. By utilizing the expertise of social and behavioral researchers, organizations at the forefront of international nutrition are using sound formative research methods to develop large-scale interventions to address undernutrition, particularly in South Asia and sub-Saharan Africa. While no single strategy will ever be able to promote or change health-seeking nutrition behavior, the continued exploration of new strategies can improve the effectiveness of public health programs. The nutrition community is moving in a positive direction by using more community-led and culturally appropriate intervention strategies to positively impact the immeasurably complex determinants of nutritional status.

References

1 UNHCR. (2009). Micronutrient powder (MixMe™) use in Kakuma Refugee Camp in Kenya (AFRICA). *Implementing, Improving Nutrition, Improving Lives, 2(3)*, 1-4. Retrieved from http://www.unhcr.org/4b7bca3c9.html

2 Goette, J. (2005, November). *Issues in nutrition for refugee children.* Paper presented at The Hopes Fulfilled or Dreams Shattered? From Resettlement to Settlement Conference. Retrieved from http://www.crr.unsw.edu.au/media/File/Nutrition_Issues.pdf

3 Goette, J. (2005, November). *Issues in nutrition for refugee children. Paper presented at the* Hopes Fulfilled or Dreams Shattered? From Resettlement to Settlement Conference. Retrieved from http://www.crr.unsw.edu.au/media/File/Nutrition_Issues.pdf

4 WHO/UNICEF/UNHCR/WFP. (2002). *Food and nutrition needs in emergencies.* Geneva: World Health Organization. Retrieved from http://whqlibdoc.who.int/hq/2004/a83743.pdf

5 WHO. (2009). *Global prevalence of vitamin A deficiency in populations at risk, 1995-2005.* WHO Global Database on Vitamin A Deficiency.

6 WHO. (2009). *Global prevalence of vitamin A deficiency in populations at risk, 1995-2005.* WHO Global Database on Vitamin A Deficiency.

7 Hansch, S. (1992). Diet and ration use in Central American refugee camps. *Journal of Refugee Studies, 5,* 300-12.

8 Weise Prinzo, Z., & de Benoist, B. (2002). Meeting the challenges of micronutrient deficiencies in emergency-affected populations. *Proceedings of the Nutrition Society, 61,* 251-57.

9 Toole, M. J. (1992). Micronutrient deficiencies in refugees. *Lancet, 339,* 1214-16.

10 Mears, C., & Young, H. (1998). *Acceptability and use of cereal-based foods in refugee camps: Case studies from Nepal, Ethiopia, and Tanzania. Oxfam Working Paper.*

11 Weise Prinzo, Z., & de Benoist, B. (2002). Meeting the challenges of micronutrient deficiencies in emergency-affected populations. *Proceedings of the Nutrition Society, 61,* 251-57.

12 Van den Briel, T., Cheung, E., & Zewari, J., & Khan, R. (2007). Fortifying food in the field to boost nutrition: case studies from Afghanistan, Angola, and Zambia. *Food and Nutrition Bulletin, 28(3),* 353-64.

13 Wahlqvist, M. L. (2008). National food fortification: A dialogue with reference to Asia: policy in evolution. *Asia Pacific Journal of Clinical Nutrition, 17*(Suppl.), 24-29.

14 WHO/UNICEF/UNHCR/WFP. (2002). *Food and nutrition needs in emergencies.* Geneva: World Health Organization. Retrieved from http://whqlibdoc.who.int/hq/2004/a83743.pdf

15 Schauer, C., & Zlotkin, S. (2003). Home fortification with micro-nutrient sprinkles: A new approach for the prevention and treatment of nutritional anemias. *Pediatric Child Health, 8*(2), 87-90.

16 De Pee, S., Moench-Pfanner, R., Martini, E., Zlotkin, S. H., Darnton-Hill, I., & Bloem, M. W. (2007). Home fortification in emergency response and transition programming: Experiences in Aceh and Nias, Indonesia. *Food and Nutrition Bulletin, 28*(2), 189-97.

17 Rah, J. H., de Pee, S., Kraemer, K., Steiger, G., Bloem, M. W., Spiegel, P., Wilkinson, C., & Bilukha, O. (2012). Program experience with micronutrient powders and current evidence. *Journal of Nutrition, 142,* 191S-96S.

18 Kodish, S., Rah, J. H., Kraemer, K., de Pee, S., & Gittelsohn, J. (2011). Understanding low usage of micronutrient powder in the Kakuma Refugee Camp, Kenya: Findings from a qualitative study. *Food and Nutrition Bulletin, 32*(3), 292-303.

19 Ndemwa, P., Klotz, C. L., Mwaniki, D., Sun, K., Muniu, E., Andango, P., Owigar, Rah, J. H., Kraemer, K., & Spiegel, P. B. (2011). Relationship of the availability of micronutrient powder with iron status and hemoglobin among women and children in the Kakuma Refugee Camp, Kenya. *Food and Nutrition Bulletin, 32,* 286-91.

20 De Pee, S., & Bloem, M. W. (2008). *Current and potential role of specially formulated foods and food supplements for preventing malnutrition among 6-23 months old and treating moderate malnutrition among 6-59 months old children.* Paper presented at the Dietary Management of Moderate Malnutrition in Under-5 Children Consultation.

21 Black, R. E., Allen, L. H., Bhutta, Z. A., Caulfield, L. E., de Onis, M., Ezzati, M., Mathers, M., Rivera, C., & Rivera, J. (2008). Maternal and child undernutrition: Global and regional exposures and health consequences. *Lancet, 371,* 243-60.

22 Bhutta, Z. A., Ahmed, T., Black, R. E., Dewey, K., Giugliani, E., Haider, B. A., . . . Shekar, M. (2008). What works? Interventions for maternal and child undernutrition and survival. *Lancet, 371,* 417-40.

23 UNICEF. (1990). *Strategy for improved nutrition of children and women in developing countries.* New York: UNICEF.

24 Haddad, L., Alderman, H., Appleton, S., Song, L., & Yishehac, Y. (2003). Reducing child malnutrition: How far does income growth take us? *World Bank Economic Review, 17*(1), 107-32.

25 Navarro, V. (2007). *Neoliberalism, globalization, and inequalities: Consequences for health and quality of life.* Amityville, NY: Baywood.

26 Bhutta, Z. A., Ahmed, T., Black, R. E., Dewey, K., Giugliani, E., Haider, B. A., . . . Shekar, M. (2008). What works? Interventions for maternal and child undernutrition and survival. *Lancet, 371,* 417-40.

27 Black, R. E., Allen, L. H., Bhutta, Z. A., Caulfield, L. E., de Onis, M., Ezzati, M., . . . Rivera, J. (2008). Maternal and child undernutrition: Global and regional exposures and health consequences. *Lancet, 371,* 243-60.

28 Bhutta, Z. A., Ahmed, T., Black, R. E., Dewey, K., Giugliani, E., Haider, B. A., . . . Shekar, M. (2008). What works? Interventions for maternal and child undernutrition and survival. *Lancet, 371,* 417-40.

29 Bhutta, Z. A., Ahmed, T., Black, R. E., Dewey, K., Giugliani, E., Haider, B. A., . . . Shekar, M. (2008). What works? Interventions for maternal and child undernutrition and survival. *Lancet, 371,* 417-40.

30 Barker, D. J. (2007). The origins of the developmental origins theory. *Journal of Internal Medicine, 261*(5), 412-17.

31 Martorell, R. (1995). The effects of improved nutrition in early childhood: The Institute of Nutrition on Central America and Panama (INCAP) follow-up study. *Journal of Nutrition, 125,* 1027S-1138S.

32 Dewey, K., & Adu-Afarwuah, S. (2008). Systematic review of the efficacy and effectiveness of complementary feeding interventions in developing countries. *Maternal & Child Nutrition, 4,* 24-85.

33 Horton, R. H. (2008). Maternal and child undernutrition: An urgent opportunity. *Lancet, 371,* 179.

34 Victora, C. G., Adair, L., Fall, C., Hallal, P. C., Martorell, R., Richter, L., & Singh Sachdev, H. (2008). Maternal and child undernutrition: Consequences for adult health and human capital. *Lancet, 371,* 340-57.

35 WHO/UNICEF/UNHCR/WFP. (2002). *Food and nutrition needs in emergencies.* Geneva: World Health Organization. Retrieved from http://whqlibdoc.who.int/hq/2004/a83743.pdf

36 Sphere Project. (2011). *Humanitarian charter and minimum standards in humanitarian response.* Northampton, UK: Practical Action Publishing.

37 Schroeder, D. G. (2008). Malnutrition. In R. D. Semba & M. W. Bloem (Eds.), *Nutrition and health: Nutrition and health in developing countries* (2nd ed.) (pp. 341-76). Totowa, NJ: Humana Press.

38 Allen, L. H. (1994). Nutritional influences on linear growth: A general review. *European Journal of Clinical Nutrition, 48,* S75-S89.

39 Ramakrishnan, U., & Huffman, S. L. (2008).Multiple micronutrient malnutrition. In R. D. Semba & M. W. Bloem (Eds.), *Nutrition and health: Nutrition and health in developing countries* (2nd ed.) (pp. 531-76). Totowa, NJ: Humana Press.

40 Dewey, K. G., Yang, Z. & Boy, E. (2009). Systematic review and meta-analysis of home fortification of complementary foods. *Maternal & Child Nutrition, 5,* 283-321.

41 UNICEF. (2009). *Workshop report on scaling up the use of multiple micronutrient powders to improve the quality of complementary foods for young children in Asia.* Retrieved from www.unscn.org/.../Summary_MNP_ workshop_3_June_2009.pdf

42 Schauer, C., & Zlotkin, S. (2003). Home fortification with micro-nutrient sprinkles: A new approach for the prevention and treatment of nutritional anemias. *Pediatric Child Health, 8*(2), 87-90.

43 Dewey, K. G., Yang, Z. & Boy, E. (2009). Systematic review and meta-analysis of home fortification of complementary foods. *Maternal & Child Nutrition, 5,* 283-321.

44 Webb, P., & Thorne-Lyman, A. (2008). Tackling nutrient deficiencies and life-threatening disease: The role of food in humanitarian relief. In R. D. Semba & M. W. Bloem (Eds.), *Nutrition and Health in Developing Countries* (2nd ed) (pp. 699-720). Totowa, NJ: Humana Press.

45 Latham, M., Jonsson, U., Sterken, E., & Kent, G. (2011). RUTF stuff: Can the children be saved with fortified peanut paste? *World Nutrition, 2*(2), 62-85.

46 Black, R. E., Allen, L. H., Bhutta, Z. A., Caulfield, L. E., de Onis, M., Ezzati, M., . . . Rivera, J. (2008). Maternal and child undernutrition: Global and regional exposures and health consequences. *The Lancet, 371,* 243-60.

47 Jones, G., Steketee, R. W., Black, R. E., Bhutta, Z. A., Morris, A. S., & Bellagio Child Survival Study Group. (2003). How many child deaths can we prevent this year? *Lancet, 362,* 65-71.

48 Navarro-Colorado, C., Mason, F., & Shoham, J. (2008). Measuring the effectiveness of supplementary feeding programmes in emergencies. *HPN Network Paper, 63,* 1-32.

49 Department for International Development (DFID). (2011). *The use of nutrition products for the prevention and treatment of undernutrition.* London, UK: DFID Human Development Resource Centre.

50 Dewey, K., & Adu-Afarwuah, S. (2008). Systematic review of the efficacy and effectiveness of complementary feeding interventions in developing countries. *Maternal & Child Nutrition, 4,* 24-85.

51 Dewey, K., & Adu-Afarwuah, S. (2008). Systematic review of the efficacy and effectiveness of complementary feeding interventions in developing countries. *Maternal & Child Nutrition, 4,* 24-85 (quote on 32-33).

52 Dewey, K., & Adu-Afarwuah, S. (2008). Systematic review of the efficacy and effectiveness of complementary feeding interventions in developing countries. *Maternal & Child Nutrition, 4,* 24-85.

53 Webb, P., & Thorne-Lyman, A. (2008). Tackling nutrient deficiencies and life-threatening disease: The role of food in humanitarian relief. In R. D. Semba & M. W. Bloem (Eds.), *Nutrition and Health in Developing Countries* (2nd ed.) (pp. 699-720). Totowa, NJ: Humana Press.

54 De Pee, S., Moench-Pfanner, R., Martini, E., Zlotkin, S. H., Darnton-Hill, I., & Bloem, M. W. (2007). Home fortification in emergency response and transition programming: Experiences in Aceh and Nias, Indonesia. *Food and Nutrition Bulletin, 28*(2), 189-97.

55 De Pee, S., Moench-Pfanner, R., Martini, E., Zlotkin, S. H., Darnton-Hill, I., & Bloem, M. W. (2007). Home fortification in emergency response and transition programming: Experiences in Aceh and Nias, Indonesia. *Food and Nutrition Bulletin, 28*(2), 189-97.

56 Menon, P., Ruel, M. T., Loechl, C. U., Arimond, M., Habicht, J., Pelto, G., & Michaud, L. (2007). Micronutrient sprinkles reduce anemia among 9- to 24-mo-old children when delivered through an integrated health and nutrition program in rural Haiti. *Journal of Nutrition, 137,* 1023-30.

57 Bilukha, O. Howard, C., Wilkinson, C., Bamrah, S., & Husain, F. (2011). Effects of multimicronutrient home fortification on anemia and growth in Bhutanese refugee children. *Food and Nutrition Bulletin, 32*(3), 264-76.

58 Rah, J. H., de Pee, S., Kraemer, K., Steiger, G., Bloem, M. W., Spiegel, P., Wilkinson, C., & Bilukha, O. (2012). Program

experience with micronutrient powders and current evidence. *Journal of Nutrition, 142,* 191S-196S.

59 Ndemwa, P., Klotz, C. L., Mwaniki, D., Sun, K., Muniu, E., Andango, P., . . . Spiegel, P. B. (2011). Relationship of the availability of micronutrient powder with iron status and hemoglobin among women and children in the Kakuma Refugee Camp, Kenya. *Food and Nutrition Bulletin, 32,* 286-91.

60 Phuka, J. C., Ashorn, U., Ashorn, P., Zeilani, M., Cheung, Y. B., Dewey, K. G., Manary, M., & Maleta, K. (2011). Acceptability of three novel lipid-based nutrient supplements among Malawian infants and their caregivers. *Maternal & Child Nutrition, 7*(4), 368-77.

61 Adu-Afarquah, S., Lartey, A., Zeilani, M., & Dewey, K. G. (2011). Acceptability of lipid-based nutrient supplements (LNS) among Ghanaian infants and pregnant or lactating women. *Maternal & Child Nutrition, 7*(4), 344-56.

62 Hess, S. Y., Bado, L., Aaron, G. J., Ouedrago, J. B., Zeilani, M., & Brown, K. H. (2010). Acceptability of zinc-fortified, lipid-based nutrient supplements (LNS) prepared for young children in Burkina Faso. *Maternal & Child Nutrition, 7*(4), 357-67.

63 Mridha, M. K., Chaparro, C. M., Matias, S. L., Hussain, S., Munira, S., Saha, S., Day, T. L., & Dewey, K. G. (2011). *Acceptability of lipid-based nutrient supplements and micronutrient powders among pregnant and lactating women and infants and young children in Bangladesh.* Final report prepared by University of California at Davis, FANTA-2, ICDDRB, LAMB. [Copy in possession of author.]

64 Kodish, S., Rah, J. H., Kraemer, K., de Pee, S., & Gittelsohn, J. (2011). Understanding low usage of micronutrient powder in the Kakuma Refugee Camp, Kenya: Findings from a qualitative study. *Food and Nutrition Bulletin, 32*(3), 292-303.

65 Ickes, S. B., Jilcott, S. B., Myhre, J. A., Adair, L. S., Thirumurthy, H., Handa, S., Bently, M. E., & Ammerman, A. S. (2011). Examination of facilitators and barriers to home-based supplemental feeding with ready-to-use food for underweight children in western Uganda. *Maternal & Child Nutrition, 8*(1), 115-29.

66 World Food Programme. (2011). *Descriptive statistics for the Burkina Faso data set.* WFP internal data. [Copy in possession of author.]

67 Flax, V. L., Phuka, J., Cheung, Y. B., Ashorn, U., Maleta, K., & Ashorn, P. (2010). Feeding patterns and behaviors during home supplementation of underweight Malawian children with lipid-based nutrient supplements or corn-soy blend. *Appetite, 54*(3), 504-11.

68 Paul, K. H., Dickin, K. L., Ali, N. S., Monterrosa, E. C., & Stoltzfus, R. J. (2008). Soy- and rice-based processed complementary food increases nutrient intakes in infants and is equally acceptable with or without added milk powder. *Journal of Nutrition, 138*(10), 1963-68.

69 Mridha, M. K., Chaparro, C. M., Matias, S. L., Hussain, S., Munira, S., Saha, S., Day, T. L., & Dewey, K. G. (2011). *Acceptability of lipid-based nutrient supplements and micronutrient powders among pregnant and lactating women and infants and young children in Bangladesh.* Final report prepared by University of California at Davis, FANTA-2, ICDDRB, LAMB. [Copy in possession of author.]

70 Shankar, A. V., Gittelsohn, J., Stalling, R., West, K. P., Gynwali, T., Dhungel, C., & Dahal, B. (2001). Comparison of visual estimates of children's portion sizes under both shared-plate and individual-plate conditions, *Journal of American Dietary Association, 101*(1), 47-52.

71 Tripp, K., Perrine, C. G., de Campos, P., Knieriemen, M., Hartz, R., Ali, F., Jefferds, M. D., & Kupka, R. (2011).Formative research for the development of a market-based home fortification programme for young children in Niger. *Maternal & Child Nutrition, 7*(Suppl. 3), 82-95.

72 Kodish, S., Rah, J. H., Kraemer, K., de Pee, S., & Gittelsohn, J. (2011). Understanding low usage of micronutrient powder in the Kakuma Refugee Camp, Kenya: Findings from a qualitative study. *Food and Nutrition Bulletin, 32*(3), 292-303.

73 Kodish, S., Rah, J. H., Kraemer, K., de Pee, S., & Gittelsohn, J. (2011). Understanding low usage of micronutrient powder in the Kakuma Refugee Camp, Kenya: Findings from a qualitative study. *Food and Nutrition Bulletin, 32*(3), 292-303.

74 De Pee, S., Moench-Pfanner, R., Martini, E., Zlotkin, S. H., Darnton-Hill, I., & Bloem, M. W. (2007). Home fortification in emergency response and transition programming: Experiences in Aceh and Nias, Indonesia. *Food and Nutrition Bulletin, 28*(2), 189-97.

75 Jefferds, M. E. D., Ogange, L., Owuor, M., Cruz, K., Person, B., Obure, A., Suchdev, P. S., & Ruth, L. J. (2010). Formative research exploring acceptability, utilization, and promotion in order to develop a micronutrient powder (Sprinkles) intervention among Luo families in western Kenya. *Food and Nutrition Bulletin, 31*(2), S179-S185.

76 Morrison, J., Osrin, D., Shreshtha, B., Tumbahangphe, K. M., Tamang, S., & Shrestha, D. (2008). How did formative research inform the development of a women's group intervention in Nepal? *Journal of Perinatology, 28*, S14-S22.

77 Tawiah-Agyemang, C., Kirkwood, B. R., Edmond, K., Bazzano, A., & Hill, Z. (2008). Early initiation of breastfeeding in Ghana: Barriers and facilitators. *Journal of Perinatology, 28*, S46-S52.

78 Steckler, A., McLeroy, K. Goodman, R. M., Bird, S. T., & McCormick, L. (1992). Toward integrating qualitative and quantitative methods: An introduction. *Health Education Quarterly, 19*, 1-8.

79 Kodish, S., Rah, J. H., Kraemer, K., de Pee, S., & Gittelsohn, J. (2011). Understanding low usage of micronutrient powder in the Kakuma Refugee Camp, Kenya: Findings from a qualitative study. *Food and Nutrition Bulletin, 32*(3), 292-303.

80 Jefferds, M. E. D., Ogange, L., Owuor, M., Cruz, K., Person, B., Obure, A., Suchdev, P. S., & Ruth, L. J. (2010). Formative research exploring acceptability, utilization, and promotion in order to develop a micronutrient powder (Sprinkles) intervention among Luo families in western Kenya. *Food and Nutrition Bulletin, 31*(2), S179-S185.

81 Tripp, K., Perrine, C. G., de Campos, P., Knieriemen, M., Hartz, R., Ali, F., Jefferds, M. D., & Kupka, R. (2011). Formative research for the development of a market-based home fortification programme for young children in Niger. *Maternal & Child Nutrition, 7*(Suppl. 3), 82-95.

82 Gittelsohn, J., Evans, M., Helitzer, D., Anliker, J., Story, M., Metcalfe, L., Davis, S., & Iron Cloud, P. (1998). Formative research in a school-based obesity prevention program for Native American school children (Pathways). *Health Education Research, 13*(2), 251-65.

83 Cortes, L. M., & Gittelsohn, J. (2001). Formative research to inform intervention development for diabetes prevention in the Republic of the Marshall Islands. *Health Education & Behavior, 28*(6), 696-715.

84 Ho, L. S., Gittelsohn, S., Harris, B., & Ford, E. (2006). Development of an integrated diabetes prevention program with First Nations in Canada. *Health Promotion International, 21*(2), 88-97.

85 Dettwyler, K. A. (1989). Styles of infant feeding: Parental/caretaker control of food consumption in young children. *American Anthropology, 9*, 696-703.

86 Gittelsohn, J., Shankar, A. V., West, K. P., Faruque, F., Gnywalf, T., & Pradhan, E. K. (1998). Child feeding and care behaviors are associated with xerophthalmia in rural Nepalese households. *Social Science and Medicine, 47*(4), 477-86.

87 Shankar, A. V., Gittelsohn, J., West, K. P., Stalling, R., Gnywali, T., & Faruque, F. (1998). Eating from a shared plate affects food consumption in vitamin A-deficient Nepali children. *Journal of Nutrition, 128*(7), 1127-33.

88 Kigutha, H. N. (1997). Assessment of dietary intake in rural communities in Africa: Experiences in Kenya. *American Journal of Clinical Nutrition, 65*, 1168-72.

89 Kitanichi, K. (2000). The Aka and Baka: Food sharing among two central Africa hunter-gatherers. *Senri Ethnological Studies*, 149-69. Retrieved from http://camel.minpaku.ac.jp/dspace/bitstream/10502/907/1/SES53_008.pdf

90 Haddad, L., & Kanbur, R. (1992). The value of intrahousehold survey data for age-based nutritional targeting. *Annales d'Economie et de Statistique, 29*, 65-81.

91 Gittelsohn, J. (1991). Opening the box: Intrahousehold food allocation in rural Nepal. *Social Science & Medicine, 33*(10), 1141-54.

92 Gittelsohn, J., & Sharma, S. (2009). Physical, consumer, and social aspects of measuring the food environment among diverse low-income populations. *American Journal of Preventative Medicine, 36*(4 Suppl.), S161-S165.

93 Ahmed, S. M., Hossain, A., Khan, M. A., Mridha, M. K., Alam, A., Choudhury, N., Sharmin, T., Afsana, K., & Bhuiya, A. (2010). Using formative research to develop MNCH programme in urban slums in Bangladesh: Experiences from MANOSHI, BRAC. *BMI Public Health, 10*, 663.

94 McKenzie-Mohr, D. (2011). *Fostering sustainable behavior: An introduction to community-based social marketing* (3rd ed.). British Columbia, Canada: New Society Publisher.

95 Kotler, P., & Zaltman, G. (1971). Social marketing: An approach to planned social change. *Journal of Marketing, 35*, 3-12.

96 Kotler, P., & Zaltman, G. (1971). Social marketing: An approach to planned social change. *Journal of Marketing, 35*, 3-12.

97 Stead, M., Hastings, G., & McDermott, L. (2007). The meaning, effectiveness, and future of social marketing. *Obesity Review, 8*(Suppl. 1), S189-S193.

98 Houston, F. S., & Gassenheimer, J. B. (1987). Marketing and exchange. *Journal of marketing, 51*, 3-18.

99 Andreasen, A. R. (1995). *Marketing social Change: Changing behavior to promote health, social development, and the environment.* San Francisco, CA: Jossey-Bass.

100 Kotler, P., Armstrong, G., Saunders, J., & Wong, V. (1996). *Principles of marketing: European edition.* United Kingdom: Oxon.

101 Lefebvre, R., & Flora, J. A. (1988). Social marketing and public health intervention. *Health Education Quarterly, 15*, 299-315.

102 MacFadyen, L., Stead, M., & Hastings, G. B. (2003). Social marketing. In M. J. Baker (Ed.), *The marketing book* (5th ed.). Oxford, UK: Butterworth Heinemann.

103 Mattson, M., & Basu, A. (2010). The message development tool: A case for effective operationalization of messaging in social marketing practice. *Health Marketing Quarterly, 27*(3), 275-90.

104 De Pee, S., Kraemer, K., Van Den Briel, T., Boy, E., Grasset, C., Moench-Pfanner, R., Zlotkin, S., & Bloem, M. W. (2008). Quality criteria for micronutrient powder products: Report of a meeting organized by the World Food Programme and Sprinkles global health initiative. *Food and Nutrition Bulletin, 29*(3), 232-41.

105 Olney, D. K., Rawat, R., Ruel, M. T. (2012). Selecting programs and delivery systems for multiple micronutrient interventions. *Journal of Nutrition, 142*, 178S-185S.

106 Sun, J., Dai, Y., Zhang, S. Huang, J., Yang, Z., Huo, J., & Chen, C. (2011). Implementation of a program to market a complementary food supplement (Ying Yang Bao) and impacts on anemia and feeding practices in Shanxi, China. *Maternal & Child Nutrition, 7*(3), 96-111.

107 Suchdev, P. S., Ruth, L., Obure, A., Were, V., Ochieng, C., Ogange, L., Owuor, M., Ngure, F., Quick, R., Juliao, P., Jung, C., Teates, K., Cruz, K., & Jefferds, M. E. (2010). Monitoring the marketing, distribution, and use of Sprinkles micronutrient powders in rural western Kenya. *Food and Nutrition Bulletin, 31*(Suppl. 2), S168-S178.

108 Paul, K. H., Muti, M., Chasekwa, B., Mbuya, M. N., Madzima, R. C., Humphrey, J. H., & Stoltzfus, R. J. (2012). Complementary feeding messages that target cultural barriers enhance both the use of lipid-based nutrient supplements and underlying feeding practices to improve infant diets in rural Zimbabwe. *Maternal & Child Nutrition, 8*, 225-38.

109 Pfeiffer, J., Gloyd, S., & Ramirez, L. L. (2001). Intrahousehold resource allocation and child growth in Mozambique: An ethnographic case-control study. *Social Science & Medicine, 53*(1), 83-97.

110 Scrimshaw, S. C. M., & Hurtado, E. (1987). *Rapid Assessment Procedures for nutrition and primary health care: Anthropological approaches to improving programme effectiveness.* Tokyo: UNU Press.

111 Vastine, A., Gittelsohn, J., Ethelbah, B., Anliker, J., & Cabellero, B. (2005). Formative research and stakeholder participation in intervention development. *American Journal of Health Behavior, 29*(1), 57-69.

112 Sharma, S., Gittlesohn, J., Rosol, R., & Beck, L. (2010). Addressing the public health burden caused by the nutrition transition through the Healthy Foods North nutrition and lifestyle intervention programme. *Journal of Human Nutrition & Diet, 23*(Suppl. 1), 120-27.

113 Bernard, H. R. (2006). *Research methods in anthropology* (2nd ed.). Thousand Oaks, CA: Sage.

114 Pfeiffer, J., Gloyd, S., & Ramirez, L. L. (2001). Intrahousehold resource allocation and child growth in Mozambique: An ethnographic case-control study. *Social Science & Medicine, 53*(1), 83-97.

115 Bernard, H. R. (2006). *Research methods in anthropology* (2nd ed.). Thousand Oaks, CA: Sage.

116 Eisenbruch, M. (1990). The cultural bereavement interview: A new clinical approach for refugees. *Psychiatric Clinics of North America, 13*(4), 715-35.

117 Bernard, H. R. (2006). *Research methods in anthropology* (2nd ed.). Thousand Oaks, CA: Sage.

118 Bernard, H. R. (2006). *Research methods in anthropology* (2nd ed.). Thousand Oaks, CA: Sage.

119 Gittelsohn, J. (1991). Opening the box: Intrahousehold food allocation in rural Nepal. *Social Science & Medicine, 33*(10), 1141-54.

120 Emerson, R. M. (2001). Part II: Fieldwork practice: Issues in participant observation. *Contemporary field research: Perspectives and formulations*, 113-52.

121 Bernard, H. R. (2006). *Research methods in anthropology* (2nd ed.). Thousand Oaks, CA: Sage.

122 Kitzinger, J. (1994). The methodology of focus groups: The importance of interaction between research participants. *Sociology of Health & Illness, 16*(1), 103-21.

123 Morgan, D. (1997). *Focus groups as qualitative research* (2nd ed.). Thousand Oaks, CA: Sage.

124 Bernard, H. R. (2006). *Research methods in anthropology* (2nd ed.). Thousand Oaks, CA: Sage.

125 Gittelsohn, J. (1998). *Rapid Assessment Procedures (RAP): Ethnographic methods to investigate women's health.* International Nutrition Foundation (INF). Retrieved from http://archive.unu.edu/unupress/food2/UIN01E/UIN01E00.HTM

126 Gittelsohn, J. (1998). *Rapid Assessment Procedures (RAP): Ethnographic methods to investigate women's health.* International Nutrition Foundation (INF). Retrieved from http://archive.unu.edu/unupress/food2/UIN01E/UIN01E00.HTM

127 Weller, S. C., & Romney, A. K. (1988). *Structured interviewing.* Newbury Park, CA: Sage.

128 Weller, S. C., & Romney, A. K. (1988). *Structured interviewing.* Newbury Park, CA: Sage.

129 Weller, S. C., & Romney, A. K. (1988). *Structured interviewing.* Newbury Park, CA: Sage.

130 Anthropac (Version 4.98) [Computer Software]. Columbia: Analytic Technologies.

Chapter 7

The Role of National Community-Based Programs in Improving Nutritional Status in Thailand

Pattanee Winichagoon, PhD

"Villagers did not trust VHVs [village health volunteers] in the early time, but over time, they prove themselves working for the community and gain trust. Sometimes, when villagers do not follow the advice, they felt discouraged, but support from the VHV team was helpful."–Villager from a community near Mahidol University, Salaya campus, describing the village health volunteer program begun in 1982 in rural Thailand, quoted in 2011

Learning Objectives

- Recognize clinical signs of common nutritional deficiencies in developing countries. Include protein-energy malnutrition, vitamin A deficiency, iron-deficiency anemia, and iodine deficiency disorders.

- Identify causes and consequences of undernutrition in women and children common in developing countries.

- Appreciate the wide variety of determinants of malnutrition and recognize the interdisciplinary nature of successful interventions to reduce malnutrition.

- Describe direct and indirect interventions that can alleviate undernutrition in communities.

Case Studies: Developments in Thailand

Introduction to the Case Studies

Although Thailand is a well-known rice exporter, the scientific community determined in the 1970s that malnutrition was prevalent in the country. Five case studies below depict three decades of evolution of Thailand's nutritional situation, beginning with scenarios common to poor developing countries and evolving through industrialization and economic development, reflecting rapid changes in living culture and environment influenced by global trends of urbanization, Westernization, and technological development. During this time, the **double (dual) burden of malnutrition** also emerges.

Case Study 1: Malnutrition and Infections in Young Children: 1981

In northeast Thailand, rural villages contrast the concrete houses that are familiar sights in the capital city Bangkok. Noy, a 15-month-old girl, was living with her parents and grandparents. She had always been small for her age, and her mother said that she did not eat much. She often had diarrhea from March to June, during the hot season when food was scarce, and had respiratory infections from July to October, during the rainy season. Her height of 69 centimeters (27 inches) and weight of 9 kilograms (20 pounds) indicated stunting and wasting, she had scars on the corners of her lips, and her inner eyelids were pale. Her mother, Nim, reported her parents were not pleased to have a girl for their first grandchild. When Noy was very ill, Nim walked 2 miles across the rice fields to the health center to get medicine.

Discussion Questions

- Why does Noy suffer from frequent diarrhea and respiratory infections?
- How might gender disparities contribute to Noy's poor nutritional status and health?

Case Study 2: Maternal and Child Dyads and Consequences During Early Life: 1990s

Another case in the same region involved a poor family that lived in isolation from the other villagers. Since becoming pregnant with her now-30-month-old son, the mother had **goiter** and **anemia**. Her son had cognitive impairment, or mild **cretinism**, and could not talk and walk, although his father made a wooden rail for him to practice walking. He appeared happy. His mother said that she received iron supplements and an iodine solution to add to their drinking water, but was too busy working to comply.

Discussion Questions

- Which nutrient deficiencies cause goiter and anemia? What health consequences have resulted or are likely to result in the mother and son?
- How can public health interventions be modified to increase compliance with supplement recommendations?

Case Study 3: Continuation of Anemia Among Pregnant Women Despite an Iron Supplementation Program: 1990s

Traditional rural Thai diets are rice- and plant-based. Animal-source foods (ASF) are traditionally expensive and unavailable. Iron-deficiency anemia due to iron deficiency threatens children, young girls, and women before and during pregnancy, when demand is three to five times higher. Iron supplementation is inevitably needed. Similar to other developing countries, peripheral health services and the transportation network serving this Thai village were very limited. The antenatal care (ANC) service coverage was only around 30%. Each health center covers a tambon, or a cluster of 5 to 10 villages. People from the tambon often had to walk 2 to 3 miles to the health center, resulting in a perception that trips to the health center for prenatal care were low priority. The central ministry did not always provide an adequate supply of iron tablets.

Discussion Questions

- Which nutrients are provided by ASF that are commonly deficient in plant-based diets in developing nations?
- How can ANC coverage be increased?

Millennium Development Goal 5: Improve Maternal Health. Target 5.B: Achieve universal access to reproductive health

Reproduced from the United Nations. (n.d.). 2015 Millennium Development Goals. Retrieved from http://www.un.org/millenniumgoals/. Accessed August 13, 2013. This source is used for all Millennium Development Goals in this chapter.

Case Study 4: Active Role of Health Volunteers and Community Participation in Alleviating Malnutrition in Children: 1990s

The implementation of primary health care in the 1980s coincided with development of a village health volunteer system (VHV). Growth monitoring and promotion (GMP) is a monitoring of growth and provision of education to mothers/caretakers; iron supplementation during pregnancy was the other contribution. VHVs were trained to use weighing scales for GMP, and decisions for individuals and groups were based on this data. VHVs also encouraged pregnant women to receive prenatal services. Routine data reporting and periodic surveys found reduced prevalence of anemia.

Discussion Questions

- What role does surveillance play in public health nutrition?
- What are the benefits and limitations of using community volunteers?

Case Study 5: Coexistence of Stunting/Mild Micronutrient Deficiency and Obesity and Noncommunicable Diseases

Industrialization leads to less physical activity through **urbanization** and the use of mechanized assistance for crop production. Dietary patterns also change. In the 1980s and 1990s, among children in Thailand, overweight and obesity increased while undernutrition decreased, with stunting and underweight prevalence at 10% and wasting at 5% or less.[1] Subclinical deficiencies of vitamin A, iron, and iodine were commonly reported. Among adults, overnutrition and diet-related chronic diseases now have higher public health priority than undernutrition. Considering the significance of "early life nutrition," known as the "1,000-day" **critical period** of life, maternal and child nutrition should receive equal attention as obesity and noncommunicable diseases (NCDs) in other age groups.

Discussion Questions

- Which factors have contributed to the improvements noted among Thai populations?
- Which problems remain to be addressed? How should they be addressed?

Introduction

Inability to meet requirements for specific nutrients leads to **malnutrition**, with forms including **undernutrition** and **protein–energy malnutrition** (PEM). Malnutrition is underreported since undernutrition is not always recognized when it is a factor in child morbidity and mortality from diarrhea, pneumonia, and measles. However, malnutrition is an urgent public health problem among children and women in developing countries, with 52.5% of all child

deaths attributable to undernutrition, and 44.8% and 60.7% of child deaths due to measles and diarrhea, respectively.[2]

Key Nutritional Deficiencies of Public Health Significance in Developing Countries

Protein–energy malnutrition, vitamin A deficiency, iron-deficiency anemia (IDA), and iodine-deficiency disorders (IDD) are common nutritional deficiencies among young children and women in developing countries. They occur in both rural and urban poor populations. Zinc deficiency is a concern where infections, diarrhea, and anemia are common; deficiencies of various B vitamins can also occur.

Protein-Energy Malnutrition

Cecily Williams recognized **kwashiorkor** as a form of PEM in the 1930s. First attributed to protein deficiency, known as a **protein gap**,[3] kwashiorkor was later also associated with a severe energy deficit, leading to a shift from using protein for growth to using it for energy. Protein–energy malnutrition, whose forms include kwashiorkor and **marasmus**, is commonly referred to as a nutritional problem of young children. Kwashiorkor is more of a protein deficiency, while marasmus refers to a relatively greater energy deficit. Clinical features include edema, poor growth or stunting, wasting, and skin lesions. Deficiencies of micronutrients, such as B vitamins, vitamin A, and iron, often accompany PEM. Also, children with PEM are likely to have frequent infections, especially diarrheal diseases and respiratory tract infections.[4]

Assessment of PEM and the International Growth Reference/Standard

Anthropometry is an approach for assessing nutritional status. Head and chest circumferences are common in clinics, while arm circumference is common in the field, where instruments are limited. More common are anthropometric measurements of weight and height to help assess children's growth and PEM. These measurements are compared against **growth standards** derived from healthy populations of the same ages. The National Center for Health Statistics (NCHS) "**growth reference**," developed from measurements of healthy American children from the 1960s and 1970s,[5] was adopted by the World Health

Organization (WHO) as the international **growth reference** in 1979.[6] Some question its appropriateness for use among diverse populations, where growth may be different due to differences in genetic background, feeding practices, and other environmental factors.

Many countries lack the technical and financial resources to develop their own growth standards. However, Thailand developed its own growth standards and observed a trend of increasing weight and height among both genders. The median trajectory of the currently used Thai standard is almost identical to that of the WHO **growth standard** from birth to 7 years.[7]

In 2006, WHO recommended an initiative to develop an international growth standard based on "an international sample of healthy breastfed infants and young children raised in environments that do not constrain growth" to be used for assessing children of any ethnicity, socioeconomic status, and feeding practice.[8] In the longitudinal Multicentre Growth Reference Study (MGRS), infants from international sites were assessed at weeks 1, 2, 4, and 6 and then monthly through 24 months. These data, together with cross-sectional measurements of children 18 to 60 months, were used to make international growth standards.

Stunting, **wasting**, and **underweight** are individual and population-level indicators used for international comparisons, setting priorities for interventions and monitoring trends. Stunting, or low height-for-age, indicates long-term or chronic undernourishment and/or repeated illnesses. Underweight, or low weight-for-age, reflects severe malnourishment. Wasting, or low weight-for-height, reflects acute malnutrition from poor nourishment or illness, such as diarrhea or respiratory infection.

The common method for classifying children's nutritional status is the extent that a child departs from the median for a specific age. Children falling below two *z*-**scores** are considered malnourished and in need of intervention.[9] At the population level, these indicators are used for screening to identify at-risk populations.

Discrepancies Between NCHS Growth References and WHO Standards

The magnitude of malnutrition determined using WHO standards often differs from that determined using the older NCHS references. The largest differences in prevalence of stunting, underweight, and wasting were found among infants up to 6 months,[10,11,12,13] with WHO standards

identifying higher prevalence for all indicators, particularly wasting. After that, WHO standards identified lower prevalence of underweight and wasting and higher prevalence of stunting and overweight. The WHO growth standard is technically superior, but it magnifies the burden of this public health problem, especially in developing countries.

Growth faltering during early infancy is another indicator of poor nutrition and the need for intervention.[14,15] Anthropometric data from WHO child anthropometrics from 39 national surveys and NCHS demonstrated growth faltering in both weight and length from 6 to 18 months of age. Another analysis with data from 54 countries found more alarming results, with growth faltering before 4 months. A more recent survey, from 2010, found faltering in height to remain similar to that of the 2001 study, while weight faltering was less drastic. Also evident was an increasing trend in overweight. Public health attention is necessary to improve prenatal and postnatal growth through improved maternal nutritional status and infant nutrition.

WHO derived **growth references** based on body mass index (BMI)-for-age growth curves for school-aged children and adolescents using the 1977 NCHS reference for 1 to 24 years, the WHO Child Growth Standards for preschool children aged 18 to 61 months, and the body mass index (BMI) cutoffs for adults. The merge was successful, with only negligible differences between the two data sets for BMI-for-age across all percentiles. The BMI-for-age cutoffs at 19 years old corresponded to the cutoffs for overweight (BMI >25 kg/m^2) and obesity (BMI >30 kg/m^2) in adults.[16]

Global Trends in Malnutrition

The two main approaches to identifying population-level childhood malnutrition are estimation of prevalence, based on the WHO Child Growth Standards discussed above, and estimation of number of undernourished people, based on estimated dietary energy availability using national food balance sheets by the Food and Agriculture Organization (FAO).

Data from the WHO Global Database on Child Growth and Malnutrition and the Child Growth Standards show trends since 1990 and estimated prevalence through 2025 of stunting (**Figure 7-1**) and underweight (**Figure 7-2**). Globally, the proportion of undernutrition has declined, but the number of affected children remains stagnant due to increased population (**Figure 7-3**). The greatest declines are in stunting and underweight in Asia and stunting in

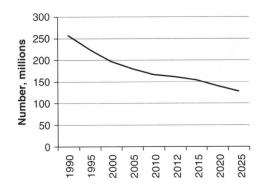

Figure 7-1 Global trends and projections for childhood stunting, 1990-2025

Data from Global Health Observatory Data Repository. (2012). Joint malnutrition estimates (UNICEF-WHO-WB): global and regional trends by UN regions, 1990-2025. Stunting: 1990-2025. Accessed October 16, 2013, from http://apps.who.int/gho/data/view.main.NUTUNSTUNTINGv?lang=en.

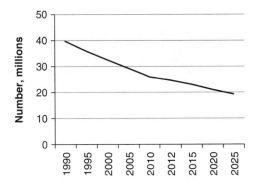

Figure 7-2 Global trends and projections for childhood underweight, 1990-2025

Data from Global Health Observatory Data Repository. (2012). Joint malnutrition estimates (UNICEF-WHO-WB): global and regional trends by UN regions, 1990-2025. Stunting: 1990-2025. Accessed October 16, 2013, from http://apps.who.int/gho/data/view.main.NUTUNSTUNTINGv?lang=en.

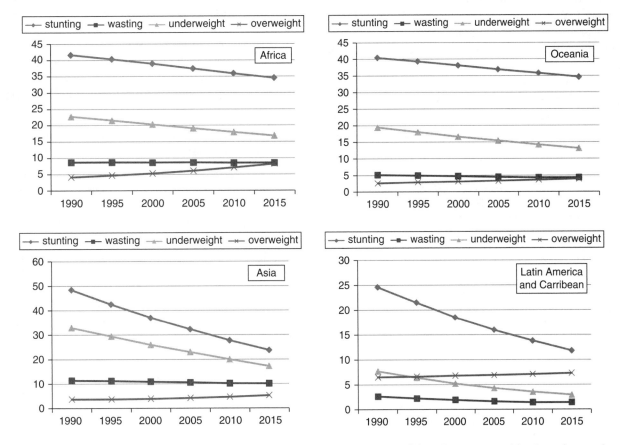

Figure 7-3 Trends of prevalence of various forms of malnutrition by geographical regions of the world

Data from the World Health Organization (WHO). (n.d.). Global database on Child growth and Malnutrition. UNICEF-WHO-The World Bank: Joint child malnutrition estimates: Levels and trends. Retrieved from http://www.who.int/nutgrowthdb/estimates/en/.

Table 7-1 Prevalence and number of under-5 child malnutrition, 2011

| Malnutrition | Prevalence and Number | | Change from Number in 1990 |
	%	Number, millions	%
Stunting	26	165	−35
Underweight	16	101	−36
Wasting	8	52	−11
Overweight	7	43	+54

Data from United Nation's Children's Fund, World Health Organization, The World Bank: Joint child malnutrition estimates – levels and trends. (2012). Available at http://www.who.int/nutgrowthdb/statistical_tables.pdf. Accessed September 6, 2013.

Latin America and the Caribbean. The increase in obesity is another concern, and stunting, underweight, and overweight coexist in many regions (**Table 7-1** and Figure 7-3). The Millennium Development Goal (MDG) to eradicate global hunger by 2015 is unlikely to be achieved.

While WHO uses anthropometry to measure undernutrition, FAO uses national **food balance sheets** and other food production data. Undernourishment is considered present when per capita energy availability is below cutoffs that represent energy needs. The *State of the Food Insecurity in the World YEAR* progress report[17] presents this information (**Figure 7-4**). Undernourishment in developing nations declined from approximately 30% in the late 1960s to about 16% in 2010, despite a sharp rise in 2009 due to short-term spikes in food prices.

Birth Weight as an Indicator for Maternal Nutrition Status

Appropriate gestational weight gain based on prepregnancy BMI can help evaluate maternal nutrition status, but prepregnancy weight can be difficult to obtain in developing countries where prenatal care starts late or is irregular. Birth weight is an alternative reflection of maternal nutrition on a public health level when assessing nutritional status or designing appropriate interventions. Since birth weight is an outcome of pregnancy, measuring it is not useful for measuring an individual's nutritional status during pregnancy.

Low birth weight (LBW) is defined as birth weight less than 2,500 grams regardless of gestational age at term.

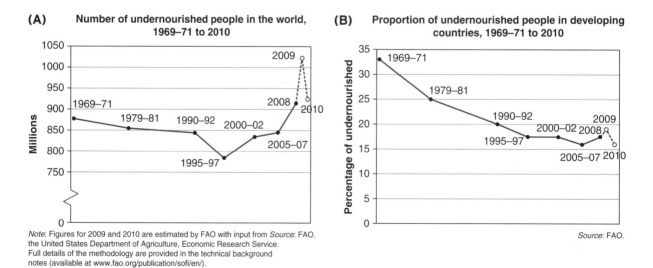

(A) Number of undernourished people in the world, 1969–71 to 2010

(B) Proportion of undernourished people in developing countries, 1969–71 to 2010

Note: Figures for 2009 and 2010 are estimated by FAO with input from *Source*: FAO. the United States Department of Agriculture, Economic Research Service. Full details of the methodology are provided in the technical background notes (available at www.fao.org/publication/sofi/en/).

Source: FAO.

Figure 7-4 (A) Number of undernourished people in the world, 1969-1971 to 2010 (B) Proportion of undernourished people in developing countries, 1969-1971 to 2010

Reproduced from Food and Agriculture Organization of the United Nations. (2010). The State of Food Insecurity in the World 2010: Addressing food insecurity in protracted crises. Rome: Author.

This facilitates assessment of maternal nutrition because gestational age is not always known. As a result, LBW is sometimes due to premature birth. In developing countries, reported prevalence of LBW can be underestimated because it may include data only from deliveries in healthcare facilities.

Undernutrition in Adults

In adults, malnutrition is assessed using **body mass index**. A BMI under 18.5 is considered **underweight**, or a chronic energy deficit, and BMI over 25, or over 23 for Asians, is overweight. The lower BMI to define overweight among Asians is due to findings that at the same BMI as other populations, Asian populations have more body fat and higher risk of cardiovascular disease.[18,19]

Iodine, Iron, and Vitamin A Deficiencies

In addition to PEM, **micronutrient** deficiencies are also common in low-income countries. These deficiencies are also referred to as "hidden hunger" because their health and functional consequences may not be directly obvious.[20] Overt clinical signs and symptoms are recognized only when the deficiency is quite severe. Iodine, vitamin A, and iron deficiencies are the most common. They are recognized as major global public health problems in developing countries, and global efforts have been made to alleviate them. Established by WHO, the Micronutrients Database of Vitamin and Mineral Nutrition Information System compiles data from national representative surveys on common indicators for iodine deficiency, anemia, and vitamin A deficiency.[21,22,23]

Iodine Deficiency Disorders

Iodine is the essential constituent of thyroid hormones, which affect all cells in the body. It contributes to metabolism, growth, and development. Iodine deficiency can cause goiter, physical and mental impairment, stillbirth, and spontaneous abortion. Consequences of iodine deficiency disorders (IDD) can be irreversible.[24]

Seafood and seaweed are rich sources of iodine in sea water, but consumption of seafood may be low due to cost and accessibility. Plants and ASF can provide iodine when grown or raised on iodine-rich food. However, iodine depletion can occur through leaching from soils by rain and deforestation. Mountains and plains that have been exposed for longer are more likely to be deficient.

Before 2007, goiter prevalence in school-aged children was a traditional proxy indicator for IDD at the community level, because schoolchildren are easily targeted and palpation of the thyroid gland to assess goiter is noninvasive and does not require equipment. The measurement is subjective, however, and thyroid gland enlargement occurs only in severe deficiency. In 2007, the International Council for Control of Iodine Deficiency Disorders (ICCIDD) and WHO recommended the use of urinary iodine concentration (UIC), which reflects dietary intake, as a population-level indicator. However, serum thyroglobulin is a more accurate indicator than UIC.[25]

Universal salt iodization (USI), or adding iodine to all salt used in the food industry, households, and livestock feed, was recommended as a global strategy in 1993. A USI fortification program can be successful because salt is commonly consumed by all individuals in any population, and the iodization technology is simple and cost effective, costing only $0.05 per person per year. In industrialized countries, processed foods contribute significantly to habitual diets and are potentially significant vehicles for fortified salt. The Netherlands and Switzerland have seen success with this strategy,[26] but the United States does not permit iodized salt in processed foods. In developing countries, salt used in the household remains the main source of iodine. However, the presence of numerous small salt producers makes quality assurance difficult. In addition, choices such as soy sauce and fish sauce are common alternatives to salt in some countries, including Thailand. Along with UIC, the percentage of households using iodized salt is used to monitor USI within regions.

WHO does not recommend supplementation when USI has been established for more than two years and household use of iodized salt is over 90%. In moderate-to-severe iodine-deficient areas, iodine supplementation prior to or during early pregnancy reduces perinatal and infant mortality, eliminates new cases of cretinism, and increases development scores by 10–20%.[27] The effects in populations with mild to moderate IDD are not yet certain.

Switzerland provides an example of a long-standing, cost-effective, and successful salt iodization program. To reduce the prevalence of cretinism and goiter, salt iodization was introduced in 1922. Indicators of IDD virtually disappeared by 1930. By 1988, 92% of retail salt and 76% of salt for human consumption, including in the food industry, was iodized. Adverse effects of iodization are minimal.[28] However, despite sufficient intakes among schoolchildren and pregnant women, recent national surveys found weaning infants and lactating women to be at risk of inadequate intake based on UIC.[29] Because household coverage is high and processed foods contribute significantly to iodine intake, the risk of inadequacy of iodine among lactating women could be explained by loss into breastmilk, as well as depletion of thyroid iodine stores during pregnancy and lactation when the requirement is highest.

> *Public Health Core Competency 1: Analytical and Assessment Skills 5: Identifies sources of public health data and information*
>
> Reproduced from Council on Linkages Between Academia and Public Health Practice. 2010 May. Core Competencies for Public Health Professionals. Washington, DC: Public Health Foundation. http://www.phf.org/resourcestools/Documents/Core_Competencies_for_Public_Health_Professionals_2010May.pdf. Accessed August 13, 2013. This source is used for all Public Health Core Competencies in this chapter.

Iodine intake remains insufficient for 285 million school-aged children and nearly two billion people globally (**Figure 7-5**).[30] Deficiency is highest in Southeast Asia, but it is also noticeably high in Europe. Because of higher physiological needs, UIC among pregnant women is lower than that of school-aged children living in the same families.[31,32]

Iron-Deficiency Anemia

Iron is a constituent of **hemoglobin** and a catalyst for various enzymes involved in respiration and energy metabolism, and it plays a role in immune functions. Moderate anemia reduces aerobic function, leading to shortness of breath and compromising the ability to perform physical work.[33,34] Severe anemia is associated with perinatal maternal mortality. Iron also plays critical roles in neurological development and cognitive functions during early life.[35]

Iron is in its **heme** form in ASF, and its less absorbable, **non-heme**, form in plant sources. Iron-deficiency anemia (IDA) is common in developing countries where diets are plant-based. Not only is heme iron intake low, but also intake of compounds that inhibit non-heme iron absorption is high.[36] Phytate, for example, is an inhibitor in most staple grains, such as wheat, corn/maize, rice, and legumes, and polyphenols are inhibitory compounds in green leafy vegetables. In contrast, vitamin C and animal protein are enhancers of non-heme iron absorption. Food-based strategies to meet population needs must consider quantity and bioavailability of dietary iron.

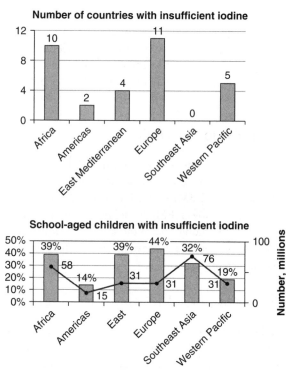

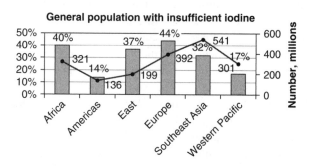

Figure 7-5 Proportion and number of school-aged children and general population having insufficient iodine intakes by urinary iodine concentration (UIC) by WHO region and global, 2011

Data from Andersson, M., Karumbunathan, V., & Zimmermann, M. B. (2012). Global iodine status in 2011 and trends over the past decade. *Journal of Nutrition, 142*(4), 744-750.

To prevent anemia and meet increased physiological needs, iron supplementation is recommended during pregnancy, before age 2, and among reproductive-aged women where the prevalence is very high (over 40%).[37] Although several countries have adopted this measure as a national policy, barriers to success include disruption of supplies and services, especially at the peripheral health functionaries, and lack of adherence to daily supplementation regimens among pregnant women who do not recognize the need for supplementation, have a fear of giving birth to big babies, or forget.[38] In addition, short-term supplementation does not appear effective for women who enter pregnancy with poor iron status and begin prenatal care late. WHO also recommends weekly iron and folic acid supplementation for menstruating women to improve iron status.[39]

Although anemia can have causes aside from iron deficiency, it is useful for assessing population-level iron status in public health. The technique requires only a finger-prick blood sample and a simple piece of equipment called a hemocue. About half of anemia in developing countries is caused by iron deficiency; the other cases of anemia are attributed to deficiencies of other nutrients and other causes. Conversely, not all iron-deficient individuals have severe enough deficiency to have anemia. Worldwide, two billion people have iron deficiency, making it the most common nutrient deficiency. Southeast Asia and Africa have the highest prevalence (**Table 7-2**). Anemia is also widely present even in developed countries where diets contain more ASF than in most developing countries.

Vitamin A Deficiency

Vitamin A is essential for growth, vision, immune function, and cellular differentiation and proliferation.[40] Vitamin A deficiency (VAD) leads to **xerophthalmia**, progressing from night blindness and dryness of the conjunctiva and cornea, to ulceration, keratomalacia, and blindness.[41] Children with mild VAD have higher mortality than their healthy counterparts. Studies in Asia and Africa have found that vitamin A supplementation can reduce child mortality by 16–54%. VAD often coexists with severe PEM and infections, such as diarrheal diseases, pneumonia, and measles.

Vitamin A is present in foods as preformed vitamin A in ASF, such as liver and dairy products, and as provitamins, mainly carotenoids, in fruits and vegetables. While preformed vitamin A is readily available for utilization by the body, carotenoids must be converted to retinol in the body, with 6 to 21 units of carotenoids required to produce each unit of active vitamin A. In Asia and Africa, young children and pregnant and lactating women are at risk for VAD due to low intake of ASF. Moreover, as a fat-soluble vitamin, vitamin A absorption requires sufficient dietary fat, but habitual diets in some populations, such as rural Thailand in early 1960s, contribute only 8–9% of total energy.[42]

Public health recommendations include vitamin A supplementation programs for children under 5 in more than 70 developing countries where VAD is prevalent. Supplements can be given once every six months by organizing a national immunization day or child day. To reduce VAD among women in poor developing countries, WHO recommends increasing dietary diversity and biofortification strategies rather than vitamin A supplementation among both pregnant and lactating women.[43,44] In addition, biofortification

Table 7-2 Worldwide prevalence of anemia and number (millions) of population affected by geographical region, 1993-2005

WHO Region	Preschool Children		Pregnant Women		Reproductive-Age Women	
	Prevalence %	# millions	Prevalence %	# millions	Prevalence %	# millions
Africa	67.6	83.5	57.1	17.2	47.5	69.9
Americas	29.3	23.1	24.1	3.9	17.8	39.0
Europe	21.7	11.1	25.1	2.6	19.0	40.8
Eastern Mediterranean	46.7	0.8	44.2	7.13	2.4	39.8
Southeast Asia	65.5	115.3	48.2	18.1	45.7	182.0
Western Pacific	23.1	27.4	30.7	7.6	21.5	97.0
Global	47.4	293.1	41.8	56.4	30.2	468.4

Reproduced from the WHO. (2008). Worldwide prevalence of anemia 1993-2005, WHO global database on anemia, 2008.

Table 7-3 Worldwide prevalence and number of young children and pregnant women affected by vitamin A deficiency by geographical region

WHO Region	Night Blindness				S Retinol < 0.7 ↔mol/L			
	Preschool Children		Pregnant Women		Preschool Children		Pregnant Women	
	Prevalence %	# millions	Prevalence %	# millions	Prevalence %	# millions	Prevalence %	# millions
Africa	2	2.55	9.8	3.02	44.4	56.4	13.5	4.18
Americas	0.6	0.36	4.4	0.5	15.6	8.68	2	0.23
Europe	0.8	0.24	3.5	0.22	19.7	5.81	11.6	0.72
Eastern Mediterranean	1.2	0.77	7.2	1.09	20.4	13.2	16.1	2.42
Southeast Asia	0.5	1.01	9.9	3.84	49.9	91.5	17.3	6.69
Western Pacific	0.2	0.26	4.8	1.09	12.9	14.3	21.5	4.9
Global	0.9	5.17	7.8	9.75	33.3	190	15.3	19.1

Reproduced from the World Health Organization. (2009). Global prevalence of vitamin A deficiency in populations at risk 1995-2005: WHO global database on vitamin A deficiency. Geneva.

of orange-flesh sweet potatoes effectively improved vitamin A status among young children in Africa.[45]

VAD in young children and pregnant women continues to require attention (**Table 7-3**). Night blindness and serum retinol, a **biochemical** indicator, are used to assess VAD. Although night blindness affects fewer than 1% of children globally, pregnant women are more affected. Greater proportions in all regions have marginal vitamin A deficiency.

Zinc, Vitamin D, and Calcium Deficiencies

Additional micronutrients can also be of public health concern, although current limitations include identifying appropriate indicators that are feasible and have functional significance. Zinc, vitamin D, and calcium are among the micronutrients that may have global public health importance, including in Thailand.

Zinc Deficiency

Zinc is an essential mineral for immune function, growth, and development, and deficiency is often suspected where soil zinc concentrations are low. No appropriate indicator for assessing zinc status among populations yet exists,[46,47] although some research studies have used serum zinc as an indicator.[48,49] Due to its efficacy in lessening diarrhea incidence and duration, zinc supplementation is recommended in the treatment of diarrhea.[50,51]

Calcium and Vitamin D

Calcium and vitamin D are two nutrients important for bone health. They are also involved in muscle function, immunity, and the circulatory system, although their roles are less well defined.[52,53] The main food sources of calcium are dairy products, small bony fish, and some green leafy vegetables. Fatty fish and fortified foods are the main sources of vitamin D, which can also be obtained through **endogenous** skin synthesis with adequate sunlight exposure.[54]

Calcium intakes are generally low when milk consumption is low, as is characteristic of many Asian populations.[55,56] In Thailand, the school milk program has led to increased calcium intakes among young children through adolescents for the past two decades. Daily calcium intakes of older adults and pregnant women, remain at half of recommendations.[57] Favorable vitamin D receptor genotypes and less urinary calcium losses due to small body build may imply lower optimal calcium intakes for Thais than Caucasians.[58] Recent evidence suggests the presence of vitamin D deficiency even in tropical areas with abundant sunshine.[59] Avoidance of sun exposure and lack of dietary vitamin D are likely causes.

Multiple Micronutrient Deficiencies and Nutrient Interactions

Multiple nutrient deficiencies often occur in populations with widespread malnutrition. High diet quality helps ensure nutritional adequacy, and plant-based, monotonous diets can lack essential nutrients. Deficiency in one nutrient may result in a compromised function that involves another. For example, iron deficiency can interfere with iodine status, and restoration of iron status can improve the response to iodine intervention.[60] Likewise, excess of one nutrient may interfere with the utilization of another. Interactions are generally stronger when the nutrients are provided as supplements than when they are from fortified foods.[61,62]

Based on successful programs, WHO recommends multiple micronutrient powder containing at least iron, vitamin A, and zinc for children 6–23 months old where prevalence of anemia is over 20%.[63] In randomized controlled studies among school children, noodles or biscuits fortified with multiple micronutrients were provided in school lunches or snacks. Results were improved micronutrient status, cognition, and morbidity in children.[64,65,66]

Maternal micronutrient status in preconception, pregnancy, and lactation is often treated separately in public health programs.[67] Furthermore, most developing nations include only iron and folic acid supplementation. In comparison, multiple micronutrient supplementation can improve maternal micronutrient status,[68,69] increase birth weight, and reduce prevalence of LBW, but has not been shown to increase birth length or gestational length[70,71] or prevalence of stillbirth or neonatal death.[72] During lactation, maternal status and intake of the B vitamins (except folate), vitamin A, selenium, and iodine affect the breastmilk's contents of these nutrients.[73]

Global Movements to Address Malnutrition

The 1990 World Summit for Children was organized by the United Nations Children's Fund (UNICEF) and WHO as an opportunity for United Nations (UN) member states to address children's needs, including education, health, and nutrition. The 1992 International Conference on Nutrition organized by FAO and WHO and the World Food Summit in 1995 further defined goals and strategies, and national progress was monitored in systems such as the Global Database on Child Growth and Malnutrition, which is a compilation of anthropometric, birth-weight, and key micronutrient deficiency data collected by individual nations or regions.

Addressing Malnutrition in Developing Nations

Impacts of undernutrition, including stunting, on the health and function of young children have been recognized, and recent decades have seen efforts to reduce malnutrition in developing nations, although undernutrition persists. Overnutrition is an increasing concern, contributing to the double burden of malnutrition, particularly where economic growth is rapid. Formerly considered a problem of adults, overnutrition in the womb and early life increases the risk of chronic diseases later. Improving maternal and young child nutrition in the first two years could be critical in reducing obesity and diet-related chronic diseases in developing countries.[74]

Multilevel Causes of Malnutrition in Children and Women

Multiple, often interrelated, determinants affect maternal and child nutrition (**Figure 7-6**). These factors can be categorized as immediate, underlying, and basic causes. Rather than simply treating malnutrition through provision of supplements, recognizing the complexity of these determinants of malnutrition encourages more holistic approaches. Both direct, or **nutrition-specific**, and indirect, or **nutrition-sensitive**, interventions should be implemented for a long-term sustainable impact (**Box 7-1**).[75,76]

Interventions for improving childhood nutrition include the promotion of **exclusive breastfeeding** for six months and appropriate **complementary feeding (CF)** from 6 to 23 months. During this period, no other foods or water should be given, as breastmilk provides both nutrients and other constituents, such as immunoglobulin, which helps to protect the child from common infection. After six months, it is essential that proper quality and quantity of CF are provided, as breastmilk alone is not adequate to meet the rapid increases in the nutrient requirements. Plant-based diets in developing nations can prevent children from meeting energy, protein, and other micronutrient needs. In Asia, for example, the staple food, rice, is very low in fat, protein, and micronutrients, and its protein quality is low. Traditional complementary foods are therefore often inadequate in micronutrients. Increasing ASF and food fortification are strategies to improve the bioavailability and adequacy of micronutrients in diets of young children.

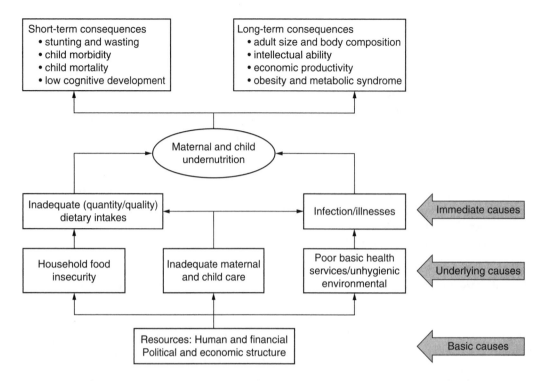

Figure 7-6 Determinants and consequences of maternal and child malnutrition

Modified from Black, R. E., Allen, L. H., Bhutta, Z. A., Caulfield, L. E., Onis, M., Ezzati, M.,. . . Rivera, J. (2008). Maternal and child undernutrition: global and regional exposures and health consequences. Maternal and Child Undernutrition Study Group. *Lancet 371*, 243-60.

Box 7-1 Direct nutrition intervention with sufficient evidence of efficacy for implementation in high stunting burden countries

Maternal and Birth Outcomes

Iron-folate supplementation

Maternal supplementation of multiple micronutrients

Maternal iodine through iodization of salt

Maternal calcium supplementation

Reduction of tobacco consumption and indoor air pollution

Newborn Babies

Promotion of breastfeeding (individual and group counseling)

Infants and Children

Promotion of breastfeeding (individual and group counseling)

Behavioral change communications for improved complementary feeding

Zinc supplementation

Zinc supplementation in management of diarrhea

Universal salt iodization

Hand washing and hygiene

Treatment of severe acute malnutrition

Modified from Bhutta, Z. A., Ahmed, T., Black, R. E., Cousens, S., Dewey, K., Giugliani, E., ... Shekar, M., for the Maternal and Child Undernutrition Study Group. (2008). What works? Interventions for maternal and child undernutrition and survival. *Lancet, 371*(9610), 417-440.

Malnutrition in Thailand: Past, Present, and the Way Forward

Thailand has been the world's major rice exporter for decades. Before 1960, agriculture was the major sector, with rice being the main dietary staple. Classified as a low-income nation in the 1960s, Thailand formulated its first five-year development plan, the National Economic Development Plan (NEDP), in 1962. The first three NEDPs focused primarily on economic development.

In 1960, the first U.S. Interdepartmental Committee on Nutrition for National Development (ICNND), in collaboration with Thai scientists in the Ministry of Health and at universities, conducted the first national nutrition survey of the civilian population and military personnel. Although hospitals routinely treated children for diarrhea or pneumonia, malnourishment had not been a concurrent focus. The nutrition survey exposed malnutrition among young children in various parts of the country, identifying undernutrition, IDA, IDD, deficiencies of B vitamins, and urinary bladder stone disease, later explained by low phosphate intakes and high intakes of oxalate foods, resulting in crystalluria and bladder stone formation.[77,78] While these findings triggered concern among scientists and those involved in the study, the information was neither disseminated to the public nor brought to the attention of high-level policy makers, thereby delaying progress in correcting these problems. The process and progress in Thailand from the 1970s to the 1990s is presented in the following sections.[79,80,81]

Impetus for the Formulation of the First National Food and Nutrition Policy/Plan

In the 1970s, Thailand already had trained professionals in the fields of medicine and food sciences. Researchers studied dietary intakes and the extent of malnutrition among young children and women in rural areas. In the early 1970s, after the ICNND exposed widespread malnutrition, advocates attempted to include a national nutrition plan for inclusion in the third National Economic and Social Development Plan (NESDP; 1972–76). Although the advocates failed to get nutrition into the plan due to political instability, the plan did include family planning, an important social program, in order to control population growth. Advocates therefore argued that nutrition should be included in the fourth NESDP because malnutrition due to low income and social disparity hinders national development, and investment in prevention and control of malnutrition promotes healthier children and a better national future.

Also in the 1970s, the international community recognized the multifactorial causes of malnutrition and the significance of multisectoral policy and programs. Officers from relevant ministries in Thailand attended a training workshop on multisectoral planning in the United States. This core group of officers worked with other national experts to formulate the National Food and Nutrition Policy (NFNP) to be included in the fourth NESDP (1977–81). Progress was facilitated by the established presence of nutrition and related expertise (though mainly in academia and the health ministry), nutrition advocacy aimed at high-level planners, and consensus building among agencies. Also, UN agencies provided expert technical support to national committees.

Implementing the NFNP at scale required an appropriate entry point for nutrition improvement in children and women to be successful.[82] Strategies included increasing protein and energy food sources and mobilizing stakeholders and sectors, including at the grassroots level. In addition, a community-based integrated nutrition project, the Nong-hai Project, was used as a World Bank–supported model for broader pilot implementation.[83]

Nutrition Policy and Program in the 1970s

Capacity development in nutrition was needed in different sectors, with early focus on specific nutrition interventions. Short trainings were provided for doctors and nurses at district hospitals and agriculture extension personnel. Primary education teachers and supervisors were trained to teach nutrition in the schools. Preservice training included nutrition in community medicine for medical and nursing students, and strengthening undergraduate degree programs in public health nutrition. The first graduate program in nutrition was developed to prepare nutritionists to conduct research and to plan and supervise national nutrition programs planned for scaling up to national levels.

Seven major nutritional problems were targeted as the basis for goal-setting, with emphasis on children under 5, schoolchildren, and pregnant and lactating women. As the poorest and most malnourished regions, northeast rural areas received priority.[84] The multisectoral national-level master plan required relevant ministries to include nutrition activities in their respective sector plans. Therefore, each subprogram had to compete for priority within the sector.

As a result, nutrition budgets varied greatly among sectors, and nutrition programming was inadequate overall.

Evaluation is essential for assessing effects of and improving public health programs. The midterm evaluation of the first NFNP in 1979 found disappointing progress toward nutritional goals. The healthcare sector was the main implementer, partly due to its established network down to the grassroots. The master NFNP did not have a clear mechanism for aligning sectoral activities. Interventions were therefore implemented vertically, and thus were fragmented and curative rather than preventive in nature. Moreover, frontline health personnel were without adequate training in nutrition planning. In the education sector, nutrition was not a distinct subject in the curriculum of formal, vocational, or nonformal education. In the agriculture sector, the outreach to the periphery was not extensive. In addition, the government system and the infrastructure and capacity were not yet sufficient.

Food and Nutrition Policy and Planning in the Fifth and Sixth NESDPs

The midterm review of the first period of NFNP implementation revealed poverty to be an underlying cause of malnutrition. Poverty is a result of social disparity, economic inequity, and unequal distribution or ineffective basic services in health and other areas. Nutrition should be integrated into the nation's broader social and health development, and the strategy and policy instrument for its implementation in Thailand were modified. Two of the nation's key programs contributing to more effective nutrition programming in Thailand are (1) the poverty alleviation plan (PAP) and (2) primary health care (PHC).

Poverty Alleviation Plan

Previously, based on the concept of economic growth and its trickle-down effect, more than 200 committees were appointed for different tasks, making duplications of efforts inevitable. The poverty alleviation plan targeted 288 districts in 38 provinces, mainly in northeastern and northern Thailand, in the first year, and expanded over the next five years. Such targeting allows integration of efforts and resources. Harmonization of macro- and micro-level structures was a reform to better align top-down macro-policy and bottom-up local planning. The goals were to improve the standard of living to a subsistence level by provision of basic services and appropriate technology, to encourage

participation and to support people to gradually take care of their own needs.

Intensive government support was provided for high-poverty areas, defined as having four or five of these criteria: transportation difficulties, lack of agricultural landholdings, inadequate agricultural productivity or low income, poor health, inadequate clean drinking water, and lack of knowledge on how to improve quality of life. "Intermediate areas" had two to three of the above problems and required less government support, and "advanced areas" had very few problems and received far less government support. Government support included: (1) rural job creation programs to provide employment opportunities during the dry season; (2) village development projects and activities, such as fish ponds, water sources, and vaccines for prevention of livestock diseases, to increase family incomes; (3) provision of basic services such as health care, clean water supply, and a literacy program; and (4) agricultural programs, including nutritious food production emphasizing foods for young children, upland rice and soil improvement projects, household food security, and income generation.

Millennium Development Goal 1: Eradicate Extreme Poverty and Hunger. Target 1.A: Halve, between 1990 and 2015, the proportion of people whose income is less than $1.25 a day

Target 1.B: Achieve full and productive employment and decent work for all, including women and young people

Primary Health Care in Thailand

The concept of PHC emerged from the field operational studies in rural northern communities with the goal of promoting self-help care, which is the core of preventive care. In these communities, roles of health officers went from service providers to "facilitators," as volunteers became active "mobilizers." After the Alma Ata declaration in 1978, Thailand adopted and implemented PHC, including aspects such as health education, endemic disease control, maternal and child care, immunization, provision of essential drugs, disease treatments, nutrition promotion, sanitation, and a safe water supply.

Nationwide implementation of PHC required new community-level organization and management. The three necessary components were community organization, financing, and manpower development, in the form of village volunteers organized by the health sector. The ministry of the interior also established community organizations or committees to plan, monitor, and evaluate program activities. PHC development had three stages.

1. Human resources and community organization development

   Village-based volunteers ("mobilizers") were responsible for health development activities in the community with support from frontline health officers. An initial two-week training session prepared volunteers to be village health communicators (VHCs). Training included grassroots-level and in-service training, and eventually exchange visits between communities. Select volunteers received additional training and became village health volunteers (VHVs). Each VHC was responsible for a cluster of 10 to 20 households, with a total of 10 to 20 volunteers per village. These VHCs were expected to communicate various health messages between health functionaries and the community. The ratio of facilitators to mobilizers was 1:100.

   The process of selecting volunteers began with a sociogram in which villagers identified whom they turn to for advice. Identified leaders were then trained to work in their own communities, receiving, as incentives, free medical services for themselves and later for their families. Still, attrition rates were high in the early phase of PHC, and replacements were necessary to maintain the cadre of volunteers.

   The volunteers promoted preventive health care through programs such as growth monitoring and encouraging childhood immunization and prenatal care. By the end of the 1980s, over 700,000 VHCs and 50,000 VHVs had been trained in nearly all villages in the country. The system remains dominant in Thailand rural areas. Volunteers receive peer acceptance and respect from their communities, and volunteerism has been passed on to the next generation, who may be children or other relatives of the volunteers. Generally, younger generations are more educated and better able to keep records than older adults.

   The success of community-based nutrition improvement activities depends on strong community participation with support from facilitators from health and other sectors. The focus of the interface between community leaders and facilitators is to define problems and plan solutions. The interface between facilitators and mobilizers focuses on specific skills training,

supervision, and quality assurance. Specific programs that were strengthened through primary health care included maternal and child health care and family planning, nutrition, environmental health, and control and eradication of communicable diseases.

2. Community self-financing and management

   Financing was the most challenging aspect of PHC. The health budget in 1969 to 2000 was 2.7–7.5% of the fiscal budget in Thailand, or 0.4–1.1% of gross domestic product (GDP). This was insufficient to fully cover PHC costs. The essential drug fund demonstrates the co-op-like model of village PHC funding. The government provided a small amount of seeding funds or provision of essential drugs, and the fund could be established when at least 60% of village households agreed to contribute by buying a share of 10 baht ($0.3) per household. Similar models were tried for sanitation, clean drinking water, and nutrition, but success was less than for the drug funds. Next, a health card was used as a health insurance scheme to replace the co-op system. It was available to families for 500 baht and pregnant women for 100 baht. The system evolved to its current system of universal coverage for health care.

3. Restructuring the health system and multisectoral approach

   Before the PHC, the few hospitals in Thailand were at the provincial level and located only in large districts. The public health system was extensive, but curative services were provided mainly by midwives or junior sanitarians. The PHC scale-up included more district-level hospitals with at least 10 beds, and improvements in quality of service and the referral system. Further improvements included increasing numbers of healthcare centers and personnel.

   When new programs show potential to be feasible and beneficial, the Ministry of Health includes them in the fiscal budget for the following year. This allows external funding to gradually decrease for that specific activity to allow support for newer activities. Thus, aid from international agencies was crucial early in the PHC, since local budgets did not yet cover new nutrition programs. When primary health care was implemented and scaled up as a national program in 1982, the communities assumed responsibility to volunteer labor (in kind) or any materials available in the community, as well as funds as described above.

Growth Monitoring Program

The scale-up of the Thai growth-monitoring and promotion program (GMP) relied on village volunteers and maternal participation. Simple and practical indicators, a weighing scale, and nutrition education were provided. VHVs and VHCs were responsible for weighing children, interpreting the results, and communicating them to mothers. Weighing was conducted quarterly, and children were classified according to the severity of malnutrition using Gomez's classification. Moderately and severely malnourished children received more attention, including infection management, provision of free complementary foods, and monthly weight monitoring. If there was no or slow improvement, then causes would be further analyzed by health personnel. Nutrition education was provided for children who were healthy or mildly malnourished, but supplemental food for these children was not provided unless agreed on by the community.

The government provided seed money or equipment so that villages could provide supplementary food for undernourished children. Community members contributed by purchasing shares in the co-op. Surplus food could be sold to needy communities, and the income was dedicated to a nutrition fund. Villagers further modified the complementary food to various snack products to provide saleable goods. The success of the GMP varied by village. Although there was no proper documentation, increased availability of volunteers, maternal understanding of benefits, and home visits for children who did not attend scheduled sessions likely contributed to better GMP effectiveness, but no proper evaluation has yet incorporated child growth monitoring and village food processing in this context. Evaluation of the growth monitoring and promotion

elsewhere did not show convincingly that this intervention was effective.[85] Despite some drawbacks, GMP continued for years, with coverage reaching one million children in 1982, and increasing after that. The GMP ceased after two decades, when it was deemed unnecessary due to only a mild degree of malnutrition remaining.

The GMP demonstrates that community-level monitoring can be implemented with limited training and simple equipment and indicators. Data were quickly made available for use in program planning. However, one limitation is lack of precision due to simple weighing and possible biases in the self-selection for mothers and children who choose to attend GMP. In addition, community volunteers might not be able to include all children in each round of weighing, resulting in a possible underestimate of undernutrition. Periodic national representative surveys or other national health surveys are preferred where resources and technical expertise are available.

Strengthening of Community-Integrated Programs: Basic Minimum Needs

During the second NFNP, in the fifth NESDP, intersectoral collaboration was inadequate because many sectors saw nutrition as a problem within the health sector. The combined efforts of the social indicators exercise and PHC led to development of the basic minimal needs (BMN), which include nutrition as one of eight components contributing to "quality of life." BMN components were translated into 32 practical indicators (**Box 7-2**). The proposed scoring system and criteria for success were adjustable according to the community's level of development. Multisectoral teams at the district and tambon level supervised community

---

Box 7-2 Basic Minimum Needs (BMN) Indicators

BMN Components	Indicators	Criteria of Success
I. Adequate food and nutrition	1. Proper nutrition from birth to 5 years, % prevalence of malnutrition (MN) below criterion levels:	
	• Third-degree MN	0
	• Second-degree MN	< 2
	• First-degree MN	< 25
	2. School-age children receiving adequate food for nutrition, % prevalence of malnutrition below criterion level	< 8
	3. Pregnant women receiving adequate and proper food, % prevalence of infant birthweight > 3,000 g	60

BMN Components	Indicators	Criteria of Success
II. Proper housing and environment	4. % HH proper housing, lasting at least five years	84
	5. % HH with tidy and hygienic living quarters	60
	6. % HH having proper latrines	75
	7. % HH having adequate drinking water for family members all year round (estimated at 2 liters/person/day)	95
III. Access to necessary basic services for good living and occupation	8. % infants < 1 year old having complete vaccination for BCG, DPT, OPV, and measles	90
	9. % school children with primary education	99
	10. % primary-school children with immunization for BCG, DPT	90
	11. % of 14- to 50-year-old people who are literate	95
	12. % family access to occupational, health, legal, and other information at least once a month	85
	13. % pregnant women with adequate antenatal services	70
	14. % pregnant women with adequate delivery and postpartum services	70
IV. Security and safety	15. Security in life and property	100
V. Efficient food production and gathering	16. % HH growing alternate crops or soil-preserving crops	30
	17. % HH using fertilizer to increase yield	50
	18. % HH using pest prevention and control	60
	19. % HH using prevention and control of animal diseases	40
	20. % HH using plants and breeds recommended by agriculture specialists	60
VI. Family planning	21. % family having no more than two children and free choice of family planning methods	75
VII. Participation in community development	22. % family members participating in self-help groups in the community	50
	23. % family participating in self-help community development	100
	24. % family participating in care of public properties	100
	25. % family preserving and promoting tradition/culture	100
	26. % family preserving natural resources	100
	27. % family eligible members active in voting	50
	28. Village committee being able to make and implement community projects	100
VIII. Spiritual and ethical morality	29. % family participating in cooperative and sharing concerns	100
	30. % family participating in religious ceremonies/events once a month	90
	31. % family members neither gambling nor addicted to alcohol or other narcotics	85
	32. % HH with modest living and spending on social events	90

Abbreviations: BCG, bacillus Calmette-Guerrin (tuberculosis); DPT, diphtheria, pertussis, tetanus; HH, households; OPV, oral polio vaccine.

Reproduced from Piyaratn, P. Basic Minimum Needs: Concepts and Practice. (1992). In P. Winichagoon, Y. Kachondham, G. Attig, & K. Tontisrin (Eds.), Integrating Food and Nutrition into Development: Thailand's Experiences and Future Visions. Institute of Nutrition Mahidol University at Salaya, Thailand and UNICEF/EAPRO, Bangkok 1992.

data collection, analysis and interpretation, and action plan development. The first level of the action plan included actions readily performed by villagers using available resources and know-how. The next level included actions that required guidance and support of local personnel. The last level included actions requiring external inputs, such as from the provincial or national level, awarded based on review of competitive proposals prepared by the community. Each community used the BMN indicators to annually plan, monitor progress, and evaluate achievement through an iterative process including establishing priorities, setting goals to be achieved, planning actions, implementing the plan, and reassessing, or by monitoring and evaluating.

Although distinct causes are not certain due to multiple simultaneous elements of national nutrition programs, Thailand's improvement in nutritional status is undeniable. Likely contributors in addition to these programs include the rapid reduction of common infections, increased immunization, and increased ANC coverage.

Key Findings from Thailand's Community-Based Nutrition Program

1. Programs require continuous support and adequate time to be established, and another two to three years to show effects.

2. Scaling up nutrition programs requires a strategic policy instrument that aligns macro- and micro-level policy, allowing for both top-down service delivery and bottom-up community participation in corrective actions.

3. Nutrition indicators are important for defining and evaluating actions.

4. Basic services and individual participation are essential elements for increased coverage.

5. Empowerment and decentralization create community responsibility and accountability.

6. Nutrition is the link between food and health, and food-based intervention should be a sustainable strategy.

7. The unit of operation for pilot programs or starting points for implementation was the district level, which also makes it possible to identify barriers to scaling up. In Thailand, the district is the nearest frontline level at which personnel from all sectors are available to provide both technical and financial support to community programs.

Specific Micronutrient Programs

Micronutrient malnutrition can require different programs than those addressing PEM. Programs in Thailand, described below, have led to reduced vitamin A deficiency. Prevalence of anemia is still mild to moderate, with prevalence of 20%,[86] and IDD persists.

IDD Policy and Program

WHO identified endemic goiter in Thailand in 1955 when a survey found low environmental concentrations of iodine and lower dietary iodine among rural residents than in residents of the capital city, Bangkok. The survey triggered salt and oil iodization programs in the severely deficient north and northeastern regions. Iodized oil capsules were given to pregnant women and women of childbearing age through the primary healthcare system, and schoolchildren with enlarged thyroid glands received iodized oil capsules through the school health program. Iodination of drinking water was also promoted, especially in primary schools. Nutrition education occurred in media campaigns, television advertisements, and radio spots, and primary school teachers monitored goiter in schoolchildren.

In 1994, the Thai Food and Drug Administration (FDA) encouraged private large and small salt producers to iodize salt at 30 parts per million (ppm), which had an excess cost of only 2–20% over non-iodized salt production. UNICEF and the Ministry of Public Health supported the use of potassium iodate as a fortificant.

The quality and concentration of iodized salt varied due to different scales and methods of production. Other challenges are that non-iodized salt is still widely available at a cheaper price, and iodized salt can have an undesirable color. The food industry and agricultural sectors can be resistant to using iodized salt. Furthermore, fish and soy sauce are common alternatives to salt in Thai cooking. In 2010, the Thai FDA revised legislation to accelerate USI and made fortification of fish and soy sauces mandatory. Innovative quality assurance schemes, particularly for small producers, will be necessary to ensure the quality and consistency of iodized salt sauces. Sustainability of iodine programs requires continued political commitment, advocacy, and a public awareness program. Community participation is crucial, and effective communication on the use of iodized salt, particularly for target populations, should continue.

Good indicators and effective monitoring and surveillance systems are necessary to ensure any resurgence of IDD. Monitoring of UIC of pregnant women is conducted in five-year cycles, and the national health examination survey includes UIC of children 1 to 14 years. The 2008 survey found that Thai children have sufficient iodine intakes, although pregnant women have lower intakes.[87]

IDA Policy and Program

Implemented as a national program for prevention and control of anemia during pregnancy, universal iron supplementation is a part of the public health system's antenatal care services. Common forms of iron provided are hydrated ferrous sulphate containing 60 milligrams of elemental iron, and a multivitamin/mineral supplement produced by the Government Pharmaceuticals Organization (GPO). Commercial multivitamin tablets were provided when the fiscal budget allowed, but these tablets cost 10 times more than the GPO's ferrous sulphate supplements.

The annual budget allocation for iron tablets is based on anemia prevalence in each province at the time of planning. An allocation for the indigent, such as mothers, children under 12, and the elderly, is provided. This allocation is provided both at the departmental level in the ministry's headquarters and at the provincial level. In case of an unexpected shortage of supply, additional iron tablets can be purchased using income generated at the local health functionaries (usually a district hospital). Because iron tablets can be produced domestically and are inexpensive, there is no cost or only minimal cost to women obtaining the prenatal services.

Program success depended on increasing the reach of ANC from its baseline of 20–30% of the population before the 1980s. VHVs and VHCs helped identify pregnant women and inform health personnel of new pregnancy cases.[88] Supplements with 50–70 mg elemental iron were to be taken daily until birth; women received their iron in packets of 30 tablets in monthly ANC visits. Usually, advice is general, with no emphasis on nutrition during pregnancy.

Compliance is a major challenge to the success of iron supplementation programs worldwide, since iron must be taken daily for extended periods of time. Compliance also depends on cultural, contextual, and health service factors. Side effects, such as nausea, upset stomach, constipation, and diarrhea, and lack of perception of need are common reasons for low compliance. Continuation of iron

supplementation is also largely related to ANC attendance. Verbal advice from health personnel reassures mothers that the supplement is useful and that side effects will diminish within one to two weeks.

Monitoring of situations and trends has been done in the routine health reporting system and reported as prevalence of anemia during pregnancy. At the individual level, the data are used by physicians to determine doses of iron tablets and the need for follow-up of anemic cases. With this curative approach, moderate to severe anemia cases are more likely to be referred and followed up closely by local personnel at the subdistrict health center, hospital staff, or both. For public health purposes, the data on anemia from the health system allow for tracking the prevalence of anemia. However, there are several limitations. First, data from the health system are likely to be self-selected, and not representative of pregnant women. Second, women who have blood taken may belong to higher socioeconomic strata because they can afford to attend hospitals where laboratory services are possible. Finally, pregnant women tend to have their first prenatal visit early within the first trimester of pregnancy. The reported prevalence of anemia could easily underestimate the true magnitude of anemia during pregnancy, especially if compliance with iron supplementation is low.

The holistic nature of iron supplementation in Thailand has contributed to improved iron status in the population. Supplementation for pregnant women is integrated into existing ANC, and VHVs promote program participation. Methods of evaluating compliance in large-scale programs are still needed, and Thailand does not yet have a universal program for adolescent girls or women before pregnancy. However, a food-based approach can eventually be effective and more sustainable for a larger female population.

Vitamin A Deficiency

Thailand does not have specific policies or large-scale programs specifically for VAD, which is often related to PEM. For VAD, a food-based approach is an appropriate long-term strategy, requiring effective communication of appropriate eating practices. For infants, breastfeeding provides an important source of vitamin A when mothers are not VAD. Mandatory vitamin A fortification of sweetened condensed milk improved vitamin A status, especially among poor people. In 1991, hospital records in the lower southern provinces of Thailand revealed 31 cases of childhood blindness that were later confirmed to be due to VAD.[89,90] After supplement and dietary diversification programs, subsequent surveys showed improvement.

Emergence of Childhood Obesity and Adult Obesity, Metabolic Syndrome, and Noncommunicable Diseases

The demographic and epidemiological transitions in Thailand create a dual challenge in malnutrition. National health examination surveys have identified obesity, **metabolic syndrome,** and diet-related noncommunicable diseases (NCDs) among adults since 1990. Other surveys suggest a rise in childhood obesity. Gestational diabetes, another concern linked to obesity, was also sporadically reported. Urban households increasingly rely on processed and prepared foods. In urban or semiurban settings, local fresh food markets still exist, but convenience stores and supermarkets are becoming more common. Processed foods contribute fat, sugar, and salt to Thai diets. Identifying determinants of the double burden of malnutrition among children in the context of rapid economic transition will permit formulation of appropriate policy and interventions.

Conclusion

Undernutrition in children and women has been a common public health problem in most developing countries, with conditions including PEM, IDD, IDA, and VAD. As some countries progress in their economic development and industrialization, problems of obesity and diet-related chronic noncommunicable diseases emerge, and rapidly become a public health problem. As a result, these countries are facing the so-called double burden of malnutrition. The challenges are greater for countries that are facing high prevalences on both ends of the spectrum.

Thailand is an example of a country that has implemented effective programs to alleviate undernutrition of children and women. The strong community-based nature of the multisectoral nutrition improvement program is an example of how preventive and promotive actions can be successfully implemented along with curative health services. The model of village volunteers in Thailand is sustained, but questions of how to build on the past success for the future generation are still being addressed. Case examples from other successful national programs at different stages of development and international movement to support nutrition improvement efforts are being documented, and more lessons will be forthcoming to benefit the field of public health nutrition. The immediate impacts are improvements in the nutrition status of the people in these countries.

References

1 Winichagoon, P. (2013). Thailand nutrition in transition: Situation and challenges of maternal and child nutrition. *Asia Pacific Journal of Clinical Nutrition, 22*(1), 6-15.

2 Caulfield, L. E., de Onis, M., Blössner, M., & Black, R. E. (2004). Undernutrition as an underlying cause of child deaths associated with diarrhea, pneumonia, malaria, and measles. *American Journal of Clinical Nutrition, 80*(1), 193-98.

3 Shetty, P. (2003). Malnutrition and undernutrition. *Medicine, 31*(4), 18-22.

4 Gibson, R. S. (2005). *Principles of Nutritional Assessment* (2nd ed.). New York, NY: Oxford University Press.

5 Hamill, P. V., Drizd, T. A., Johnson, C. L., Reed, R. B., Roche, A. F., & Moore, W. M. (1979). Physical growth: National Center for Health Statistics percentiles. *American Journal of Clinical Nutrition, 32*(3), 607-29.

6 Waterlow, J. C., Buzina, R., Keller, W., Lane, J. M., Nichaman, M. Z., & Tanner, J. M. (1977). The presentation and use of height and weight data for comparing the nutritional status of groups of children under the age of 10 years. *Bulletin of the World Health Organization, 55*(4), 489-98.

7 Chavalittamrong, B., & Tantiwongse, P. (1987). Height and weight of Thai children: Update. *Journal of the Medical Association of Thailand, 70*(Suppl. 1), 1-40.

8 World Health Organization Multicentre Growth Reference Study Group. (2006). WHO Child Growth Standards based on length/height, weight and age. *Acta, 450*(Suppl.), 76-85.

9 Gibson, R. S. (2005). *Principles of Nutritional Assessment* (2nd ed.). New York, NY: Oxford University Press.

10 de Onis, M., Onyango, A. W., Borghi, E., Garza, C., & Yang, H., for the WHO Multicentre Growth Reference Study Group. (2006). Comparison of the World Health Organization (WHO) Child Growth Standards and the National Center for Health Statistics/WHO international growth reference: Implications for child health programmes. *Public Health Nutrition, 9*(7), 942-47.

11 Wright, C., Lakshman, R., Emmett, P., & Ong, K. K. (2008). Implications of adopting the WHO Growth Standard in the UK: Two prospective cohort studies. *Archives of Disease in Childhood, 93*(7), 566-69. doi:10.1136/adc.2007.126854

12 Hui, L. L., Schooling, C. M., Cowling, B. J., Leung, S. S. L., Lam, T. H., & Leung, G. M. (2008). Are universal standards

for optimal infant growth appropriate? Evidence from a Hong Kong Chinese birth cohort. *Archives of Disease in Childhood, 93*(7), 561-65. doi:10.1136/adc.2007.119826

13 Kerac, M., Blencowe, H., Grijalva-Eternod, C., McGrath, M., Shoham, J., Cole, T. J., & Seal, A. (2011). Prevalence of wasting among under 6-month-old infants in developing countries and implications of new case definitions using WHO growth standards: A secondary data analysis. *Archives of Disease in Childhood, 96*(11), 1008-13. doi:10.1136/adc.2010.191882

14 Shrimpton, R., Victora, C. G., de Onis, M., Lima, R. C., Blössner, M., & Clugston, G. (2001). Worldwide timing of growth faltering: Implications for nutritional interventions. *Pediatrics 107*(5), e75. doi:10.1542/peds.107.5.e75

15 Victora, C. G., de Onis, M., Hallal, P. C., Blössner, M., & Shrimpton, R. (2010). Worldwide timing of growth faltering: Revisiting implications for interventions. *Pediatrics, 125*(3), e473-80. doi:10.1542/peds.2009-1519

16 World Health Organization Expert Consultation. (2004). Appropriate body-mass index for Asian populations and its implications for policy and intervention strategies. *Lancet, 363*(9403), 157-63.

17 Food and Agriculture Organization of the United Nations. (2010). *The state of food insecurity in the world 2010: Addressing food insecurity in protracted crises.* Rome: FAO.

18 Deurenberg-Yap, M., Schmidt, G., van Staveren, W. A., & Deurenberg, P. (2000). The paradox of low body mass index and high body fat percentage among Chinese, Malays and Indians in Singapore. *International Journal of Obesity and Related Metabolic Disorders: Journal of the International Association for the Study of Obesity, 24*(8), 1011-17.

19 Pan, W. H., Yeh, W. T., & Weng, L. C. (2008). Epidemiology of metabolic syndrome in Asia. *Asia Pacific Journal of Clinical Nutrition, 17*(Suppl. 1), 37-42.

20 Flour Fortification Initiative, Global Alliance for Improved Nutrition, Micronutrient Initiative, USAID, The World Bank, and UNICEF. (2009). *Investing in the future: A united call to action for vitamin and mineral deficiencies. Global Report.* Retrieved from http://www.unitedcalltoaction.org/documents/Investing_in_the_future.pdf

21 Andersson, M., Karumbunathan, V., & Zimmermann, M. B. (2012). Global iodine status in 2011 and trends over the past decade. *Journal of Nutrition, 142*(4), 744-50. doi:10.3945/jn.111.149393

22 World Health Organization. (2011). *Guideline: Intermittent iron and folic acid supplementation in menstruating women.* Geneva: World Health Organization.

23 World Health Organization. (2011). *Guideline: Vitamin A supplementation in pregnant women.* Geneva: World Health Organization.

24 Zimmermann, M. B., Jooste, P. L., & Pandav, C. S. (2008). Iodine deficiency disorders. *Lancet, 372*(9645), 1251-62. doi:10.1016/S0140-6736(08)61005-3

25 Zimmermann, M. B., Aeberli, I., Andersson, M., Assey, V., Yorg, J. A., Jooste, P., . . . Timmer, A. (2013). Thyroglobulin is a sensitive measure of both deficient and excess iodine intakes in children and indicates no adverse effects on thyroid function in the UIC range of 100-299 µg/L: A UNICEF/ICCIDD Study Group Report. *Journal of Clinical Endocrinology and Metabolism, 98*(3), 1271-80. doi:10.1210/jc.2012-3952

26 Zimmermann, M. B. (2010). Symposium on "Geographical and geological influences on nutrition": Iodine deficiency in industrialized countries. *Proceedings of the Nutrition Society, 69,* 133-43.

27 Zimmermann, M. B. (2012). The effects of iodine deficiency in pregnancy and infancy. *Pediatric and Perinatal Epidemiology, 26*(Suppl. 1), 108-17. doi:10.1111/j.1365-3016.2012. 01275.x

28 Bürgi, H., Supersaxo, Z., & Selz, B. (1990). Iodine deficiency diseases in Switzerland one hundred years after Theodor Kocher's survey: A historical review with some new goitre prevalence data. *Acta Endocrinologica, 123*(6), 577-90.

29 Andersson, M., Aeberli, I., Wüst, N., Piacenza, A. M., Bucher, T., Henschen, I., . . . Zimmermann, M. B. (2010). The Swiss iodized salt program provides adequate iodine for school children and pregnant women, but weaning infants not receiving iodine-containing complementary foods as well as their mothers are iodine deficient. *Journal of Clinical Endocrinology and Metabolism, 95*(12), 5217-54. Epub 2010 Sep 1. doi:10.1210/jc.2010-0975

30 Andersson, M., Karumbunathan, V., & Zimmermann, M. B. (2012). Global iodine status in 2011 and trends over the past decade. *Journal of Nutrition, 142*(4), 744-50. doi:10.3945/jn.111.149393

31 Gowachirapant, S., Winichagoon, P., Wyss, L., Tong, B., Baumgartner, J., Melse-Boonstra, A., & Zimmermann, M. B. (2009). Urinary iodine concentrations in pairs of pregnant women and their school-aged children from Thai households indicate iodine sufficiency in the children but iodine deficiency in the women. *Journal of Nutrition, 139*(6), 1169-72.

32 Andersson, M., Aeberli, I., Wüst, N., Piacenza, A.M., Bucher, T., Henschen, I., . . . Zimmermann, M. B. (2010). The Swiss iodized salt program provides adequate iodine for school children and pregnant women, but weaning infants not receiving iodine-containing complementary foods as well as their mothers are iodine deficient. *Journal of Clinical Endocrinology and Metabolism, 95*(12), 5217-24. Epub 2010 Sep 1. doi:10.1210/jc.2010-0975

33 Lynch, S. (2011). Case studies: Iron. *American Journal of Clinical Nutrition, 94*(2), 673S-678S.

34 Beard, J. L. (2001). Iron biology in immune function, muscle metabolism and neuronal functioning. *Journal of Nutrition 131*(2), 568S-580S.

35 Beard, J. L. (2007). Recent evidence from human and animal studies regarding iron status and infant development. *Journal of Nutrition, 137*(2), 524S-530S.

36 Hurrell R., & Egli I. (2010). Iron bioavailability and dietary reference values. *American Journal of Clinical Nutrition, 91*(5), 1461S-1467S. Epub 2010 Mar 3. doi:10.3945/ajcn.2010.28674F

37 Stoltzfus, R. J., & Dreyfuss, M. L., International Nutritional Anemia Consultative Group (INACG). (1998). *Guidelines for the use of iron supplements to prevent and treat iron deficiency anemia.* Washington, DC: ILSI Press.

38 Galloway, R. (2003). *Anemia prevention and control: What works*. Washington, DC: USAID. Retrieved from http://siteresources.worldbank.org/NUTRITION/Resources/281846-1090335399908/Anemia_Part1.pdf

39 World Health Organization. (2011). *Guideline: Intermittent iron and folic acid supplementation in menstruating women*. Geneva: World Health Organization.

40 Gropper, S. S., Smith, J. L., & Groff, J. L. (2013). *Advanced nutrition and human metabolism* (5th ed.) (pp. 373–90). Belmont, CA: Wadsworth Cengage Learning.

41 Sommer, A. (2008). Vitamin A deficiency and clinical disease: An historical overview. *Journal of Nutrition, 138*(10), 1835–39.

42 Interdepartmental Committee on Nutrition for National Defense. (1962). *Thailand: Nutrition Survey of the Armed Forces* (pp. 1–285). Bethesda, MD: U.S. Department of Health Education and Welfare, Public Health Service, National Institutes of Health.

43 World Health Organization. (2011). *Guideline: Intermittent iron and folic acid supplementation in menstruating women*. Geneva: World Health Organization.

44 World Health Organization. (2011). *Guideline: Vitamin A supplementation in pregnant women*. Geneva: World Health Organization.

45 Low, J. W., Arimond, M., Osman, N., Cunguara, B., Zano, F. & Tschirley, D. (2007). A food-based approach introducing orange-fleshed sweet potatoes increased vitamin A intake and serum retinol concentrations in young children in rural Mozambique. *Journal of Nutrition, 137*(5), 1320–27.

46 International Zinc Nutrition Consultative Group (IZiNCG). (2004). Assessment of the risk of zinc deficiency in populations and options for its control. In C. Hotz & K. H. Brown (Eds.), *Food and Nutrition Bulletin, 25*, S91–S202. Retrieved from http://archive.unu.edu/unupress/food/fnb25-1s-IZiNCG.pdf

47 Gibson, R. S. (2012). A historical review of progress in the assessment of dietary zinc intake as an indicator of population zinc status. *Advances in Nutrition, 3*, 772–82. doi:10.3945/an.112.002287

48 Wasantwisut, E., Winichagoon, P., Chitchumroonchokchai, C., Yamborisut, U., Boonpraderm, A., Pongcharoen, T., . . . Russameesopaphorn, W. (2006). Iron and zinc supplementation improved iron and zinc status, but not physical growth, of apparently healthy, breast-fed infants in rural communities of northeast Thailand. *Journal of Nutrition, 136*(9), 2405–11.

49 Thurlow, R. A., Winichagoon, P., Pongcharoen, T., Gowachirapant, S., Boonpraderm, A., Manger, M. S., . . . Gibson, R. S. (2006). Risk of zinc, iodine and other micronutrient deficiencies among school children in North East Thailand. *European Journal of Clinical Nutrition, 60*(5), 623–32.

50 Agarwal, R., Sentz, J., & Miller, M. A. (2007). Role of zinc administration in prevention of childhood diarrhea and respiratory illnesses: A meta-analysis. *Pediatrics, 119*(6), 1120–30.

51 Haider, B. A., & Bhutta, Z. A. (2009). The effect of therapeutic zinc supplementation among young children with selected infections: A review of the evidence. *Food and Nutrition Bulletin, 30*(Suppl. 1), S41–S59.

52 Jones, A. P., Tulic, M. K., Rueter, K., & Prescott, S. L. (2012). Vitamin D and allergic disease: Sunlight at the end of the tunnel? *Nutrients, 4*(1), 13–28. doi:10.3390/nu4010013

53 Norman, A. W., & Bouillon, R. (2010). Vitamin D nutritional policy needs a vision for the future. *Experimental Biology and Medicine, 235*(9), 1034–45. doi:10.1258/ebm.2010.010014

54 Holick, M. F. (2007). Vitamin D deficiency. *New England Journal of Medicine, 357*, 266–81. doi:10.1056/NEJMra070553

55 Lee, W. T., & Jiang, J. (2008). Calcium requirements for Asian children and adolescents. *Asia Pacific Journal of Clinical Nutrition, 17*(Suppl. 1), 33–36.

56 Bailey, R. L., Dodd, K. W., Goldman, J. A., Gahche, J. J., Dwyer, J. T., Moshfegh, A. J., . . . Picciano, M. F. (2010). Estimation of total usual calcium and vitamin D intakes in the United States. *Journal of Nutrition, 140*(4), 817–22.

57 Sukchan, P., Liabsuetrakul, T., Chongsuvivatwong, V., Songwathana, P., Sornsrivichai, V., & Kuning M. (2010). Inadequacy of nutrients intake among pregnant women in the deep south of Thailand. *BMC Public Health, 10*:572. doi:10.1186/1471-2458-10-572

58 Ongphiphadhanakul, B. (2002). Osteoporosis in Thailand. *Clinical Calcium, 12*(6), 822–26.

59 Chailurkit, L., Aekplakorn, W., & Ongphiphadhanakul, B. (2011). Regional variation and determinants of vitamin D status in sunshine-abundant Thailand. *BMC Public Health, 11*, 853. Retrieved from http://www.biomedcentral.com/1471-2458/11/853

60 Zimmermann, M. B., Adou, P., Torresani, T., Zeder, C., & Hurrell, R. F. (2000). Iron supplementation in goitrous, iron deficient children improves their response to oral iodized oil. *European Journal of Endocrinology/European Federation of Endocrine Societies, 142*(3), 217–23.

61 Wasantwisut, E., Winichagoon, P., Chitchumroonchokchai, C., Yamborisut, U., Boonpraderm, A., Pongcharoen, T., . . . Russameesopaphorn W. (2006). Iron and zinc supplementation improved iron and zinc status, but not physical growth, of apparently healthy, breast-fed infants in rural communities of northeast Thailand. *Journal of Nutrition, 136*(9), 2405–11.

62 Wieringa, F. T., Berger, J., Dijkhuizen, M. A., Hidayat, A., Ninh, N. X., Utomo, B., . . . Winichagoon, P., for the SEAMTIZI (South-East Asia Multi-country Trial on Iron and Zinc supplementation in Infants) Study Group. (2007). Combined iron and zinc supplementation in infants improved iron and zinc status, but interactions reduced efficacy in a multicountry trial in southeast Asia. *Journal of Nutrition, 137*(2), 466–71.

63 World Health Organization. (2011). *Guideline: Vitamin A supplementation in postpartum women*. Geneva: World Health Organization.

64 Winichagoon, P., McKenzie, J., Chavasit, V., Pongcharoen, T., Gowachirapant, S., Boonpraderm, A., . . . Gibson, R. S. (2006). A multimicronutrient-fortified seasoning powder enhances the hemoglobin, zinc and iodine status of primary school children in North East Thailand: A randomized controlled trial of efficacy. *Journal of Nutrition, 136*(6), 1617–23.

65 Manger, M. S., McKenzie, J. E., Winichagoon, P., Gray, A., Chavasit, V., Pongcharoen, T., & Gibson, R. S. (2008). A

micronutrient-fortified seasoning powder reduces morbidity and improves short-term cognitive function, but has no effect on anthropometric measures in primary school children in northeast Thailand: A randomized controlled trial. *American Journal of Clinical Nutrition, 87*(6), 1715-22.

66 Nga, T. T., Winichagoon, P., Dijkhuizen, M. A., Khan, N. C., Wasantwisut, E., Furr, H., & Wieringa, F. T. (2009). Multi-micronutrient-fortified biscuits decreased prevalence of anemia and improved micronutrient status and effectiveness of deworming in rural Vietnamese school children. *Journal of Nutrition, 139*(5), 1013-21. Epub 2009 Mar 25. doi:10.3945/jn.108.099754

67 Allen, L. H. (2005). Multiple micronutrients in pregnancy and lactation: An overview. *American Journal of Clinical Nutrition, 81*(5 Suppl.), 1206S-1212S.

68 Allen, L. H., Peerson, J. M., & the Maternal Micronutrient Supplementation Study Group (MMSSG). (2009). Impact of multiple micronutrient versus iron-folic acid supplements on maternal anemia and micronutrient status in pregnancy. *Food and Nutrition Bulletin, 30*(4 Suppl.), S527-S532.

69 Shrimpton, R., Huffman, S. L., Zehner, E. R., Darnton-Hill, I., & Dalmiya, N. (2009). Multiple micronutrient supplementation during pregnancy in developing-country settings: Policy and program implications of the results of a meta-analysis. *Food and Nutrition Bulletin, 30*(4 Suppl.), S556-S573.

70 Fall, C. H. D., Fisher, D. J., Osmond, C., Margetts, B. M., & the Maternal Micronutrient Supplementation Study Group (MMSSG). (2009). Multiple micronutrient supplementation during pregnancy in low-income countries: A meta-analysis of effects on birth size and length of gestation. *Food and Nutrition Bulletin, 30*(4) (Suppl.), S533-546.

71 Haider, B. A., Yakoob, M. Y., & Bhutta, Z. A. (2011). Effect of multiple micronutrient supplementation during pregnancy on maternal and birth outcomes. *BMC Public Health 11*(Suppl. 3), S19-S27. doi:10.1186/1471-2458-11-S3-S19

72 Ronsmans, C., Fisher, D. J., Osmond, C., Margetts, B. M., Fall, C. H., & the Maternal Micronutrient Supplementation Study Group (MMSSG). (2009). Multiple micronutrient supplementation during pregnancy in low-income countries: A meta-analysis of effects on stillbirths and on early and late neonatal mortality. *Food and Nutrition Bulletin, 30*(4 Suppl.), S547-S555.

73 Allen, L. H. (2005). Multiple micronutrients in pregnancy and lactation: An overview. *American Journal of Clinical Nutrition, 81*(5 Suppl.), 1206S-1212S.

74 Gluckman, P. D., Hanson, M. A., Cooper, C., & Thornburg, K. L. (2008). Effect of in utero and early-life conditions on adult health and disease. *New England Journal of Medicine, 359*(1), 61-73.

75 Bhutta, Z. A., Ahmed, T., Black, R. E., Cousens, S., Dewey, K., Giugliani, E., . . . Shekar, M., for the Maternal and Child Undernutrition Study Group. (2008). What works? Interventions for maternal and child undernutrition and survival. *Lancet, 371*(9610), 417-40. doi:10.1016/S0140-6736(07)61693-6

76 Bryce, J., Coitinho, D., Darnton-Hill, I., Pelletier, D., & Pinstrup-Andersen, P., for the Maternal and Child Undernutrition Study Group. (2008). Maternal and child undernutrition: Effective action at national level. *Lancet, 371*(9611), 510-26.

77 Valyasevi, A., & Dhanamitta, S. (1974). Study of bladder stone disease in Thailand. XVII. Effect of exogenous source of oxalate on crystalluria. *American Journal of Clinical Nutrition, 27*(8), 877-82.

78 Interdepartmental Committee on Nutrition for National Defense (ICNND). (1962). *Thailand: Nutrition Survey of the Armed Forces* (pp. 1-285). Bethesda, MD: U.S. Department of Health Education and Welfare, Public Health Service, National Institutes of Health.

79 Valyasevi, A., Winichagoon, P., & Dhanamitta, S. (1995). Community-based surveillance for action towards health and nutrition: Experience in Thailand. *Food and Nutrition Bulletin, 16*(2), 120-25.

80 Tontisirin, K., Attig, G. A., & Winichagoon, P. (1995). An eight stage process for national nutrition development. *Food and Nutrition Bulletin, 16*(1), 8-16.

81 Tontisirin, K., & Winichagoon, P. (1999). Community-based programmes: Success factors for public nutrition derived from the experience of Thailand. *Food and Nutrition Bulletin, 20*(3), 315-22.

82 Dhanamitta, S., Virojsailee, S., & Valyasevi, A. (1981). Implementation of a conceptual scheme for improving the nutritional status of the rural poor in Thailand. *Food and Nutrition Bulletin, 3*(3), 11-15.

83 Tontisirin, K., Attig, G. A., & Winichagoon, P. (1995). An eight-stage process for national nutrition development. *Food and Nutrition Bulletin, 16*(1), 8-16.

84 Interdepartmental Committee on Nutrition for National Defense (ICNND). (1962). *Thailand: Nutrition Survey of the Armed Forces* (pp. 1-285). Bethesda, MD: U.S. Department of Health Education and Welfare, Public Health Service, National Institutes of Health.

85 Heaver, R., & Kachondam, Y. (2002). *Thailand's national nutrition program: Lessons in management and capacity development*. Health, nutrition and population (HNP) discussion paper. Washington, DC: The International Bank for Reconstruction and Development/The World Bank.

86 Winichagoon, P. (2002). Prevention and control of Anemia: Thailand experiences. *Journal of Nutrition, 132*(4), 862S-866S.

87 Gowachirapant, S., Winichagoon, P., Wyss, L., Tong, B., Baumgartner, J., Melse-Boonstra, A., & Zimmermann, M. B. (2009). Urinary iodine concentrations in pairs of pregnant women and their school-aged children from Thai households indicate iodine sufficiency in the children but iodine deficiency in the women. *Journal of Nutrition, 139*(6), 1169-72.

88 Winichagoon, P. (2002). Prevention and control of Anemia: Thailand experiences. *Journal of Nutrition, 132*(4), 862S-866S.

89 Wasantwisut, E., Chittchang, U., & Sinawat, S. (2000). Moving a health system from a medical towards a dietary approach in Thailand. *Food and Nutrition Bulletin, 21*(2), 157-60.

90 Wasantwisut, E. (2002). A combined approach to vitamin A deficiency in Thailand. *Sight and Life Newsletter, 3*, 63-67.

Part III

Infant and Young Child Nutrition: Foundations of a Healthy Population

Chapter 8

Infant and Young Child Feeding: Strategies and Lessons Learned in Bangladesh

Tina G. Sanghvi, PhD
Rukhsana Haider, MBBS, MSc, IBCLC, PhD

"We talk about the different healthcare priorities and problems our families face. And with the help of the health professionals in our community, we learn to adopt a more useful approach to tackle any problems."–Grandmother from Senegal, Maimouna Mbengue

Quoted in http://www.npr.org/2011/08/11/139543928/in-senegal-the-grandmas-are-in-charge

Learning Objectives

- Describe the significance of infant and young child feeding (IYCF).

- Understand how breastfeeding and complementary feeding practices influence health status and well-being.

- Explain the technical basis of global IYCF recommendations and what barriers families and countries face in following the recommendations.

- Suggest ways to design program strategies to reduce barriers to desirable IYCF.

Case Study: Undernutrition in Infants and Young Children in Bangladesh

While many health and economic indicators have improved in Bangladesh in the past decade, undernutrition remains high, with a 41% prevalence of **stunting** among children under 5 years of age.[1] Inappropriate feeding among children below 2 years of age is an important cause of continued undernutrition and lack of progress toward achieving Millennium Development Goal (MDG) 1 throughout South Asia.[2] While exclusive breastfeeding levels for infants below 6 months of age have recently improved in Bangladesh, from 43% in 2007 to 64% in 2011, **complementary feeding** practices remain extremely poor, and only 21% of all children in the 6- to 23-month-old age group receive an adequate diet.[3] Even in the wealthiest 20% of Bangladeshi families, only 30% of 6- to 23-month-old children receive an adequate diet. They develop frequent illnesses partly caused by unhygienic complementary food preparation. The results include rapid declines in linear growth rates compared with well-nourished children. The presence of stunting increases from less than 20% at 6 months of age to 28% at 9 to 11 months, 46% at 12 to 17 months, and 52% at 18 to 23 months. Stunting can have permanent consequences, but it can be largely prevented through improving **infant and young child feeding (IYCF)**.[4,5]

Public health programs in Bangladesh have the potential to improve IYCF and health outcomes. The Integrated Management of Childhood Illness (IMCI) strategy was launched in the mid-1990s by the World Health Organization (WHO) and the United Nations Children's Fund (UNICEF). It is a holistic approach to reducing childhood mortality and morbidity and to improving growth and development.[6] Focus is on improving healthcare systems, case management skills of healthcare workers, and home health practices, including nutrition. Reports assessing its effects in Brazil, Peru, Uganda, and Tanzania were published by 2005, and results from Bangladesh were published in 2009, after six years of follow-up. In Bangladesh, healthcare quality improved, and use of healthcare facilities and rates of exclusive breastfeeding increased, although mortality rates were not significantly lower in IMCI groups than in control groups.

The global incidence of low birth weight (LBW), or babies born under 2,500 grams, is 23.8%,[7] and it is higher in resource-poor settings. Bangladesh, for example, has an incidence of LBW of 37% in rural areas and 29% in urban regions.[8] Compared with normal-weight infants, LBW infants have a mortality rate that is three times higher, and the rate is eight times higher for very low birth weight (VLBW) infants, or those under 1,500 grams at birth. Breastfeeding is an example of a nutritional strategy that can reduce mortality and improve weight and length gain among LBW infants. Providing education for mothers can be an effective public health strategy to increase breastfeeding and improve infant health outcomes.

Programs such as IMCI and nutrition education demonstrate the potential for public health to improve IYCF and children's health in Bangladesh and globally.

Discussion Questions

- How does childhood nutritional status in Bangladesh compare with that in the surrounding region and in developing nations worldwide?

- Which features of the IMCI strategy have led to improved outcomes in Bangladesh?

- How might differences in cultural, economic, and other factors lead to differences in effective IMCI implementation in different nations?

- What are some possible explanations for the lack of decline in mortality rates in Bangladesh? Which future strategies might help reduce childhood mortality?

Introduction

Feeding of infants and young children has become a public health priority as evidence increases regarding substantial health, cognitive, and behavioral short-term and long-term benefits.[9] Some experts estimate that optimal breastfeeding and complementary feeding together could prevent 19% of childhood deaths globally (**Figure 8-1**).[10] The WHO

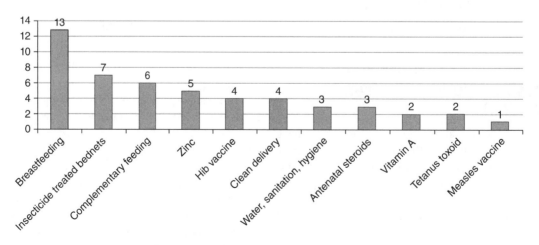

Figure 8-1 Percent of preventable deaths with known interventions

Data from Jones, G., Steketee, R. W., Black, R. E., Bhutta, Z. A., & Morris, S. S. (2003). How many child deaths can we prevent this year? *Lancet, 362*(9377), 65-71.

promotes infant and young child feeding (IYCF) as a priority intervention for achieving MDG 4.[11]

Millenium Development Goal 4: Reduce Child Mortality. Target 4.A: Reduce by two-thirds, between 1990 and 2015, the under-five mortality rate

This chapter discusses the scientific basis of global IYCF recommendations, describes common barriers to improving IYCF, and, using Bangladesh as an example, illustrates efforts to increase rates of exclusive breastfeeding and improve complementary feeding.

Importance of IYCF

The period of about 1,000 days from conception to 24 months is considered a critical window of opportunity for ensuring children's appropriate growth and development through optimal feeding.[12] Children are most vulnerable to lifelong damage when they experience poor nutrition during this period.[13] Undernutrition is responsible, directly or indirectly, for about one-half of the estimated 11 million child deaths occurring before the age of 5 years.[14] Nearly 20% of deaths are preventable through improved IYCF. No other approach provides this level of child survival impact. Additional benefits of better IYCF include reducing the effects of undernutrition, such as stunting, **wasting**, and micronutrient deficiencies, preventing overnutrition, improving maternal health, and building healthy dietary habits.

Public Health Core Competency 6A5: Describes the scientific evidence related to a public health issue, concern, or intervention

Reproduced from Council on Linkages Between Academia and Public Health Practice. 2010 May. Core Competencies for Public Health Professionals. Washington, DC: Public Health Foundation. http:// www.phf.org/resourcestools/Documents/Core_Competencies_for_ Public_Health_Professionals_2010May.pdf. Accessed August 13, 2013. This source is used for all Public Health Core Competencies in this chapter.

Importance of Breastfeeding

One in five newborn deaths can be prevented by starting breastfeeding within the first hour after birth.[15] In developing countries, infants who are not breastfed are 14 times more likely to die before 6 months than breastfed infants.[16] Breastfeeding is also protective against frequency and severity of diarrhea and pneumonia,[17] even in situations with adequate hygiene, as in Portugal.[18] Other acute infections, including otitis media, *Haemophilus influenzae* meningitis, and urinary tract infection, are less common and less severe in breastfed infants.

Even among undernourished mothers, when proper breastfeeding techniques are used, exclusive breastfeeding provides all the energy, most of the critical nutrients, and all the fluid needs of the vast majority of infants for the first six months of life.[19] No other foods or even water is necessary for proper growth, development, and functioning.[20] Breastmilk contains antibodies, and it continues to protect infants and young children against deaths and diseases in the first 2 years of life when accompanied by adequate complementary foods.[21]

Breastfeeding also confers long-term benefits. Formula-fed children have an increased risk of chronic diseases with an immunological basis, including asthma and other atopic conditions, type 1 diabetes, celiac disease, ulcerative colitis, and Crohn disease. Artificial or formula feeding is also associated with a greater risk of childhood leukemia.[22] Evidence suggests a dose–response relationship between duration of breastfeeding and lower risk of obesity.[23] Artificial feeding is linked to increased blood pressure, altered blood cholesterol levels, and atherosclerosis in adulthood.

Importance of Complementary Feeding

After 6 months, a combination of breastfeeding and complementary foods is needed for optimally meeting nutrient needs and protecting the immune system. Proper IYCF helps to avoid the cycle of malnutrition and infection in which young children experience recurrent illnesses, and they eventually become undernourished or severely ill, with increasing chances of mortality with each bout of infection.

Brain Development and Cognitive Performance

Proper nutrition during the 1,000-day window supports normal brain development, laying the foundation for future cognitive, motor, and social ability; school success; and productivity. Undernutrition interferes with brain development and cognition, both directly, through impaired anatomical development and functional processes, and indirectly, as undernourished children interact less and are less able to learn from their environments.

Gestation and infancy are periods of rapid brain development. The neural tube begins to form 16 days after conception and, within seven months, increasingly resembles the adult brain. Energy, protein, fatty acids, and micronutrients are needed for the creation of new neurons, axons, and dendrites; formation of synapses; and covering of axons with myelin, the fatty matter that allows rapid transmission of nerve impulses.

Beyond directly impairing the brain's physical development, undernourishment indirectly interferes with cognitive development. Undernourished children are fussy, irritable, frequently ill, and withdrawn. They have limited interactions with caregivers and conduct less exploration of the environment. These behaviors further delay motor and cognitive development, and are clearly seen in children with iron-deficiency anemia, iodine-deficiency disorders, and protein–energy malnutrition. Children who suffer undernutrition at an early age or are stunted have reduced school achievement, have impaired motor development, and exhibit more behavioral problems. On average, scores of cognitive function are lower among children who were breastfed than those who were formula fed, with a greater difference among LBW children.[24] Increased duration of breastfeeding and improved cognitive development can increase individuals' ability to contribute to society as adults. If women were malnourished as children, their reproductive capacity is affected, their infants may have lower birth weight, and they tend to have more complicated deliveries. A high prevalence of malnourished children therefore not only is a drain on health resources, but also has implications for national development.

Growth and Nutrition

Inadequate IYCF can lead to growth faltering. The peak incidence occurs during the time of complementary feeding from 6 to 23 months, when micronutrient deficiencies and infectious illnesses also peak. Through 2 years of age, breastfeeding remains a critical source of energy and nutrients in developing countries, where low-income families can have difficulties procuring food as nutritious as breastmilk. When recommended feeding practices are followed, breastmilk provides about one-half of an infant's energy needs from 6 to 12 months, and one-third of energy through 24 months of age. Since breastmilk continues to supply protective factors tailored to the pathogens in the child's immediate environment, and it is free from allergens, breastfeeding on demand along with adequate complementary feeding should continue through 2 years or beyond.

Proper complementary feeding for optimal growth provides energy and nutrients to bridge the gaps between the content of breastmilk and the child's nutritional needs.

A critical component of proper nutrition is preventing microbial contamination through proper handwashing and hygiene practices. Another consideration is that children of this age experience frequent infections. Ensuring increased breastmilk intake and continued feeding of complementary foods during each illness is important to maintain good growth. To make up for lost nutrients and prevent growth faltering, young children should be fed extra foods as they recover and as appetite returns.

Nutritional Needs and IYCF Recommendations from Birth to 2 Years

Considering the importance of IYCF, the World Health Organization developed recommendations for the appropriate feeding of infants and young children in 2001 and a global strategy to facilitate actions for developed and developing countries to take to support appropriate feeding practices. The Global IYCF Strategy and feeding recommendations (**Table 8-1**) are evidence-based.[25]

Characteristics of Breastmilk

Breastmilk contains all the energy and fluid and almost all of the nutrients that a healthy infant needs in the first 6 months of life.[26] It also contains bioactive factors that augment the infant's immature immune system, providing protection against infection, and other factors that help digestion and absorption of nutrients. Breastmilk is easily digested and efficiently used.

Early Breastmilk or Colostrum

Colostrum is the thick, yellowish breastmilk that women produce in the first few days after delivery. It contains more antibodies, white blood cells, and other anti-infective proteins than mature milk. These immune factors help prevent the bacterial infections that threaten newborn babies.

Composition of Breastmilk

- **Fats**: Breastmilk contains 3.5 grams of fat per 100 milliliters (about 8 grams per 8-ounce cup) of milk, therefore providing 30 fat calories per 100 milliliters, and about half of its energy, from fat. The concentration of fat increases throughout each feed, so **foremilk** is lower in fat and has a bluish-gray color, while **hindmilk** is rich in fat and creamy white. Fat in breastmilk

Table 8-1 Recommended IYCF feeding practices by age of child

0-6 Months of Age	7-8 Months of Age	9-11 Months of Age	12-24 Months of Age
Initiate breastfeeding immediately, within first hour after birth			
In the first few days feed only colostrum			
Do not give pre- or post-lacteal feeds			
....No bottle feeding.............................			
Exclusive breastfeeding (no liquids or foods other than breastmilk)	Continue breastfeeding on demand during the day and night.........		
Do not start complementary feeding	Feed ½ bowl (250 ml size) mashed semisolid/solid family foods 2 times a day plus snacks	Feed ½ bowl (250 ml size) solid family foods 3 times a day plus snacks	Feed 1 bowl (250 ml size) small solid pieces of family foods 3 times a day plus snacks
	Increase the frequency, amount, and variety of complementary foods, including animal foods, fruits and vegetables, solid part of lentils/dal, oils/fat. Complete the transition from mashed to usual family foods soon after 12 months.		

Data from the World Health Organization (WHO) & UNICEF. (2003). *Global strategy for infant and young child feeding.* Geneva: WHO.

fat contains long-chain polyunsaturated fatty acids that are not available in other milks. These fatty acids, known as **docosahexaenoic acid**, or **DHA**, and **arachidonic acid**, or **AA**, are important for the neurological development of a child. These fatty acids may be added to formula milk.

- **Carbohydrates**: The main carbohydrate is a **disaccharide** called lactose, or "milk sugar." Breastmilk contains about 7 grams of lactose per 100 milliliters (17 grams per cup), which is equivalent to 28 calories per 100 milliliters (70 calories per cup). The amount is higher than in most other milks, and is another important source of energy. Oligosaccharides, or sugar chains, are additional carbohydrates in breastmilk. They provide protection against infection.

- **Protein**: Protein in breastmilk is more suitable for infants than animal milk proteins because of its higher quality, or particular composition of amino acids. The concentration of protein in breastmilk (0.9 grams per 100 milliliters) is lower than in animal milks and less likely than animal milk to overload the infant's immature kidneys with waste nitrogen products. Breastmilk contains less of the protein casein, and it forms softer,

more easily digested curds than casein in other milks. Artificially fed babies may develop intolerance to protein from animal milk, and may have diarrhea, abdominal pain, and rashes.

- **Vitamins and minerals**: Breastmilk normally contains sufficient vitamins for an infant, unless the mother herself is deficient. To ensure sufficient vitamin D, however, mothers and children should receive vitamin D supplements or adequate exposure to sunlight.[27] The minerals iron and zinc are present in relatively low concentration, but their bioavailability and absorption is high. LBW infants may need supplements before 6 months. Delaying clamping of the cord until pulsations have stopped, or three minutes, can improve infant iron status during the first six months of life.[28]

- **Anti-infective factors**: Anti-infective factors in breastmilk include substances that coat the intestinal mucosa and prevent bacteria from entering cells; white blood cells that can kill micro-organisms; antibodies that can kill bacteria, viruses, and fungi; and carbohydrates that prevent bacteria from attaching to mucosal surfaces. These valuable factors are protective without being inflammatory and causing fever. Also, since the antibodies are formed in the mother's body in response to bacteria in her gut, they are protective against bacteria that are particularly likely to be in the baby's environment.

- **Other bioactive factors**: Substances in breastmilk facilitate the complete digestion of fat droplets in the small intestine. The less-digested fat in substitutes can cause gastric distress. Breastmilk factors stimulate the maturation of the gut lining to improve nutrient digestion and absorption and reduce sensitivity to foreign proteins and allergies. Other growth factors present in human milk promote nerve and retinal development and maturation.

Requirements for Successful Breastfeeding

The WHO recommendations on breastfeeding promotion and support are based on the physiology of lactation. Prolactin and oxytocin are maternal hormones that regulate the supply and flow of breastmilk. Reflexes in the baby that are important for appropriate breastfeeding are rooting, suckling, and swallowing. To stimulate the nipple and remove milk from the breast, and to ensure an adequate supply and a good flow of milk, a baby's mouth needs to be well attached to the mother's breast. Breastmilk production increases with increased demand.

To ensure adequate milk production and flow for six months of exclusive breastfeeding, a baby needs to feed as often and for as long as desired, both day and night. This is called demand feeding, unrestricted feeding, or baby-led feeding. Even undernourished mothers can breastfeed successfully if they practice good techniques of position, attachment, and frequent suckling unless the mother is extremely malnourished.

Technical Basis of Complementary Feeding Recommendations

Public Health Core Competency 6A5: Describes the scientific evidence related to a public health issue, concern, or, intervention

Hygienically prepared, age-appropriate complementary foods must provide sufficient energy and nutrients to complement

breastmilk after six months. The rationale for complementary feeding recommendations includes the following:

- Physiological need for energy and nutrients required for healthy growth and development of the child
- Prevention of growth failure and specific deficiencies
- Developmental level from 6 months to 24 months of age, including the child's ability to chew and swallow, dentition, stomach size, taste preferences, emerging independence from the mother, fine and large motor development related to handling foods, and social interactions
- Impact of characteristics of food ingredients on appetite, taste, density, and nutrient absorption
- Impact of caregiver behaviors on the child's interest in eating
- Feeding patterns and methods used for optimizing breastfeeding during the period of complementary feeding from 6 to 23 months
- Common gaps, hazards, or pitfalls observed in traditional complementary feeding practices
- Cultural adaptation for locally available foods and diets in each community or country

Desirable Characteristics of Complementary Foods

Energy

Additional energy from complementary foods must supplement breastmilk (**Table 8-2**), with greater energy needs after illness or if the child has become malnourished. Complementary foods should have sufficient energy density. They must be thick and contain fat, oil, or animal foods, which are the energy-rich foods. Diluted cow's milk, thin gruels made of semolina and sugar, and watery lentil soup are low energy-dense, but common complementary foods. They fill up children's small stomachs and predispose children to undernutrition by reducing appetite and displacing breastmilk without providing sufficient energy and nutrients for growth.

Protein

Protein is required for synthesis of muscle tissue, enzymes, hormones, and blood cells. Animal-source foods (ASF) are the main sources of high-quality protein. In general,

Table 8-2 Recommended consistency, frequency and amount of complementary food by age

Age	Energy Needed per Day in Addition to Breastmilk	Texture	Frequency	Amount of Food an Average Child Will Usually Eat at Each Meal
6-8 months	200 calories (kcal) per day	Start with thick porridge, well-mashed foods; continue with mashed family foods	2-3 meals per day Depending on the child's appetite, 1-2 snacks may be offered	Start with 2-3 tablespoons per feed, increasing gradually
9-11 months	300 kcal per day	Finely chopped or mashed foods and foods that baby can pick up	3-4 meals per day Depending on the child's appetite, 1-2 snacks may be offered	½ of a 250 ml cup/bowl
12-23 months	550 kcal per day	Family foods, chopped or mashed if necessary	3-4 meals per day Depending on the child's appetite, 1-2 snacks may be offered	½ to full 250 ml cup/bowl

Data from the World Health Organization. Dewey, K. (2001). Guiding principles for complementary feeding of the breastfed child. Accessed August 25, 2013, from http://www.who.int/nutrition/publications/guiding_principles_compfeeding_breastfed.pdf

children whose diets contain adequate energy and a variety of foods, protein deficits are rare. Eggs, seafood, meat, chicken, and milk are examples of sources of high-quality protein.

Fats

Fat should provide 35% of total calories for children 6 to 23 months. One gram of fat provides nine calories of energy, while protein and carbohydrates each provide only four calories per gram. Fats therefore increase energy density and allow adequate intake in the limited space of their stomach. However, excess fat can interfere with appetite and breastmilk intake, and predispose infants to hyperlipidemia.

Essential fatty acids are critical for development of the immune system and brain, which is more than 50% fat by weight. Omega-3 fatty acids and total amount of fats in diets of young children in developing countries are generally below recommended levels.[29] Walnuts, soybean oil, rapeseed (canola) oil, and oily fish, such as salmon, sardines, herring, trout, and tuna, are good sources and should be used in complementary foods.

Vitamins

Vitamin A supports immune function and aids in nutrient absorption and utilization. Dark-green leafy vegetables and orange fruits and vegetables are good sources. Clinical vitamin A deficiency, including night blindness and corneal damage, is associated with higher mortality rates. Vitamin A deficiency was widespread in Bangladesh among young children until a nationwide campaign in the 1990s to distribute high-dose supplements to children aged 6 to 59 months. Coverage with vitamin A supplements in Bangladesh has been maintained at over 85% for almost a decade, and the country's rapid fall in child mortality is attributed in part to this intervention. Vitamin C is another critical vitamin during complementary feeding.

Minerals

Iron, zinc, and calcium are frequently deficient in diets of young children. ASF are rich in these minerals, but the necessary quantities to meet iron needs are too large to meet daily needs. To prevent and treat anemia, experts recommend iron supplements that provide 10–12 milligrams daily for 6- to 23-month-old children. Iron drops, syrups, or powders should be used under the guidance of a health provider.

Complementary Feeding Recommendations

The following are global recommendations that have been adapted and included in national nutrition strategies of many countries.

1. ***Introduce complementary foods at 6 months of age while continuing to breastfeed.***

   At 6 months, an infant requires foods other than breastmilk, and is developmentally ready for chewing, swallowing, and digesting other foods. The digestive system is mature enough to digest the starch, protein, and fat in a nonmilk diet. Very young infants push foods out with their tongues, but by 6 to 9 months, they can receive and hold semisolid food in their mouths.

2. ***Continue frequent on-demand breastfeeding until 2 years of age or beyond.***

   Breastfeeding should continue with complementary feeding up to 2 years of age or beyond. It should be on demand to allow the child's optimized intake of nutrients. Children tend to breastfeed less often after complementary foods are introduced, and breastfeeding needs to be actively encouraged during the day and night. Meals and snacks should be spaced to encourage breastfeeding.

3. ***Practice responsive feeding by applying the principles of psychosocial development.***

   Optimal complementary feeding depends not only on what, but also on how, when, where, and by whom a child is fed. Responsive complementary feeding includes considering the child's interests in food and feeding, giving enough time for children to feed properly, and offering healthy choices. Children should have their own plates or bowls so caregivers can know whether the child is eating enough. Children should be fed with clean utensils, such as spoons, or thoroughly washed hands. Feeding should be slow, patient, and encouraging but not forceful. Caregivers should wait until the child is ready and offer different tastes, textures, and varieties of food to interest the child. Caregivers should allow children to pick up foods for self-feeding, but continue to supervise. They should keep the focus on feeding rather than distractions. The child should be seated facing the mother or caregiver to allow frequent eye contact, and the caregiver should show positive emotions with each mouthful. Refusal by children is normal from time to time, but caregivers can maintain interest by waiting and offering new foods.

4. ***Practice good hygiene and proper food handling.***

   Safe preparation and storage of complementary foods can prevent microbial contamination, a major cause of diarrheal disease. Diarrhea peaks at the time of complementary feeding at 6–11 months of age as children eat increasing amounts and varieties of foods. Diarrhea in the first 2 years is associated with nutrient losses and stunting. Nutritional status also suffers during fevers and respiratory infections, due to appetite loss and increased nutrient needs for fighting infections in addition to growth.

   Tropical, or environmental, enteropathy is common in developing countries and does not exhibit clinical signs. It is associated with poor hygiene and sanitation and causes damage to the absorptive capacity of the small intestine. Washing hands with soap and water has been found to reduce diarrhea. In Bangladesh, mothers of children under 2 years improved handwashing with soap before handling the child's food by locating soap and water close to the place of feeding, when this was accompanied by home visits and community groups where the causation of illness due to poor handwashing practices was discussed.[30]

5. ***Starting at 6 months of age, increase the quantity of solid and semisolid foods as the child gets older, while maintaining frequent breastfeeding.***

   Recommendations for the quantity of food needed to meet caloric needs of young children have been developed for the ages of 6 to 8 months, 9 to 11 months, and 12 to 24 months (Table 8-2). Adequacy of nutrients is assured by choosing concentrated sources, such as ASF.

6. ***Change the consistencies or texture of foods as the infant grows older, adapting to the infant's requirements and abilities.***

   Appropriate consistency for complementary food depends on the child's age and neuromuscular development. Beginning at 7 months, infants can eat mashed or semisolid family foods. By 8 months, most infants can start picking up and eating small pieces of food. By 9 months, most children want to feed themselves. Caregivers should encourage this, but continue to supervise during meal times. By 12 months, most children can eat the same foods as the rest of the family. A complementary food should be thick enough to stay on a spoon without dripping off. These foods are also generally more energy- and nutrient-dense than thin, watery, or soft foods, and more likely to allow nutrient needs to be met.

7. *Increase the number of times that the child is fed complementary foods as the child gets older.*

As children grow and need larger total quantities of food, meal frequency and size should be increased. The number of meals needed depends on children's energy needs and the capacity or size of the child's stomach, which is usually 30 milliliters per kilogram of the child's body weight. A child who weighs 8 kilograms will have a stomach capacity of 240 milliliters, about one large cupful, and cannot be expected to eat more than that at one meal. If the child has the appetite, one to two nutritious, convenient snacks, often self-fed finger foods, should be offered.

8. *Feed a variety of nutrient-rich foods to meet all nutrient needs.*

Diet diversity is associated with better nutritional status and lower stunting. Four or more varieties fed in a day are associated with better nutrition indicators and likelihood of meeting nutrient needs. In addition to ASF, pulses (peas, beans, lentils, nuts), served with vitamin C-rich foods to aid iron absorption, provide important nutrients.

Common mistakes in complementary feeding include providing overdiluted foods and water; too much rice, potatoes, or banana that contains mainly starch; and highly sweetened or salty processed foods like juice, biscuits, chocolates, and chips that reduce appetite for healthy family foods. Sugar and sugary drinks, such as soda, should be avoided because they decrease the child's appetite for more nutritious foods. Tea and coffee are not recommended because they contain compounds that can interfere with iron absorption.

9. *Use vitamin and mineral supplements for the infant as needed.*

Plant-based complementary foods are unlikely to provide sufficient amounts of certain nutrients, such as iron, zinc, vitamin B6, and vitamin B12, to meet recommended nutrient intakes. Inclusion of ASF can help fulfill needs, and fortified foods or micronutrient supplements may also be necessary.

10. *During illness, increase fluid intake through more frequent breastfeeding, and encourage the child to eat soft, favorite foods. After illness, give food more often and encourage the child to eat more.*

To meet increased fluid needs during illness, children should be encouraged to take more breastmilk. Appetite often decreases and the desire to breastfeed increases, so breastmilk may become the main source of both fluid and nutrients. Children should be encouraged to eat some complementary food to maintain nutrient intake and enhance recovery. Intake is usually better when children are offered their favorite foods, and when foods are soft and appetizing. To make up for a smaller appetite, caregivers must offer more frequent, smaller meals than usual. During recovery, caregivers should offer an extra portion at each meal or provide an extra meal or snack each day.

Current Patterns of Infant and Young Child Feeding

Actual IYCF practices are largely inconsistent with recommendations, and high levels of undernutrition persist in many developing nations. Efforts to improve IYCF have resulted in some improvements, but much remains to be done.

Twenty-seven countries have documented increases in exclusive breastfeeding since 1990, according to UNICEF (**Figure 8-2**).[31] However, globally, as the level of exclusive breastfeeding for six months has remained below 40% since 1990, further improvements are both possible and necessary.

Barriers to Good IYCF Practices

Public Health Core Competency 4A2: Recognizes the role of cultural, social, and behavioral factors in the accessibility, availability, acceptability, and delivery of public health services

Public Health Core Competency 5A1: Recognizes community linkages and relationships among multiple factors (or determinants) affecting health

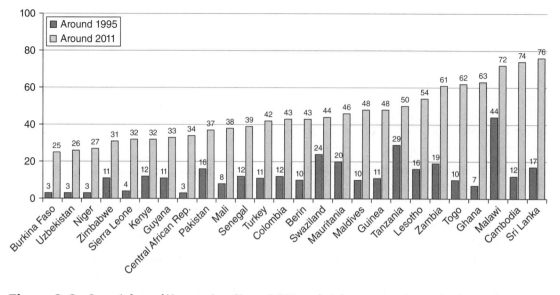

Figure 8-2 Countries with greater than 20% point increases in exclusive breastfeeding levels

Reproduced from Childinfo (United Nations Children's Fund). (2012). Statistics by area: child nutrition: progress. Accessed September 10, 2013, from http://www.childinfo.org/breastfeeding_progress.html

---

> *Public Health Core Competency 6A2: Identifies prominent events in the history of the public health profession*

Most mothers and caregivers of young children remain unaware about the "what" and "why" of proper IYCF. Low income and lack of time are common barriers, although even well-to-do families can display poor feeding practices. Reducing poverty and overcoming gaps in awareness can help address challenges, but progress has been hindered, around the world, by lack of resources and sustained commitment to implement programs for IYCF on a large scale. Although numerous policies, strategies, and guidelines exist, political and financial investment in delivering one of public health's most cost-effective preventive interventions has been inadequate. Perhaps the case for investing in IYCF has not been made effectively. Regional differences may also be barriers. For example, in Africa, concern about HIV transmission through breastmilk has been a barrier to increasing breastfeeding rates. Insufficient policy and implementation guidelines for countries, indicators for tracking status and progress, and consensus on what constitutes adequate complementary feeding in developing countries are additional barriers. Advice on optimal complementary feeding has expanded to include recommendations to increase protein intake and total energy consumption, and to improve the micronutrient density of complementary foods. Changing recommendations created confusion, and frontline programs and personnel could not keep pace with changing knowledge in this area.[32,33,34] Today, however, the renewed interest in trying to improve complementary feeding to achieve better health stems from: (1) new scientific evidence on how this should be done,[35] (2) updated guidelines from WHO with concrete recommendations,[36,37] (3) new data on the effectiveness of fortified therapeutic foods for moderately and severely malnourished children, and (4) many new products to enrich children's diets. For example, a micronutrient powder commonly referred to as "sprinkles" has been developed as a home-based fortificant for complementary foods and is widely used in Africa and Asia.[38]

According to global authorities,[39] reasons for lagging progress in IYCF worldwide include the lack of a common agenda with a shared vision of change. IYCF appears to be an "orphan issue" not owned in a cohesive and passionate advocacy community. Forces of the infant formula industry counter efforts to promote breastfeeding. The importance of IYCF is only beginning to be recognized. The absence of effective, comprehensive approaches at scale and lack of fully implemented interventions have added to delays in progress.

Additional barriers to breastfeeding are at the individual or community level. Mothers may be discouraged by cracked nipples, engorgement, and mastitis. Support to the mother for early initiation, proper technique, and ongoing breastfeeding is effective. Marketing of infant formula, workplace policies, and education also affect breastfeeding. Social support and degree of confidence influence a mother's choice to continue or discontinue breastfeeding.

Examples of Feeding Constraints in Bangladesh

In Bangladesh, infants are frequently fed a diluted gruel made of semolina, sugar, and water. BRAC (formerly the Bangladesh Rural Advancement Committee), the largest nongovernmental organization (NGO) working to improve IYCF, promotes the addition of fried food to increase fat content and ASF, such as fish, to provide essential fatty acids. The program includes home visits by trained community workers to coach mothers on selecting appropriate foods for children 6 to 23 months of age from what is cooked for the family. An accompanying television campaign places advertisements in the favorite drama serials and movies watched by women in Bangladesh. Results have shown a significant increase in use of the complementary foods being promoted after two years.

The casual style of feeding that predominates in some areas of Bangladesh is another barrier to proper IYCF. Young children are left to feed themselves, and encouragement to eat is rare. In such settings, a more active style of feeding can improve dietary intake. In other regions, caregivers try to force young children to eat. Rural mothers may be busy with household chores, such as house cleaning, laundry, cooking, and caring for poultry and small animals, and they may lack time to prepare appropriate types of foods and slowly teach young children to eat them. Mothers may push or force food into the child's mouth, or grandparents and school-age children may have responsibility for complementary feeding. Mothers may not be available to feed when the child is ready to eat, and other family members may feed nonnutritious foods such as chips, sugary drinks, and biscuits. Children can become disinterested in consuming healthy family foods at meal times.

In Bangladesh, national hygiene promotion programs raised levels of handwashing after using the toilet, but less than 20% of mothers reported washing hands with soap before feeding young children after a national campaign in 2010. Obstacles include lack of social pressure, water and soap not being conveniently located where young children are fed, and lack of belief that washing hands properly can protect children, although most children are fed by mashing the food by hand and feeding by hand. A new initiative is now linking handwashing with complementary feeding, and health workers are trained to help families locate a water container and soap close to the place where the young child is fed. Reminders are also delivered through television advertisements and by distributing stickers that can be placed inside the home.

Setting Up Country Programs

The Global Strategy for Infant and Young Child Nutrition[40] includes evidence-based suggestions and approaches for scaling up public health interventions to improve nutrition and health outcomes. Three main approaches are involved in setting up country programs:

- Improve the policy and regulatory environment to support IYCF interventions.

- Shape, create, and support demand for the means to provide proper IYCF, with a focus on early and exclusive breastfeeding and appropriate complementary feeding.

- Increase demand for and supply and use of nutrient-rich, safe complementary foods and related products, including family foods and fortified foods.

The following programmatic interventions are considered effective for improving IYCF:[41]

- The **International Code of Marketing of Breast-milk Substitutes**, which limits the promotion of breastmilk substitutes in ways that discourage breastfeeding.

- The **Baby-Friendly Hospital Initiative** (BFHI).[42,43] The hospital environment can be highly influential in ensuring timely initiation and supporting mothers to start up breastfeeding successfully. BFHI contains 10 steps that hospitals can take for supporting mothers to breastfeed. The lack of continued monitoring of the 10 steps allows decline of quality of breastfeeding support in hospitals designated as Baby Friendly. BFHI principles should be extended to community health clinics. However, in nations where home delivery is common, other means of support are needed, such as counseling during pregnancy in preparation for early breastfeeding. In Bangladesh, for example, a far higher proportion of pregnant women are seen at least once for antenatal checkups as compared with the proportion who deliver in health facilities, underscoring the need for prenatal counseling.[44] In Latin America, where a large proportion of births occur in hospitals, countries have developed monitoring mechanisms to ensure that pro-breastfeeding practices are being followed in hospitals.[45] Recommendations for optimal feeding in the United States include supporting breastfeeding in the hospital after delivery through education and practice.[46]

- Advocacy and policy changes for giving higher priority to nutrition in medical and nursing education, in-service training, and pre-service education of health professionals to implement proven IYCF interventions as part of routine maternal and child health. Currently, most health service providers in developing countries do not obtain information or skills training on IYCF and counseling techniques during their medical and nursing education.

- Community-based promotion and support. Mothers need ongoing support to deal with a changing array of feeding-related situations as they move from initiation to maintaining exclusive breastfeeding over a six-month period, to the introduction of complementary feeding.[47] In many communities, feeding chores shift to other family members if mothers go back to work. As children grow from 6 months to 2 years, mothers and other caregivers need to be prepared to deal with a new range of issues such as fussy eaters, continuation of breastfeeding in the older infant, feeding during and after illness, food preferences, and so on. Health workers, social workers, and extension agents have shown impacts by counseling mothers through direct interpersonal contact.

- Maternity legislation and workplace support, which are increasingly necessary as more mothers of infants and young children enter the workforce.[48] Increasing numbers of nations, including Bangladesh, Chile, and Vietnam, are mandating six months of maternity leave, including job security and in some cases benefits, to mothers who stay home to be able to breastfeed exclusively. Some are providing breastfeeding rooms and breaks so that women can express and store breastmilk. In the United States, for example, the 2010 Patient Protection and Affordable Care Act mandates that companies provide private spaces where mothers can breastfeed, as well as adequate break time to do so.[49]

- Public awareness and mass media initiatives. Results from previous mass media campaigns[50] and recent program experiences from the Alive & Thrive project in Bangladesh, Ethiopia, and Vietnam are showing that public awareness and mass media reaching mothers and other family members, plus social mobilization to engage community-level opinion leaders, are key program actions to support large-scale shifts in IYCF.

Scaling Up IYCF Programs: Emphasis on Bangladesh

Public Health Core Competency 3A4: Communication Skills: Conveys public health information using a variety of approaches (e.g., social networks, media, blogs)

With the acceptance of IYCF as a high global priority for public health investments,[51,52] several countries have begun the process of **scaling up**, which requires modifications to ensure that interventions will remain consistent and sustainable on the national level. Several significant program reviews and frameworks helped inform the development of fresh approaches with a focus on bringing about behavior change and scaling up. For example, a review of country case studies highlighted the importance of policies, legislation, large-scale communication activities, and community support for mothers.[53] A review of interventions for infant and child feeding highlighted the importance of dietary diversity, micronutrient content, and continuation of breastfeeding.[54] Partnerships and coordination across sectors were highlighted in a review of successful programs in 2005 from Africa and Latin America.[55] Complementary feeding interventions related to maternal education were reviewed and showed evidence that programs can be effective when tailored to local settings and available resources.[56,57] A global framework for the integration of IYCF in routine health programs was developed in 1999 and adopted by multiple countries.[58]

A national coalition of government and NGO agencies are applying lessons learned in Bangladesh and elsewhere to expand the geographic coverage of effective interventions. Multiple community-based interventions showed positive results, and main challenges identified through situational analysis and formative research in 2008–2009 involved the lack of large-scale programs to reach more mothers. In addition, no cohesive strategy existed to focus on the various barriers that influence feeding choices made by mothers. Recent increases in breastfeeding in Bangladesh have built on many favorable conditions, such as the presence of successful NGO programs, improved access to and utilization of basic health services by the population, high exposure to mass media, and a common national language, which facilitates communications. National IYCF policies are largely consistent with current global WHO recommendations. In 2007, the Institute of Public Health Nutrition of the ministry of health of Bangladesh prepared a National IYCF Strategy, and in 2010, the National Communication Framework and Plan for IYCF was prepared with the support of Alive & Thrive and more than 20 other stakeholders. An active Nutrition Working Group of donors and NGO partners that facilitates exchange of information about broader nutrition programs, and formation in 2010 of an Alliance for IYCF composed of implementing agencies specifically for IYCF, such as UNICEF, CARE, Save the Children, various governmental departments, and others, helped give momentum to a cohesive national program for IYCF. Childhood malnutrition has been highlighted for special attention by the ministry of health of Bangladesh as part of the planning process for the 2011–2016 health sector strategy. Maternal Newborn and Child Health (MNCH) programs are especially well suited to integrating IYCF counseling for mothers into existing programs because they come in frequent contact with pregnant women and children under 2 years of age.

Role of a Collaborative Public Health Program: Alive & Thrive

Alive & Thrive is a six-year initiative being implemented in Ethiopia, Vietnam, and Bangladesh during 2009–2014. Its focus is improving infant and child nutrition by promoting early initiation of breastfeeding, exclusive breastfeeding for six months, and improved complementary feeding. In each country, several agencies work together to achieve the project objectives. The lead global managing agency of Alive & Thrive is FHI 360, which also implements the communication component. Another collaborating organization is BRAC, which implements the community component consisting of home visits to coach and support mothers and social mobilization to obtain community support for the program and mothers. Governmental agencies include IPHN (Institute of Public Health Nutrition Bangladesh), which coordinates implementation, and GMMB, which leads advocacy efforts to raise policy makers' awareness of IYCF and child nutrition and promotes implementation of the national policies and strategies for IYCF in collaboration with journalists. The International Food Policy Research Institute (IFPRI) is responsible for measurement

and evaluation, and the University of California at Davis manages a small research grant program.

To address barriers and motivations identified in the formative research conducted to understand maternal perceptions,[59,60] a practical and effective community model was developed through BRAC's Essential Health Care and MNCH programs in Bangladesh. This provides direct hands-on support to mothers of under-2-year-old children and is reinforced by a multimedia communication strategy. The basis for designing the Alive & Thrive Bangladesh program is a theory of change model (**Table 8-3**), whose main program components are:

Multiple communication channels and media. These reach mothers and key influential decision makers, and mobilize thousands of BRAC and other NGO community-based volunteers and NGO/government health workers so that they can support mothers in following IYCF desirable practices through home visits and group meetings.

Dialogue and forums with policymakers and community leaders. Ongoing dialogue is maintained with selected categories of national, district, and community leaders on the importance of nutrition and IYCF and to encourage each category of opinion leaders to contribute to improving IYCF.

Enhanced skills and performance of frontline workers and health providers. To enable community workers to support mothers, several performance-enhancing strategies are used: basic training on IYCF, supervision, ongoing refresher training, job aids, monthly meetings, recognition of good work, and simple monitoring methods. Medical and nursing colleges are also being engaged to update medical and nursing curricula so that health providers and public health professionals are pro-IYCF in their practice.

Innovations. Innovations being tested in Bangladesh include cash incentives provided to frontline workers based on their performance, as well as handwashing linked with complementary feeding and phone counseling to supplement home visits.

Strategic prioritization. Priority is given to strengthening coalitions, alliances, and champions for building leadership and to broaden stakeholder ownership of the IYCF interventions within and outside the nutrition sector. For sustainability, the project makes a special effort to create widespread awareness and generate commitment to investing in IYCF.

Table 8-3 Alive & Thrive Theory of Change in Bangladesh

Barriers to address	Absence of proven nutrition interventions
	Use of ineffective practices in health facilities
	Lack of skill and knowledge in health workers
	Unawareness of efforts by general population
	Lack of social support
	No clear leadership
Diverse strategies to use	Target advocacy at all levels: national, organizational, private, and professional sectors
	Mobilize trained health workers into communities
	Implement multi-channel communications
	Hold organizations accountable for results
	Build investment and strategies for stakeholders
Desired outcomes	Exclusive breastfeeding for infants under 6 months
	Improvement of diet and feeding practices for children under 2 years
	Political support to mainstream, invest in, and enforce policies
Measurable impact	4.3 million DALYs
	299,000 fewer children with stunted growth
	Additional 844,000 infants exclusively breastfed

Data from Alive & Thrive (n.d.). Alive & Thrive's strategies for improving infant and young child feeding practices. http://www.aliveandthrive.org/sites/default/files/A&T%20strategies%20and%20theory%20of%20change%20June%202011.pdf. Accessed September 6, 2013.

Conclusion

Proper IYCF supports proper childhood growth and development, while inappropriate practices increase morbidity and mortality among infants and young children. Suboptimal breastfeeding and complementary feeding practices remain widespread globally, for reasons such as lack of resources, inadequate nutrition knowledge, and unsupportive policies. As recognition of the economic and health consequences of poor IYCF increases, public health nutrition programs can gain leverage among nonprofit organizations and in the political arenas, the private sector, and the community. As seen in the Alive & Thrive initiative in Bangladesh, Ethiopia, and Vietnam, a holistic approach based on theories of change, along with strong multisector collaboration and careful scaling up, can lead to improved IYCF policy and programs. Future concerns include sustainability and reaching all segments of society.

References

1 National Institute of Population Research and Training (NIPORT), Mitra and Associates, & ICF International. (2013). *Bangladesh demographic and health survey 2011*. Dhaka, Bangladesh, and Calverton, MD: NIPORT, Mitra and Associates & ICF International.

2 Senarath, U., Agho, K. E., Akram, D. E., Godakandage, S. S., Hazir, T., Jayawickrama, H., Joshi, N., . . . Dibley, M. J. (2012). Comparisons of complementary feeding indicators and associated factors in children aged 6-23 months across five South Asian countries. *Maternal & Child Nutrition*, (Suppl. 1), 89-106. doi:10.1111/j.1740-8709.2011.00370.x

3 World Health Organization. (n.d.). Feto-maternal nutrition and low birth weight. Retrieved from http://www.who.int/nutrition/topics/feto_maternal/en/index.html

4 National Institute of Population Research and Training (NIPORT), Mitra and Associates, & ICF International. (2013). *Bangladesh demographic and health survey 2011*. Dhaka, Bangladesh, and Calverton, MD: NIPORT, Mitra and Associates & ICF International.

5 Senarath, U., Agho, K. E., Akram, D. E., Godakandage, S. S., Hazir, T., Jayawickrama, H., Joshi, N., . . . Dibley, M. J. (2012). Comparisons of complementary feeding indicators and associated factors in children aged 6-23 months across five South Asian countries. *Maternal & Child Nutrition*, (Suppl. 1), 89-106. doi:10.1111/j.1740-8709.2011.00370.x

6 Arifeen, S. E., Hogue, D. M., Akter, T., Rahman, M., Hoque, M. E., Begum, K., . . . & Black, R. E. (2009). Effect of the Integrated Management of Childhood Illness (IMCI) strategy on childhood

mortality and nutrition in a rural area in Bangladesh: A random-ized controlled trial. *Lancet, 374*(9687), 393-403.

7   World Health Organization. (n.d.). Feto-maternal nutrition and low birth weight. Retrieved from http://www.who.int/nutrition/topics/feto_maternal/en/index.html

8   Thakur, S. K., Roy, S. K., Paul, K., Khanam, M., Khatun, W., & Sarker, D. (2012). Effect of nutrition education on exclusive breastfeed-ing for nutritional outcome of low birth weight babies. *European Journal of Clinical Nutrition, 66*(3), 376-81.

9   Lutter, C. K., & Lutter, R. (2012). Fetal and early childhood undernu-trition, mortality, and lifelong health. *Science, 337*(6101), 1495-99.

10 Jones, G., Steketee, R. W., Black, R. E., Bhutta, Z. A., & Morris, S. S. (2003). How many child deaths can we prevent this year? *Lancet, 362*(9377), 65-71.

11 United Nations. (n.d.). *The Millennium Development Goals report 2013*. New York, NY: United Nations.

12 World Health Organization. (2009). *Infant and young child feeding: Model chapter for textbooks for medical students and allied health professionals*. Geneva: World Health Organization.

13 Scaling Up Nutrition. (n.d.). Website, http://scalingupnutrition.org

14 UNICEF. (n.d.). *The big picture*. Retrieved from http://www.unicef.org/nutrition/index_bigpicture.html

15 Lutter, C. K., & Chaparro, C. M. (2009). Neonatal period: Linking best nutrition practices at birth to optimize maternal and infant health and survival. *Food and Nutrition Bulletin, 30* (2 Suppl.), S215-24.

16 *Scientific rationale: Benefits of breastfeeding*. (2012). Retrieved from UNICEF website, http://www.unicef.org/nutrition/files/Scientific_rationale_for_benefits_of_breasfteeding.pdf

17 Lamberti, L. M., Fischer Walker, C. L., Noiman, A., Victora, C., & Black, R. E. (2011). Breastfeeding and the risk for diarrhea morbidity and mortality. *BMC Public Health, 11*(Suppl. 3), S15. doi:10.1186/1471-2458-11-S3-S15

18 Aguiar, H., & Silva, A. I. (2011). Breastfeeding: The importance of intervening. *Acta Médica Portuguesa, 24*(Suppl. 4), 889-96.

19 World Health Organization (WHO). (2002). *Report of the expert consultation on the optimal duration of exclusive breastfeeding*. Geneva: World Health Organization. Retrieved from http://www.who.int/nutrition/publications/optimal_duration_of_exc_bfeed-ing_report_eng.pdf

20 Kramer, M. S., & Kakuma, R. (2012). Optimal duration of exclu-sive breastfeeding. *Cochrane Database of Systematic Reviews, 8*, Art. CD003517. doi:10.1002/14651858.CD003517.pub2

21 Pan American Health Organization & World Health Organization. (2003). *Guiding principles for complementary feeding of the breastfed child*. Washington, DC: Pan American Health Organization.

22 Aguiar, H., & Silva, A. I. (2011). Breastfeeding: The importance of intervening. *Acta Médica Portuguesa, 24*(Suppl. 4), 889-96.

23 Harder, T., Bergmann, R., Kallischnigg, G., & Plagemann A. (2005). Duration of breastfeeding and risk of overweight: A meta-analysis. *American Journal of Epidemiology, 162*(5), 397-403.

24 Aguiar, H., & Silva, A. I. (2011). Breastfeeding: The importance of intervening. *Acta Médica Portuguesa, 24*(Suppl. 4), 889-96.

25 World Health Organization & UNICEF. (2003). *Global strat-egy for infant and young child feeding*. Geneva: World Health Organization.

26 Lutter, C. K., & Lutter, R. (2012). Fetal and early childhood under-nutrition, mortality, and lifelong health. *Science, 337*(6101), 1495-99.

27 World Health Organization. (2009). *Infant and young child feeding: Model chapter for textbooks for medical stu-dents and allied health professionals*. Geneva: World Health Organization. Retrieved from http://whqlibdoc.who.int/publica-tions/2009/9789241597494_eng.pdf

28 Garofalo, M., & Abenhaim, H. A. (2012). Early versus delayed cord clamping in term and preterm births: A review. *Journal of Obstetrics and Gynaecology Canada (JOGC), 34*(6), 525-31.

29 Huffman, S. L., Harika, R. K., Eilander, A., Osendarp, S. J. (2011). Essential fats: how do they affect growth and development of infants and young children in developing countries? A literature review. *Maternal and Child Nutrition,* (Suppl 3), 44-65.

30 Ghosh, P. K., for the Center for Communicable Diseases. (2012). *Handwashing and nutrition practices in rural Bangladesh*. Retrieved from Alive & Thrive website, http://www.aliveandthrive.org/sites/default/files/Handwashing%20and%20nutriton%20practices-Probir%20Kumar%20Ghosh-April%2019%202012.pdf

31 Cai, X., Wardlaw, T., & Brown, D. W. (2012). Global trends in exclu-sive breastfeeding. *International Breastfeeding Journal, 7*, 12.

32 Thakur, S. K., Roy, S. K., Paul, K., Khanam, M., Khatun, W., & Sarker, D. (2012). Effect of nutrition education on exclusive breastfeed-ing for nutritional outcome of low birth weight babies. *European Journal of Clinical Nutrition, 66*(3), 376-81.

33 Lutter, C. K., & Lutter, R. (2012). Fetal and early childhood under-nutrition, mortality, and lifelong health. *Science, 337*(6101), 1495-99.

34 Jones, G., Steketee, R. W., Black, R. E., Bhutta, Z. A., & Morris, S. S. (2003). How many child deaths can we prevent this year? *Lancet, 362*(9377), 65-71.

35 United Nations. (n.d.) *The Millennium Development Goals report 2013*. New York, NY: United Nations.

36 World Health Organization. (2009). *Infant and young child feed-ing: Model chapter for textbooks for medical students and allied health professionals*. Geneva: World Health Organization.

37 Scaling Up Nutrition. (n.d.). Website, http://scalingupnutrition.org

38 Zlotkin, S., Arthur, P., Antwi, K. Y., & Yeung G. (2001). Treatment of anemia with microencapsulated ferrous fumarate plus ascorbic acid supplied as sprinkles to complementary (wean-ing) foods. *American Journal of Clinical Nutrition, 74*(6), 791-95.

39 Alipui, N. (2012). *Breastfeeding on the worldwide agenda: Successes, challenges and the way forward*. PowerPoint presen-tation at the World Breastfeeding Conference, December 6-9, 2012. Retrieved from http://www.worldbreastfeedingconference.org/images/128/Dr_%20Nicholas%20Alipui.pdf

40 World Health Organization & UNICEF. (2003). *Global strategy for infant and young child feeding.* Geneva: World Health Organization.

41 World Health Organization. (2013). *Essential nutrition actions: Improving maternal, newborn, infant and young child health and nutrition.* Geneva: World Health Organization. Retrieved from http://apps.who.int/iris/bitstream/10665/84409/1/9789241505550_eng.pdf

42 Saadeh, R. J. (2012). The baby-friendly hospital initiative 20 years on: Facts, progress, and the way forward. *Journal of Human Lactation, 28*(3), 272-75. doi:10.1177/0890334412446690

43 World Health Organization & UNICEF. (2009). *Baby-friendly hospital initiative: Revised, updated and expanded for integrated care.* Geneva: World Health Organization. Retrieved from http://www.who.int/nutrition/topics/bfhi/en/index.html

44 Pervin, J., Moran, A., Rahman, M., Razzaque, A., Sibley, L., Streatfield, P. K., . . . Rahman, A. (2012). Association of antenatal care with facility delivery and perinatal survival: A population-based study in Bangladesh. *BMC Pregnancy and Childbirth, 12*, 111.

45 Pérez-Escamilla, R. (2007). Evidence based breast-feeding promotion: The Baby-Friendly Hospital Initiative. *Journal of Nutrition, 137*(2), 484-47.

46 Baby Friendly USA. (n.d.). *The ten steps to successful breastfeeding.* Retrieved from http://www.babyfriendlyusa.org/about-us/baby-friendly-hospital-initiative/the-ten-steps

47 Lassi, Z. S., Haider, B. A., & Bhutta, Z. A. (2010). Community-based intervention packages for reducing maternal and neonatal morbidity and mortality and improving neonatal outcomes. *Cochrane Database of Systemic Reviews, 11*, Art. CD007754. doi:10.1002/14651858.CD007754.pub2

48 Ogbuanu, C., Glover, S., Probst, J., Liu, J., & Hussey, J. (2011). The effect of maternity leave length and time of return to work on breastfeeding. *Pediatrics, 127*(6), e1414-27. doi:10.1542/peds.2010-0459

49 Rogers, H. R., & Hartman, K. V. (2010). Nursing mothers in the workplace: New federal law creates new obligations for employers. *Bloomberg Law Reports: Labor & Employment, 4*(43).

50 McDivitt, J. A., Zimicki, S., Hornik, R., & Abulaban, A. (1993). The impact of the Healthcom mass media campaign on timely initiation of breastfeeding in Jordan. *Studies in Family Planning, 24*(5), 295-309.

51 Scaling Up Nutrition. (n.d.). Website, www.scalingupnutrition.org

52 One Thousand Days. (n.d.). Website, www.thousanddays.org

53 Mangasaryan, N., Martin, L., Brownlee, A., Ogunlade, A., Rudert, C., & Cai, X. (2012). Breastfeeding promotion, support and protection: Review of six country programmes. *Nutrients, 4*(8), 990-1014. doi:10.3390/nu4080990

54 Dewey, K. G., & Adu-Afarwuah, S. (2008). Systematic review of the efficacy and effectiveness of complementary feeding interventions in developing countries. *Maternal & Child Nutrition, 4* (Suppl. s1), 24-85. doi:10.1111/j.1740-8709.2007.00124.x

55 Quinn, V. J., Guyon, A. B., Schubert, J. W., Stone-Jiménez, M., Hainsworth, M. D., & Martin, L. H. (2005). Improving breastfeeding practices on a broad scale at the community level: Success stories from Africa and Latin America. *Journal of Human Lactation, 21*(3), 345-54.

56 Huffman, S. L., Green, C. P., Caulfield, L. E., & Piwoz, E. G. (2000). Improving infant feeding practices: Programs can be effective! *Malaysian Journal of Nutrition, 6*(2), 139-46.

57 Shi, L., & Zhang, J. (2011). Recent evidence of the effectiveness of educational interventions for improving complementary feeding practices in developing countries. *Journal of Tropical Pediatrics, 57*(2), 91-98. doi:10.1093/tropej/fmq053

58 World Health Organization, BASICS, & UNICEF. (1999). *Nutrition essentials: A guide for health managers.* Retrieved from http://whqlibdoc.who.int/hq/1999/a81547.pdf

59 Rasheed, S., Haider, R., Hassan, N., Pachón, H., Islam, S., Jalal, C. S., & Sanghvi, T. G. (2011). Why does nutrition deteriorate rapidly among children under 2 years of age? Using qualitative methods to understand community perspectives on complementary feeding practices in Bangladesh. *Food and Nutrition Bulletin, 32*(3), 192-200.

60 Haider, R., Rasheed, S., Sanghvi, T. G., Hassan, N., Pachon, H., Islam, S., & Jalal, C. S. (2010). Breastfeeding in infancy: Identifying the program-relevant issues in Bangladesh. *International Breastfeeding Journal, 5*, 21-32. doi:10.1186/1746-4358-5-21

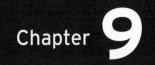
Global Perspectives on the Promotion, Protection, and Support of Breastfeeding

Heather Wasser, PhD, MPH, RD, IBCLC

"Each mother's decision about how she feeds her baby is a personal one. Because of the ramifications of her decision on her baby's health as well as her own, every mother in our nation deserves information, guidance, and support with this decision from her family and friends, the community where she lives, the health professionals on whom she relies, and her employer."–Kathleen Sebelius, Secretary, U.S. Department of Health and Human Services

Reproduced from the U.S. Department of Health and Human Services. (2011). The Surgeon General's Call to Action to Support Breastfeeding. Washington, DC: U.S. Department of Health and Human Services, Office of the Surgeon General. Available at: http://www.surgeongeneral .gov/library/calls/breastfeeding/index.html.

Learning Objectives

- List the recommendations for breastfeeding by the World Health Organization and the American Academy of Pediatrics.
- Explain the differences between breastfeeding, predominant breastfeeding, and exclusive breastfeeding.
- Describe current trends in breastfeeding, based on data from global and domestic surveys.
- List benefits of breastfeeding for infants and children, for women, and for society.
- Identify at least three barriers to achieving optimal breastfeeding practices.
- Describe at least three public health approaches that can help women initiate and maintain breastfeeding.

Case Study: Mothers and Others

In the United States, African American mothers are less likely than Caucasian or Hispanic mothers to meet national breastfeeding objectives. Despite this **disparity**, few **evidence-based** interventions target this racial group specifically. To fill this gap, public health researchers at the University of North Carolina at Chapel Hill designed an **efficacy trial** of a multicomponent, tailored intervention focused on African American infants, mothers, and families.

The Infant Care, Feeding, and Risk of Obesity (Infant Care) study was an earlier trial conducted by the same set of researchers, among 217 African American mothers living in central North Carolina. Infant Care data showed that many mothers were feeding formula and introducing **complementary foods** as early as the first month, with half of the infants fed complementary foods by 3 months of age. The World Health Organization (WHO) and the American Academy of Pediatrics (AAP)[1] recommend exclusive breastfeeding through 6 months. The most common food given was infant cereal, which was often added to the infant's bottle. Feeding cereal in the bottle is a common practice to soothe infants. Caregivers may perceive that infant crying is due to hunger and the need for more than breastmilk or formula.[2,3] Consistent with this belief, mothers in the Infant Care study were more likely to have introduced complementary foods if their infants were perceived as "fussy."[4]

Development of the Mothers and Others program was influenced by **peer-reviewed** studies on the barriers to breastfeeding for African American mothers and by lessons learned from Infant Care. First, the intervention needed to begin during pregnancy to prevent switching to formula and/or introducing complementary foods as early as the first month of life. Second, the intervention needed to address infant fussing and crying. The Baby Behavior Campaign was an existing effective breastfeeding intervention developed by researchers at the Human Lactation Center at the University of California, Davis, and piloted in the California **Special Supplemental Nutrition Program for Women, Infants, and Children (WIC)**.

The literature also documented the impact of fathers' and grandmothers' attitudes and opinions on breastfeeding. For example, negative paternal attitudes toward breastfeeding are associated with lower likelihood of initiating and maintaining breastfeeding.[5,6] Similarly, inclusion of fathers or grandmothers in educational components tends to increase initiation and duration of breastfeeding.[7,8] Given these findings, the Mothers and Others intervention was designed to include these influential people by asking mothers multiple times throughout the intervention to identify the person they want to be included in the intervention. The use of **focus groups** is planned to adapt the California Baby Behavior Campaign and other materials to specific needs of local fathers and grandmothers. If successful in promoting breastfeeding, Mothers and Others will have public health relevance for future breastfeeding promotion efforts.

Discussion Questions

- Which social determinants can lead to disparities in breastfeeding rates?
- Why was the Infant Care study an important precursor to Mothers and Others?
- In which ways did Mothers and Others address the specific target population?
- Describe the importance of social support in breastfeeding.

Introduction

Ensuring optimal breastfeeding practices is critical in achieving various Millennium Development Goals (MDGs). Suboptimal breastfeeding practices result in 1.4 million annual deaths of children under 5, account for 10% of the annual disease burden,[9] and have further health and economic benefits for children, women, and society. Consequently, the research and support of promotion, protection, and support of breastfeeding has surged among the public health community. Lasting change requires public health interventions that address all levels of society, including women and families, healthcare facilities, employers, child care centers, and the policy arena.

Millennium Development Goal 1: Eradicate Extreme Poverty and Hunger. Target 1.A: Halve, between 1990 and 2015, the proportion of people who suffer from hunger

Reproduced from the United Nations. (n.d.). 2015 Millennium Development Goals. Retrieved from http://www.un.org/millenniumgoals/. Accessed August 13, 2013. This source is used for all Millennium Development Goals in this chapter.

Millennium Development Goal 4: Reduce Child Mortality. Target 4.A: Reduce by two-thirds, between 1990 and 2015, the under-five mortality rate

Millennium Development Goal 5: Improve Maternal Health. Target 5.A: Reduce by three quarter, between 1990 and 2015, the maternal mortality ratio

Breastfeeding Recommendations and Definitions

WHO and AAP recommend that mothers **exclusively breastfeed** for the first 6 months of life and continue breastfeeding for at least one (AAP recommendation) or two (WHO recommendation) years.[10,11] Establishment and use of standardized definitions of breastfeeding are critical to the protection, promotion, and support of breastfeeding (**Table 9-1**).[12]

Table 9-1 Criteria that define selected infant feeding practices

Feeding Practice	Requires That the Infant Receive	Allows the Infant to Receive	Does Not Allow the Infant to Receive
Exclusive breastfeeding	Breastmilk (including milk expressed or from a wet nurse)	Oral rehydration salts (ORS), drops, syrups (vitamins, minerals, medicines)	Anything else
Predominant breastfeeding	Breastmilk (including milk expressed or from a wet nurse) as the predominant source of nourishment	Certain liquids (water and water-based drinks, fruit juice), ritual fluids and ORS, drops or syrups (vitamins, minerals, medicines)	Anything else (in particular, nonhuman milk, food-based fluids)
Breastfeeding	Breastmilk (including milk expressed or from a wet nurse)	Anything else: any food or liquid including nonhuman milk and formula	N/A

Reproduced from the World Health Organization (WHO). (2008). Indicators for assessing infant and young child feeding practices: Conclusions of a consensus meeting held 6-8 November 2007 in Washington D.C. Geneva: Author.

They enable the interpretation of **epidemiological** data in surveillance and research and the development, implementation, and evaluation of breastfeeding programs and curricula for caregivers or community health workers.

Breastfeeding Goals, Objectives, and Current Practices

Global Estimates

The World Health Organization recommends that all women breastfeed, except in rare circumstances in which **human milk substitutes** may be appropriate (**Table 9-2**).[13] According to the United Nations Children's Fund (UNICEF), many countries have witnessed improvements in breastfeeding patterns, yet all **indicators** remain far below recommended levels (**Table 9-3**).[14] Worldwide, the percentage of infants under the age of 6 months that were exclusively breastfed increased from 34% in 1995 to 43% in 2011. Progress was slightly greater in the least developed countries, increasing from 34% of infants 0–6 months that were exclusively breastfed in 1995 to 48% in 2011. In 26 countries, exclusive breastfeeding rates rose by more than 20% (**Figure 9-1**). However, fewer than half of all infants are breastfed within one hour of birth or exclusively breastfed for six months (**Figure 9-2**).

United States

In the United States, the Centers for Disease Control and Prevention (CDC) annually publishes data on progress toward all five outcome indicators and three **Healthy People 2020 Objective** (HP 2020) indicators related to breastfeeding.[15,16]

HP 2020 Objectives

Maternal, Infant, and Child Health (MICH)-21: Increase the proportion of infants who are breastfed

21.1: Increase the proportion of infants who were ever breastfed

21.2: Increase the proportion of infants who are breastfed at 6 months

21.3: Increase the proportion of infants who are breastfed at 1 year

21.4: Increase the proportion of infants who are breastfed exclusively through 3 months

21.5: Increase the proportion of infants who are breastfed exclusively through 6 months

MICH-22: Increase the proportion of employers that have worksite lactation support programs

MICH-23: Reduce the proportion of breastfed newborns who receive formula supplementation within the first 2 days of life

MICH-24: Increase the proportion of live births that occur in facilities that provide recommended care for lactating mothers and their babies

Centers for Disease Control and Prevention. (Page last updated: June 6, 2013). Breastfeeding report card: U.S., 2012. Available at: http://www.cdc.gov/breastfeeding/data/reportcard.htm. Accessed March 11, 2013 and U.S. Department of Health and Human Services. Office of Disease Prevention and Health Promotion. (Page last updated: Wednesday, April 24, 2013). Healthy People 2020. Maternal, Infant, and Child Health. Washington, DC. Available at http://www.healthypeople.gov/2020/topicsobjectives2020/objectiveslist.aspx?topicid=26. Accessed March 11, 2013.

Table 9-2 Acceptable medical reasons for use of breastmilk substitutes

---

Infants who should not receive breastmilk or any other milk except specialized formula

- Infants with classic galactosemia: a special galactose-free formula is needed.
- Infants with maple syrup urine disease: a special formula free of leucine, isoleucine, and valine is needed.
- Infants with phenylketonuria: a special phenylalanine-free formula is needed (some breastfeeding is possible, under careful monitoring).

Infants for whom breastmilk remains the best feeding option but who may need other food in addition to breastmilk for a limited period

- Infants born weighing less than 1,500 grams (very low birth weight).
- Infants born at less than 32 weeks of gestation (preterm).
- Newborn infants who are at risk of hypoglycemia by virtue of impaired metabolic adaptation or increased glucose demand (such as those who are preterm, are small for gestational age or have experienced significant intrapartum hypoxic/ischemic stress; those who are ill; and those whose mothers are diabetic) if their blood sugar fails to respond to optimal breastfeeding or breastmilk feeding.

Maternal conditions that may justify temporary avoidance of breastfeeding

- Severe illness that prevents a mother from caring for her infant (e.g., sepsis).
- Herpes simplex virus type 1 (HSV-1): direct contact between lesions on the mother's breasts and the infant's mouth should be avoided until all active lesions have resolved.
- Maternal medication
  - Sedating psychotherapeutic drugs, antiepileptic drugs and opioids, and their combinations may cause side effects such as drowsiness and respiratory depression and are better avoided if a safer alternative is available.
  - Radioactive iodine-131 is better avoided given that safer alternatives are available—a mother can resume breastfeeding about two months after receiving this substance.
  - Excessive use of topical iodine or iodophors (e.g., povidone-iodine), especially on open wounds or mucous membranes, can result in thyroid suppression or electrolyte abnormalities in the breastfed infant and should be avoided.
  - Cytotoxic chemotherapy requires that a mother stops breastfeeding during therapy.

Maternal conditions during which breastfeeding can still continue, although health problems may be of concern

- Breast abscess: breastfeeding should continue on the unaffected breast; feeding from the affected breast can resume once treatment has started.
- Hepatitis B: infants should be given hepatitis B vaccine, within the first 48 hours or as soon as possible thereafter.
- Hepatitis C.
- Mastitis: if breastfeeding is very painful, milk must be removed by expression to prevent progression of the condition.
- Tuberculosis: mother and baby should be managed according to national tuberculosis guidelines.
- Substance use
  - Maternal use of nicotine, alcohol, ecstasy, amphetamines, cocaine, and related stimulants has been demonstrated to have harmful effects on breastfed babies.
  - Alcohol, opioids, benzodiazepines, and cannabis can cause sedation in both the mother and the baby.

Reproduced from the World Health Organization. (2009). Infant and young child feeding: Model chapter for textbooks for medical students and allied health professionals. Geneva: WHO.

Table 9-3 Recommended indicators for assessing breastfeeding practices

Recommended core indicators

Early initiation of breastfeeding: Proportion of children born in the past 24 months who were put to the breast within 1 hour of birth

Children born in the last 24 months who were put to the breast within 1 hour of birth

$\div$

Children born in the last 24 months

Exclusive breastfeeding under 6 months: Proportion of infants 0-5 months of age who are fed exclusively with breastmilk

Infants 0-5 months of age who received only breastmilk during the previous day

$\div$

Infants 0-5 months of age

Continued breastfeeding at 1 year: Proportion of children 12-15 months of age who are fed breastmilk

Children 12-15 months of age who received breastmilk during the previous day

$\div$

Children 12-15 months of age

Optional indicators

Children ever breastfed: Proportion of children born in the past 24 months who were ever breastfed

Children born in the past 24 months who were ever breastfed

$\div$

Children born in the past 24 months

Continued breastfeeding at 2 years: Proportion of children 20-23 months of age who are fed breastmilk

Children 20-23 months of age who received breastmilk during the previous day

$\div$

Children 20-23 months of age

Age-appropriate breastfeeding: Proportion of children 0-23 months of age who are appropriately breastfed

The indicator is calculated from the following two fractions:

Infants 0-5 months of age who received only breastmilk during the previous day

$\div$

Infants 0-5 months of age

and

Children 6-23 months of age who received breastmilk, as well as solid, semisolid, or soft foods, during the previous day

$\div$

Children 6-23 months of age

Predominant breastfeeding under 6 months: Proportion of infants 0-5 months of age who are predominantly breastfed

Infants 0-5 months of age who received breastmilk as the predominant source of nourishment during the previous day

$\div$

Infants 0-5 months of age

Duration of breastfeeding: Median duration of breastfeeding among children less than 36 months of age

The age in months when 50% of children 0-35 months did not receive breastmilk during the previous day

Bottle feeding: Proportion of children 0-23 months of age who are fed with a bottle

Children 0-23 months of age who were fed with a bottle during the previous day

$\div$

Children 0-23 months of age

Modified from the World Health Organization (WHO). (2008). Indicators for assessing infant and young child feeding practices: Conclusions of a consensus meeting held 6-8 November 2007 in Washington D.C. Geneva: Author.

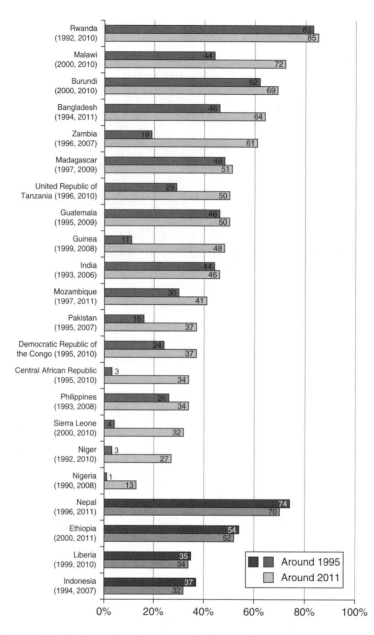

Figure 9-1 Percentage of infants under the age of 6 months who are exclusively breastfed

Reproduced from UNICEF. ChildInfo. Monitoring the situation of children and women. (Last update: Feb 2013.) Statistics by area: Child nutrition: Progress. Retrieved from http://www.childinfo.org/breastfeeding_progress.html. Accessed September 4, 2013.

Nationally, breastfeeding rates have been on the rise (**Figure 9-3**),[17] with greater initiation and longer duration of breastfeeding and more breastfeeding exclusively at three and six months postpartum; however, substantial **disparities** persist. Breastfeeding rates are lowest for mothers who live in the southeastern United States, are African American, are under 20 years old, have less than a high school education, are unmarried, live in households with an income below 100% of the poverty level, and/or participate in WIC.[18] While multiple disparities often co-occur, little research examines the degree to which these risk factors "cluster." Regardless, the data are helpful in identifying segments of society with greater needs for targeted breastfeeding programs.

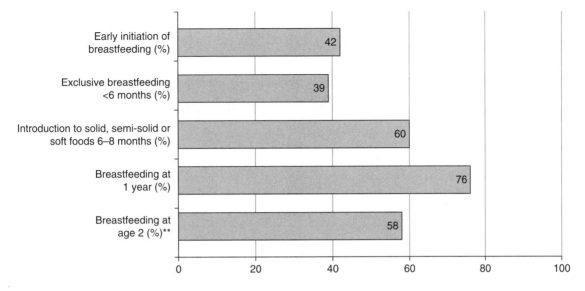

Figure 9-2 Global averages of key breastfeeding indicators (%), 2007-2011

Reproduced from UNICEF. ChildInfo. Monitoring the situation of children and women. (Last update: Feb 2013.) Statistics by area: Child nutrition: Status. Retrieved from http://www.childinfo.org/breastfeeding_status.html. Accessed September 4, 2013.

The Public Health Importance of Breastfeeding

Breastmilk contains numerous biologically active molecules that are not present in infant formula.[19,20] Its immune factors help protect infants from early exposures to environmental microorganisms, and its **epidermal growth factor** helps the lining of the gut prepare to receive subsequent, more mature breastmilk.

Breastmilk is dynamic. Its composition changes with the **gestational** age of the infant. Milk from mothers of preterm babies (less than 37 weeks' gestation) is higher in

---

Box 9-1 The Special Supplemental Nutrition Program for Women, Infants, and Children (WIC)

The WIC program is a U.S. Department of Agriculture federal nutrition assistance program. Each year, Congress budgets funds to provide to states to administer WIC. WIC is operated through local entities, such as local health departments, and services are examples of locations where participants may go to receive benefits. The program is for low-income pregnant, postpartum, and lactating women, infants, and children through age 5. Household income must be less than 185% of the poverty level, and participants must have a nutritional risk factor, such as anemia, poor growth, or obesity. Because WIC is not an entitlement program, not all eligible applicants are accepted to the program.

WIC benefits include food packages, nutrition education and screenings, and referrals to healthcare providers. Foods are meant to fill in gaps in intake of nutrients of concern, such as iron and calcium. Food packages include cereal, tuna, eggs, fruit juice, and peanut butter, as well as vouchers for fresh fruits and vegetables. Food packages for infants include infant cereal and baby food meat. To encourage breastfeeding, lactating women are permitted to stay in the program longer after birth than mothers who do not breastfeed, and their food packages are larger. In addition, they receive breastfeeding support, such as information, peer-to-peer counseling, and breast pumps.

Data from the Food and Nutrition Service, USDA. (n.d.). Women, Infants and Children (WIC). Retrieved from http://www.fns.usda.gov/wic/

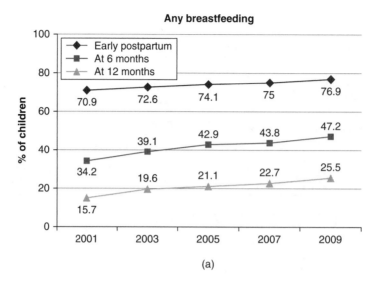

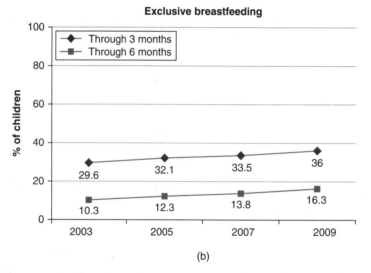

Figure 9-3 Breastfeeding trends among U.S. children

Modified from the Centers for Disease Control and Prevention. Breastfeeding among U.S. children born 2000–2009, CDC National Immunization Survey. http://www.cdc.gov/breastfeeding/data/nis_data/. Last updated: August 1, 2012. Accessed March 11, 2013.

energy, lipids, protein, nitrogen, fatty acids, and some vitamins and minerals. After birth, milk begins as **colostrum** and becomes mature milk within the first two weeks. Breastmilk is also dynamic because its fat composition increases over the course of a feeding as the infant reaches the **hindmilk**.[21]

The **bioactive** substances in breastmilk that are not present in infant formula are significant. While commercial infant formula successfully mimics the energy, macronutrients, and micronutrients composition of breastmilk, a variety of immunologic and anti-inflammatory substances remain absent from formula.

Child Health

Strong evidence from both developed and developing countries demonstrates that breastfeeding reduces the **incidence** and/or severity of many infectious diseases, including bacterial meningitis, bacteremia, diarrhea, respiratory tract infections, necrotizing enterocolitis (intestinal cell death due to severe bacterial infection), otitis media (ear infections), and urinary tract infections.[22,23,24,25] Breastfeeding also reduces the risk of **sudden infant death syndrome** (SIDS) and provides protection from chronic conditions occurring later in life, including diabetes mellitus, certain cancers (lymphoma, leukemia, and Hodgkin disease), overweight and obesity, high cholesterol, and asthma.[26,27,28,29] Breastfeeding is also associated with better cognitive development outcomes, such as better performance on standardized tests.

Maternal Health

Mothers also receive multiple health benefits from breastfeeding.[30,31,32,33] Breastfeeding speeds the healing process after delivery by decreasing postpartum bleeding and promoting faster uterine involution, or the return of the uterus to its prepregnancy state. Breastfeeding may help mothers return more quickly to their prepregnancy weight and decrease risk of breast and ovarian cancers, osteoporosis after menopause, and postpartum depression.

Breastfeeding is also an important family planning method.[34] The lactational amenorrhea method (LAM) (**Table 9-4**) can be used by all women, regardless of economic, social, or other barriers to using other forms of birth control. When LAM is implemented correctly, a woman's risk of becoming pregnant is less than 2%, comparable to risks using other contraceptives, such as condoms, intrauterine devices, and hormonal birth control pills.

Societal Health

Benefits of breastfeeding extend to the economy and the environment.[35,36,37] In the United States, families could save between $1,200 and $1,500 per child by optimizing breastfeeding. Furthermore, due to reductions in associated illnesses and diseases, the United States could save $10.5 billion annually if 80% of women breastfed according to the recommendations. Unlike infant formula, breastmilk is also a natural and renewable food that doesn't require disposable packaging. On average, 150 containers of formula are consumed per infant.

Barriers and Facilitators to Meeting National and International Breastfeeding Goals and Objectives

Given all the research on the benefits of breastfeeding, why don't all mothers choose to breastfeed? Why do so few exclusively breastfeed until 6 months or continue to breastfeed beyond 1 year as recommended? The issue is complex and influenced by history and current context. This section presents key historical events from the initial decline in breastfeeding practices to the resurgence of breastfeeding internationally and in the United States. The final section summarizes barriers to breastfeeding and identifies the strategies recommended by WHO/UNICEF and the U.S. Surgeon General to promote, protect, and support breastfeeding.

Major Historical Events Related to Breastfeeding

Development of Formula and the Decline of Breastfeeding

Until the 20th century, breastfeeding was the norm worldwide.[38,39,40] In rare cases when woman could not breastfeed, or chose not to breastfeed (as was common among wealthy European women), wet nurses were "hired" to breastfeed the infant. However, events beginning in the 18th century led to a gradual decline of breastfeeding.

Jean Charles Des-Essartz's 1760 publication *Treatise of Physical Upbringing of Children* included some of the first compositional comparisons between human and animal

Table 9-4 The lactational amenorrhea method

No other method needed if:	Use another method if:
• No menstruation	• Menstruation has returned
AND	*OR*
• Baby LESS than 6 months old	• Baby MORE than 6 months old
AND	*OR*
• Baby exclusively breastfed	• Other foods and fluids have been introduced

Reproduced from the World Health Organization. (2009). Infant and young child feeding: Model chapter for textbooks for medical students and allied health professionals. Geneva: WHO.

milks.[41] By 1865, the first modern infant formula was developed, patented, and released by Justus von Liebig. By 1883, 27 patented brands of infant foods were available. In 1912, the first modern feeding bottle with an easy-to-clean rubber nipple became available. Women and families now had access to artificial human milk substitutes and a sanitary vessel for feeding them.

In the United States, feeding of breastmilk substitutes remained limited to the upper classes, due to the expense of "complete" infant formulas fortified with vitamins and minerals.[42] Evaporated milk, an inexpensive cow's milk product that could be stored at room temperature, became available in 1885, but was not commonly used to feed infants because it lacked essential micronutrients. This changed by the mid-1920s with the discovery that fruit juices could prevent scurvy, or vitamin C deficiency, among nonbreastfed infants. Physicians began promoting an evaporated milk recipe as an alternative to breastmilk. Breastfeeding rates plummeted, with fewer than 20% of U.S. women breastfeeding during the 1950s to 1970s.

The Resurgence of Breastfeeding

By the early to mid-1970s, similar declines in breastfeeding were documented worldwide, particularly in developing countries where formula companies were aggressively marketing their products to women and families.[43,44] Concern over these marketing practices emerged among governments, **nongovernmental organizations** (NGOs), and civic groups. Since the late 1970s, multiple resolutions by WHO/UNICEF and the **World Health Assembly** and policy documents from the office of the U.S. Surgeon General have been published.

The International Code of the Marketing of Breast-milk Substitutes (The Code) was adopted by Member States of the World Health Assembly in 1981.[45] Its aim is to regulate marketing practices surrounding breastmilk substitutes. The Code also has provisions for the marketing of feeding bottles and teats. A few examples of specific provisions in the Code include:

- No advertising of breastmilk substitutes and no provision of free samples of breastmilk substitutes to mothers.

- No promotion of breastmilk substitutes through healthcare facilities.

- No words or pictures idealizing the use of breastmilk substitutes, including pictures of infants on product labels of the products.

- Information on the labels of breastmilk substitutes explaining the benefits of breastfeeding and the risks associated with artificial feeding.

The Convention on the Rights of the Child (CRC) was adopted by the World Congress in 1989.[46] The CRC was among the first legally binding international documents encompassing the full range of human rights, including basic rights of children: the right to survival; to develop to the fullest potential; to protection from harmful influences, abuse, and exploitation; and to participate fully in family, cultural, and social life. The CRC protects children's rights by setting standards in healthcare, education, and legal, civil, and social services. It is an important policy document that holds governments accountable to making progress in the area of infant and young child feeding (IYCF). Article 24 states the following:

> States Parties shall pursue full implementation of this right and, in particular, shall take appropriate measures to ensure that all segments of society, in particular parents and children, are informed, have access to education, and are supported in the use of basic knowledge of child health and nutrition, the advantages of breastfeeding, hygiene and environmental sanitation, and the prevention of accidents.

The Innocenti Declaration was adopted in 1991 by participants at the WHO/UNICEF policy makers' meeting entitled "Breastfeeding in the 1990s: A Global Initiative."[47] The meeting, held at the Spedale degli Innocenti in Florence, Italy, in the summer of 1990, was cosponsored by the United States Agency for International Development (USAID) and the Swedish International Development Authority (SIDA). The Declaration contained the following four operational targets: (1) appoint a national breastfeeding coordinator with appropriate authority; (2) ensure that every facility providing maternity services fully practices all the "Ten Steps to Successful Breastfeeding" (**Table 9-5**); (3) enact legislation protecting the breastfeeding rights of working women and establish means of its enforcement; and (4) support the principles and aims of the Code.

The Global Strategy for Infant and Young Child Feeding (Global Strategy) was published in 2003 by the WHO and UNICEF after a two-year **participatory** process involving input from leading experts, nongovernmental organizations (NGOs), professional associations, country office staff, and the food industry.[48] The Global Strategy built on previous achievements, including the Code, the Innocenti Declaration, and the Ten Steps, also called the Baby-Friendly

Table 9-5 The Baby-Friendly Hospital Initiative: The Ten Steps to Successful Breastfeeding

1. Have a written breastfeeding policy that is routinely communicated to all healthcare staff.
2. Train all healthcare staff in skills necessary to implement this policy.
3. Inform all pregnant women about the benefits and management of breastfeeding.
4. Help mothers initiate breastfeeding within one half-hour of birth.
5. Show mothers how to breastfeed and how to maintain lactation even if they should be separated from their infants.
6. Give newborn infants no food or drink other than breastmilk, unless medically indicated.
7. Practice rooming-in: allow mothers and infants to remain together 24 hours a day.
8. Encourage breastfeeding on demand.
9. Give no artificial teats or pacifiers (also called dummies or soothers) to breastfeeding infants.
10. Foster the establishment of breastfeeding support groups and refer mothers to them on discharge from the hospital or clinic.

Reproduced from UNICEF. (n.d.). The Baby-Friendly Hospital Initiative. Available at: http://www.unicef.org/programme/breastfeeding/baby.htm#10. Accessed March 11, 2013.

Hospital Initiative (BFHI). The Global Strategy was a call to action outlining obligations and responsibilities for a variety of stakeholders, including governments, NGOs, healthcare providers, employers, and commercial producers of infant feeding products. The specific objectives of the Global Strategy were as follows:

- To raise awareness of the main problems affecting infant and young child feeding, identify approaches to their solution, and provide a framework of essential interventions;

- To increase the commitment of governments, international organizations, and other concerned parties for optimal feeding practices for infants and young children;

- To create an environment that will enable all mothers, families, and other caregivers in all circumstances to make—and implement—informed choices about optimal feeding practices for infants and young children.

Released in 2011, the U.S. Surgeon General's Call to Action to Support Breastfeeding (Call to Action)[49] provides a comprehensive overview of the health effects of breastfeeding, barriers to breastfeeding in the United States, and public health recommendations for increasing breastfeeding and achieving breastfeeding goals. The strategies are organized according to those for (1) mothers and families, (2) communities, (3) health care, (4) employers, (5) research and surveillance, and (6) public health infrastructure (**Table 9-6**). The Call to Action was preceded by the first Surgeon General's Workshop on Breastfeeding, convened by C. Everett Koop in 1984, and the *Blueprint for Action on Breastfeeding*, published by the U.S. Department of Health and Human Services in 1999.[50,51]

Current Barriers to Breastfeeding: A Social Ecological Framework

While progress has been made, much remains to be done to achieve recommended rates of exclusive and continued breastfeeding.[52,53] This section uses the Social Ecological Framework to present barriers and promising public health approaches to promote, protect, and support breastfeeding at each level.[54,55]

The Individual Sphere

A woman's knowledge about breastfeeding, her attitudes and beliefs about breastfeeding, and her self-efficacy impact her choice to initiate and sustain breastfeeding.[56,57,58,59,60] In the United States, approximately 75% of women are unaware of specific benefits of breastfeeding, such as reducing the infant's risk of diarrheal disease or another illness. Women with low confidence in their ability to breastfeed are likely to continue breastfeeding for less time than women with greater confidence in their abilities. Women with negative attitudes about breastfeeding or positive attitudes about feeding formula are also less likely to continue breastfeeding. A particularly important factor is a woman's perception of her milk supply. The most commonly reported reason for early **weaning** is insufficient milk production, despite data showing fewer than 5% of women unable to fully lactate for a biological reason, such as an anatomic breast abnormality or hormonal insufficiency. Other reasons for actual or perceived insufficient milk supply are related to

Table 9-6 Recommended actions for protecting, promoting, and supporting breastfeeding in the United States

---

Mothers and Their Families

Action 1. Give mothers the support they need to breastfeed their babies.

Action 2. Develop programs to educate fathers and grandmothers about breastfeeding.

Communities

Action 3. Strengthen programs that provide mother-to-mother support and peer counseling.

Action 4. Use community-based organizations to promote and support breastfeeding.

Action 5. Create a national campaign to promote breastfeeding.

Action 6. Ensure that the marketing of infant formula is conducted in a way that minimizes its negative impacts on exclusive breastfeeding.

Health Care

Action 7. Ensure that maternity care practices throughout the United States are fully supportive of breastfeeding.

Action 8. Develop systems to guarantee continuity of skilled support for lactation between hospitals and healthcare settings in the community.

Action 9. Provide education and training in breastfeeding for all health professionals who care for women and children.

Action 10. Include basic support for breastfeeding as a standard of care for midwives, obstetricians, family physicians, nurse practitioners, and pediatricians.

Action 11. Ensure access to services provided by International Board Certified Lactation Consultants.

Action 12. Identify and address obstacles to greater availability of safe banked donor milk for fragile infants.

Employment

Action 13. Work toward establishing paid maternity leave for all employed mothers.

Action 14. Ensure that employers establish and maintain comprehensive, high-quality lactation support programs for their employees.

Action 15. Expand the use of programs in the workplace that allow lactating mothers to have direct access to their babies.

Action 16. Ensure that all child care providers accommodate the needs of breastfeeding mothers and infants.

Research and Surveillance

Action 17. Increase funding of high-quality research on breastfeeding.

Action 18. Strengthen existing capacity and develop future capacity for conducting research on breastfeeding.

Action 19. Develop a national monitoring system to improve tracking of breastfeeding rates as well as policies and environmental factors that affect breastfeeding.

Public Health Infrastructure

Action 20. Improve national leadership on the promotion and support of breastfeeding.

Reproduced from DHHS. (2010). The Surgeon General's Call to Action to Support of Breastfeeding. Available at: http://www.surgeongeneral.gov/library/calls/breastfeeding/index.html. Accessed March 11, 2013.

improper breastfeeding management, such as poor hospital practices or lack of knowledge of normal breastfeeding physiology and infant behavioral states, such as crying and sleep patterns.

A wide variety of free, downloadable materials for increasing maternal knowledge and fostering more positive breastfeeding attitudes and breastfeeding confidence is available. *Your Guide to Breastfeeding* is a comprehensive breastfeeding guide for mothers maintained by the U.S. Department of Health and Human Services Office of Women's Health and free for download, with versions targeted to specific races/ethnicities. Another downloadable and comprehensive resource is the *Feeding Your Baby* magazine series produced by the National WIC Association. *The Community Infant and Young Child Feeding Counselling Package (IYCF Counselling Package)*, produced by UNICEF, is helpful for developing nations.[61]

The Interpersonal Sphere

Women's breastfeeding practices are affected by interpersonal relationships, especially those with fathers, grandmothers, friends and peers.[62,63,64,65,66] A woman's intention to breastfeed and her breastfeeding self-efficacy are two of the strongest predictors of breastfeeding duration and are influenced by her social network.[67] Strategies aimed at increasing women's knowledge, attitudes, or self-efficacy about breastfeeding have limited impact on breastfeeding outcomes if these other social influences remain unsupportive. Lack of lay, or peer-to-peer, support for breastfeeding can also decrease a mother's likelihood of meeting her breastfeeding goals. Randomized controlled trials in both low/middle- and high-income countries have tested the effect of lay support for breastfeeding on breastfeeding duration outcomes and found that women receiving lay support had higher rates of any and exclusive breastfeeding.

The Texas WIC program implemented a peer-to-peer support pilot program that involved training fathers of WIC participants to be "peer dads."[68] Training was designed to increase the peer dads' knowledge and counseling skills, with topics including the advantages of breastfeeding, breastmilk composition and immunological properties, anatomy and physiology of the breast, and recommended infant feeding and weaning practices. Peer dads performed one-on-one counseling with other fathers, conducted group sessions, and made public speaking appearances. The majority of fathers in the pilot sites rated the information received from peer dads as "very important" and likely to help them support breastfeeding. Breastfeeding initiation rates in the WIC pilot sites were higher after the peer dad program.

The Community Sphere

A woman's immediate environment, or community, affects breastfeeding. Factors most noted in the literature are the degrees to which healthcare and employment practices and policies are supportive of breastfeeding. The body of

research on the importance of child care practices and policies is also growing.

Healthcare

The Ten Steps are based on research associating selected policies and practices with women's breastfeeding success.[69,70,71,72,73] The Maternity Care Practices Survey (mPINC), developed and implemented by the Centers for Disease Control and Prevention (CDC), annually reports the extent to which U.S. hospitals and birthing centers implement the Ten Steps.[74] In 2011, the majority of hospitals surveyed provided prenatal education and taught breastfeeding techniques and infant feeding cues, but few hospitals had a breastfeeding policy, placed limits on breastmilk supplements or pacifiers, practiced rooming-in, or provided breastfeeding support after discharge (**Figure 9-4**).

mPINC is both an assessment and intervention tool for healthcare facilities, and it can be used as a model for providing feedback to healthcare programs and providers. For each participating facility, CDC prepares a **benchmark** report, comparing the facility's scores to those of other facilities in the country, that are in the same state, and that are similar in size or other characteristics. Facilities can therefore use the benchmark reports as a means of identifying the maternity care practices that they need to change to fully support women to breastfeed. Sample benchmark reports are available on the CDC's website.

Other resources and tools available for educating and training health workers are the WHO textbook for medical staff, *Infant and Young Child Feeding: Model Chapter for Textbooks for Medical Students and Allied Health Professionals (Model Chapter)*, and the previously mentioned IYCF Counselling Package by UNICEF.[75] The comprehensive *Model Chapter* is written from a public health perspective and covers all recommended topic areas in the Global Strategy. The IYCF Counselling Package contains all the tools needed to plan for and implement evidence-based training for community health workers, including a planning guide, a guide for adapting key breastfeeding messages to the local country/regional context, a facilitator's guide, training aids, counseling cards for community health workers, a key messages booklet, and brochures.

The International Lactation Consultant Association (ILCA) is a source of breastfeeding information. International Board Certified Lactation Consultants (IBCLC), certified by the International Board of Lactation Consultant Examiners, Inc., are trained to assist in the initiation and sustenance of breastfeeding in homes and healthcare

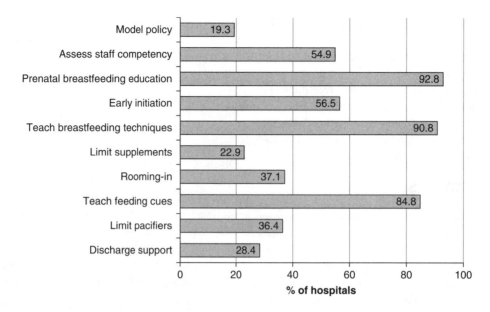

Figure 9-4 Percent of U.S. hospitals with recommended policies and practices consistent with the Ten Steps to Successful Breastfeeding

Data from the Centers for Disease Control and Prevention. (2011). Breastfeeding: mPINC results, 2011. Available at: http://www.cdc.gov/breastfeeding/data/mpinc/results.htm. Accessed March 11, 2013.

facilities around the world.[76] La Leche League International is another resource for mothers and public health professionals. Its mission is "to help mothers worldwide to breastfeed through mother-to-mother support, encouragement, information, and education, and to promote a better understanding of breastfeeding as an important element in the healthy development of the baby and mother."[77]

Employment

Mothers' work expectations and routines can interfere with breastfeeding.[78,79,80] Women, particularly those of lower **socioeconomic status**, work long hours in laborious activities, while also maintaining responsibilities for the care of children within the home.[81] Mothers may be separated from their infants for long periods and may not be supported in expressing their breastmilk while working. Lack of refrigeration can also be a problem. Unrefrigerated breastmilk can be kept for up to eight hours, but must be discarded thereafter.[82] Even if breastmilk must be discarded, mothers should continue hand expression (**Box 9-2**) in order to prevent breastmilk supply from decreasing.

Maternal participation in the labor force has more than doubled in the United States in recent decades.[83] This is significant because lower breastfeeding initiation rates and

shorter breastfeeding durations are likely among employed mothers.[84] Longer maternity leaves, part-time versus full-time work, and breastfeeding-friendly workplace environments are associated with better breastfeeding outcomes among employed women.[85,86,87] In 2011 in the United States, 24 states had laws supporting women's right to breastfeed in the workplace.[88]

No **randomized trials** or **quasi-experimental trials** evaluating the effectiveness of workplace interventions in promoting breastfeeding among women are known.[89] To help meet this need, the U.S. Health Resources and Services Administration (HRSA) developed *The Business Case for Breastfeeding*.[90] This comprehensive toolkit contains two booklets for business executives and human resource managers, which detail the benefits of a workplace breastfeeding support program to a company's return on investment, and an employee's guide to breastfeeding and working. The accompanying lactation support toolkit contains sample policies, a lactation program assessment form, a timeline for implementing the program, and promotional flyers. The *Business Case* has been put into action in Kansas, where the Norton County Health Department and the Kansas Breastfeeding Coalition have teamed up to offer one-day training sessions to local employers and other community agencies and/or groups. The goal of the

---

Box 9-2 Instructions for expressing breastmilk by hand

The mother should:

- Have a clean, dry, wide-necked container for the expressed milk.
- Wash her hands thoroughly.
- Sit or stand comfortably and hold the container under her nipple and areola.
- Put her thumb on top of her breast and her first finger on the underside of her breast so that they are opposite each other, about 4 centimeters from the tip of the nipple.
- Compress and release her breast between her finger and thumb a few times. If milk does not appear, reposition her thumb and finger a little closer or further away from the nipple and compress and release a number of times as before. This should not hurt—if it hurts, the technique is wrong. At first no milk may come, but after compressing a few times, milk starts to drip out. It may flow in streams if the oxytocin reflex is active.
- Compress and release all the way around her breast, with her finger and thumb the same distance from the nipple.
- Express each breast until the milk drips slowly.
- Repeat expressing from each breast five to six times.
- Stop expressing from each breast when milk drips slowly from the start of compression and does not flow.
- Avoid rubbing or sliding her fingers along the skin.
- Avoid squeezing or pinching the nipple itself.

Reproduced from the World Health Organization. (2009). Infant and young child feeding: Model chapter for textbooks for medical students and allied health professionals. Geneva: WHO.

---

project is "to increase workplace lactation support for employed breastfeeding women by equipping breastfeeding advocates to conduct effective outreach and education activities with employers."[91] Participants are given a copy of the *Business Case* resource kit and taught ways to communicate effectively with employers.

Child Care

Child care arrangements affect breastfeeding. In developing countries, a caregiver may be a grandmother, sibling, or other mother, although more formal child care settings, such as preschools and child care centers, are increasing.[92] Little published work examines the influence of child care on breastfeeding outcomes in these settings, although some information comes from studies conducted in the United States.

In the United States, paralleling the rise in maternal employment rates, the number of formal/licensed child care facilities increased from 25,000 in 1977 to 116,000 in 2004.[93] Enrollment in formal child care is associated with a *decreased* likelihood of breastfeeding.[94,95] While multiple factors are likely at play, the extent to which the policies and environments in these facilities are supportive of breastfeeding may influence a mother's ability to continue

breastfeeding while working. Benjamin and colleagues analyzed child care regulations related to infant feeding practices in all U.S. states and census regions and found that only 11 states (22%) had regulations specific to breastfeeding promotion or support.[96] In another survey of breastfeeding policies and practices in 101 child care centers in North Carolina, only 21.7% of facilities encouraged mothers to come to the facility to breastfeed, 20.8% had a written policy that encouraged breastfeeding, 13.9% provided staff training on breastfeeding promotion and support, 3% displayed breastfeeding images and posters, and 1% referred families to community resources.[97]

To facilitate improved nutrition and physical activity practices in child care facilities, in 2001 First Lady Michelle Obama announced the Let's Move! Child Care program, a joint effort of the government, private, and nonprofit communities. Infant feeding, specifically breastfeeding, is one of the five target areas. The website provides a self-assessment of existing policies and practices, and resources for creating a breastfeeding-friendly child care facility. Patterned after the BFHI, one such resource is the Ten Steps to Breastfeeding Friendly Child Care Centers: Resource Kit produced by the Wisconsin Department of Health Services (**Table 9-7**).

Table 9-7 Ten steps to breastfeeding friendly child care centers

Step 1. Designate an individual or group who is responsible for development and implementation of the 10 steps.
Step 2. Establish a supportive breastfeeding policy and require all staff be aware of and follow the policy.
Step 3. Establish a supportive worksite policy for staff members who are breastfeeding.
Step 4. Train all staff so that they are able to carry out breastfeeding promotion and support activities.
Step 5. Create a culturally appropriate breastfeeding friendly environment.
Step 6. Inform expectant and new families and visitors about your center's breastfeeding friendly policies.
Step 7. Stimulate participatory learning experiences with the children, related to breastfeeding.
Step 8. Provide a comfortable place for mother to breastfeed or pump their milk in privacy, if desired. Educate families and staff that a mother may breastfeed her child wherever they have a legal right to be.
Step 9. Establish and maintain connections with local breastfeeding coalition or community breastfeeding resources.
Step 10. Maintain an updated resource file of community breastfeeding services and resources kept in an accessible area for families.

Reproduced from the Wisconsin DHS, Division of Public Health, Nutrition, Physical Activity and Obesity Program, Wisconsin Partnership for Activity and Nutrition Breastfeeding Committee. Ten steps to breastfeeding friendly child care centers. http://www.dhs.wisconsin.gov/publications/P0/P00022.pdf. Updated May 2013. Accessed March 11, 2013.

Policy

Some national or international policies are **correlated** with suboptimal breastfeeding practices. One of the best examples is the U.S. Special Supplemental Nutrition Program for Women, Infants, and Children, commonly referred to as WIC. Data on breastfeeding practices have consistently shown lower rates among women participating in WIC, even lower than rates for women who are eligible to participate, but choose not to **(Figure 9-5)**.[98] As part of a larger review process of the WIC food packages, several expert recommendations were made to enhance breastfeeding promotion in the WIC program.[99] Relevant changes included (1) postponing the age at which complementary foods are given (from 4 months to 6 months), (2) reducing the amount of infant formula in the package for partially breastfeeding

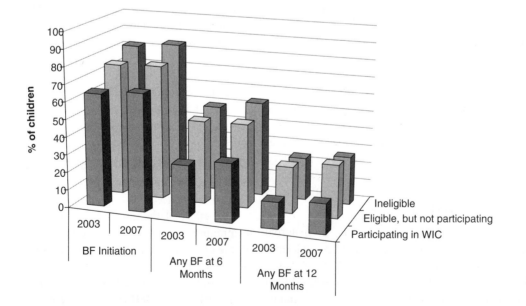

Figure 9-5 Breastfeeding rates in the U.S. by participation in the Special Supplemental Nutrition Program for Women, Infants, and Children (WIC)

Data from the Centers for Disease Control and Prevention. Breastfeeding among U.S. children born 2000–2009, CDC National Immunization Survey. http://www.cdc.gov/breastfeeding/data/nis_data/. Accessed September 11, 2013.

mothers, and (3) providing exclusively breastfeeding mothers that do not accept infant formula from WIC the largest amount and variety of foods for themselves, as well as their infants when they turn 6 months of age.

Thus far, the changes to the food package appear to have had a limited impact on breastfeeding-related outcomes.[100] Results from a national random sample of 17 WIC agencies showed the following differences in food-package assignments before versus after implementation of the new rules: more mothers received the exclusive breastfeeding package (9.8% before vs. 17.1% after), fewer received the partially breastfeeding package (24.7% vs. 13.8%), and more received the fully formula-feeding package (24.7% vs. 13.8%). There were no changes in breastfeeding initiation rates. The findings are therefore mixed.

The addendum to the Patient Protection and Affordable Care Act, signed March 23, 2010, is another example of a national policy that affects breastfeeding.[101] The first provision requires that employers with more than 50 employees provide "reasonable break time" for breastfeeding mothers to express their milk. This provision lasts up until the child's first birthday. The second provision requires that employers have a private place, other than a bathroom, for mothers to express their breastmilk.

Family medical leave policies can indirectly affect women's breastfeeding efforts. All countries except the United States, Liberia, Papua New Guinea, and Swaziland have a national policy requiring paid maternity leave.[102] The minimum recommendation by the International Labor Organization (ILO) is 18 weeks of paid maternity leave,[103] which 13 European countries currently meet.[104] In the United States, under the Family and Medical Leave Act (FMLA), employees can take up to 12 months of unpaid, job-protected leave for certain family and medical reasons, including for the birth of a child and for the care for a newborn child up until the first year of life.[105] During this time, employees retain group health insurance coverage but receive no monetary compensation.

Only 22% of U.S. employers currently offer paid maternity leave beyond that of short-term disability benefits.[106]

To assist countries in developing a *national* breastfeeding strategy—among other optimal infant and young child feeding practices—the Global Strategy was accompanied by a planning document, *Infant and Young Child Feeding: A Tool for Assessing National Practices, Policies and Programmes,* and followed more recently by the *Planning Guide for National Implementation of the Global Strategy for Infant and Young Child Feeding.* The *Planning Guide,* written for government and/or NGO program managers working in the areas of maternal and child health and nutrition, outlines seven steps for moving countries from the Global Strategy to country-specific strategies and actions: (1) identify and orient key **stakeholders** and prepare for developing a comprehensive strategy, (2) assess and analyze the local situation (3) define preliminary national objectives, (4) identify and prioritize actions, (5) develop a national strategy, (6) develop a national plan of action, and (7) implement and monitor. While there are no comprehensive examples of how governments have applied all the steps of the *Planning Guide,* similar examples of situational analyses of IYCF practices in six countries in the Sahel region of Africa have been published.[107]

Conclusion

The support of breastfeeding is an important strategy for achieving several of the MDGs. Breastfeeding can reduce child **undernutrition** and mortality and has a multitude of other health and economic benefits for children, women, and society. While current breastfeeding rates are below the levels recommended by WHO/UNICEF and HP 2020, they are far improved from the lowest rates documented in the 1950s to 1970s. While the work is not over, research over the past few decades has illuminated many barriers to women's breastfeeding success. In response, public health researchers and practitioners are developing programs and resources that can help to make a difference.

References

1 Wasser, H., Bentley, M., Borja, J., et al. (2011). Infants perceived as "fussy" are more likely to receive complementary foods before 4 months. *Pediatrics, 127*(2), 229-37.

2 Bentley, M., Gavin, L., Black, M. M., & Teti, L. (1999). Infant feeding practices of low-income, African-American, adolescent mothers: An ecological, multigenerational perspective. *Social Science & Medicine, 49*(8), 1085-1100.

3 Corbett, K. S. (2000). Explaining infant feeding style of low-income black women. *Journal of Pediatric Nurs*ing, *15*(2), 73-81.

4 Wasser, H., Bentley, M., Borja, J., et al. (2011). Infants perceived as "fussy" are more likely to receive complementary foods before 4 months. *Pediatrics, 127*(2), 229-37.

5 Arora, S., McJunkin, C., Wehrer, J., & Kuhn, P. (2000). Major factors influencing breastfeeding rates: Mother's perception of father's attitude and milk supply. *Pediatrics, 106*(5), E67.

6 Bar-Yam, N. B., & Darby, L. (1997). Fathers and breastfeeding: A review of the literature. *Journal of Human Lactation, 13*(1), 45-50.

7 Morrow, A. L., Guerrero, M. L., Shults, J., Calva, J. J., Lutter, C., Bravo, J., . . . Butterfoss, F. D. (1999). Efficacy of home-based peer counselling to promote exclusive breastfeeding: A randomised controlled trial. *Lancet, 353*(9160), 1226-31.

8 Shi, L., Zhang, J., Wang, Y., Caulfield, L. E., & Guyer, B. (2010). Effectiveness of an educational intervention on complementary feeding practices and growth in rural China: A cluster randomised controlled trial. *Public Health Nutrition, 13*(4), 556-65.

9 Black, R. E., Allen, L. H., Bhutta, Z. A., Caulfield, L. E., de Onis, M., & Ezzati, M., Maternal and Child Undernutrition Study Group. (2008). Maternal and child undernutrition: Global and regional exposures and health consequences. *Lancet, 371*(9608), 243-60.

10 World Health Organization & United Nations Children's Fund. (2003). *Global strategy for infant and young child feeding*. Geneva: UNICEF/WHO.

11 American Academy of Pediatrics, Section on Breastfeeding. (2012). Breastfeeding and the use of human milk. *Pediatrics, 129*, e827-841.

12 United Nations Children's Fund & World Health Organization. (2008). *Indicators for assessing infant and young child feeding practices. Part I: Definitions*. Geneva: UNICEF/WHO.

13 Bentley, M., Gavin, L., Black, M. M., & Teti, L. (1999). Infant feeding practices of low-income, African-American, adolescent mothers: An ecological, multigenerational perspective. *Social Science & Medicine, 49*(8), 1085-1100.

14 United Nations Children's Fund. (n.d.). *Childinfo: Monitoring the situation of children and women*. Retrieved from http://www.childinfo.org/breastfeeding_progress.html

15 Centers for Disease Control and Prevention. (2012). *Breastfeeding report card—U.S., 2012*. Retrieved from http://www.cdc.gov/breastfeeding/data/reportcard.htm

16 U.S. Department of Health and Human Services, Office of Disease Prevention and Health Promotion. (n.d.). *Healthy People 2020*. Retrieved from http://www.healthypeople.gov/2020/topicsobjectives2020/objectiveslist.aspx?topicid=26

17 Centers for Disease Control and Prevention. *Breastfeeding among U.S. children born 2000-2009: CDC national immunization survey*. Retrieved from http://www.cdc.gov/breastfeeding/data/nis_data

18 Centers for Disease Control and Prevention. (2010). Racial and ethnic differences in breastfeeding initiation and duration, by state, CDC national immunization survey, United States, 2004-2008. *MMWR Morbidity and Mortality Weekly Report, 59*, 327-34.

19 Lawrence, R. A., & Lawrence, R. M. (2010). *Breastfeeding: A guide for the medical profession* (7th ed.). Philadelphia, PA: Saunders.

20 World Health Organization. (2009). *Infant and young child feeding: Model chapter for textbooks for medical students and allied health professionals*. Geneva: World Health Organization.

21 Lawrence, R. A., & Lawrence, R. M. (2010). *Breastfeeding: A guide for the medical profession* (7th ed.). Philadelphia, PA: Saunders.

22 American Academy of Pediatrics, Section on Breastfeeding. (2012). Breastfeeding and the use of human milk. *Pediatrics, 129*, e827-41.

23 Ip, S., Chung, M., Raman, G., Chew, P., Magula, N., DeVine, D., & Lau, J. (2007). Breastfeeding and maternal and infant health outcomes in developed countries. *Evidence report/technology Assessment* (153), 1-186.

24 Chien, P. F., & Howie, P. W. (2001). Breast milk and the risk of opportunistic infection in infancy in industrialized and non-industrialized settings. *Advances in Nutritional Research, 10*, 69-104.

25 Bachrach, V. R., Schwarz, E., & Bachrach, L. R. (2003). Breastfeeding and the risk of hospitalization for respiratory disease in infancy: A meta-analysis. *Archives of Pediatrics & Adolescent Medicine, 157*(3), 237-43.

26 American Academy of Pediatrics, Section on Breastfeeding. (2012). Breastfeeding and the use of human milk. *Pediatrics, 129*, e827-41.

27 Kwan, M. L., Buffler, P. A., Abrams, B., & Kiley, V. A. (2004). Breastfeeding and the risk of childhood leukemia: A meta-analysis. *Public Health Reports, 119*(6), 521-35.

28 Owen, C. G., Martin, R. M., Whincup, P. H., Smith, G. D., & Cook, D. G. (2006). Does breastfeeding influence risk of type 2 diabetes in later life? A quantitative analysis of published evidence. *American Journal of Clinical Nutrition, 84*(5), 1043-54.

29 World Health Organization. (2007). *Evidence on the long-term effects of breastfeeding: Systematic reviews and meta-analyses*. Geneva: World Health Organization.

30 Lawrence, R. A., & Lawrence, R. M. (2010). *Breastfeeding: A guide for the medical profession* (7th ed.). Philadelphia, PA: Saunders.

31 World Health Organization. (2009). *Infant and young child feeding: Model chapter for textbooks for medical students and allied health professionals*. Geneva: World Health Organization.

32 Bernier, M. O., Plu-Bureau, G., Bossard, N., Ayzac, L., & Thalabard, J. C. (2000). Breastfeeding and risk of breast cancer: A meta-analysis of published studies. *Human Reproduction Update, 6*(4), 374-86.

33 Dennis, C. L., & McQueen, K. (2009). The relationship between infant-feeding outcomes and postpartum depression: A qualitative systematic review. *Pediatrics, 123*(4), e736-51.

34 World Health Organization. (2009). *Infant and young child feeding: Model chapter for textbooks for medical students and allied health professionals*. Geneva: World Health Organization.

35 World Health Organization. (2009). *Infant and young child feeding: Model chapter for textbooks for medical students and allied health professionals*. Geneva: World Health Organization.

36 Ball, T. M., & Wright, A. L. (1999). Health care costs of formula-feeding in the first year of life. *Pediatrics, 103*(4 Pt. 2), 870-76.

37 Bartick, M., & Reinhold, A. (2010). The burden of suboptimal breastfeeding in the United States: a pediatric cost analysis. *Pediatrics, 125*(5), e1048-56.

38 Fomon, S. (2001). Infant feeding in the 20th century: Formula and beikost. *Journal of Nutrition, 131*(2), 409S-20S.

39 Stevens, E. E., Patrick, T. E., & Pickler, R. (2009). A history of infant feeding. *Journal of Perinatal Education, 18*(2), 32-39.

40 Fildes, V. A. (1985). *Breasts, bottles and babies: A history of infant feeding.* Edinburgh: Edinburgh University Press.

41 Stevens, E. E., Patrick, T. E., & Pickler, R. (2009). A history of infant feeding. *Journal of Perinatal Education, 18*(2), 32-39.

42 Fomon, S. (2001). Infant feeding in the 20th century: Formula and beikost. *Journal of Nutrition, 131*(2), 409S-20S.

43 Fomon, S. (2001). Infant feeding in the 20th century: Formula and beikost. *Journal of Nutrition, 131*(2), 409S-20S.

44 Stevens, E. E., Patrick, T. E., & Pickler, R. (2009). A history of infant feeding. *Journal of Perinatal Education, 18*(2), 32-39.

45 World Health Organization. (1981). *International Code of Marketing of Breast-Milk Substitutes.* Geneva: World Health Organization.

46 United Nations Treaty Collection. (1989). *Convention on the Rights of the Child.* Retrieved from http://treaties.un.org/Pages/ViewDetails.aspx?src=TREATY&mtdsg_no=IV-11&chapter=4&lang=en

47 United Nations Children's Fund & World Health Organization. (1990). *Innocenti Declaration on the Protection, Promotion, and Support of Breastfeeding.* Retrieved from http://www.unicef.org/programme/breastfeeding/innocenti.htm

48 World Health Organization & United Nations Children's Fund. (2003). *Global strategy for infant and young child feeding.* Geneva: UNICEF/WHO.

49 U.S. Department of Health and Human Services. (2011). *The Surgeon General's Call to Action to Support Breastfeeding.* Washington, DC: U.S. Department of Health and Human Services, Office of the Surgeon General.

50 U.S. Department of Health and Human Services. (1984). *Report of the Surgeon General's Workshop on Breastfeeding and Human Lactation.* Washington, DC: U.S. Department of Health and Human Services.

51 U.S. Department of Health and Human Services. (2000). *HHS Blueprint for Action on Breastfeeding.* Washington, DC: U.S. Department of Health and Human Services, Office on Women's Health.

52 United Nations Children's Fund. *Childinfo: Monitoring the situation of children and women.* Retrieved from http://www.childinfo.org/breastfeeding_progress.html

53 Centers for Disease Control and Prevention. (2012). *Breastfeeding report card–U.S., 2012.* Retrieved from http://www.cdc.gov/breastfeeding/data/reportcard.htm

54 Bentley, M. E., Dee, D. L., & Jensen, J. L. (2003). Breastfeeding among low income, African-American women: Power, beliefs and decision making. *Journal of Nutrition, 133*(1), 305S-309S.

55 Sallis, J. F., Owen, N., & Fisher, E. B. (2008). Ecological models of health behavior. In K. Glanz, B. K. Rimer, & K. Viswanath (Eds.), *Health behavior and health education: Theory, research, and practice* (4th ed., pp. 465-520). San Francisco, CA: Jossey-Bass.

56 Bertino, E., Varalda, A., Magnetti, F., Di Nicola, P., Cester, E., Occhi, L., Prandi, G. (2012). Is breastfeeding duration influenced by maternal attitude and knowledge? A longitudinal study during the first year of life. *Journal of Maternal-Fetal & Neonatal Medicine, 25*, 32-36.

57 Blyth, R., Creedy, D. K., Dennis, C. L., Moyle, W., Pratt, J., & De Vries, S. M. (2002). Effect of maternal confidence on breastfeeding duration: an application of breastfeeding self-efficacy theory. *Birth, 29*(4), 278-84.

58 Dungy, C. I., McInnes, R. J., Tappin, D. M., Wallis, A. B., & Oprescu, F. (2008). Infant feeding attitudes and knowledge among socioeconomically disadvantaged women in Glasgow. *Maternal & Child Health Journal, 12*(3), 313-22.

59 Kronborg, H., & Vaeth, M. (2004). The influence of psychosocial factors on the duration of breastfeeding. *Scandinavian Journal of Public Health, 32*(3), 210-16.

60 Thulier, D. & Mercer, J. (2009) Variables associated with breastfeeding duration. *Journal of Obstetric, Gynecologic, & Neonatal Nursing, 38*, 259-68.

61 United Nations Children's Fund. (2012). The community infant and young child feeding package. Retrieved from http://www.unicef.org/nutrition/index_58362.html

62 Arora, S., McJunkin, C., Wehrer, J., & Kuhn, P. (2000). Major factors influencing breastfeeding rates: Mother's perception of father's attitude and milk supply. *Pediatrics, 106*(5), E67.

63 Bentley, M. E., Caulfield, L. E., Gross, S. M., Bronner, Y., Jensen, J., Kessler, L. A., & Paige, D. M. (1999). Sources of influence on intention to breastfeed among African-American women at entry to WIC. *Journal of Human Lactation, 15*(1), 27-34.

64 DiGirolamo, A., Thompson, N., Martorell, R., Fein, S., & Grummer-Strawn, L. (2005). Intention or experience? Predictors of continued breastfeeding. *Health Education & Behavior, 32*(2), 208-26. doi:10.1177/1090198104271971

65 Meedya, S., Fahy, K., & Kable, A. (2010). Factors that positively influence breastfeeding duration to 6 months: A literature review. *Women and Birth: Journal of the Australian College of Midwives, 23*(4), 135-45.

66 Britton, C., McCormick, F. M., Renfrew, M. J., Wade, A., & King, S. E. (2007). Support for breastfeeding mothers. *Cochrane Database of Systematic Reviews* (Online), (1), CD001141.

67 Meedya, S., Fahy, K., & Kable, A. (2010). Factors that positively influence breastfeeding duration to 6 months: A literature review. *Women and Birth: Journal of the Australian College of Midwives, 23*(4), 135-45.

68 Stermler, J., & Lovera D. (2004). Insight from a breastfeeding support pilot program for husbands and fathers of Texas WIC participants. *Journal of Human Lactation, 20*(4), 417-22.

69 DiGirolamo, A. M., Grummer-Strawn, L. M., & Fein, S. B. (2008). Effect of maternity-care practices on breastfeeding. *Pediatrics, 122*(Suppl. 2), S43-49.

70 Rajan, L. (1994). The impact of obstetric procedures and analgesia/anaesthesia during labour and delivery on breast feeding. *Midwifery, 10*(2), 87-103.

71 Riordan, J., Gill-Hopple, K., & Angeron, J. (2005). Indicators of effective breastfeeding and estimates of breast milk intake. *Journal of Human Lactation, 21*(4), 406-12.

72 Rowe-Murray, H. J., & Fisher, J. R. (2002). Baby friendly hospital practices: Cesarean section is a persistent barrier to early initiation of breastfeeding. *Birth, 29*(2), 124-31.

73 Taveras, E. M., Li, R., Grummer-Strawn, L., Richardson, M., Marshall, R., Rego, V. H., & Lieu, T. A. (2004). Opinions and practices of clinicians associated with continuation of exclusive breastfeeding. *Pediatrics, 113*(4), e283-90.

74 Centers for Disease Control and Prevention. (n.d.). *CDC national survey of maternity practices in infant nutrition and care (mPINC)*. Retrieved from http://www.cdc.gov/breastfeeding/data/mpinc/index.htm

75 United Nations Children's Fund. (n.d.). *The community infant and young child feeding package: Adaptation guide.* Retrieved from http://www.unicef.org/nutrition/index_58362.html

76 International Lactation Consultant Association. (n.d.). *International Lactation Consultant Association.* Retrieved from http://www.ilca.org/i4a/pages/index.cfm?pageid=1

77 La Leche League International. (n.d.). *La Leche League Mission.* Retrieved from http://www.llli.org/mission.html?m=1,0,2

78 Johnston, M. L., & Esposito, N. (2007). Barriers and facilitators for breastfeeding among working women in the United States. *Journal of Obstetric, Gynecologic, and Neonatal Nursing, 36*(1), 9-20.

79 Kosmala-Anderson, J., & Wallace, L. M. (2006). Breastfeeding works: The role of employers in supporting women who wish to breastfeed and work in four organizations in England. *Journal of Public Health, 28*(3), 183-91.

80 Rojjanasrirat, W. (2004). Working women's breastfeeding experiences. *Maternal Child Nursing, 29*(4), 222-27.

81 United Nations. (2009). *Rural women in a changing world: Opportunities and challenges.* Retrieved from http://www.un.org/womenwatch/daw/public/Women%202000%20-%20Rural%20Women%20web%20English.pdf

82 World Health Organization. (2009). *Infant and young child feeding: Model chapter for textbooks for medical students and allied health professionals.* Geneva: World Health Organization.

83 Bianchi, S. M., & Casper, L. M. (2000). American Families. *Population Bulletin, 55*(4).

84 Johnston, M. L., & Esposito, N. (2007). Barriers and facilitators for breastfeeding among working women in the United States. *Journal of Obstetric, Gynecologic, and Neonatal Nursing, 36*(1), 9-20.

85 Johnston, M. L., & Esposito, N. (2007). Barriers and facilitators for breastfeeding among working women in the United States. *Journal of Obstetric, Gynecologic, and Neonatal Nursing, 36*(1), 9-20.

86 Kosmala-Anderson, J., & Wallace, L. M. (2006). Breastfeeding works: The role of employers in supporting women who wish to breastfeed and work in four organizations in England. *Journal of Public Health, 28*(3), 183-91.

87 Rojjanasrirat, W. (2004). Working women's breastfeeding experiences. *Maternal & Child Nursing, 29*(4), 222-27.

88 National Council of State Legislatures. (2011). *Breastfeeding laws.* Retrieved from http://www.ncsl.org/issues-research/health/breastfeeding-state-laws.aspx

89 Abdulwadud, O. A., & Snow, M. E. (2012). Interventions in the workplace to support breastfeeding for women in employment. *Cochrane Database of Systematic Reviews* (Online), (10), CD006177.

90 U.S. Department of Health and Human Services. (2008). *The business case for breastfeeding: Employee's guide to breastfeeding and working.* Retrieved from http://www.womenshealth.gov/breastfeeding/government-in-action/business-case-for-breastfeeding

91 Kansas Breastfeeding Coalition, Inc., Kansas Business Case for Breastfeeding. Retrieved from http://www.kansasbusinesscase.com

92 Global Monitoring Report Team. (2004). *EFA Global Monitoring Report 2005: Education for All: The Quality Imperative.* Paris, France: UNESCO.

93 Story, M., Kaphingst, K. M., & French, S. (2006). The role of child care settings in obesity prevention. *The Future of Children, 16*(1), 143-68.

94 Kim, J., & Peterson, K. E. (2008). Association of infant child care with infant feeding practices and weight gain among US infants. *Archives of Pediatric and Adolescent Medicine, 162*(7), 627-33.

95 Pearce, A., Li, L., Abbas, J., Ferguson, B., Graham, H., Law, C., & Millennium Cohort Study Child Health Group. (2012). Childcare use and inequalities in breastfeeding: Findings from the UK millennium cohort study. *Archives of Disease in Childhood, 97*(1), 39-42.

96 Benjamin, S. E., Taveras, E. M., Cradock, A. L., Walker, E. M., Slining, M. M., & Gillman, M. W. (2009). State and regional variation in regulations related to feeding infants in child care. *Pediatrics, 124*(1), e104-11.

97 Cameron, B., Javanparast, S., Labbok, M., Scheckter, R., & McIntyre, E. (2012). Breastfeeding support in child care: An international comparison of findings from Australia and the United States. *Breastfeeding Medicine, 7*(3), 163-66.

98 Centers for Disease Control and Prevention. (n.d.). *Breastfeeding among U.S. children born 2000-2009: CDC national immunization survey.* Retrieved from http://www.cdc.gov/breastfeeding/data/nis_data

99 Institute of Medicine. (2005). *WIC food packages: Time for a change.* Washington, DC: National Academies Press.

100 Wilde, P., Wolf, A., Fernandes, M., & Collins, A. (2012). Food-package assignments and breastfeeding initiation before and after a change in the special supplemental nutrition program for women, infants, and children. *American Journal of Clinical Nutrition, 96*(3), 560-66.

101 United States Breastfeeding Committee. (n.d.). *Workplace support in federal law.* Retrieved from http://www.usbreastfeeding.org/Workplace/WorkplaceSupport/WorkplaceSupportinHealthCareReform/tabid/175/Default.aspx

102 Heymann, J., Earle, A., & Hayes, J., for the Project on Global Working Families and the Institute for Health and Social Policy. (n.d.). *The work, family, and equity index: How does the United States measure up?* Retrieved from http://www.mcgill.ca/files/ihsp/WFEI2007.pdf

103 International Labour Organization. (n.d.). *R191 Maternity Protection Recommendation, 2000* (No. 191). Retrieved from http://www.ilo.org/ilolex/cgi-lex/convde.pl?R191

104 European Commission. (2008, October 3). *Commission improves work-life balance for millions with longer and better maternity leave*. Retrieved from http://europa.eu/rapid/press-release_IP-08-1450_en.htm

105 U.S. Department of Labor. (2003). *Leave benefits: Family & Medical Leave*. Retrieved from http://www.dol.gov/dol/topic/benefits-leave/fmla.htm

106 Society for Human Resource Management. (2012). *Employee benefits: The employee benefits landscape in a recovering economy*. Retrieved from http://www.shrm.org/research/surveyfindings/articles/documents/2012_empbenefits_report.pdf

107 Wuehler, S. E., & Ly Wane, C. T. (2011). Situational analysis of infant and young child nutrition policies and programmatic activities in Senegal. *Maternal & Child Nutrition, 7*(Suppl. 1), 157–81.

Chapter 10

Improving Infant and Young Child Feeding in Low-Resource Communities: Case Studies from Ghana, West Africa

Grace S. Marquis, PhD, LLD (*hc*)

"Famine is a characteristic of some people not having enough food; it is not a characteristic of there being not enough food."–Amartya Sen

World Development. (1980) Vol. 8, pp. 613–621.

Learning Objectives

- Become familiar with international feeding recommendations for infants and young children and the tools with which these are assessed.

- Examine the concept of food entitlement in relation to child nutrition and the individual, societal, and environmental factors that determine food entitlement.

- Evaluate diverse approaches to improve infants' and young children's diets and nutritional status through a food entitlement framework, using case studies.

Case Study: Improving Support for Optimal Infant and Young Child Nutrition in Ghana

Despite Ghana's economic growth, the prevalence of childhood malnutrition remains high. The Demographic and Health Survey (DHS) reports a 29% prevalence of wasting among 6- to 8-month-old infants and 40% stunting rate among 18- to 23-month-olds.[1] Breastfeeding initiation is almost universal, but 37% of mothers reported early termination of **exclusive breastfeeding** before 6 months of age, which is associated with increased morbidity and mortality.[2] The poor quality of infants' first foods, usually a thin maize or millet porridge (*Koko*) with low energy and micronutrient density, contributes to high rates of **wasting**.[3] Diets are based on cereals and roots, and the 2008 DHS reported that 29% of breastfed Ghanaian children 6–23 months of age consumed no micronutrient-rich animal product in the past day.[4]

The Ghanaian government's principal mechanisms to address childhood malnutrition have been through (1) legislative and educational support of breastfeeding, including the **Baby-Friendly Hospital Initiative (BFHI)** to promote optimal breastfeeding practices in healthcare facilities, and (2) growth monitoring and promotion activities, including nutrition education, carried out through Ghana Health Services' child welfare clinics. Child welfare clinics may be rural children's only access to primary health care and therefore must be effective. Health workers are an important source of information on infant and young child (IYC) feeding for young mothers. Ghana Health Services staff are generally knowledgeable about breastfeeding, but less competent in complementary feeding education. A recent evaluation found that healthcare staff had poor technical knowledge and unsupportive attitudes toward caregivers' problems with IYC feeding, poor communication skills, inadequate follow-up of problem cases, and unstable community volunteers.[5] Rural families may have more contact with community health volunteers and agricultural extension agents than Ghana Health Services professionals, so these human resources should be strengthened.

Individual project interventions in Ghana have demonstrated that collaboration across sectors can improve IYC nutritional status through national policies, community resources, intra-household food distribution norms, maternal income and education, child feeding behaviors, caregiving practices, and child health. Bilateral[6] and multinational efforts[7] to improve child nutrition integrate these approaches.

Discussion Questions

- Which common infant feeding practices in Ghana can lead to suboptimal nutrient status and health outcomes?
- What role has the Ghanaian government played in improving nutritional practices in Ghana?
- How can intersectoral collaboration support better nutrition?

Introduction

Nutritional status reflects the balance between dietary intake and energy and nutrient needs. Diets provide the energy, **macronutrients**, **micronutrients,** and nonnutritive factors necessary for normal growth and a healthy, active life. Nutrient status can be compromised by poor-quality diets, with effects such as mineral losses associated with high phytate diets, and by effects of illnesses, such as increased metabolic rates, urinary nutrient losses, gastrointestinal malabsorption, and illness-related anorexia.[8] Poor diets and illness are of concern especially in poor communities. Applied nutritional scientists aim to help families achieve optimal diets for IYC when extreme poverty diminishes intakes and morbidity augments nutrient losses.

The 1990 publication of UNICEF's *Strategy for Improved Nutrition of Children and Women in Developing Countries* recognized the complexity of issues involved in childhood malnutrition in low-resource communities.[9] The framework categorized influencing factors as immediate, underlying, and basic causes by their proximity to the child outcome. The inclusion of community- and national-level factors recognized that malnutrition is not just a household problem, but an indicator of society-wide dysfunction.[10] To achieve the Millennium Development Goal (MDG)[11] of reducing childhood underweight by half, countries must address how immediate causes, such as diet and illness, are influenced by underlying household and community causes, such as food insecurity, insufficient maternal and child care, poor-quality health services, and health environment.

> *Millennium Development Goal 1: Eradicate Extreme Poverty and Hunger. Target 1.C: Halve, between 1990 and 2015, the proportion of people who suffer from hunger*
>
> Reproduced from the United Nations. (n.d.). 2015 Millennium Development Goals. Retrieved from http://www.un.org/millenniumgoals/. Accessed August 13, 2013. This source is used for all Millennium Development Goals in this chapter.

Lack of Access to Food

The condition of famine[12] illustrates the influence on individual nutrition of basic societal-level causes, including organization of society and development of policies that affect resource distribution. Economist Amartya Sen argued that famines have been associated primarily *not* with shortages of food, but with people's **access** to food.[13] Lack of access to food can occur when individuals neither produce their own food nor have the ability to purchase or barter for food in the market system. During the Irish famine, for example, food was available but inaccessible because of its cost. As noted by Sen in his paper *Famines*, in late 1846, Major Parker, the local relief inspector, wrote, "On Saturday, notwithstanding all this distress, there was a market plentifully supplied with meat, bread, fish, in short everything." The ability to establish entitlement is determined by societal factors. Legal and political systems include land ownership laws and democratic rule. Economic and social policies include market price control, minimum wages, social safety nets, and education reforms. Cultural practices include sharing resources among extended families. Public health nutrition programs must consider these factors.

Additional Causes of Infant and Young Children Malnutrition

As with famine, IYC malnutrition does not always have absence of food as the primary cause. This is evident when one considers households in which adult overweight/obesity and child undernutrition coexist.[14] In low-income countries, an estimated one-fifth to two-thirds of households with an underweight individual may also have an overweight individual.[15]

Child malnutrition commonly arises because there is a failure in entitlement to access the requisite amount and quality of food needed by the child. Barriers to **entitlement** can include availability in the community, household accessibility, and utilization by the child.[16] Availability of food in communities may be limited by ecology, national agriculture, and market policies and land ownership laws. Accessibility incorporates home production, purchasing power in the markets, and knowledge about food. Finally, utilization includes resource allocation within the family and reflects child allocation practices, feeding behaviors, as well as individual child characteristics. Some factors may influence entitlement at multiple levels. Cultural beliefs, for example, may affect which foods are offered to children, influence which foods are sold in markets, and define gender roles that impact agricultural production.

This chapter reviews dietary recommendations for IYC and examines effective strategies that address the three levels of impediments to food entitlement and use legal, economic, social, and cultural approaches to enhance diets, diminish losses, and improve children's nutritional status. Case studies from Ghana are presented as illustrations.

Breastfeeding Infants and Young Children

The World Health Organization (WHO) recommends **exclusive breastfeeding** for the first 6 months of life, followed by the introduction of nutritionally adequate and safe **complementary foods** while continuing to breastfeed for up to 2 years of age or more.[17] Breastfeeding has both nutritional and immunological roles that contribute to children's growth and development. Human milk generally meets requirements for fluid, energy, macronutrients, and most micronutrients until about 6 months of age. However, vitamin D supplementation from birth is recommended for infants in conditions where dietary factors and inadequate sun exposure may lead to low vitamin D concentration in human milk.[18] Some concern exists regarding adequacy of iron and zinc among exclusively breastfed infants,[19] but given the benefit of lactational amenorrhea for women,[20] the lack of evidence of clinical consequences of zinc deficiency before 6 months,[21] and alternative means of addressing the iron needs through delayed cord clamping[22] and/or supplements, exclusive breastfeeding for six months is recommended in both low- and high-income countries.[23]

Benefits of Breastfeeding

Mortality among nonbreastfed infants is 4-fold higher than that of those breastfed.[24,25] This protective effect is greatest in early infancy. Late initiation of breastfeeding, after the first day, increases risk of death compared with early initiation.[26] Exclusivity of breastfeeding is also significant. Introducing other liquids in predominant breastfeeding, or of other liquids or solids in partial breastfeeding, increases risk for all-cause mortality in early infancy.[27] Among nonbreastfed infants under 6 months, all-cause mortality increased by 14-fold compared with exclusively breastfed infants, with pneumonia-related deaths 6-fold higher than among partially breastfed infants. In most cases, the benefits of breastfeeding outweigh the risk of transmission of human immunodeficiency virus (HIV). The World Health Organization's infant feeding recommendations for communities affected by HIV have changed over time as testing and access to drug therapy has improved (**Box 10-1**).[28] For mothers, benefits of breastfeeding include cost savings and reduced risk of type 2 diabetes, certain cancers, and postpartum depression.

The WHO developed eight core IYC feeding indicators to standardize IYC feeding methodology, thus permitting comparisons across communities and over time. Three of these indicators are focused on breastfeeding behaviors at key transition moments: birth, 6 months, and 1 year.[29,30,31,32] Suggested questionnaires also help standardize data collection.

Improving Breastfeeding Behaviors in Ghana Through Coordinated Institutional Activities

Despite improvements in recent decades, exclusive breastfeeding (EBF) is not universal.[33] The lowest income countries reported the rate of EBF among infants under 6 months to be 32% in 1995, and 43% by 2010. Nations in west and central Africa continue to have the lowest EBF

Box 10-1 WHO infant feeding recommendation for HIV-infected mothers

HIV-infected mothers whose infants are HIV uninfected or of unknown HIV status should exclusively breastfeed their infants for the first 6 months of life. Introduction of appropriate complementary foods should then begin, with continuation of breastfeeding for the first 12 months of life.

Breastfeeding should then only stop once a nutritionally adequate and safe diet without breastmilk can be provided.

Modified from the World Health Organization. (2010). Guidelines on HIV and Infant Feeding, Geneva: Author. Retrieved from http://www.who.int /child_adolescent_health/documents/9789241599535/en/index.html. Accessed August 12, 2013.

---

rates, with a rate of 24% in 2010. Despite the poor regional statistics, the West African country of Ghana has shown greater improvements, with rates of EBF among children under 6 months old increasing from 7% in 1993 to 63% in 2008.[34] Increases may be due to social pressure and the Baby-Friendly Hospital Initiative.[35]

Public Health Approaches to Encourage Breastfeeding in Ghana

This national public health success story[36] resulted from integrated factors supporting breastfeeding. They included (1) focused, common public health messages, (2) multiple actors/activities that supported the same messages, and (3) important, measureable health outcomes, such as lower infant morbidity and mortality and improved infant growth, that could be clearly linked to the promoted behavior change (**Table 10-1**).

Progress via Policy and Communication

In 1992, the Ghanaian legislative branch adopted the World Health Assembly's International Code of Marketing of Breast-milk Substitutes,[37] which led to the cessation of free distribution of formula in the country and the promotion of breastfeeding. The Ministry of Health reassessed program priorities and made control of diarrheal diseases its primary goal. Promotion of breastfeeding, which strengthens infants' immune systems directly and through nutritional adequacy, became part of the program. The Baby-Friendly Hospital Initiative[38] began two years later, helping to encourage breastfeeding in hospital environments and through training of health staff. In 2000, Ghana Health Services, the applied arm of the Ministry of Health, implemented the Integrated Management of Childhood Illness[39] program. Additional legislation in 2000 and 2003 included the Breastfeeding Promotion Regulation and the Maternity

---

Table 10-1 Changes in national legislation and Ministry of Health policies on infant feeding in Ghana

Year Adopted	Policy or Program Implemented
1992	Code on Breastmilk Substitutes
1992	Control of Diarrheal Diseases Program
1993	Baby-Friendly Hospital Initiative
1998	National Breastfeeding Policy
1998	Integrated Management of Childhood Illness adopted
2000	Community implementation of Integrated Management of Childhood Illnesses
2000	Breastfeeding Promotion Regulation (L.I.1667)
2003	Maternity Protection law

Data from Timpo, O. M. (2007). Programs and policies associated with improved exclusive breastfeeding rates in Ghana: 1989-2003. MSc Thesis. Storrs CT: University of Connecticut.

Protection Law, which addressed maternity and lactation leave concerns by providing at least 12 weeks of maternity leave and one-hour breaks for lactation for one year.

Public Health Core Competency 3: Communication Skills 4: Conveys public health information using a variety of approaches

Reproduced from Council on Linkages Between Academia and Public Health Practice. 2010 May. Core Competencies for Public Health Professionals. Washington, DC: Public Health Foundation. http://www.phf.org/resourcestools/Documents/Core_Competencies_for_Public_Health_Professionals_2010May.pdf. Accessed August 13, 2013. This source is used for all Public Health Core Competencies in this chapter.

Nutrition education occurred through train-the-trainer approaches. The US-AID LINKAGES project (1997–2004) contributed directly or indirectly to the training of thousands of governmental and nongovernmental organization staff and community workers on breastfeeding and related topics.[40] Consistent breastfeeding messages reached families through diverse routes, such as mass media, counseling at health centers, and discussion groups. Efforts to integrate infant nutrition into medical and paramedical training curricula resulted in breastfeeding questions becoming part of national qualifying exams for nurses and midwives. The project contributed to the expansion of the number of health and community-based workers who were knowledgeable about breastfeeding counseling.

This case study demonstrates that promotion of positive health behaviors can be successful when the behaviors are simultaneously protected by legislation, encouraged by the local infrastructure and social environment, and amply supported by well-trained staff.

Complementary Feeding for Infants and Young Children

Complementary feeding allows a child to transition from exclusive breastfeeding to no breastfeeding. International child feeding recommendations focus on the age at introduction of foods and liquids; frequency of feeding; quantity, quality, and safety of the diet; and interactions with the caregiver during feeding.[41] WHO's indicators of IYC feeding facilitate assessment of behaviors across countries and time (**Box 10-2**).[42,43,44] Minimum dietary diversity is an indicator of diet quality. The current definition was derived from the analysis of data sets from 10 countries.[45,46]

A separate indicator evaluates iron intake by measuring consumption of iron-rich foods or iron-fortified IYC foods. Feeding frequency is a good indicator of energy intake among breastfed infants. The WHO indicator "minimum meal frequency" incorporates both meals and snacks and reflects recent research on energy requirements, which are likely lower than previously estimated.[47]

Feeding Frequency Among Infants and Young Children in Ghana

Information from a recent DHS allows estimation of some of the new WHO complementary feeding indicators. The 2008 Ghana DHS survey asked about the number of times solid, semisolid, or soft foods were eaten yesterday, and mothers responded to a **food frequency questionnaire**, with 17 different foods and liquids used to estimate diet diversity.[48] While 73% of infants had received foods by 6 to 8 months of age, only 47% and 50% of the 6- to 23-month-old children met the dietary diversity and meal frequency recommendations, respectively, and 27% met both.

Factors Influencing Feeding Frequency

In rural southern Ghana, breastfeeding was the most influential factor in determining low feeding frequency.[49] The mean frequency was 2.2 meals, compared with a recommended three times for breastfed 9-month-old infants. In interviews, Ghanaian caregivers reported that young children should eat three times per day, the same as other family members. When probed, some mothers admitted using breastfeeding to substitute for meals if they were busy with work (**Box 10-3**).

Birk[50] reported that eating frequency among 2- to 5-year-old rural Ghanaian children, most of whom were weaned, was associated strongly with geographic location, a crude indicator of economic status, and caregiver time demands. The average number of daily feedings was 3.7 among those living in the north, a poor, dry savannah region, and 5.0 among those living in the "breadbasket" center of the country. Eighty-eight percent of the breastfed children consumed less frequently than the Ghanaian Ministry of Health's recommendation of four times per day.

Feeding frequency was also lower during the preharvest season, when food stockpiles are low, and when maternal occupations required substantial time outside the home. This is common in rural Ghanaian communities, where older siblings or adult relatives care for young children

---

Box 10-2 Complementary feeding indicators for breastfed IYC

Introduction of solid, semi-solid, or soft foods: Proportion of infants 6-8 months of age who receive solid, semi-solid or soft foods

Minimum dietary diversity: Proportion of children 6-23 months of age who receive foods from four or more food groups: grains, roots, and tubers; legumes and nuts; dairy products; flesh foods; eggs; vitamin-A rich fruits and vegetables; other fruits and vegetables

Minimum meal frequency: Proportion of children 6-23 months of age who receive solid, semisolid, or soft foods the minimum number of times or more (two times for 6-8 months; three times for 9-23 months)

Minimum acceptable diet: Proportion of children 6-23 months of age who receive a minimum acceptable diet: at least minimum dietary diversity and at least minimum meal frequency

Consumption of iron-rich or iron-fortified foods: Proportion of children 6-23 months of age who receive an iron-rich food or iron fortified food that is specially designed for infants and young children, or that is fortified in the home.

Modified from: World Health Organization, UNICEF, United States Agency for International Development, Academy for Educational Development, University of California, Davis, International Food Policy Research Institute. (2008). *Indicators for assessing infant and young child feeding practices: Part 1: Definitions.* Geneva: World Health Organization; World Health Organization. (2010). *Indicators for assessing infant and young child feeding practices: Part 2: Measurement.* Geneva: World Health Organization; and World Health Organization. (2010). *Indicators for assessing infant and young child feeding practices: Part 3: Country profiles.* Geneva: World Health Organization.

---

as women farm and trade. Studies in other settings have documented poor child dietary outcomes with suboptimal caregiving substitutions.[51] Community-based day care centers can offer child care alternatives and opportunities to improve children's diets.

Potential for Day Care Centers to Increase Nutrient Intake

Day care centers are increasingly common in rural Ghana. Nongovernmental organizations or enterprising residents assist in initiation of these private centers. Some centers provide meals for children through communal feeding programs, in which children bring a small amount of a staple food, such as yam, firewood, and/or cash for additional ingredients, food processing costs, and staff. The children share the lunch meal. One study found that the lunch provided through a communal feeding program was higher in energy but lower in some micronutrients, such as calcium, iron, and zinc, than lunches of children with home-prepared meals.[52] Since mothers did not consider the center meal to be lunch, their children ate a second meal after school, resulting in a meal frequency of 4.2 per day compared with 3.4 for children without shared meals. Despite the lower nutritional quality of the center lunch, the additional meal led to increased dietary diversity and total intakes of energy, calcium, iron, and zinc. In this setting, communal feeding programs improved dietary intakes by offering an additional feeding event in school that did not replace a home meal.

Box 10-3 Feeding frequency among 2- to 5-year-old children in northern Ghana

Question: How many times does the child normally eat?

Response: The child is fed two times since I waste time when feeding. I feed her three times on non-working days.

(Caregiver, Eastern region, Ghana)

Reproduced from Birk, K. A. (2013). Making child feeding frequency a priority: An evaluation of current practices and perceptions in Ghana MSc thesis. McGill University Montreal Canada.

This case study demonstrates the importance of understanding the environmental, social, and cultural factors that influence feeding behaviors. Enhancing economic activities increases caregivers' buying power, but increasing women's working time away from home can harm children's diets. Community programs may counterbalance these effects.

Public Health Core Competency 5: Community Dimensions of Practice Skills 8: Identifies community assets and resources

Improving Nutrient Quality of the Diets for Better Growth Among Children Younger Than 5 Years of Age

In low-resource communities, young children's diets are plant-based, with cereals, roots, and tubers, and little to no animal source foods (ASF). Micronutrient **bioavailability** is low. Approaches to improve children's diet quality and nutritional status include diet supplementation, nutrition education, increasing household production, and integrated interventions.

Supplemental Feeding Programs

Supplemental feeding programs provide energy and nutrients in addition to the home diet.[53] Programs have distinct recipients, nutrients, and modes of delivery. Examples include using feeding centers versus home distribution, community-wide coverage versus targeting of high-risk individuals, provision of staples versus specific nutrient-rich preparations versus micronutrient powders for home fortification, family versus child rations, and long-term versus short-term programs. Program effectiveness is modulated by the relative contribution of diet to malnutrition, the specific nutritional deficiencies, and the extent of supplement sharing within the family. Interventions of direct provision of food or nutrient supplements to the child or the child's household do not always resolve childhood malnutrition, even after careful targeting. In a recent study in southern Ethiopia, 30% of malnourished children failed to recover after four months of fortified corn-soya blend (CSB, World Food Programme rations); the comparison group that received ready-to-use therapeutic food

(RUTF) also had a high, although lower, nonresponsive rate (24%). This difference may reflect the perception of RUTF as a medicine and a lower likelihood of being shared in the family.[54]

The cumulative experience of supplementation programs is disappointing. A recent meta-analysis of eight randomized controlled trials in nine countries assessed the effectiveness of community-based supplementary feeding in promoting the growth of children younger than 5 years of age.[55] Treatments varied widely, and control groups received no supplement or a low-energy/low-nutrient supplement. Treatment had small effect on linear growth, with the average effect being an additional 1.3 centimeters after 12 months of intervention. The study concluded that "clinicians and public health policy makers should not place undue expectations on the effectiveness of supplementary feeding for promoting the growth of children under five years of age living in low and middle income countries."

Efforts by the Codex Alimentarius Commission of the Food and Agriculture Organization to improve the quality of formulated complementary foods will help develop market products that can be used in supplementary food programs to meet energy and nutrient requirements of infants and young children.[56] The role of these products to improve the diets of infant and young children is potentially large, since even in rural Ghana, market foods compose a substantial portion of preschool-aged children's diets.[57]

Nutrition Education for Caregivers

Nutrition education[58] programs with no supplementary feeding can be effective, especially in regions where poverty and food scarcity are not the primary determinants of child malnutrition. A randomized controlled trial in peri-urban communities in northern Peru investigated diet quality and nutritional status outcomes of infants and young children.[59] The nutrition education intervention improved caregiver nutrition knowledge and feeding practices, such as use of nutrient and energy-dense paps, or common infant cereal-based complementary food, and child's dietary quality, with 26% and 34% increased daily intakes of zinc and calcium, respectively. At 18 months of age, the adjusted group difference in linear growth was significant but small, while the effect on stunting was large, suggesting the intervention's effectiveness in preventing extreme cases of malnutrition. The project's success was linked mainly to high intervention implementation (50–90% of expected frequency) and not intervention fidelity (only 28–70% of expected).

Integration of nutrition throughout the health center, with the same message repeated by all staff, was beneficial.[60] In an evaluation of a **Positive Deviance/Hearth** intervention in Ecuador,[61,62,63] nutrition education activities increased dietary intakes of iron, zinc, vitamin A, protein, and energy; improved weight-for-age z scores; and eliminated the risk of severe underweight. Both of these examples demonstrate that nutrition education programs can successfully change feeding behaviors and contribute to improved IYC diets and growth.

A systematic review of young child feeding interventions analyzed studies that used only an educational intervention approach in six theme areas: (1) continuation of breastfeeding after six months, (2) consistency of food, (3) inclusion of ASF, (4) dietary diversity, (5) responsive feeding, and (6) hygiene.[64] The effect of education alone on increasing micronutrient intakes was mixed. However, effects on weight and linear growth were modest but positive. Results suggested that nutrition education may be more effective when messages focus on increasing use of ASF or other nutrient-rich foods.

Household Animal Production and Diet Quality

Another approach to increase the availability and accessibility of ASF in IYC diets is to increase household animal production. One review[65] examined the effectiveness of 14 agriculture production interventions, focusing on aquaculture (4), dairy (3), poultry (3), or integrated production and nutrition education (4) to increase intakes of ASF in children or the households. The interventions led to increased production but did not necessarily improve household income or diets. When ASF intake increased, whether the increase was due to increased home production or income was unclear. In a study of interventions with the explicit aim to improve nutritional status of children,[66] most interventions had a positive effect on diets. Increased intake was associated with the specific agriculture target; for example, dairy endeavors led to increased dairy intakes. This suggests that increased production directly affected children's diets.

Individually, these diverse intervention approaches are each limited in what they can accomplish. In the following case study, an integrated approach includes (1) nutrition education sessions to address caregivers' knowledge gaps on children's dietary needs and provide participatory demonstrations on food preparation, (2) entrepreneurial training to improve knowledge and skills needed to increase profitability of women's small businesses, and (3) microcredit loans that opened up access to financial resources and increased women's financial capacity needed to expand their enterprises. The project's success was due not only to addressing multiple layers of impediments to food entitlement, but also to the inclusion of multiple partners, as government, nongovernment, private, and community entities who worked together to improve child nutrition.

Case Study: Improving Children's Diets Through Integrated Programs: The ENAM Project in Ghana

The 2003 Ghanaian DHS found that an estimated 42% of children 20–23 months of age consumed no ASF during the previous day.[67] To improve ASF intakes, the US-AID-funded Enhancing Child Nutrition through Animal Source Food Management (ENAM) project introduced a 16-month intervention. Women's microenterprise development activities were the focus.[68] ENAM worked to improve profits by providing business development services, including group support, microcredit services (initially through the project and later through local private banks), and technical training specific to enterprises, such as poultry rearing and fish smoking. Financial services were organized through formation of women's Credit and Savings Associations (CSA), with loan repayment, obligatory savings deposits, and all training events occurring at weekly CSA meetings. The Ministries of Food and Agriculture and Health, the nongovernmental organizations Freedom from Hunger–Ghana and Heifer International–Ghana, local private rural banks, diverse departments at the University of Ghana, and the local communities were key stakeholders.

Since economic gains do not automatically improve child nutrition, the project's activities integrated nutrition and health education, addressing the six principal constraints to the inclusion of ASF in young children's diets in rural Ghana that were identified through formative research (**Table 10-2**). The project was implemented in six rural communities in three agro-ecological zones (Guinea Savannah, Forest-Savannah Transitional, and Coastal Savannah), and included 181 caregivers of children 2 to 5 years of age. Six matched communities from the same ecological zones in Ghana served as comparison sites.

Table 10-2 Barriers to food entitlement and corresponding ENAM project activities

Barrier	Activity
Poor producer-consumer linkages	Small business training
Low income	Microcredit loans and small business training
Poor skills of extension staff	Training/skill building
Low nutrition knowledge	Training/skill building
Restrictive cultural beliefs	Group discussions
Preferential food distribution for adults/older children	Training/group discussions

Data from: Colecraft, E., Marquis, G. S., Aryeetey, R., Sakyi-Dawson, O., Lartey, A., Ahunu, B., ... Huff-Lonergan, E. (2006). Constraints on the Use of Animal Source Foods for Young Children in Ghana: A Participatory Rapid Appraisal Approach. *Ecology of Food and Nutrition, 45*(5), 351–377.

The integration of financial and educational activities helped women increase profits and become more knowledgeable about children's nutritional requirements. Diet quality and children's nutritional status improved. One study[69] found that more intervention caregivers expanded and diversified their businesses compared with nonintervention controls. They also had higher average enterprise profits and greater savings than comparison caregivers. Participants tended to spend a higher percentage of income to household food expenses and purchase more ASF. Although the consumption of nonpurchased ASF was similar between groups, intervention households consumed more total ASF. Number of children, wealth, and being involved in an ASF-related small business increased children's ASF diversity.[70] Increased ASF intakes may result from direct access to that product from small businesses or from higher profits associated with ASF-related business that increase household capacity to purchase ASF in the market.

This case study demonstrates the importance of understanding the physical and social environment, including local cultural beliefs, and the value of engaging all stakeholders in planning an intervention.[71] The formative phase worked closely with stakeholders to identify the main obstacles to consumption of ASF and pointed out necessary intervention activities. Income was considered only one of many barriers by the women, program staff, and policy leaders who worked with the project. In addition, the project depended on local partners (governmental and nongovernmental organizations and the private sector) to share substantial experience in working in the rural communities. Finally, the intensity of the intervention, with 16 months of weekly or more frequent meetings, strengthened group dynamics and individual responses.

Conclusion

The UNICEF framework introduced at the beginning of this chapter and the presented case studies in Ghana suggest that the responsibility for child nutrition lies with all institutions that address determinants of nutrition. Agriculture, health, education, finance, and other sectors need to be cognizant of the potential for their institution's policies and programs to improve children's lives and make the commitment to integrate activities to achieve the MDGs. Cross-sector and cross-institutional programming need staff with common knowledge and understanding about the determinants of child malnutrition, and similar values that help to prioritize child nutrition and health in the country.[72] Training of personnel across sectors is essential to developing the interest and collaboration needed to move forward. The Scaling Up Nutrition (SUN) movement began in 2010 as an effort to improve the commitment to nutrition at the national level and encourage cross-sector collaborations.[73] This network of governments, institutions, civic groups, and private industry is pushing for the rapid expansion of interventions that have been shown to be effective in improving nutritional outcomes. The implementation of indicators of undernutrition as part of the measurement of success of programs across the diverse sectors will help secure a level of commitment of society to child nutrition that reaches beyond just the health sector and provides the opportunity to improve child nutrition worldwide.

References

1 Du Bois, E. F. (1936). *Basal metabolism in health and disease.* Philadelphia, PA: Lea & Febiger.

2 Stephensen, C. B., Alvarez, J. O., Kohatsu, J., Hardmeier, R., Kennedy, J. I., Jr., & Gammon, R. B., Jr. (1994). Vitamin A is excreted in the urine during acute infection. *American Journal of Clinical Nutrition, 60,* 388-92.

3 Brown, K. H. (2003). Diarrhea and malnutrition. *Journal of Nutrition, 133,* 328S-332S.

4 Du Bois, E. F. (1936). *Basal metabolism in health and disease.* Philadelphia, PA: Lea & Febiger.

5 Martorell, R., Yarbrough, C., Yarbrough, S., & Klein, R. E. The impact of ordinary illnesses on the dietary intakes of malnourished children. *American Journal of Clinical Nutrition, 33,* 345-50.

6 Marquis, G. S., Lopez, T., Peerson, J. M., & Brown, K. H. (1993). Effect of dietary viscosity on energy intake by breast-fed and non-breast-fed children during and after acute diarrhea. *American Journal of Clinical Nutrition, 57,* 218-23.

7 United Nations Children's Fund. (1990). *Strategy for improved nutrition of children and women in developing countries: A policy review.* New York, NY: UNICEF.

8 Marquis, G. S., Lopez, T., Peerson, J. M., et al. (1993). Effect of dietary viscosity on energy intake by breast-fed and non-breast-fed children during and after acute diarrhea. *American Journal of Clinical Nutrition, 57,* 218-23.

9 United Nations Children's Fund. (1990). *Strategy for improved nutrition of children and women in developing countries: A policy review.* New York, NY: Author.

10 Pelletier, D. L. (2002). *Toward a common understanding of malnutrition: Assessing the contributions of the UNICEF framework.* Background paper. World Bank/UNICEF Nutrition Assessment Background Paper. Retrieved from Tulane University website at http://tulane.edu/publichealth/internut/resources.cfm

11 United Nations. (n.d.). Millennium Development Goals. Retrieved from http://www.un.org/millenniumgoals

12 IPC Global Partners. (2008). *Integrated food security phase classification technical manual (Version 1.1).* Rome: Food and Agriculture Organization.

13 Sen, A. (1980). Famines. *World development, 8,* 613-21.

14 Gittelsohn, J., Haberle, H., Vastine, A. E., Dyckman, W., & Palafox, N. (2003). Macro and micro-level processes affect food choice and nutritional status in the Republic of the Marshall Islands. *Journal of Nutrition, 133*(1), 310S-313S.

15 Doak, C. M., Adair, L. S., Bentley, M., & Popkin, B. M. (2005). The dual burden household and the nutrition transition paradox. *International Journal of Obesity and Related Metabolic Disorders, 29,* 129-36. doi:10.1038/sj.ijo.0802824

16 Colecraft, E., Marquis, G. S., Aryeetey, R., Sakyi-Dawson, O., Lartey, A., Ahunu, B., . . . Huff-Lonergan, E. (2006). Constraints on the use of animal source foods for young children in Ghana:

A participatory rapid appraisal approach. *Ecology of Food and Nutrition, 45*(5), 351-77. doi:10.1080/03670240600985464

17 World Health Organization. (2003) *Global strategy on infant and young child feeding.* Geneva: World Health Organization.

18 Wagner, C. L., Greer, F. R., American Academy of Pediatrics Section on Breastfeeding, & American Pediatrics Committee on Nutrition. (2008). Prevention of rickets and vitamin D deficiency in infants, children, and adolescents. *Pediatrics, 122*(5), 1142-52. doi:10.1542/peds.2008-1862

19 Michaelsen, K. F., Larnkjaer, A., Lauritzen, L., & Molgaard, C. (2010). Science base of complementary feeding practice in infancy. *Current Opinion in Clinical Nutrition and Metabolic Care, 13*(3), 277-83.

20 Ramos, R., Kennedy, I. K., & Visness, C. M. (1996). Effectiveness of lactational amenorrhoea in prevention of pregnancy in Manila, the Philippines: Non-comparative prospective trial. *BMJ, 313,* 909-12.

21 Krebs, N. F., Mazariegos, M., Chomba, E., Sami, N., Pasha, O., Tshefu, A., . . . Hambidge, K. M. (2012). Randomized controlled trial of meat compared with multimicronutrient-fortified cereal in infants and toddlers with high stunting rates in diverse settings. *American Journal of Clinical Nutrition, 96,* 840-47.

22 Andersson, O., Hellström-Westas, L., Andersson, D., & Domellöf, M. (2011). Effect of delayed versus early umbilical cord clamping on neonatal outcomes and iron status at 4 months: A randomised controlled trial. *BMJ, 343,* d7157. doi:10.1136/bmj.d7157

23 American Academy of Pediatrics. (2012). Breastfeeding and the use of human milk [policy statement]. *Pediatrics, 129*(3), e827-e841.

24 Effect of breastfeeding on infant and child mortality due to infectious diseases in less developed countries: A pooled analysis. WHO Collaborative Study Team on the Role of Breastfeeding on the Prevention of Infant Mortality. (2000). *Lancet, 355*(9202), 451-55.

25 Black, R. E., Allen, L. H., Bhutta, Z. A., Caulfield, L. E., de Onis, M., Ezzati, M., . . . Maternal and Child Undernutrition Study Group. (2008). Maternal and child undernutrition: Global and regional exposures and health consequences. *Lancet, 371,* 243-60. doi:10.1016/S0140-6736(07)61690-0

26 Edmond, K. M., Zandoh, C., Quigley, M. A., Amenga-Etego, S., Owusu-Agyei, S., & Kirkwood, B. R. (2006). Delayed breastfeeding initiation increases risk of neonatal mortality. *Pediatrics, 117,* e380-86.

27 Black, R. E., Allen, L. H., Bhutta, Z. A., Caulfield, L. E., de Onis, M., Ezzati, M., . . . Maternal and Child Undernutrition Study Group. (2008). Maternal and child undernutrition: Global and regional exposures and health consequences. *Lancet, 371,* 243-60. doi:10.1016/S0140-6736(07)61690-0

28 World Health Organization. (2010). *Guidelines on HIV and infant feeding.* Geneva: World Health Organization. Retrieved from http://www.who.int/child_adolescent_health/documents /9789241599535/en/index.html

29 World Health Organization. (2010). *Guidelines on HIV and infant feeding*. Geneva: World Health Organization. Retrieved from http://www.who.int/child_adolescent_health /documents/9789241599535/en/index.html

30 World Health Organization, UNICEF, United States Agency for International Development, Academy for Educational Development, University of California, Davis, International Food Policy Research Institute. (2008). *Indicators for assessing infant and young child feeding practices. Part 1: Definitions*. Geneva: World Health Organization.

31 World Health Organization. (2010). *Indicators for assessing infant and young child feeding practices. Part 2: Measurement*. Geneva: World Health Organization.

32 World Health Organization. (2010). *Indicators for assessing infant and young child feeding practices. Part 3: Country profiles*. Geneva: World Health Organization.

33 UNICEF. (2012). Introduction to UNICEF's work on statistics and monitoring. Retrieved from http://www.unicef.org/statistics /index.html

34 Ghana Statistical Service (GSS), Ghana Health Service (GHS), & ICF Macro. (2009). *Ghana demographic and health survey, 2008*. Accra, Ghana: GSS, GHS, and ICF Macro.

35 Laar, A. K., Ampofo, W., Tuakli, J. M., & Quakyi, I. A. (2009). Infant feeding choices and experiences of HIV-positive mothers from two Ghanaian districts. *Journal of AIDS and HIV Research, 1*(2), 23-33.

36 Timpo, O. M. (2007). *Programs and policies associated with improved exclusive breastfeeding rates in Ghana: 1989-2003* (master's thesis). University of Connecticut, Storrs, CT.

37 World Health Organization. (1981). *The International Code of Marketing of Breast-milk Substitutes*. Geneva: World Health Organization. Retrieved from http://www.who.int/nutrition /publications/code_english.pdf

38 World Health Organization & UNICEF. (2009). *Baby-Friendly Hospital Initiative: Revised, updated and expanded for integrated care*. Geneva: World Health Organization. Retrieved from http://www.who.int/nutrition/publications/infantfeeding /9789241594950/en/index.html

39 World Health Organization. (n.d.). *Integrated Management of Childhood Illness (IMCI)*. Retrieved from http://www.who.int /maternal_child_adolescent/topics/child/imci/en

40 LINKAGES Project Ghana. (2004). *Final report (1997-2004)*. Washington, DC: Academy for Educational Development.

41 Pan American Health Organization. (2003). *Guiding principles for complementary feeding of the breastfed child*. Washington, DC: Pan American Health Organization. Retrieved from http:// www.who.int/child_adolescent_health/documents/a85622/en /index.html

42 World Health Organization, UNICEF, United States Agency for International Development, Academy for Educational Development, University of California, Davis, & International Food Policy Research Institute. (2008). *Indicators for assessing infant and young child feeding practices. Part 1: Definitions*. Geneva: World Health Organization.

43 World Health Organization. (2010). *Indicators for assessing infant and young child feeding practices. Part 2: Measurement*. Geneva: World Health Organization.

44 World Health Organization. (2010). *Indicators for assessing infant and young child feeding practices. Part 3: Country profiles*. Geneva: World Health Organization.

45 Working Group on Infant and Young Child Feeding Indicators. (2006). *Developing and validating simple indicators of dietary quality and energy intake of infants and young children in developing countries: Summary findings from analysis of 10 data sets*. Washington, DC: Food and Nutrition Technical Assistance (FANTA) Project, Academy for Educational Development (AED).

46 Working Group on Infant and Young Child Feeding Indicators. (2007). *Developing and validating simple indicators of dietary quality and energy intake of infants and young children in developing countries: Additional analysis of 10 data sets*. Washington, DC: Food and Nutrition Technical Assistance (FANTA) Project, Academy for Educational Development (AED).

47 Butte, N. F. (2005). Energy requirements of infants. *Public Health Nutrition, 8*, 953-67.

48 Ghana Statistical Service (GSS), Ghana Health Service (GHS), & ICF Macro. (2009). *Ghana demographic and health survey, 2008*. Accra, Ghana: GSS, GHS, and ICF Macro.

49 Birk, K. A. (2013). *Making child feeding frequency a priority: An evaluation of current practices and perceptions in Ghana* (master's thesis). McGill University, Montreal, Canada.

50 Birk, K. A. (2013). *Making child feeding frequency a priority: An evaluation of current practices and perceptions in Ghana* (master's thesis). McGill University, Montreal, Canada.

51 Lamontagne, J. F., Engle, P. L., & Zeitlin, M. F. (1998). Maternal employment, child care, and nutritional status of 12-18-month-old children in Managua, Nicaragua. *Social Science & Medicine, 46*(3), 403-14.

52 Harding, K. B., Marquis, G. S., Colecraft, E. K., Lartey, A., & Sakyi-Dawson, O. (2012). Participation in communal daycare centre feeding programs is associated with improved diet quantity but not quality among rural Ghanaian children. *African Journal of Food, Agriculture, and Nutrition, 12*(1), 5802-21.

53 Beaton, G. H. (1982). Evaluation of nutrition interventions: Methodologic considerations. *American Journal of Clinical Nutrition, 35*, 1280-89.

54 Karakochuk, C., van den Briel, T., Stephens, D., & Zlotkin, S. (2012). Treatment of moderate acute malnutrition with ready-to-use supplementary food results in higher overall recovery rates compared with a corn-soya blend in children in southern Ethiopia: An operations research trial. *American Journal of Clinical Nutrition, 96*(4), 911-16.

55 Sguassero, Y., de Onis, M., Bonotti, A. M., & Carroli, G. (2012). Community-based supplementary feeding for promoting the growth of children under five years of age in low and middle income countries. *Cochrane Database of Systematic Reviews*, (6), CD005039. doi:10.1002/14651858.CD005039.pub3

56 Huffman, S. L., & Schofield D. (2012). Enhancing young child nutrition and development in developing countries. *Maternal and Child Nutrition, 9*(Suppl. 1), 6-11. doi:10.1111/mcn.12009

57 Colecraft, E. K., Marquis, G. S., Bartolucci, A. A., Pulley, L., Owusu, W. B., & Maetz, H. M. (2004). A longitudinal assessment of the diet and growth of malnourished children participating in nutrition rehabilitation centres in Accra, Ghana. *Public Health Nutrition. 7*(4), 487-94.

58 Contento, I. R., Balch, G. I., Bronner, Y. L., Lytle, L. A., & Maloney, S. K. (1995). The effectiveness of nutrition education and implications for nutrition education policy, programs, and research: A review of research. *Journal of Nutrition Education, 27*, 277-422.

59 Penny, M. E., Creed-Kanashiro, H. M., Robert, R. C., Narro, M. R., Caulfield, L. E., & Black, R. E. (2005). Effectiveness of an educational intervention delivered through the health services to improve nutrition in young children: A cluster-randomised controlled trial. *Lancet, 365*(9474), 1863-72.

60 Robert, R. C., Gittelsohn, J., Creed-Kanashiro, H. M., Penny, M. E., Caulfield, L. E., Narro, M. R., . . . Black, R. E. (2007). Implementation examined in a health center-delivered, educational intervention that improved infant growth in Trujillo, Peru: Successes and challenges. *Health Education Research, 22*(3), 318-31.

61 Roche, M. L. (2011). *A community-based positive deviance /hearth intervention to improve infant and young child nutrition in the Ecuadorian Andes* (doctoral dissertation). Retrieved from http://catalogue.mcgill.ca.proxy2.library.mcgill .ca/F/KSYMERIEGYG8YJ8GJGX4U22II2HC782EVKIFNGSFTAH 2NATGBV-45098?func=full-set-set&set_number=004693&set _entry=000001&format=999.

62 Marsh, D. R., Schroeder, D. G., Dearden, K. A., Sternin, J., & Sternin, M. (2004). The power of positive deviance. *BMJ, 329,* 1177-79. doi:10.1136/bmj.329.7475.1177

63 McNulty, J., & CORE Group. (2005). *Positive deviance /Hearth essential elements: A Resource Guide for Sustainably Rehabilitating Malnourished Children* (Addendum). Retrieved from http://www.positivedeviance.org/pdf/manuals/addendum.pdf.

64 Dewey, K. G., & Adu-Afarwuah, S. (2008). Systematic review of the efficacy and effectiveness of complementary feeding interventions in developing countries. *Maternal and Child Nutrition, 4,* 24-85. doi:10.1111/j.1740-8709.2007.00124.x

65 Leroy, J. L., & Frongillo, E. A. (2007). Can interventions to promote animal production ameliorate undernutrition? *Journal of Nutrition, 137*(10), 2311-16.

66 Masset, E., Haddad, L., Cornelius, A., & Isaza-Castro, J. (2012). Effectiveness of agricultural interventions that aim to improve nutritional status of children: Systematic review. *British Medical Journal, 344,* d8222. doi:10.1136/bmj.d8222

67 Ghana Statistical Service (GSS), Noguchi Memorial Institute for Medical Research (NMIMR), & ORC Macro. (2004). *Ghana demographic and health survey, 2003.* Calverton, MD: GSS, GHS, and ICF Macro.

68 Colecraft, E., Marquis, G. S., Aryeetey, R., Sakyi-Dawson, O., Lartey, A., Ahunu, B., . . . Huff-Lonergan, E. (2006). Constraints on the use of animal source foods for young children in Ghana: A participatory rapid appraisal approach. *Ecology of Food and Nutrition, 45*(5), 351-77. doi:10.1080/03670240600985464

69 Homiah, P. A., Sakyi-Dawson, O., Bonsu, A. M., & Marquis, G. S. (2012). Microenterprise development coupled with nutrition education can help increase caregivers' incomes and household accessibility to animal source foods. *African Journal of Food, Agriculture, Nutrition and Development, 12*(1), 5725-45.

70 Christian, A. K., Lartey, A., Colecraft, E. K., Marquis, G. S., Sakyi-Dawson, O., Ahunu, B., & Butler, L. M. (2012). Relationship between caregivers' income generation activities and their children's animal source food intake. *African Journal of Food, Agriculture, Nutrition and Development, 12*(1), 5746-58.

71 Marquis, G. S., & Colecraft, E. K. (2012). The Nutrition-microcredit synergy: A case for multiple interventions and strategies. *African Journal of Food, Agriculture, Nutrition and Development, 12*(1), 5674-86.

72 Pelletier, D. L. (2002). *Toward a common understanding of malnutrition: Assessing the Contributions of the UNICEF framework.* World Bank/UNICEF Nutrition Assessment Background Paper. Retrieved from Tulane University website at http://tulane.edu /publichealth/internut/resources.cfm..

73 *Scaling Up Nutrition (SUN) movement strategy, 2012-2015.* (2012). Retrieved from www.scalingupnutrition.org.

Chapter 11

Nutrition of Women and Children: Focus on Ghana and HIV/AIDS

Amos Laar, PhD, MPH
Richmond Aryeetey, PhD, MPH

"If you take away my food, you will kill me faster than my HIV."—HIV-positive woman from Ghana

Learning Objectives

- Discuss the relevance of maternal and child malnutrition as part of a broader discussion of human development.

- Discuss the key nutritional status challenges affecting women and children in Ghana as a representation of the situation in low-income sub-Saharan African countries.

- Describe the diets of Ghanaian women and children in terms of quality and adequacy.

- Discuss the determinants of poor nutrition among women and children in Ghana.

- Explain the rationale for nutrition interventions currently implemented in low-income settings to address maternal and childhood undernutrition.

- Discuss the nutrition situation of women and children in the context of human immunodeficiency virus (HIV) and acquired immune deficiency syndrome (AIDS).

- Describe the impact of the HIV epidemic on women and children living in a resource-poor setting.

- Justify the use of nutrition as a tool for preventing HIV in a resource-poor setting.

Case Studies

Two case studies drawn from research and professional practice illustrate salient concepts on this subject. The first case study is about local efforts to manage **severe acute malnutrition (SAM)** in a non-emergency setting in Ghana. The second communicates nutrition and HIV-related challenges of women and children in a resource-poor setting.

Case Study: Supplementary Feeding and Management of Severe Acute Malnutrition

Severe acute malnutrition can occur in children exposed to poor care, infections, and poor dietary quality, especially inadequate **micronutrient** intake. These risk factors and SAM can exist in emergency and non-emergency settings. In Ghana in the early 2000s, 2% of children below age 5 had SAM, and management was mainly clinic-based and restricted to 42 nutrition rehabilitation centers in various locations in the country. In June 2007, the Ghana Health Services, in partnership with the Food and Nutrition Technical Assistance project, implemented a community-based intervention to manage SAM (CMAM). Under this program, facility staff and community volunteers are trained and become collaborators. Community volunteers actively search for SAM among children and refer cases to selected facilities for assessment. Fortified food supplements can be provided for home use, and children at high risk for mortality can be admitted to the facility for treatment. Five of Ghana's 10 administrative regions had CMAM programs in 2012, and all regions are expected to participate by 2016.

Discussion Questions

- What is the advantage of treating noncomplicated acute malnutrition at home rather than in a facility?
- What is the role of facility-based treatment in acute malnutrition management as community care is expanded?
- What skills do community volunteers need to identify acute malnutrition?

Case Study: Experiences of an HIV-Positive Mother from a Resource-Poor Setting

Mamunatu from Accra, Ghana, is a 34-year-old HIV-positive widow whose husband died in 2007. Mamunatu only learned that she had been infected with HIV when she tested positive during a routine antenatal care exam. She decided not to disclose her status to her family members, and her first instinct was to abort the fetus. However, she decided to keep the pregnancy after counseling from her healthcare provider. With further counseling, she learned that her baby could become infected through breastfeeding. The counselor told her that she could feed the child either exclusively with formula or exclusively with breastmilk, and explained the constraints of both options. Knowing the high cost of formula and the risk of infection resulting from water of uncertain quality as a risk for other infections, she made her decision and started exclusive breastfeeding of her child. However, at the fourth month postpartum, her fear of transmitting HIV to her child forced her to switch abruptly to formula.

Discussion Questions

- Why did Mamunatu not disclose her HIV serostatus to her family members?
- Given Mamunatu's circumstance, which of the two feeding options would be appropriate for her infant?
- Was her abrupt cessation of breastfeeding at four months a sensible action?
- What other information do you need from Mamunatu to assess the suitability of the formula feeding option she switched to?
- Can you think of other dilemmas that other women in Mamunatu's circumstances face?

Introduction

Despite advances in nutrition knowledge and technology, hunger and malnutrition remain significant developmental challenges, particularly in low-income countries like Ghana. News about famines and starvation in Africa, especially in nations experiencing civil strife and natural disasters, is familiar, but widespread and often hidden hunger affecting millions of vulnerable women and children on the continent receives less exposure. This chapter discusses the nutrition situation of women and children living in Ghana as a representation of low-income countries, especially in sub-Saharan Africa. The chapter will also discuss the determinants of undernutrition, as well as current actions to address malnutrition in Ghana. The next part of the chapter provides an overview of the relationship between nutrition and HIV. The chapter argues for a vigorous implementation of the concept of "nutrition as prevention" as part of multilevel HIV response strategies in a resource-poor setting.

Introduction to Maternal and Child Malnutrition

Malnutrition is a state of suboptimal nourishment ranging from **undernutrition** to **overnutrition**. Malnutrition influences development failure, and it is increasingly recognized to hinder socioeconomic development and nonproductivity through multiple pathways.[1] Economists and other development scientists attempt to objectively describe the negative impacts of widespread population undernutrition across the **life cycle**. Furthermore, the 2012 Copenhagen Consensus validated these relationships by ranking nutrition interventions as having higher cost–benefit ratios than many interventions related to infectious diseases, climate change, water and sanitation, and natural disasters.[2]

Undernutrition can directly or indirectly limit national capacity for economic growth.[3] Direct effects arise from reduced individual physical work output. Indirect effects include suppressing cognitive capacity, school and work performance, and achievement. A supplemental intervention in Guatemala found that improving nutrition in young boys led to higher-wage earnings as adults.[4] This finding showed that improved **nutritional capital** early in life can translate to subsequent developmental dividends and a favorable cost–benefit ratio. Undernutrition can limit economic growth by increasing the disease burden, leading to increased healthcare expenditures and more downtime due to illness.[5] For this reason, the first Millennium Development Goal (MDG) seeks to eradicate extreme poverty and hunger by the year 2015.[6] Achieving the other MDGs depends on a well-nourished global population.

Malnutrition remains critical, with almost one billion people undernourished globally.[7] The most vulnerable groups include women and children. This is partly because women of reproductive age must satisfy nutritional requirements not only for themselves, but also for their children, beginning from conception. Women are also likely to eat less when household food resources are insufficient, a coping mechanism to protect children. An undernourished mother is likely to deliver an undernourished child. Childhood vulnerability to malnutrition is also linked to dependence on adults to provide food and, during infancy, to feed them. Malnourished children are less likely to survive and grow and develop healthfully. They lack adequate nutritional capital needed for healthy and productive

living. In low-income settings, a high burden of infectious disease further limits opportunity for adequate nutrition.

The Importance of Diets in Health and Adequate Nutrition

Diet must be present in any discussion of nutrition. To support health, all individuals must consume adequate amounts of all essential nutrients. Current food production is sufficient to meet the nutrient needs of all seven billion humans, but nearly one billion individuals are **food insecure**. Poor access to optimal diets in developing countries has been widely reported.[8,9,10] Nutritional status and services in countries with high burdens of undernutrition often have inequities across education levels, wealth, and gender.

Suboptimal diets can be low in energy, or calories, and are also lacking in sufficient **essential nutrients** needed for health and well-being. These diets can result from poverty and the inability to afford sufficient, high-quality food. Limited food access can be worsened during periods of seasonal drought, floods, or other natural disasters. Additionally, the nonavailability of essential social services and infrastructure, such as transportation, communication, and markets, limits distribution of available agricultural produce to where it is needed. Furthermore, lack of security and the breakdown of infrastructure and services in conditions of civil strife may further limit access to food.

Plant-Based Diets and Nutrient Content

As in many African countries, Ghanaian diets are mainly plant-based. Such diets can be low in bioavailable essential nutrients and high in factors that inhibit nutrient absorption.[11] Some diets supply adequate energy but inadequate micronutrients. Young children are particularly susceptible to micronutrient deficiencies.

Sociocultural Factors and Nutrition

In developing nations, deeply rooted sociocultural factors strongly influence dietary choices. Cultural beliefs and practices may prohibit the consumption of healthy foods even when they are available. For example, feeding eggs to young children is taboo in some Ghanaian communities due to the belief that young children will learn to crave eggs and begin to steal eggs in the future.[12] Another harmful practice due to cultural beliefs is the discarding of **colostrum** because it is considered "unclean."[13] In some societies, adult males may receive food first and thus place children at higher risk for malnutrition. Understanding the cultural context is thus important for devising culturally sensitive dietary interventions.

> *Public Health Core Competency 4A: Cultural Competency Skills: Describes the dynamic forces that contribute to cultural diversity*

Ghanaian Diets: Availability, Access, and Quality

Ghana is a mostly tropical country with a traditionally agrarian economy. Except for a few imported food crops, such as rice and wheat flour, most typical foods in Ghanaian diets are indigenous and locally cultivated across the multiple ecological zones of the country (**Figure 11-1**). The many ethnic groups in Ghana display a diversity of food-related cultural practices. Although the Akans form the largest ethnic group in Ghana, members have many dialects and a variety of culinary methods and meals. As is true worldwide, food is part of cultural identity in Ghana. Traditional ethnic festivals, such as the annual "new yam" and *homowo* harvest celebrations, often demonstrate food diversity in Ghana. Additionally, food is central to many social events, including funerals, births, and marriages, in which food is served and exchanged as a sign of goodwill.

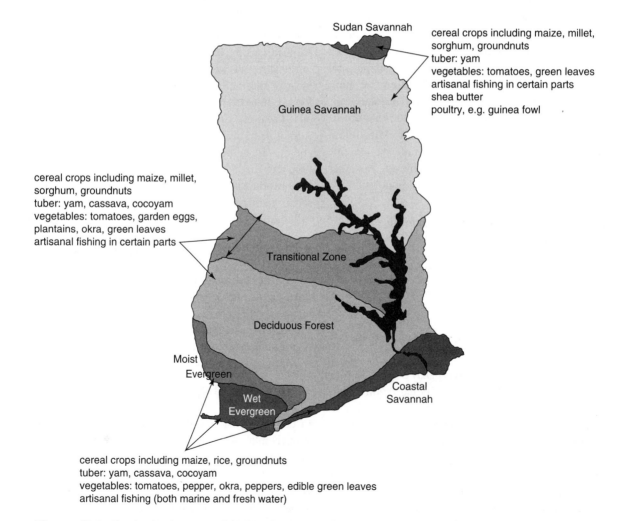

Figure 11-1 Ecological zones and the foods cultivated

Data from: Dixon, J. Gulliver, A., & Gibbon, D. (2001). Farming Systems and Poverty. Food and Agriculture Organization. Available at http://www.fao.org/docrep/003/Y1860E/y1860e00.htm. Accessed September 5, 2013.

Traditional Beliefs Versus Scientific Nutrition Knowledge

Traditional cultural definitions of an adequate diet do not always align with established scientific knowledge. The Akan adage that "any food that fills the tummy satisfies hunger" suggests an emphasis on quantity and not nutritional quality of food. The adage may explain why typical Ghanaian meals are focused on quantity while diet quality can be poor.

Commonly Consumed Foods in Ghana

Generally, the adult Ghanaian diet has a main energy-dense component served with either a soup or a stew.[14] Carbohydrates provide the majority of energy. Common sources in northern Ghana include yams, maize, millet, and black-eyed peas, while maize, cassava, yams, cocoyam, and plantains are main sources in southern Ghana.

Contributions of Animal-Source Foods

Stews and soups can be prepared with fish, beef, poultry, pork, chevon (goat), snails, or crabs, as available. Since animal-source foods (ASFs) have high nutrient density, the quantity of soup or stew and its ASF content are indicative of dietary quality. In Ghana, availability and economic access limit dietary ASF.[15] The diets of children in Ghana are covered later in the chapter.

Nutritional Concerns from Scarcity of Animal-Source Foods

This dietary pattern, featuring most calories coming from starchy carbohydrates and limited ASF, is characteristic of many developing regions worldwide. Nutritional concerns include inadequate protein consumption, low **bioavailability** of essential minerals, such as iron, and poor intake of other nutrients, such as vitamin A, due to monotonous diets and insufficient consumption of fresh fruits and vegetables. Within the same country, access to ASF and therefore diet quality can vary greatly.[16]

Population Food Insecurity and Undernourishment

Representatives at the 1996 World Food Summit of the Food and Agriculture Organization (FAO) defined food security and symbolized a stronger commitment toward eliminating malnutrition worldwide. However, many nations remain food insecure. At the national level, undernourishment, or hunger, is an indicator developed by the FAO used to describe food availability.[17] One way to measure undernourishment is to estimate the proportion of people in a population who lack availability to adequate dietary energy over a specified 12-month period.

Food Balance Sheets to Assess Undernourishment

A **food balance sheet** (FBS) can estimate national undernourishment. Over a 12-month period, the FBS records a nation's food sources, including food stocks/reserves, agricultural and livestock production, and total imports. Food lost to exports, industrial use, animal feed, and pest damage during storage is then subtracted. What remains is the food available for human consumption. This value is then compared with the total food energy required to meet the population's needs. A gap between food availability and requirements indicates undernourishment.

The first MDG is for all countries to halve their estimates of the proportion of undernourished persons by 2015. In 2010, Ghana became one of six African countries to attain this target, successfully reducing its undernourishment from 40.5% to below 5% by 2012.[18,19]

Household-Level Indicators of Food Insecurity

Food insecurity at the household level or among vulnerable groups can persist despite overall national reductions in undernourishment. Household-level indicators of food insecurity include economic and physical access indicators, such as the household dietary diversity score (HDDS), proportion of household income spent on food, and frequency of food consumption from nutrient-dense food groups.

Although hunger rates in Ghana dramatically decreased overall by 2012, wide inter-regional disparities were observed in household food insecurity, ranging from 1% to 34%. Generally, urban settings had less food insecurity. These estimates suggest the need for more targeted interventions to address household-level vulnerabilities that are not visible using FBS-driven estimates of food insecurity.

Nutritional Status of Women: Maternal Undernutrition

A woman's nutritional status reflects both her recent and historical nutrition experiences. Nutritional assessment considers both acute and chronic indicators.

Impaired Stature

Among adults, attained height or **stature** is an indicator of nutrition status.[20] Maternal short stature (less than 1.45 meters, or 57 inches) is associated with obstructed labor and the need for cesarean section, which is often unavailable in poor settings.[21] Globally, about 10% of women of reproductive age have a short stature. Ghanaian women of reproductive age have low prevalence of short stature: 1.5%,[22] compared with 13% in Sierra Leone, another nation in the sub-Saharan African region.

Underweight

Underweight, or **body mass index (BMI)** under 18.5 kg/m², can indicate acute or recent maternal undernutrition. BMI is particularly useful in public health assessments since it is rapid, noninvasive, and inexpensive. Maternal underweight increases the risk of **intrauterine growth restriction** and **low birth weight (LBW)**, which are risk factors for neonatal morbidity and stunting. Globally, 10–20% of women are underweight. In Ghana, 9% of women are underweight, with higher risk among those living in rural areas or in the three northern regions, or those who are below age 20.

Overweight and Obesity

In contrast, women with BMI of at least 25 kg/m² are considered overweight, and a BMI greater than or equal to 30 kg/m² indicates obesity. Obesity is a risk factor for many noncommunicable diseases as well as adverse **obstetric** outcomes, such as lower fertility, **gestational hypertension** and **diabetes**, **breech presentation** at delivery, and increased need for cesarean delivery.

The 2008 Demographic and Health Survey (DHS) estimates that 30% of Ghanaian women are overweight or obese, with rates up to 45% in the Greater Accra region. A separate study in this region found overweight prevalence exceeding 65%.[23] This finding is similar to findings of prevalence of 20–50% elsewhere in sub-Saharan Africa.[24] Notably, in sub-Saharan Africa, the transition to overweight status is occurring rapidly, especially among the poor and uneducated, and simultaneously high rates of underweight and overweight among women are also noteworthy.

Iron Deficiency

The most common nutrient deficiency in Ghana and the world, iron deficiency is especially severe in developing nations. Severe iron deficiency leads to anemia, which is commonly used as an indicator of iron deficiency. However, anemia lacks specificity as an indicator of iron deficiency, because possible causes, besides low dietary iron intake, include genetic disorders, malaria, parasitic worms, and other systemic or chronic infections, as well as deficiencies of other nutrients, such as vitamins A, B2, B12, C, and folate.[25] Iron deficiency is a significant cause of anemia in malaria-endemic settings like Ghana.[26]

Globally, an estimated 42% of pregnant women and 47% of preschool children are anemic.[27] Anemia contributes to 20% of maternal and perinatal **mortality** in developing countries. Anemia additionally limits childhood cognitive and learning abilities.

About 59% of women of reproductive age were anemic in 2008,[28] compared with 45% in 2003.[29] Prevalence is greater in rural communities.

Vitamin A Deficiency

Vitamin A is another micronutrient of concern among women, and requirements increase during pregnancy. Important for maintaining epithelial integrity, vision, regulation of gene expression, and normal performance of the immune system, vitamin A is also related to iron metabolism. Vitamin A deficiency impairs iron status in women. Furthermore, vitamin A content of breastmilk reflects maternal vitamin A status.

Due to high costs and technological needs of determining vitamin A status, only proxy indicators of dietary vitamin A and supplemental vitamin A coverage are used to monitor population vitamin A status in Ghana. Only 60% of mothers receive postpartum vitamin A supplements.[30]

Determinants of Maternal Malnutrition

Current and past factors contribute to perinatal malnutrition. Some influences of nutritional status are related to high fertility and childbearing, harmful cultural practices, poor education and illiteracy, and food insecurity.

Previous Malnutrition

Poor nutritional status early in life is a risk factor for maternal malnutrition; adult malnutrition can have fetal origins and may start with intrauterine growth restriction.[31] Without intervention during the first two years of life, children with low birth weight fail to reverse growth deficits, and may enter adolescence and adulthood with chronic undernutrition. Females are likely to enter pregnancy undernourished and transmit malnutrition to their offspring.

High Fertility Rates

Pregnancy increases requirements for energy and micronutrients, particularly iron, folate, and vitamin A. High fertility and inadequate birth spacing can deplete the nutrient reserves of women and also lead to malnourishment of their fetuses. Reducing fertility rates contributes to the achievement of the fifth Millennium Development Goal.

Millennium Development Goal 5: Improve Maternal Health

The global average fertility rate is 2.5 children per woman. Values are typically lower in industrialized nations and higher in developing nations. In 2009, the lifetime fertility of sub-Saharan African women was estimated at 5.4 children, down from 6.1 a decade earlier.[32] Excluding South Africa, which has a fertility rate of 2.3, the rate in Africa is 5.5. The value of four children per women in Ghana[33] is high compared with developed countries, and is associated with elevated risk of maternal morbidity and mortality.

Low Education

Low education is associated with poor nutrition outcomes. Conversely, poor nutrition limits educational potential and achievement. For these reasons, the premise of the second MDG is that universal primary education is a basic requirement for human development. In 2008, sub-Saharan Africa had the lowest net enrollment ratio in primary education, and also accounted for almost half of children worldwide who were out of school. In Ghana, the primary education net enrollment ratio is estimated at 95%.[34]

Millennium Development Goal 2: Achieve Universal Basic Education

High caregiver literacy is beneficial for child nutrition because it improves capacity to acquire and process child care information and to learn from their peers who exhibit healthful behaviors.[35] In the 2008 DHS in Ghana, childhood underweight prevalence was higher among the least educated women versus those with more education.[36] Interventions that improve maternal education can likely improve nutrition outcomes.

Food Insecurity

Although women are actively engaged in agriculture in Ghana and other sub-Saharan countries, they are often exposed to food insecurity due to their low empowerment status, unfair intra-household food distribution, and the willingness of women to forego meals in order to give more food to children during periods of food scarcity. In some ethnic groups, women eat meals only after men have been served, and in some Ghanaian communities, nutrient-rich ASFs are largely served to male household members.[37]

Infant and Young Child Nutrition

Childhood undernutrition remains a major public health challenge, especially in low-income settings. Among children under age 5, growth faltering indicates undernutrition. **Stunting** is low **height for age**, and is used to identify **chronic** undernutrition in children, just as for adults. **Wasting**, or low **weight for height**, is useful for identifying **acute** malnutrition. Underweight, or low **weight for age**, does not on its own differentiate between chronic and acute undernutrition. These anthropometric indicators are simple, noninvasive, and relatively inexpensive. Of the three indicators, underweight is typically used in screening programs, because it requires only measurement of weight.

Adequate nutritional status is important for early child survival and well-being. An estimated seven million children die annually of preventable causes; half of these deaths and 35% of the related disease burden are related to malnutrition. Further, childhood undernutrition contributes about 11% of disability adjusted life years (DALY). A DALY is an indicator of productive years lost to death, disability, or disease.

Global Status and Trends in Infant and Young Child Undernutrition

In 2012, the United Nations Children's Fund (UNICEF) State of the World's Children report indicated that 16% of children under age 5 were underweight,[38] but this global estimate conceals wide subregional disparities ranging from as low as 4% in the Latin America and Caribbean region to a high of 42% in South Asia. Nevertheless, sub-Saharan Africa and South Asia together have the highest burden of undernutrition. Between 1998 and 2012, underweight prevalence has declined from 30% to 19% in sub-Saharan Africa, but the decline in South Asia during the same period has declined only from 51% to 42%.

The prevalence of stunting is declining only slowly, and it remains unacceptably high in developing nations. Values are 15%, 23%, and 39% in Latin America and the Caribbean, Asia, and sub-Saharan Africa, respectively. Similar to underweight, stunting prevalence remains highest in both South Asia and sub-Saharan Africa. The majority of the 36 nations with the highest rates of stunting are in sub-Saharan Africa.[39]

In Ghana, stunting prevalence is still high, at 28% in 2008, compared with 34% in 1988. Underweight has declined more rapidly, from 23% to 14% in those two decades. Progress is slow given the numerous interventions that have been implemented, but Ghana is close to achieving the MDG target of halving underweight prevalence among under-5s.

A further challenge to nutritional status of Ghanaian children is the persistent high burden of LBW. Although the rate of 10% is comparable to the 8% rate in the United States, the survival rate in Ghana is lower. Since less than half of births are captured in vital statistics, many children do not have their birth weights recorded. As a result, the estimated LBW prevalence of 10% in Ghana may be low. The 2008 DHS reported that 15% of women believe their babies are smaller than average, at birth.[40] In sub-Saharan Africa, LBW is estimated at 13%, and in South Asia, the estimate is 27%.

In Ghana, as in many other developing countries, most childhood mortality results from exposure to infections and suboptimal diets. Vaccine-preventable diseases, malaria, and inadequate breastfeeding and complementary feeding are further barriers to adequate nourishment.[41] Improvements in the nutritional status of children in the past decade may partly be due to improved breastfeeding practices, increased prevalence of immunization, and expanded access to disease prevention and treatment services.

Concurrent Increases in Overnutrition Among Children Worldwide

Even as childhood undernutrition remains devastating, childhood overnutrition is an increasing public health threat. Overnutrition, leading to weight gain and obesity, increases the risk of diet-related noncommunicable diseases, such as diabetes mellitus, orthopedic and endocrine disorders, and cognitive and psychosocial deficits.[42] Globally, more than 170 million children under age 18 are overweight or obese, including 40 million under age 5.[43,44] Although low-income countries and rural areas continue to have lower prevalence of overweight, they have the fastest rates of increase. Across Africa, overweight among children under 5 was estimated at 8.5%,[45] including 17% in northern Africa and 10% in the remainder of Africa.

In 2008, under-5 overweight prevalence in Ghana was 5%, a dramatic increase from 1% in 1988.[46] Data among school-aged children are lacking, but preliminary results from a recent survey in urban Ghana suggest that overweight prevalence among school-age children and adolescents is increasing.

The rapid increase in childhood overweight and obesity is the result of changes in diet and physical activity.[47] There has been an increase in availability of and access to energy-dense foods that are often nonindigenous, processed, and imported.[48] Increased access to technology for transportation and leisure has allowed reduced energy expenditure. The underlying rapid urbanization and improving standard of living that are driving these diet and physical activity changes in developing countries are likely occurring at faster rates than was observed in industrialized countries. Comprehensive interventions incorporating prevention and management actions have therefore been recommended by the World Health Organization to address childhood overweight.[49]

Micronutrient Deficiency

Similar to their mothers, Ghanaian children younger than 5 have a high anemia rate of 78%,[50] which is far higher than the prevalence of 47% among preschool children globally and 68% in Africa.[51] Anemia and likely iron deficiency imply potential adverse impacts on physical and cognitive development, and indicate poor dietary quality and frequent infections. In Ghana, the 2008 DHS reported that only 27% of children reported having received iron supplements within the past seven days, partly because iron supplementation is not a routine intervention for addressing anemia in Ghana.

Vitamin A deficiency in children is also a major global public health challenge, particularly in low-income settings. Night blindness is an outcome of vitamin A deficiency exhibited by 2% of children in Africa (2.5 million).[52] With coverage for postnatal vitamin A supplementation remaining below 60%, large-scale interventions to address micronutrient malnutrition are urgently needed in Ghana.

Infant and Young Child Feeding

Adequate and appropriate child feeding is essential for preventing and controlling **malnutrition**. Children whose diets are suboptimal are at increased risk for growth retardation, micronutrient malnutrition, and vulnerability to infections. In low-income settings like Ghana, poor feeding practices and inadequate dietary quality and quantity deprive children of the nutrients needed to ensure a well-functioning immune system and to grow. As a result, children are exposed to repeated episodes of infectious diseases, which further depletes their nutrient stores and retards growth.

WHO Recommendations for Infant and Young Child Feeding

The World Health Organization's Global Strategy for Infant and Young Child Feeding[53] promotes initiation of exclusive breastfeeding as soon as possible after birth and continuation throughout the first 6 months of life. With the exception of medicines and micronutrient supplements prescribed by

a qualified healthcare practitioner, no other food or fluid, including water, is recommended for six months.

Ghana's endorsement of the WHO recommendations is evident in the National Strategy Document on infant and young child feeding[54] and the national policy on breastfeeding. Further, in 2000, the Parliament of Ghana passed the Breastfeeding Promotion Regulations (Legislative Instrument 1667). This law supports breastfeeding as the appropriate feeding practice for young children and is designed to prevent and control inappropriate marketing and promotion of breastmilk substitutes.

Complementary Foods

Once an infant is 6 months old, appropriate **complementary** foods should be gradually introduced while continuing to breastfeed until the child is 24 months. During this period of complementary feeding, breastfeeding should continue because breastmilk continues to provide important immune-active components.

Infant Feeding in Ghana

Breastfeeding is a culturally accepted norm in Ghana, and nearly all children receive at least some breastmilk (**Figure 11-2**). Ghanaian children are breastfed for a

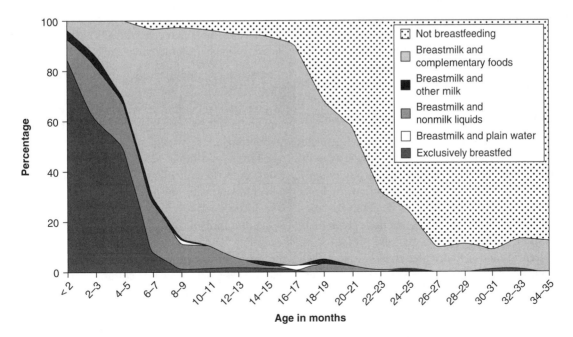

Figure 11-2 Infant feeding practices by age in Ghana

Reproduced from Ghana Statistical Service, G., Ghana Health Services, G., & ICF Macro. (2009). *Ghana Demographic and Health Survey 2008*. Accra: GSS, GHS, ICF Macro.

median of 20 months. Exclusive breastfeeding, however, was rare until the 1990s. The current exclusive breastfeeding rate of 63% is thus a dramatic improvement over the rate of 2% in 1988.[55]

Despite this improvement, breastfeeding practices are far from optimal. The current median duration of exclusive breastfeeding is 3.2 months, indicating that many children start receiving other foods and fluids much earlier than the recommended sixth month. In sub-Saharan Africa, a wide range of exclusive breastfeeding duration has been observed in recent years, ranging from a low of 0.5 months in Nigeria to 5.4 months in Rwanda. Reasons given for early cessation of exclusive breastfeeding include caregiver perception of child thirst, inadequacy of breastmilk, social influence, and inappropriate marketing of commercial complementary foods.[56]

The timing of breastfeeding initiation is an important marker of adequate child feeding. Currently, only an estimated 52% of infants start breastfeeding within the first hour of birth.[57] Thus, nearly half of mothers delay **initiation**. Reasons given include lack of infant crying for milk and the infant or mother needing to rest.[58] Conversely, 27% of children 6 to 9 months had delayed introduction of complementary feeding, increasing risk of undernutrition and weakening of the immune system.

Among 18% of children, a **prelacteal** feed is given during the first few hours before breastmilk is introduced.[59] This practice is fueled by the belief among some groups in Ghana that colostrum is "unclean" and thus discarded, although it is a nutritious substance. In these cases, children are fed with a variety of fluids, including coconut juice, water mixed with sucrose, or just plain water. This practice can expose children to infections, especially where water quality is uncertain.

Ensuring adequacy of complementary feeding is a major challenge. Local recommendations are to provide a diverse diet with foods from a minimum of three food groups daily; to include ASF, vitamin A–rich foods, and fats and oils; to breastfeed on demand and to provide complementary foods three or more times daily. Meeting these recommendations is more challenging than exclusive breastfeeding. First, children in food-insecure households are less likely to be fed nutritionally adequate diets. Second, caregivers, especially those caring for their first children, need to learn how to prepare nutritionally adequate diets, when and how often to feed, and how to deal with feeding challenges, such as food rejection by the child, or preference for only one type of food.

Typically, the first complementary food for Ghanaian children is a fermented high-carbohydrate maize porridge called *koko*. Because *koko* provides sufficient energy but has low micronutrient density, children fed on *koko* can develop deficiencies of multiple micronutrients, including iron, calcium, zinc, riboflavin, and niacin.[60] The 2008 DHS shows that among children between 6 and 23 months, about 85% are fed grain-based liquids.[61] Only 36% of children were fed appropriately based on complementary feeding recommendations.

Additionally, Ghana does not support the use of a bottle with nipple for feeding children. However, about 13% of children were reported to be fed with a bottle in 2008.[62] Bottle feeding increases the risk of transmitting infectious pathogens to the child because bottles are more difficult to keep clean and sterilized compared with cups and spoons.

Public- and Private-Sector Actions to Address Maternal and Childhood Malnutrition

Addressing malnutrition requires understanding of the multiple factors that affect the nutritional status of women and children and how these factors interact with each other. In 1990, UNICEF proposed a framework for mapping the determinants of malnutrition.[63] This framework categorized malnutrition determinants into three hierarchical levels: immediate, underlying, and basic (**Figure 11-3**).

Inadequate quality and quantity of diets, diseases, and their interactions constitute immediate determinants, whose frequency and severity are affected by underlying determinants, such as household food insecurity, suboptimal care, inadequate access to health care, water, sanitation, and other social services. Poverty, especially, contributes to immediate determinants of malnutrition, which, along with infectious diseases, is more evident in low-income settings. Basic determinants affecting underlying and immediate determinants are the sociopolitical, economic, and institutional arrangements that directly or indirectly influence access to livelihood resources and services. These factors include cultural and traditional practices, leadership arrangements, policies, and technologies that affect communities' access to services and resources needed for optimum nutrition. Understanding the profile of determinants allows development of appropriate nutrition interventions.

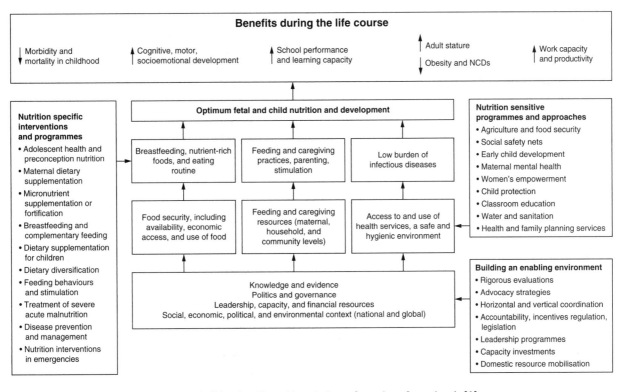

Benefits during the life course

| Morbidity and mortality in childhood | Cognitive, motor, socioemotional development | School performance and learning capacity | Adult stature / Obesity and NCDs | Work capacity and productivity |

Optimum fetal and child nutrition and development

Nutrition specific interventions and programmes
- Adolescent health and preconception nutrition
- Maternal dietary supplementation
- Micronutrient supplementation or fortification
- Breastfeeding and complementary feeding
- Dietary supplementation for children
- Dietary diversification
- Feeding behaviours and stimulation
- Treatment of severe acute malnutrition
- Disease prevention and management
- Nutrition interventions in emergencies

Breastfeeding, nutrient-rich foods, and eating routine

Feeding and caregiving practices, parenting, stimulation

Low burden of infectious diseases

Food security, including availability, economic access, and use of food

Feeding and caregiving resources (maternal, household, and community levels)

Access to and use of health services, a safe and hygienic environment

Knowledge and evidence
Politics and governance
Leadership, capacity, and financial resources
Social, economic, political, and environmental context (national and global)

Nutrition sensitive programmes and approaches
- Agriculture and food security
- Social safety nets
- Early child development
- Maternal mental health
- Women's empowerment
- Child protection
- Classroom education
- Water and sanitation
- Health and family planning services

Building an enabling environment
- Rigorous evaluations
- Advocacy strategies
- Horizontal and vertical coordination
- Accountability, incentives regulation, legislation
- Leadership programmes
- Capacity investments
- Domestic resource mobilisation

Figure 11-3 UNICEF framework illustrating the determinants of malnutrition

Reproduced from the 2013 Lancet Maternal and Child Nutrition Series (Executive Summary). Available at http://download.thelancet.com/flatcontentassets/pdfs/nutrition-eng.pdf. Accessed August 12, 2013.

Nutrition-Specific and Nutrition-Sensitive Interventions

Based on this framework, population nutrition interventions can be categorized into nutrition-specific and nutrition-sensitive. Nutrition-specific, or direct, interventions address immediate determinants of malnutrition. Dietary interventions seek to improve micronutrient status, promote optimal dietary practices, and ensure access to quality health services and treatment for malnutrition. Interventions are coordinated by public health specialists with training in nutrition, dietetics, nursing, medicine, and related backgrounds. Leadership comes from health and nutrition departments.

Nutrition-sensitive, or indirect, interventions complement direct interventions by addressing underlying and basic determinants of undernutrition, and include strategies to improve food security, water and sanitation, social protection and mitigation of vulnerability, education and empowerment, advocacy and civil action, and family planning. Nutrition-sensitive interventions are not specifically designed to improve nutrition, but their successful implementation has measurable and sustainable benefits for nutrition. Indirect interventions often span multiple public and private sectors, including education, health, transport, agriculture, finance and trade, business, and civil society. Various sector activities must be coordinated to maximize benefits for nutrition.

Successful implementation of these strategies recognizes the unique nutrition needs across the life cycle and addresses the needs of the highest-risk groups, including women of reproductive age, infants, and children under 5.

Assessment of Nutritional Risk and Need

Needs assessment helps identify the risks for malnutrition across the levels of determinants for malnutrition to help develop the appropriate mix of interventions that maximizes outcomes for the most vulnerable in a population. In Ghana, nutrition status evidence is obtained mainly from the DHS, other nationally representative surveys, and program data generated and reported routinely by the Ghana

Health Service. Nutrition surveys constitute a useful part of a broader surveillance system to identify vulnerability. Information obtained from needs assessment is then used to design appropriate strategies to address challenges at different causal levels and among identified vulnerable groups. The successes of these interventions are then routinely monitored and also evaluated at specified periods to assess impact against set targets.

In 2008, the *Lancet* published a series on undernutrition that identified 11 evidence-based nutrition-specific interventions with potential for reducing chronic malnutrition in the world's 36 high-burden countries, including Ghana (**Table 11-1**).[64] These interventions are available and implemented in many of the 36 high-burden countries, but the scale of implementation remains low.[65,66]

A recent landscape analysis of nutrition in Ghana identified several interventions already in place:

- *Government-endorsed policies:* Policies address infant and young child feeding, food security and agriculture, micronutrient malnutrition, growth promotion, safe motherhood, and child health and protection.

- *Regulations and laws:* Parliament supports mass fortification of salt, cooking oil, and wheat flour; breastfeeding and marketing of breastmilk substitutes; and labeling, promotion, and distribution of food products.

- *Public health programs and projects:* These include good manufacturing procedures (GMP), integrated management of neonatal and childhood illness (IMNCI), infant and young child feeding (IYCF), food fortification, and programs listed in Table 11-1. Micronutrient powders and lipid-based dietary supplementation are also being tested for efficacy. Community-based management of acute malnutrition using supplementary feeding is being piloted in selected regions in Ghana among children with SAM, and among individuals with HIV or receiving tuberculosis treatment.

These interventions are challenged, however, by institutional arrangements and leadership issues, including:

1. The low priority that nutrition has on the development agenda. Currently, nutrition remains underfunded. At the district and community levels, scarce

Table 11-1 Nutrition-specific and nutrition-sensitive interventions by vulnerability group

Category of Vulnerable Group	Nutrition-Specific	Nutrition-Sensitive
Children	Behavior change communication promoting exclusive breastfeeding, complementary feeding, as part of growth monitoring and promotion	Integrated management of childhood and neonatal illnesses
	Vitamin A supplementation after six months	Zinc supplements for diarrhea treatment
	School feeding targeted at children living in poor communities	Kangaroo mother care
Women of reproductive age	Iron and folic acid supplementation	Malaria prevention and control strategies: intermittent preventive treatment for malaria (IPT), bed net use promotion
	Postnatal vitamin A supplementation	Focused antenatal care
		Family planning interventions to limit and space births
All vulnerable groups	Universal iodization of salt for human and animal consumption	Unconditional cash transfers: Livelihood Empowerment Assistance Program (LEAP)
	Mass/mandatory multiple micronutrient fortification of vegetable cooking oil and wheat flour	Deworming of schoolchildren
	Dietary diversification	Insecticide-treated bed nets promotion
		Handwashing with soap and hygiene promotion
		Home gardening

Data from: Bhutta et al. (2008). What works? Interventions for maternal and child undernutrition and survival. *Lancet, 371*, 417-440.

health budgets are allocated in favor of infectious disease programming, leaving little for nutrition actions.

2. Inadequate cross-sector coordination and collaboration at the national and subnational levels and lack of an intersectoral/interministerial body coordinating nutrition actions. This leads to weak integration of agencies that are implementing interventions.

3. Inadequate human resource numbers, quality, and distribution, especially at the subnational levels, limit effective implementation of nutrition interventions.

4. Inadequate civil society participation in nutrition advocacy, policy formulation, and implementation. This creates a situation lacking fulfillment of a "watchdog" role to hold relevant public and private institutions accountable.

In addition to government entities providing nutrition services in Ghana are many civil society (CS) partners and United Nations agencies, including UNICEF, WHO, the World Food Programme (WFP), the United States Agency for International Development (USAID), PLAN, CARE, World Vision, and the Adventist Development and Relief Agency (ADRA). Their direct and indirect interventions are often in collaboration with public health services and are based on the respective areas of focus and expertise.

The capacity of sub-Saharan African countries to deploy nutrition interventions depends on their policies and available resources. For example, in 2008, the WHO-commissioned landscape analysis of country readiness to scale up nutrition interventions found that Burkina Faso has strong political commitment to nutrition, as indicated by existing governance structure, policies and strategies, and resources for nutrition programming. However, the commitment has not been successfully translated into action, as key interventions have not been scaled up throughout the country. The interventions that have not been scaled up everywhere in the country include treatment of severe acute malnutrition, behavior change communication, and availability of well-trained staff. Burkina Faso's lower income in comparison to Ghana may be a factor.

Emerging Perspectives on Maternal and Childhood Nutrition

The 2008 *Lancet* series mentioned above renewed global attention to maternal and childhood undernutrition.

In 2010, Ghana was among 21 nations that committed to scaling up proven nutrition interventions to all vulnerable groups. As a result, national and local institutional, policy, and programmatic rearrangements are being implemented. Expansion of both nutrition-specific and nutrition-sensitive interventions using both public and private resources and partnerships is key. Additionally, the private sector is developing new food products and technologies to reduce undernutrition. The potential for these interventions to be effective is demonstrated; what remains unknown is their effect on long-term nutritional status, especially with the emerging burden of overnutrition.

Nutrition of Women and Children in the Context of HIV and AIDS

The chapter's opening quote from a rural Ghanaian woman underscores the relevance of nutrition in HIV. Attempts to reduce maternal and child malnutrition must acknowledge that nutritional concerns among women and children in resource-poor settings are complex and sometimes confounded by the high burden of infectious diseases. HIV in particular affects nutrition and food insecurity, infant and young child feeding, and the immune status of the infected. HIV also affects close relatives and family.

HIV and AIDS

The **human immunodeficiency virus (HIV)** was identified as the cause of **acquired immune deficiency syndrome (AIDS)** in 1984. It is a type of *lentivirus*, or "slow virus," which causes disease progression very slowly. HIV causes AIDS by progressively damaging blood cells called CD4+ T lymphocytes, or T-cells, which are infection-fighting and vital components of the **immune system**. The development of AIDS for HIV-positive individuals at least 13 years old is defined as having T-cell count below a specified level, usually less than 200 cells/μL, or a CD4+ T-lymphocyte percentage of total lymphocytes of less than 14% plus one of several AIDS-defining clinical conditions. Different definitions exist for children younger than 13 years and those younger than 18 months.[67] This low T-lymphocyte count severely compromises the immune system, and the patient has difficulty fighting infections that would ordinarily be overcome, leading to **opportunistic infections**. Other factors, such as malnutrition, can also cause immune deficiency and opportunistic infections.

During the early days of the HIV epidemic, most HIV infections progressed to AIDS in a few years, and opportunistic infections, such as pneumonia and tuberculosis, could quickly cause death. Antiretroviral therapy (ART) and maintenance of optimal nutritional status can now help persons infected with HIV live for decades. While current medications can dramatically improve the health of people living with HIV (PLHIV) and delay the progression from HIV infection to AIDS, a vaccine for HIV or cure for AIDS does not exist.

Global Prevalence of HIV/AIDS

By 2012, over 34 million people worldwide were living with HIV, with 70% in sub-Saharan Africa, including 91% of infected children.[68] In Ghana, nearly one-quarter million are infected, including 30,439 children.[69] This translates into 1% of the population. The annual HIV sentinel surveillance among pregnant women suggests a downward trend in HIV prevalence in Ghana, declining from 3.6% in 2003 to 2.0% in 2010.[70] Ghana's response to the HIV epidemic has been focused on three thematic areas: prevention, treatment care and support, and mitigation of the socioeconomic effects of HIV. Life-saving therapy is still beyond the reach of many PLHIV in Ghana due to chronic shortages and inaccessibility of medications. Therefore, complementary approaches for improving the health of HIV-infected persons are needed. Optimal nutrition is one such strategy, but food and nutrition assistance to PLHIV in Ghana is inadequate. The sole documented food and nutrition assistance program, under Opportunities Industrialization Centers International (OICI) and Catholic Relief Services (CRS), covered an insignificant proportion of those in need and was terminated due to lack of funding.

Impact of the Epidemic on Women and Children

HIV disproportionately impacts females, as confirmed by morbidity and mortality statistics. This is particularly true in resource-poor settings such as Ghana, where infection rates among young women are twice as high as among men of the same age. Women account for 58% of all people living with HIV in sub-Saharan Africa, and over 60% of young people living with HIV worldwide are young women.[71]

HIV and Mortality

HIV is the leading cause of death of women of reproductive age, causing 60,000 maternal deaths in 2008.[72] This extra risk in maternal deaths attributed to HIV is sometimes referred to as **attributable risk (AR)** or **population attributable risk (PAR)**. HIV also impacts children, with 3.4 million children younger than 15 years living with HIV in 2011. About 330,000 children were new cases of HIV, and an estimated 230,000 children died of AIDS-related illnesses in 2011.[73] The estimated annual AIDS-related child mortality in Ghana for the years 2010 and 2011 were 2,472 and 2,080, respectively.[74]

Vertical transmission, or perinatal transmission of the virus, is another concern in low-resource settings. Possible modes of vertical transmission include during pregnancy (prepartum), during labor or the birthing process (intrapartum), and via breastfeeding (postpartum). Also referred to as mother-to-child transmission (MTCT) of HIV, its rates in the absence of interventions (as is the case in most parts of the developing world) are 5–10% prepartum, 10–20% intrapartum, and 5–20% from breastfeeding.[75] It is important to note that in many respects, the impacts of HIV on women and children in resource-poor settings differ from those of their counterparts in the developed world. While the overall MTCT rate for Ghana in 2011 was estimated to be 9%,[76] rates of prenatal transmission in the United States and other developed economies are less than 2%.[77,78] This feat is attributed to widespread availability of and access to ART and elective cesarean section procedures, among other interventions.

Women are biologically more vulnerable to risk of heterosexual transmission of HIV than men,[79] but their vulnerability, particularly in resource-poor settings, is compounded by socioeconomic and sociocultural factors. In Ghana, just as in other developing nations, traditional and ingrained gender injustices exacerbate the disproportionate impact of this socioeconomic burden on women. Women, the default caregivers of the family, care for family members who are ill as well as those orphaned by AIDS. These caregiving roles sometimes make women altruistically institute certain coping strategies. Studies have demonstrated that such strategies, which include transactional sex, are often negative, undesired, unsustainable, and irreversible.[80,81] A recent survey involving a nationally representative sample of 1,745 HIV-affected households in Ghana gives an idea of the prevalence of some of these coping strategies. Sixty percent of households reported either limiting portion sizes of their meals or reducing the number of meals per day, and 30% borrowed food from friends and relatives.[82]

Breastfeeding is another caregiver role of women in Ghana. While impacts of breastfeeding on infant HIV appear relatively minimal, the impact on the HIV-positive mother is still unclear. Some studies suggest that HIV-positive mothers are exposed to an increased risk of adverse conditions when they breastfeed,[83,84] but a more recent systematic review does not support this.[85] Most of the studies reviewed attributed maternal morbidity and mortality to high levels of plasma HIV viral load.

Nutrition and HIV

Knowledge is increasing regarding the complex relationship between individual, household, and community-level factors and HIV and nutrition. Individual factors include inherent metabolic changes and gastrointestinal disorders,[86] effects of various opportunistic infections,[87] side effects of medications, and the effect of the virus itself. Household factors are related to household attributes such as poverty and food unavailability.[88] Community-level factors relate to sociopolitical, religious, cultural, and structural factors.[89,90]

Effect of HIV on Nutritional Status and Food Security

The impacts of HIV infection on the overall **nutritional status** of infected persons were characterized within the first decade of the emergence of the HIV epidemic, although recognition of the impacts on household food insecurity was slower.[91,92,93] HIV affects nutrition in at least four major ways, including increased nutrient needs, reduction in dietary intake, nutrient malabsorption, and metabolic alterations.

Increased Energy and Protein Requirements

As with other infections, HIV increases **metabolic rate** as the body struggles to maintain optimal immune function and repair damaged cells.[94,95,96,97] HIV medications also increase **resting energy expenditure** independent of viral load.[98] Among asymptomatic HIV-infected persons, needs increase by 10–15% for energy and up to 50% for protein,[99] or about an additional 300 calories and 25 grams of protein per day. Frequent snacking and consuming an extra daily meal can meet this extra need, but food intake is often reduced among HIV-infected patients.

Reductions in Food Intake

Multiple pathways explain reduction in food intake associated with HIV. Painful sores in the mouth and/or esophagus, fatigue, depression, and changes in mental state are common effects of the infection that can make eating more difficult. Nutrient deficiencies due to

HIV infection can also reduce appetite and interest in food. Additional reasons for suboptimal dietary intake include the side effects of disease-management medications; these can include nausea, vomiting, diarrhea, and abdominal cramps. A recent Ghanaian study revealed high prevalence of inadequate dietary intake among HIV-positive pregnant women with nausea, vomiting, and oral lesions.[100] Food insecurity related to HIV can also reduce food intake.

Nutrient Malabsorption

HIV's association with micronutrient deficiencies[101,102,103] is partly attributed to malabsorption. HIV infection reduces the efficiency of nutrient absorption and utilization partly because of the frequent diarrhea occasioned by compromised immunity. This may be due to increased intestinal permeability and other gut defects that occur in both symptomatic and asymptomatic stages of the infection.[104] A fundamental tenet in nutrition is that malabsorption of some nutrients can impact the absorption of others. For instance, lipid malabsorption can seriously affect the absorption and utilization of lipid-soluble vitamins.

Metabolic Alterations

Changes in metabolism among HIV-infected individuals result from severely reduced food intake and the immune response to HIV infection.[105,106] It is established in nutritional immunology that the body releases pro-oxidant **cytokines** in response to invading pathogens. The ensuing reactions result in increased utilization of **antioxidant nutrients**, such as zinc, selenium, and vitamins A, E, and C. **Oxidative stress** occurs when there is an imbalance between pro-oxidants and antioxidants,[107] resulting in damage to cells, proteins, and enzymes.[108] Other HIV-related metabolic changes include changes in the levels of the hormones insulin and glucagon. This can result in both reduced food intake and an immune response to infection, and can ultimately lead to muscle wasting.

HIV and Household Food Insecurity

Food insecurity is present among the general Ghanaian population,[109] and is more severe among HIV-affected households. A national survey found that 16% of HIV-affected Ghanaian households were food insecure.[110] In addition to its effects on the metabolism, ingestion, and digestion of food, HIV infection can disrupt livelihoods. HIV-infected persons may lose the ability to work and generate income, leading to food insecurity. The dynamics

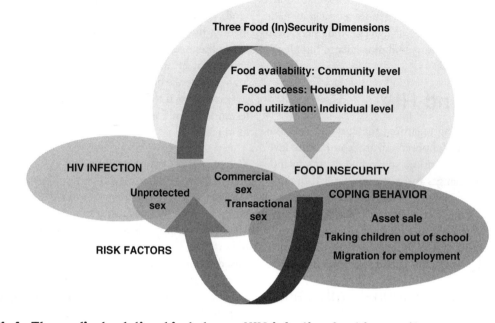

Figure 11-4 The cyclical relationship between HIV infection food insecurity

Reproduced from the World Food Programme Executive Board. (2010). Second Regular Session Rome, 8–11 November 2010 Policy issues. Agenda item 4 WFP HIV and AIDS policy. Available at http://one.wfp.org/eb/docs/2010/wfp225092~1.pdf. Accessed August 28, 2013.

that link HIV to food insecurity are complex and cyclical (**Figure 11-4**). The recognition of these casual pathways informed the recent description of the marriage of HIV and food insecurity or malnutrition in resource-poor settings as a syndemic.[111]

Effect of Malnutrition on HIV

Preexisting malnutrition weakens the immune system and exacerbates the effects of HIV. The clinical outcome of HIV is poorer in individuals with compromised nutritional status.[112] The immune system requires micronutrients, such as selenium, zinc, and vitamins A, B12, and E, to fight infections, and deficiencies thus tilt the outcome of this fight in favor of the virus. Increased oxidative stress resulting from poorer nutrient status can increase the rate of HIV replication,[113] leading to higher viral load and a weaker immune system due to faster destruction of CD4+ T lymphocytes. The progression of HIV disease from asymptomatic to symptomatic to fatal among malnourished individuals is therefore expected to be faster.

While optimal nutrition cannot prevent HIV infection, it can delay AIDS by delaying the progression from asymptomatic HIV to symptomatic AIDS. Good nutrition does this by reducing vulnerability to weight loss and wasting,

improving the effectiveness of, and adherence to, HIV medications, and enhancing the body's ability to fight opportunistic illnesses. Drawing on the current concept of **treatment as prevention**, whereby use of AIDS medications is an effective HIV prevention tool based on ART's ability to reduce community viral load, the same logic is applied to optimization of nutritional status.

Nutrition Issues of Women and Children Infected or Affected by HIV

Specific groups of HIV-infected people, such as women, men, the elderly, children, treatment-naive, and treatment-exposed, have their unique nutrition-related issues. Examined here are nutritional concerns in HIV-infected women and their infants.

Macronutrient and Micronutrient Needs

Based on pre-ART evidence, WHO in 2003 indicated that in asymptomatic HIV-infected adults and asymptomatic children, a 10% increase in energy requirements is warranted to remain physically active and to maintain body weight. In the symptomatic or advanced phase of HIV, the energy requirement is increased by 20–30%. For children who lose weight, energy needs increase by 50–100% above normal.[114]

No conclusive evidence currently supports specific protein or lipid requirements in HIV-infected persons. However, it is generally advised that protein should provide at least 10% of total energy intake. HIV-positive persons are advised to eat twice the **recommended dietary allowance (RDA)** for protein, or about 1.0–1.5 grams of protein per day per kilogram of body weight. The rule of thumb is to eat five to six 1-ounce (30-gram) servings of high-protein foods per day, plus two high-protein snacks. Sources may include meat, fish, poultry, eggs, dairy, and beans.

Maintaining adequate intake of micronutrients is also essential. In addition to being in dietary sources, micronutrients can be obtained from supplements. Useful details are given in the Food and Nutrition Technical Assistance program (FANTA) Technical Notes of 2004.[115]

Nutrition Issues in Pregnant Women Infected with HIV

Studies in animal models show that nutrient deficiencies during pregnancy affect the immune function of the next generation.[116] This may be explained by **immunosenescence**, or premature deterioration of the immune system of the nutrient-deficient immune function of a nutrient-deficient fetus. Immunosenescence in HIV is not well characterized; a review on the subject concluded that accelerated immunosenescence in HIV is associated with increased morbidity and mortality, but called for more investigation into its causes, diagnosis, and treatment.[117]

Independent of HIV status, maternal requirements for protein, folate, niacin, zinc, iron, and iodine during pregnancy are 30–50% higher than before pregnancy.[118] At present, dietary recommendations and nutrition counseling for pregnant women with HIV are similar to those for the general population.[119] Benefits of micronutrient supplementation in pregnant women with HIV include protection against adverse pregnancy outcomes.[120,121] Vitamin A supplementation, for example, is associated with significantly improved birth weight,[122] although it must be noted that hypervitaminosis, or vitamin A toxicity, can occur with intakes exceeding allowable limits. Excessive use of vitamin A supplements shortly before and during pregnancy can harm fetuses.

Feeding Options for Infants Born to HIV-Positive Women

A critical nutrition concern in HIV is what and how to feed the infant. Breastfeeding is generally recommended for infant feeding, but the recognition that HIV is transmissible through breastfeeding[123] precipitated a public health dilemma. That is, should HIV-positive mothers breastfeed, thus providing an optimally nutritious diet, or formula feed, thus avoiding the risk of HIV transmission from the mother? This question has led to heated debates.[124,125,126] The question in resource-limited settings is whether the nutritional, health, and economic benefits of breastfeeding outweigh the risk of postnatal transmission of the virus. The postnatal HIV transmission rate is estimated to be 15–20% for prolonged breastfeeding.[127,128] Feeding with infant formula instead eliminates risk of postnatal HIV transmission, but significantly increases risks of mortality and morbidity due to common childhood diseases.[129,130] The 2011 global estimate of the under-5 mortality rate is 51.4 per 1,000, while the estimate for Africa is 106.5 per 1,000.[131] The factors implicated in over half of the deaths in Africa include malnutrition and diarrheal-related infections. Given that formula feeding increases the risk of those infectious morbidities, a careful balancing act is required when making decisions as to what to feed the infant. In South Africa, cumulative three-month mortality in exclusively breastfed infants was 6.1% versus 15.1% in infants given replacement feeds.[132] A study among infants born to Ugandan HIV-positive mothers found that the cumulative 12-month probability of infant mortality was 18% among the formula-fed compared with 3% among the breastfed infants.[133] In the late 1990s, WHO and other UN agencies developed consensus declarations and guidelines that metamorphosed into recommendations and have since been revised multiple times. Revisions from 2010 were motivated by evidence that when antiretroviral drugs are administered during pregnancy and postnatally, the risk of vertical transmission is significantly reduced even with breastfeeding.[134,135] Thus, current guidelines state that "when replacement feeding is acceptable, feasible, affordable, sustainable, and safe (AFASS), as is said to be in the developed world, avoidance of all breastfeeding by HIV-infected mothers is recommended; otherwise, as is likely in resource-limited settings, exclusive breastfeeding is recommended during the first 6 months of life with antepartum and postnatal ARV prophylaxis or treatments given where available."[136] The pediatric HIV epidemic has been nearly eliminated in the United States and Europe (**Figure 11-5**).[137,138]

Based on these encouraging results, in 2009, HIV prevention and treatment organizations emphasized a new goal of "virtual elimination" of pediatric HIV infection, defined as the reduction of MTCT to less than 5%.[139]

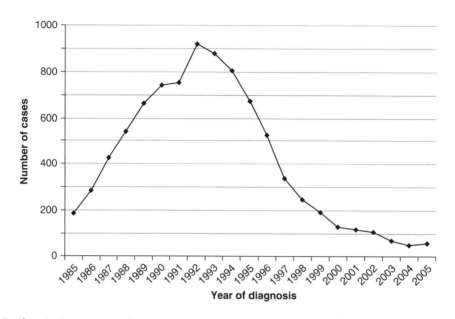

Figure 11-5 Estimated number of cases of perinatally acquired AIDS by year of diagnosis–United States, 1985-2005

Reproduced from: Branson, B.M. (n.d.). Revised recommendations for HIV screening of adults, adolescents, and pregnant women in health care settings. Centers for Disease Control and Prevention. *MMWR* 2006; vol 55: no 21. Retrieved from http://www.cdc.gov/hiv/topics/perinatal/pdf/Perinatal_Graph_2.pdfhttp://www.cdc.gov/hiv/topics/perinatal/pdf/Perinatal_Graph_2.pdf

Aside from death and perinatal transmission of HIV, HIV may impact the growth of HIV-infected as well as HIV-exposed but uninfected children. Evidence made available since 2006 show that infants born to HIV-positive mothers are likely to be malnourished.[140,141,142] This thus calls for the use of "disease-free survival," rather than simply HIV-exposed but uninfected, as a measure of success for pediatric HIV.

In a longitudinal study, researchers from the University of Ghana showed that maternal HIV is associated with reduced infant growth in weight and length throughout the first year of life.[143] A related study in Kenya found similar results and further reported a slower rate of decline in length growth during the two-year follow-up in formula-fed infants compared with breastfed infants.[144] The researchers surmised that the micronutrient or macronutrient content of infant formula might be responsible for this observation. In fact, in 2008, Agnes Binagwaho, drawing on anecdotal evidence from Rwanda, argued against universally decreeing that HIV-infected mothers and their infants in resource-poor settings are better off with breastfeeding.[145]

While the time may not be ripe to challenge the orthodoxy of HIV and infant feeding in most resource-poor settings, which favors breastfeeding, that which is long overdue is enabling health workers to effectively implement these guidelines. As observed in the Rwandan study[146] and

confirmed by a Ghanaian study,[147] some health workers fail to provide information to mothers about replacement feeding options and authoritatively prescribe breastfeeding to these mothers. And yet, the right to choose is a fundamental human right. Parents and caregivers everywhere should be permitted to choose what to feed their infant; freedom of choice is the sine qua non of informed consent.

Conclusion

Despite the plethora of scholarship on the essential role that nutrition plays in HIV, necessary actions on this evidence, particularly in resource-poor settings, are weak but urgently needed. Some of these actions, which could be taken through public–private partnerships, are identified below.

Nutrition-Specific and Nutrition-Sensitive Interventions

Governments in resource-poor settings (such as Ghana) need to integrate both nutrition-specific and nutrition-sensitive interventions into their programming. Nutrition-sensitive approaches, such as improvement of community water and sanitation, using poverty reduction strategies, and social protection policies to sustain livelihoods, could be integrated into approaches that seek to improve food security and nutrition of HIV-affected persons. Ghana's Livelihood Empowerment Against Poverty (LEAP) program could be expanded to cover particularly food-insecure PLHIV or female-headed households.

Planning and implementation of such programs should encourage cross-sector civil society engagement and PLHIV playing relevant roles. Developing relevant policies on food and nutrition that recognize the role of nutrition in HIV prevention is essential. For all PLHIV, and for those on ART in particular, providing food support can increase compliance with treatment in instances where a lack of food is contributing to nonadherence. In addition, the ministries of health of developing world countries should ensure that health workers receive appropriate training on HIV and infant feeding.

International Support

Governments of the developed world, United Nations agencies, development partners, and other multilaterals must demonstrate continued support for HIV programming that integrates nutrition, food security, livelihood support, improvement in general health literacy, as well as capacity of healthcare providers. Civil society organizations, local nongovernmental organizations, and PLHIV groups should advocate and lobby for policies and programs that incorporate nutrition and food security into universal access to prevention, treatment, and care and support. Universities and other academic institutions, particularly nursing schools, medical schools, and schools of public health, need to incorporate nutrition and HIV issues into their curricula and recognize it as an obligatory competency. Finally, lessons learned from the current concept of combination prevention (particularly the concept of "treatment as prevention") should motivate all stakeholders to appreciate and optimize nutrition as an HIV prevention tool.

Public Health Core Competency 5A: Community Dimensions of Practice Skills: Identifies stakeholders

References

1 The World Bank. (2006). *Directions in development: Repositioning nutrition as central to development: A strategy for large-scale action.* Washington, DC: The World Bank.

2 The Copenhagen Consensus Center. (2012). *The Copenhagen Consensus 2012: Solving the world's challenges.* Copenhagen, Denmark: The Copenhagen Consensus Center.

3 The World Bank. (2006). *Directions in development: Repositioning nutrition as central to development: A strategy for large-scale action.* Washington DC: The World Bank.

4 Hoddinott, J., Maluccio, J., Behrman, J., Flores, R., & Martorell, R. (2008). Effect of a nutrition intervention during early childhood on economic productivity in Guatemalan adults. *Lancet, 371,* 411-16.

5 Jesmin, A., Yamamoto, S., Malik, A., & Hague, A. (2011). Prevalence and determinants of chronic malnutrition among preschool children: A cross-sectional study in Dhaka City Bangladesh. *Journal of Health, Population, and Nutrition, 29*(5), 494-99.

6 United Nations. (2012, July 12). *The Millenium Development Goals.* Retrieved from http://www.un.org/millenniumgoals.

7 Food and Agriculture Organization, International Fund for Agricultural Development, & World Food Programme. (2012). *The state of food insecurity in the world 2012.* Rome: FAO.

8 Allen, L. (1993). The nutrition CRSP: What is marginal malnutrition, and does it affect human function? *Nutrition Review, 51*(9), 255-67.

9 Haddad, L., & Smith, L. (1999). *Explaining child malnutrition in developing countries: A cross-country analysis.* Washington, DC: International Food Policy and Research Institute.

10 Khan, Y., & Bhutta, Z. (2010). Nutritional deficiencies in the developing world: Current status and opportunities for intervention. *Pediatric Clinics of North America, 57*(6), 1409-41.

11 Food and Agriculture Organization, International Fund for Agricultural Development, & World Food Programme. (2012). *The state of food insecurity in the world 2012.* Rome: FAO.

12 Alhassan, L. (2008). *Nutritional status of pre-school children: A comparative study of two communities in Savelugu-Nanton District Northern Region* (MSc thesis). Kwame Nkrumah University of Science and Technology, Kumasi.

13 Ghana Statistical Service, & Institute for Resource Development/Macro Systems, Inc. (1989). *Ghana demographic and health survey 1988.* Accra, Ghana: GSS/Macro.

14 Amoako-Kwakye, F. A. (2010). Foods and food-related practices of cultural groups in southern Ghana. Accra: Ghana Universities Press.

15 Colecraft, E., Marquis, G., Aryeetey, R., Sakyi-Dawson, O., Lartey, A., Ahunu, B., . . . Huff-Lonergan, E. (2006). Constraints on the use of animal source foods for young children in Ghana: A participatory rapid appraisal approach. *Ecology of Food and Nutrition, 45*, 351–77.

16 Gwatkin, D., Rutstein, S., Johnson, K., Suliman, E., & Wagstaff, A. (2003). *Initial country-level information about socio-economic differences in health, nutrition, and population* (2nd ed.). Washington, DC: World Bank.

17 Food and Agriculture Organization, International Fund for Agricultural Development, & World Food Programme. (2012). *The state of food insecurity in the world 2012*. Rome: FAO.

18 Food and Agriculture Organization, International Fund for Agricultural Development, & World Food Programme. (2012). *The state of food insecurity in the world 2012*. Rome: FAO.

19 Food and Agriculture Organization, International Fund for Agricultural Development, & World Food Programme. (2012). *The state of food insecurity in the world 2012*. Rome: FAO.

20 Black, R., Allen, L., Bhutta, Z., Caulfield, L., de Onis, M., Ezzati, M., . . . Maternal and Child Undernutrition Study Group. (2008). Maternal and child undernutrition: Global and regional exposures and health consequences. *Lancet, 371*(9608), 243–60.

21 Black, R., Allen, L., Bhutta, Z., Caulfield, L., de Onis, M., Ezzati, M., . . . Maternal and Child Undernutrition Study Group. (2008). Maternal and child undernutrition: Global and regional exposures and health consequences. *Lancet, 371*(9608), 243–60.

22 Ghana Statistical Service, & Institute for Resource Development /Macro Systems Inc. (1989). *Ghana demographic and health survey 1988*. Accra, Ghana: GSS/Macro.

23 Hill, A. G., Darko, R., Seffah, J., Adanu, R. M., Anarfi, J. K., & Duda, R. B. (2007). Health of urban Ghanaian women as identified by the Women's Health Study of Accra. *International Journal of Gynaecology and Obstetrics, 99*(2), 150–56. doi:10.1016 /j.ijgo.2007.05.024

24 Ziraba, A., Fotso, J., & Ochako, R. (2009). Overweight and obesity in urban Africa: A problem of the rich or the poor? *BMC Public Health, 9*.

25 MOST USAID Micronutrient Program. (2004). *A strategic approach to anemia control programs*. Arlington, VA: MOST USAID Micronutrient Program.

26 Rastogi, R., & Mathers, C. (2000). *Global burden of iron deficiency anaemia in the year 2000*. Retrieved from http://www .who.int/healthinfo/statistics/bod_irondeficiencyanaemia .pdf.

27 World Health Organization & Centers for Disease Control and Prevention. (2008). *Worldwide prevalence of anaemia, 1993-2005: WHO Global Database on Anaemia*. Geneva: World Health Organization.

28 Ghana Statistical Service, Ghana Health Services, & ICF Macro. (2009). *Ghana Demographic and Health Survey, 2008*. Accra, Ghana: GSS, GHS, ICF Macro.

29 Ghana Statistical Service, Noguchi Memorial Institute for Medical Research, & ORC Macro. (2004). *Ghana Demographic and Health Survey 2003*. Calverton, MD: GSS, NMIMR, and ORC Macro.

30 Ghana Statistical Service, Ghana Health Services, & ICF Macro. (2009). *Ghana Demographic and Health Survey, 2008*. Accra: GSS, GHS, ICF Macro.

31 United Nations Administrative Committee on Coordination Sub-Committee on Nutrition & International Food Policy Research Institute. (2000). *Fourth report of the world nutrition situation: Nutrition throughout the life cycle*. Geneva: ACC/SCN in Collaboration with IFPRI.

32 Gribble, J., & Haffey, J. (2008). *Reproductive health in sub-Saharan Africa*. Population Reference Bureau Selected Publications. Washington, DC: Population Reference Bureau.

33 Ghana Statistical Service, Ghana Health Services, & ICF Macro. (2009). *Ghana Demographic and Health Survey, 2008*. Accra: GSS, GHS, ICF Macro.

34 United Nations Development Programme. (2012, August 12). *MDG progress in Ghana*. Retrieved from http://www.undp-gha .org/mainpages.php?page=MDG%20Progress.

35 Engle, P., Menon, P., & Haddad, L. (1999). Care and nutrition: Concepts and measurement. *World Development, 27*(8), 1309–37.

36 Ghana Statistical Service & Institute for Resource Development /Macro Systems Inc. (1989). *Ghana demographic and health survey 1988*. Accra, Ghana: GSS/Macro.

37 Colecraft, E., Marquis, G., Aryeetey, R., Sakyi-Dawson, O., Lartey, A., Ahunu, B., . . . Huff-Lonergan, E. (2006). Constraints on the use of animal source foods for young children in Ghana: A participatory rapid appraisal approach. *Ecology of Food and Nutrition, 45*, 351–77.

38 United Nations Children's Fund. (2012). *State of the the world's children 2012: Children in an urban world*. New York: UNICEF.

39 Black, R., Allen, L., Bhutta, Z., Caulfield, L., de Onis, M., Ezzati, M., . . . Maternal and Child Undernutrition Study Group. (2008). Maternal and child undernutrition: global and regional exposures and health consequences. *Lancet, 371*(9608), 243–60.

40 Ghana Statistical Service & Institute for Resource Development /Macro Systems Inc. (1989). *Ghana demographic and health survey 1988*. Accra, Ghana: GSS/Macro.

41 Lartey, A., Marquis, G. S., Mazur, R., Perez-Escamilla, R., Brakohiapa, L., Ampofo, W., Sellen, D., et al. (2012). Maternal HIV is associated with reduced growth in the first year of life among infants in the Eastern region of Ghana: The Research to Improve Infant Nutrition and Growth (RIING) Project. *Maternal & Child Nutrition*. doi:10.1111/j.1740-8709.2012.00441.x

42 Must, A., Jacques, P., Dallal, G., Bajema, C., & Dietz, W. (1992). Long-term morbidity and mortality of overweight adolescents. A follow-up of the Harvard Growth Study of 1922 to 1935. *New England Journal of Medicine, 327*, 1350–55.

43 World Health Organization. (2012, July 12). *Obesity and overweight*. WHO Fact Sheet No. 311. Retrieved from http://www .who.int/mediacentre/factsheets/fs311/en.

44 World Health Organization. (2012). *Population-based approaches to childhood obesity*. Geneva: World Health Organization.

45 De Onis, M., Blossner, M., & Borghi, E. (2010). Global prevalence and trends of overweight and obesity among preschool children. *American Journal of Clinical Nutrition, 92*, 1257–64.

46 Ghana Statistical Service, Ghana Health Services, & ICF Macro. (2009). *Ghana Demographic and Health Survey 2008*. Accra, Ghana: GSS, GHS, ICF Macro.

47 World Health Organization. (2012). *Population-based approaches to childhood obesity*. Geneva: World Health Organization.

48 Lobstein, T. (2005). Can we prevent child obesity? *SCN News, 29*, 33-38.

49 World Health Organization. (2012b). *Population-based approaches to childhood obesity*. Geneva: World Health Organization.

50 Ghana Statistical Service, Ghana Health Services, & ICF Macro. (2009). *Ghana Demographic and Health Survey 2008*. Accra, Ghana: GSS, GHS, ICF Macro.

51 World Health Organization & Centers for Disease Control and Prevention. (2008). *Worldwide prevalence of anemia, 1993-2005: WHO global database on anemia*. Geneva: World Health Organization.

52 World Health Organization. (2009). *Global prevalence of vitamin A deficiency in populations at risk, 1995-2005: WHO global database on vitamin A deficiency*. Geneva: World Health Organization.

53 World Health Organization. (2003). *Nutrient requirements for people living with HIV/AIDS: Report of a technical consultation*. Geneva: World Health Organization.

54 Ghana Health Services (GHS). (2007). *National infant and young child feeding for Ghana strategy document*. Accra, Ghana: GHS.

55 Ghana Statistical Service & Institute for Resource Development /Macro Systems Inc. (1989). *Ghana Demographic and Health Survey, 1988*. Accra, Ghana: GSS/Macro.

56 Otoo, G. E., Lartey, A. A., & Perez-Escamilla, R. (2009). Perceived incentives and barriers to exclusive breastfeeding among periurban Ghanaian women. *Journal of Human Lactation, 25*(1), 34-41.

57 Ghana Statistical Service, Ghana Health Services, & ICF Macro. (2009). *Ghana Demographic and Health Survey, 2008*. Accra, Ghana: GSS, GHS, ICF Macro.

58 Tawiah-Agyemang, C., Kirkwood, B. R., Edmond, K., Bazzano, A., & Hill, Z. (2008). Early initiation of breast-feeding in Ghana: barriers and facilitators. *Journal of Perinatology, 28*, S46-52.

59 Ghana Statistical Service, Ghana Health Services, & ICF Macro. (2009). *Ghana Demographic and Health Survey, 2008*. Accra, Ghana: GSS, GHS, ICF Macro.

60 Lutter, C., & Rivera, J. (2003). Nutritional status of infants and young children and characteristics of their diets. *Journal of Nutrition, 133*, 2941S-2949S.

61 Ghana Statistical Service, Ghana Health Services, & ICF Macro. (2009). *Ghana demographic and health survey, 2008*. Accra, Ghana: GSS, GHS, ICF Macro.

62 Ghana Statistical Service, Ghana Health Services, & ICF Macro. (2009). *Ghana Demographic and Health Survey, 2008*. Accra, Ghana: GSS, GHS, ICF Macro.

63 United Nations Children's Fund. (1998). *State of the the world's children, 1998: Focus on nutrition*. New York: UNICEF.

64 Bhutta, Z., Ahmed, T., Black, R., Cousens, S., Dewey, K., Giugliani, E., et al. (2008). What works? Interventions for maternal and child undernutrition and survival. *Lancet, 371*, 417-40.

65 Bhutta, Z., Ahmed, T., Black, R., Cousens, S., Dewey, K., Giugliani, E., et al. (2008). What works? Interventions for maternal and child undernutrition and survival. *Lancet, 371*, 417-40.

66 Brantuo, M., Okwabi, W., Adu-Afuawuah, S., Agyepong, E., Attafuah, N., Brew, G., . . . Ashong, J. (2009). Landscape analysis of readiness to accelerate the reduction of maternal and child undernutrition in Ghana. *SCN News, 37*, 31-37.

67 Centers for Disease Control and Prevention. (2008). Revised surveillance case definitions for HIV infection among adults, adolescents, and children aged <18 months and for HIV infection and AIDS among children aged 18 months to <13 years: United States. *Morbidity and Mortality Weekly Report, 57*(RR10), 1-8. Retrieved from http://www.cdc.gov/mmwr/preview /mmwrhtml/rr5710a1.htm

68 UNAIDS. (2012). *UNAIDS report on the global AIDS epidemic, 2011*. United Nations Programme on HIV/AIDS. Geneva: UNAIDS.

69 National AIDS/STI Control Programme (NACP). (2011). *The 2010 HIV sentinel survey report*. Accra, Ghana: Ghana Health Service, Ministry of Health.

70 National AIDS/STI Control Programme (NACP). (2011). *The 2010 HIV sentinel survey report*. Accra, Ghana: Ghana Health Service, Ministry of Health.

71 UNAIDS. (2012). *UNAIDS report on the global AIDS epidemic, 2011*. United Nations Programme on HIV/AIDS. Geneva: UNAIDS.

72 Hogan, M. C., Foreman, K. J., Naghavi, M., Ahn, S. Y., Wang, M., Makela, S. M., Lopez, A. D., Lozano, R., & Murray, C. J. (2010). *Lancet, 375*(9726), 1609-23. doi:10.1016/S0140-6736(10)60518-1

73 UNAIDS. (2012). *UNAIDS report on the global AIDS epidemic, 2011. United Nations Programme on HIV/AIDS*. Geneva: UNAIDS.

74 Ghana AIDS Commission. (2012). *Ghana Country AIDS progress report: Reporting period January 2010-December 2011* (p. 153). Retrieved from UNAIDS website, http://www.unaids.org/en /dataanalysis/knowyourresponse/countryprogressreports /2012countries/ce_GH_Narrative_Report[1].pdf

75 De Cock, K. M., Fowler, M. G., Mercier, E., de Vincenzi, I., Saba, J., Hoff, E., Alnwick, D. J., Rogers, M., & Shaffer, N. (2000). Prevention of mother-to-child HIV transmission in resource-poor countries: Translating research into policy and practice. *Journal of the American Medical Association, 283*(9), 1175-82.

76 Ghana AIDS Commission. (2012). *Ghana Country AIDS progress report: Reporting period January 2010-December 2011* (p. 153). Retrieved from UNAIDS website, http://www.unaids.org/en /dataanalysis/knowyourresponse/countryprogressreports/201 2countries/ce_GH_Narrative_Report[1].pdf

77 European Collaborative Study. (2005). Mother-to-child transmission of HIV infection in the era of highly active antiretroviral therapy. *Clinical Infectious Diseases, 40*(3), 458-65.

78 Centers for Disease Control and Prevention. (2013). *HIV among pregnant women, infants, and children*. Retrieved from http://www.cdc.gov/hiv/risk/gender/pregnantwomen/facts /index.html

79 Nicolosi, A., Corrêa Leite, M. L., Musicco, M., Arici, C., Gavazzeni, G., & Lazzarin, A. (1994). The efficiency of male-to-female and female-to-male sexual transmission of the human immunodeficiency virus: A study of 730 stable couples. Italian Study Group on HIV Heterosexual Transmission. *Epidemiology*, 5(6), 570-57.

80 Ivers, L. C., & Cullen, K. A. (2011). Food insecurity: Special considerations for women. *American Journal of Clinical Nutrition*, 94(Suppl.), 1740S-1744S. doi:10.3945/ajcn.111.012617

81 Oldewage-Theron, W. H., Dicks, E. G., & Napier, C. E. (2006). Poverty, household food insecurity and nutrition: Coping strategies in an informal settlement in the Vaal Triangle, South Africa. *Public Health*, 120(9), 795-804.

82 Laar, A., Manu, A., Fiaveh, D., & Laar, M. (2012, September 30-October 4). *Vulnerability to food insecurity and negative coping strategies of HIV-affected households in Ghana*. Presented at the 24th Congress of the Nutrition Society of South Africa and the 5th African Nutrition Epidemiology Conference University of Free State, Bloemfontein, South Africa.

83 Nduati, R., Richardson, B. A., John, G., Mbori-Ngacha, D., Mwatha, A., Ndinya-Achola, J., Bwayo, J., et al. (2001). Effect of breastfeeding on mortality among HIV-1 infected women: a randomised trial. *Lancet*, 357(9269), 1651-55. doi:10.1016/S0140-6736(00)04820-0

84 Otieno, P. A. (2009). Breast-feeding and HIV-1 infection: Maternal health. *Advances in Experimental Medicine and Biology*, 639, 313-18. doi:10.1007/978-1-4020-8749-3_22

85 Laar, M., & Laar, A. (2012). Does infant feeding modality have an impact on the health of mothers infected with human immunodeficiency virus in sub-Saharan Africa? A systematic literature review. *Journal of AIDS and HIV Research*, 4(1), 1-7.

86 Kotler, D. P. (2005). HIV infection and the gastrointestinal tract. *AIDS*, 19(2), 107-17.

87 Villamor, E., Saathoff, E., Mugusi, F., Bosch, R. J., Urassa, W., & Fawzi, W. W. (2006). Wasting and body composition of adults with pulmonary tuberculosis in relation to HIV-1 coinfection, socioeconomic status, and severity of tuberculosis. *European Journal of Clinical Nutrition*, 60(2), 163-71. doi:10.1038/sj.ejcn.1602281

88 Lemke, S. (2005). Nutrition security, livelihoods and HIV/AIDS: Implications for research among farm worker households in South Africa. *Public Health Nutrition*, 8(7), 844-52.

89 Fields-Gardner, C., & Fergusson, P. (2004). Position of the American Dietetic Association and Dietitians of Canada: Nutrition intervention in the care of persons with human immunodeficiency virus infection. *Journal of the American Dietetic Association*, 104(9), 1425-41. doi:10.1016/j.jada.2004.07.012

90 Maj, M. (1990). Psychiatric aspects of HIV-1 infection and AIDS. *Psychological Medicine*, 20(3), 547-63.

91 Greene, J. B. (1988). Clinical approach to weight loss in the patient with HIV infection. *Gastroenterology Clinics of North America*, 17(3), 573-86.

92 Keating, J., Bjarnason, I., Somasundaram, S., Macpherson, A., Francis, N., Price, A. B., Sharpstone, D., et al. (1995). Intestinal absorptive capacity, intestinal permeability and jejunal histology in HIV and their relation to diarrhoea. *Gut*, 37(5), 623-29.

93 Macallan, D. (1999). Dietary intake and weight loss patterns in HIV infection. In T. I. Miller & S. L. Gorbach (Eds.), *Nutritional aspects of HIV infection*. New York: Oxford University Press.

94 Blossner, M., & De Onis, M. (2005). Malnutrition: Quantifying the health impact at national and local levels. *WHO Environmental Burden of Disease Series*, 12, 1-43.

95 Grunfeld, C., Pang, M., Shimizu, L., Shigenaga, J., Jensen, P., & Feingold, K. R. (1992). Resting energy expenditure, caloric intake, and short-term weight change in human immunodeficiency virus infection and the acquired immunodeficiency syndrome. *American Journal of Clinical Nutrition*, 55(2), 455-60.

96 Hommes, M. J., Romijn, J. A., Godfried, M. H., Schattenkerk, J. K., Buurman, W. A., Endert, E., & Sauerwein, H. P. (1990). Increased resting energy expenditure in human immunodeficiency virus-infected men. *Metabolism: Clinical and Experimental*, 39(11), 1186-90.

97 Melchior, J. C., Raguin, G., Boulier, A., Bouvet, E., Rigaud, D., Matheron, S., Casalino, E., et al. (1993). Resting energy expenditure in human immunodeficiency virus-infected patients: Comparison between patients with and without secondary infections. *American Journal of Clinical Nutrition*, 57(5), 614-19.

98 Mangili, A., Murman, D. H., Zampini, A. M., & Wanke, C. A. (2006). Nutrition and HIV infection: Review of weight loss and wasting in the era of highly active antiretroviral therapy from the nutrition for healthy living cohort. *Clinical Infectious Diseases*, 42(6), 836-42. doi:10.1086/500398

99 Woods, M. (1999). Dietary recommendations for the HIV/AIDS patient. In T. I. Miller & S. L. Gorbach (Eds.), *Nutritional Aspects of HIV Infection*. New York: Oxford University Press.

100 Laar, A., Ampofo, W., Tuakli, J., Wonodi, C., Asante, R., & Quakyi, I. (2009). Factors associated with suboptimal intake of some important nutrients among HIV-positive pregnant adolescents from two Ghanaian districts. *Journal of the Ghana Science Association*, 11(2), 25-39.

101 Allard, J. P., Aghdassi, E., Chau, J., Salit, I., & Walmsley, S. (1998). Oxidative stress and plasma antioxidant micronutrients in humans with HIV infection. *American Journal of Clinical Nutrition*, 67(1), 143-47.

102 De Waal, A., & Whiteside, A. (2003). New variant famine: AIDS and food crisis in southern Africa. *Lancet*, 362(9391), 1234-37. doi:10.1016/S0140-6736(03)14548-5

103 Haddad, L., & Gillespie, S. (2001). Effective food and nutrition policy responses to HIV/AIDS: What we know and what we need to know. *Journal of International Development*, 13(4), 487-511. doi:10.1002/jid.799

104 Keating, J., Bjarnason, I., Somasundaram, S., Macpherson, A., Francis, N., Price, A. B., Sharpstone, D., et al. (1995). Intestinal absorptive capacity, intestinal permeability and jejunal histology in HIV and their relation to diarrhoea. *Gut*, 37(5), 623-29.

105 Blossner, M., & De Onis, M. (2005). Malnutrition: Quantifying the health impact at national and local levels. *WHO Environmental Burden of Disease Series*, 12, 1-43.

106 Hommes, M. J., Romijn, J. A., Godfried, M. H., Schattenkerk, J. K., Buurman, W. A., Endert, E., & Sauerwein, H. P. (1990). Increased resting energy expenditure in human immunodeficiency

virus-infected men. *Metabolism: Clinical and Experimental, 39*(11), 1186–90.

107 Ahmed, R. (2005). Is there a balance between oxidative stress and antioxidant defense system during development? *Medical Journal of Islamic World Academy of Sciences, 15*(2), 55–63.

108 Robbins, D., & Zhao, Y. (2012). Oxidative Stress Induced by MnSOD-p53 Interaction: Pro- or anti-tumorigenic? *Journal of Signal Transduction, 2012*, 101465. doi:10.1155/2012/101465

109 World Food Programme. (2009). *Comprehensive food security and vulnerability analysis (CFSVA)* (p. 162). Accra, Ghana: World Food Programme. Retrieved from http://grad.ochaopt.org /documents/CFSVA_WBGS.pdf

110 Laar, A., Manu, A., Fiaveh, D., & Laar, M. (2012, September 30– October 4). *Vulnerability to food insecurity and negative coping strategies of HIV-affected households in Ghana*. Presented at the 24th Congress of the Nutrition Society of South Africa and the 5th African Nutrition Epidemiology Conference University of Free State, Bloemfontein, South Africa.

111 Reddi, A., Powers, M. A., & Thyssen, A. (2012). HIV/AIDS and food insecurity: Deadly syndemic or an opportunity for healthcare synergism in resource-limited settings of sub-Saharan Africa? *AIDS, 26*(1), 115–17. doi:10.1097 /QAD.0b013e32834e14ac

112 Semba, R. D., & Tang, A. M. (1999). Micronutrients and the pathogenesis of human immunodeficiency virus infection. *British Journal of Nutrition, 81*(3), 181–89.

113 Azu, O. (2012). The male genital tract in the era of highly active antiretroviral therapy (HAART): Implication for anti-oxidant therapy. *Journal of AIDS and Clinical Research, 3*(7). doi:10.4172/2155-6113.1000169

114 World Health Organization. (2003). *Nutrient requirements for people living with HIV/AIDS: Report of a technical consultation*. Geneva: World Health Organization.

115 Food and Nutrition Technical Assistance (FANTA). (2004). *HIV/AIDS: A guide for nutrition, care and support* (p. 56). Washington, DC: FANTA.

116 Friis, H., Gomo, E., Koestel, P., Ndhlovu, P., Nyazema, N., Krarup, H., & Michaelsen, K. F. (2001). HIV and other predictors of serum folate, serum ferritin, and hemoglobin in pregnancy: A cross-sectional study in Zimbabwe. *American Journal of Clinical Nutrition, 73*(6), 1066–73.

117 Deeks, S. G., Verdin, E., & McCune, J. M. (2012). Immunosenescence and HIV. *Current Opinion in Immunology, 24*(4), 501–6. doi:10.1016/j.coi.2012.05.004

118 World Health Organization & Food and Agricultural Organization. (2004). *Vitamin and mineral requirements in human nutrition: Report of a joint FAO/WHO expert consultation, Bangkok, Thailand, 21–30 September 1998* (2nd ed.). Geneva: WHO & FAO.

119 World Health Organization. (2003). *Nutrient requirements for people living with HIV/AIDS: Report of a technical consultation*. Geneva: World Health Organization.

120 Fawzi, W., Msamanga, G., Spiegelman, D., & Hunter, D. J. (2005). Studies of vitamins and minerals and HIV transmission and dis-ease progression. *Journal of Nutrition, 135*(4), 938–44.

121 World Health Organization. (2003). *Nutrient requirements for people living with HIV/AIDS: Report of a technical consultation*. Geneva: World Health Organization.

122 Wiysonge, C. S., Shey, M. S., Sterne, J. A. C., & Brocklehurst, P. (2005). Vitamin A supplementation for reducing the risk of mother-to-child transmission of HIV infection. *Cochrane Database of Systematic Reviews (Online)*, (4), CD003648. doi:10.1002/14651858.CD003648.pub2

123 Ziegler, J. B., Cooper, D. A., Johnson, R. O., & Gold, J. (1985). Postnatal transmission of AIDS-associated retrovirus from mother to infant. *Lancet, 1*(8434), 896–98.

124 Binagwaho, A. (2008). The right of children in developing coun-tries to be born and live HIV-free. *Health and Human Rights, 10*(1), 149–52.

125 Coovadia, H. M., Rollins, N. C., Bland, R. M., Little, K., Coutsoudis, A., Bennish, M. L., & Newell, M.-L. (2007). Mother-to-child trans-mission of HIV-1 infection during exclusive breastfeeding in the first 6 months of life: An intervention cohort study. *Lancet, 369*(9567), 1107–16.

126 Coutsoudis, A., Coovadia, H. M., & Wilfert, C. M. (2008). HIV, infant feeding and more perils for poor people: New WHO guide-lines encourage review of formula milk policies. *Bulletin of the World Health Organization, 86*(3), 210–14.

127 Coovadia, H. M., Rollins, N. C., Bland, R. M., Little, K., Coutsoudis, A., Bennish, M. L., & Newell, M.-L. (2007). Mother-to-child trans-mission of HIV-1 infection during exclusive breastfeeding in the first 6 months of life: An intervention cohort study. *Lancet, 369*(9567), 1107–116.

128 Kourtis, A. P., Lee, F. K., Abrams, E. J., Jamieson, D. J., & Bulterys, M. (2006). Mother-to-child transmission of HIV-1: Timing and implications for prevention. *Lancet Infectious Diseases, 6*(11), 726–32. doi:10.1016/S1473-3099(06)70629-6

129 Coutsoudis, A., Coovadia, H. M., & Wilfert, C. M. (2008). HIV, infant feeding and more perils for poor people: New WHO guide-lines encourage review of formula milk policies. *Bulletin of the World Health Organization, 86*(3), 210–14.

130 Kagaayi, J., Gray, R. H., Brahmbhatt, H., Kigozi, G., Nalugoda, F., Wabwire-Mangen, F., Serwadda, D., et al. (2008). Survival of infants born to HIV-positive mothers, by feeding modality, in Rakai, Uganda. *PLOS One, 3*(12), e3877. doi:10.1371/journal .pone.0003877

131 World Health Organization. (2011). *World health statistics, 2011* (p. 162). Geneva: World Health Organization. Retrieved from http://www.who.int/whosis/whostat/EN_WHS2011_Full.pdf

132 Coovadia, H. M., & Bland, R. M. (2007). Preserving breastfeed-ing practice through the HIV pandemic. *Tropical Medicine & International Health, 12*(9), 1116–33.

133 Kagaayi, J., Gray, R. H., Brahmbhatt, H., Kigozi, G., Nalugoda, F., Wabwire-Mangen, F., . . . Wawer, M. J. (2007). Survival of infants born to HIV-positive mothers, by feeding modality, in Rakai, Uganda. *PloS One, 3*(12), e3877. doi:10.1371/journa l.pone.0003877

134 Taha, T. E., Li, Q., Hoover, D. R., Mipando, L., Nkanaunena, K., Thigpen, M. C., Taylor, A., et al. (2011). Postexposure prophylaxis

of breastfeeding HIV-exposed infants with antiretroviral drugs to age 14 weeks: Updated efficacy results of the PEPI-Malawi trial. *Journal of Acquired Immune Deficiency Syndromes, 57*(4), 319–25. doi:10.1097/QAI.0b013e318217877a

135 The Kesho Bora Study Group. (2011). Safety and effectiveness of antiretroviral drugs during pregnancy, delivery and breastfeeding for prevention of mother-to-child transmission of HIV-1: The Kesho Bora Multicentre Collaborative Study rationale, design, and implementation challenges. *Contemporary Clinical Trials, 32*(1), 74–85. doi:10.1016/j.cct.2010.09.008

136 WHO. (2010). *Guidelines on HIV and infant feeding 2010: Principles and recommendations for infant feeding in the context of HIV and a summary of evidence.* Geneva: World Health Organization. Retrieved from http://www.who.int/child_adolescent_health/ documents/9789241599535/e

137 Centers for Disease Control and Prevention. (2010). *Diagnoses of HIV infection by age.* Atlanta, GA: Centers for Disease Control and Prevention. Retrieved from http://www.cdc.gov/hiv/topics/surveillance/basic.htm#hivaidsage

138 European Collaborative Study. (2005). Mother-to-child transmission of HIV infection in the era of highly active antiretroviral therapy. *Clinical Infectious Diseases, 40*(3), 458–65.

139 World Health Organization. (2003). *Nutrient requirements for people living with HIV/AIDS: Report of a technical consultation.* Geneva: World Health Organization.

140 Lartey, A., Marquis, G. S., Mazur, R., Perez-Escamilla, R., Brakohiapa, L., Ampofo, W., Sellen, D., et al. (2012). Maternal HIV is associated with reduced growth in the first year of life among infants in the Eastern region of Ghana: The Research to Improve Infant Nutrition and Growth (RIING) Project. *Maternal & Child Nutrition.* doi:10.1111/j.1740-8709.2012.00441.x

141 McGrath, C. J., Nduati, R., Richardson, B. A., Kristal, A. R., Mbori-Ngacha, D., Farquhar, C., & John-Stewart, G. C. (2012). The prevalence of stunting is high in HIV-1-exposed uninfected infants in Kenya. *Journal of Nutrition, 142*(4), 757–63. doi:10.3945/jn.111.148874

142 Rollins, N. C., Coovadia, H. M., Bland, R. M., Coutsoudis, A., Bennish, M. L., Patel, D., & Newell, M.-L. (2007). Pregnancy outcomes in HIV-infected and uninfected women in rural and urban South Africa. *Journal of Acquired Immune Deficiency Syndromes, 44*(3), 321–28. doi:10.1097/QAI.0b013e31802ea4b0

143 Lartey, A., Marquis, G. S., Mazur, R., Perez-Escamilla, R., Brakohiapa, L., Ampofo, W., Sellen, D., et al. (2012). Maternal HIV is associated with reduced growth in the first year of life among infants in the Eastern region of Ghana: The Research to Improve Infant Nutrition and Growth (RIING) Project. *Maternal & Child Nutrition.* Advance online publication. doi:10.1111/j.1740-8709.2012.00441.x

144 McGrath, C. J., Nduati, R., Richardson, B. A., Kristal, A. R., Mbori-Ngacha, D., Farquhar, C., & John-Stewart, G. C. (2012). The prevalence of stunting is high in HIV-1-exposed uninfected infants in Kenya. *Journal of Nutrition, 142*(4), 757–63. doi:10.3945/jn.111.148874

145 Binagwaho, A. (2008). The right of children in developing countries to be born and live HIV-free. *Health and Human Rights, 10*(1), 149–52.

146 Franke, M. F., Stulac, S. N., Rugira, I. H., Rich, M. L., Bucyibaruta, J. B., Drobac, P. C., Iyamungu, G., et al. (2011). High human immunodeficiency virus-free survival of infants born to human immunodeficiency virus-positive mothers in an integrated program to decrease child mortality in rural Rwanda. *Pediatric Infectious Disease Journal, 30*(7), 614–16. doi:10.1097/INF.0b013e31820a599e

147 Laar, A., Amankwa, B., & Asiedu, C. (2012, July). Prevention of mother-to-child transmission of HIV service providers in the Accra Metropolis and their clients face unique challenges. Presented at the 19th International AIDS Conference (AIDS 2012), Washington D.C.

Chapter 12

Pneumonia in Severely Malnourished Children in Developing Countries: Public Health Nutrition Approaches to Prevention and Early Treatment

Mohammod Jobayer Chisti, MBBS, MMed
Abu Syed Golam Faruque, MBBS, MPH
Hasan Ashraf, MBBS, MCPS, MD
Md. Iqbal Hossain, MBBS, DCH, PhD
Md. Munirul Islam, MBBS, PhD
Sumon Kumar Das, MBBS
Tahmeed Ahmed, MBBS, PhD

"Many small hospitals in the developing world have unacceptably high case-fatality rates for childhood pneumonia, often as high as 15-20%. Most of these deaths are avoidable with adequate care." – E. K. Mulholland, childhood pneumonia specialist

Reproduced from: Mulholland, E., Smith, L., Carneiro, I., Becher, H., & Lehmann, D. (2008). Equity and child-survival strategies. *Bulletin of the World Health Organization, 86*(5), 399-407.

Learning Objectives

- Define, identify, and assess severe acute malnutrition (SAM) in children.
- Link SAM to infectious disease development.
- Understand the value of rapid management of pneumonia in children with severe malnutrition and how best to implement it from a public health perspective.
- Understand the need for appropriate antimicrobial therapy depending on cause.
- Use public health approaches to decrease morbidity and mortality due to pneumonia in severely malnourished children.

- Use public health interventions to reduce SAM among children, thereby reducing mortality due to pneumonia.

- Evaluate the benefits, dangers, and costs of treatment options when making population-based decisions for public health interventions.

Case Study: Malnourished Child with Pneumonia

The following case study describes a real series of events in an intensive care unit (ICU). The table accompanying the case study identifies and explains many of the clinical terms.

Hospital Admittance, Initial Examination, and Diagnosis

An 18-month-old boy was admitted to the International Centre for Diarrheal Disease Research, Bangladesh (icddr,b), Intensive Care Unit on December 24, 2011, at 4:00 p.m., with the complaints of fever, cough, and shortness of breath for four days. He was the only child of non-consanguineous parents and had been partially breastfed since birth and was immunized as per the **Expanded Program on Immunization (EPI)** schedule.

On examination during admission, the patient was dyspnoic, or short of breath, and had severe lower chest wall in-drawing. The following were other findings upon examination:

- Temperature: 36.6 degrees Celsius (97.9 degrees Fahrenheit)

- Respiratory rate (RR): 70 breaths/minute (abnormally rapid)

- Arterial oxygen saturation (SpO2): 88% (abnormally low)

- Pulse: 140 beats/minute

- Capillary refilling time (CRT): 2 seconds

- Blood pressure (BP): 110/70 mm Hg

The child was mildly pale, but had no signs of dehydration. He weighed 7 kilograms (15 pounds) and had a height of 75 centimeters (30 inches). The weight-for-age (W/A) z score was −3.54 (low), and the z score of the weight-for-length (W/L) was −3.26 (low). His random blood glucose (RBS) was 7.5 mmol/L (normal). Examination of the respiratory system exposed lower chest wall in-drawing and bronchial breath sound with coarse rales (crackling noises) over both sides of the left lung. An urgent chest X-ray (CXR) upon admission to the ICU revealed **lobar consolidation** involving almost all of the lung fields at the left side. Other body systems appeared normal.

Based on patient history and the clinical findings, the patient was diagnosed with **severe acute malnutrition (SAM)** with severe pneumonia with **hypoxemia**.

Early Treatment and Monitoring

Upon immediate oxygen (O_2) supplementation, respiratory distress gradually improved and SpO2 saturation was maintained. Patient care included the antibiotics ampicillin and gentamycin and other supportive measures for malnutrition as per hospital protocol for the management of pneumonia and malnutrition. Continued monitoring, including **arterial blood gas (ABG) analysis (Table 12-1)**, suggested the presence of **hyperkalemia**, believed to be spurious due to hemolyzed serum, along with **hypocalcemia** and acute renal failure (ARF). Doctors repeated serum electrolyte tests the next morning, on December 25, and simultaneously administered one dose of intravenous (IV) calcium gluconate to correct hypocalcemia and also to counteract any cardiac toxicity likely in the presence of hyperkalemia.

The patient's clinical condition gradually deteriorated as the patient again developed respiratory distress with RR of 60 breaths per minute, abdominal contraction, and severe lower chest wall in-drawing, although he was maintaining SpO2 with high O_2 flow. An urgent arterial blood gas (ABG) and CXR revealed mild metabolic acidosis and more severe pneumonia, with consolidation extended to the right side.

Continued Treatment and Signs of Kidney Failure

Due to the patient's worsening condition, the antibiotics were changed to ceftriaxone and levofloxacin. The patient was maintaining SpO2 with high-flow O_2, and the ABG report did not indicate the need for intubation and mechanical ventilation. However, the patient's urine output decreased alarmingly to less than 0.5 ml/kg/hr despite stable circulation. Physicians provided more intravenous (IV) calcium gluconate, salbutamol nebulization to open the airways, and IV glucose—insulin infusion to maintain blood sugar levels. Increased airway secretion, managed with repeated oropharyngeal suction, indicated the possibility of volume depletion. To increase urine output, physicians unsuccessfully tried two doses of IV fluid of normal saline (N/S): 10 ml/kg at a one-hour interval.

Table 12-1 Parameters used in this case study

Parameters	Purpose	In this Study's Patient	Significance/Implications
Arterial oxygen saturation (SpO2)	To measure the presence or absence of hypoxemia	88% in air	Hypoxemia was present and oxygen supplementation was given
Z score against weight-for-age (W/A)	To measure the severity of malnutrition	-3.54 z score (known as severe undernutrition)	Severe form of chronic malnutrition for which the patient received protocolized management of severe malnutrition
Z score against weight-for-length/ height (W/L)	To measure the severity of malnutrition	-3.26 z score (known as severe wasting)	Severe form of acute malnutrition for which the patient received protocolized management of severe malnutrition
Fast breathing and lower chest wall in-drawing, bronchial breath sound with huge coarse rales on auscultation over both side of the whole left lung	To evaluate the severity of pneumonia	Presence of all the parameters	Very severe pneumonia for which the patient received protocolized management of very severe pneumonia
Hemoglobin (HB)	To evaluate level of HB in blood	9 gm/dl (little bit low called mild anemia)	Only required the management of ongoing above mentioned illness
White blood cell (WBC) count	To evaluate the potential existence of infection by bacteria	24,000/cmm	Very high and antibiotics were started
Neutrophil	To evaluate the potential existence of infection by bacteria	72%	High and antibiotics were started
Platelet	To evaluate the severity of infection	50,000/cmm	Low; might be due to severe bacterial infection in blood and antibiotics were started
Calcium (Ca++)	To evaluate the Ca++ level in blood	1.82 mmol/L	Low (hypocalcemia) and correction was given with supplemental calcium
Creatinine	To evaluate the kidney function	294.3 µmol/L	High (acute kidney/renal failure) and treated initially with fluid and later with furusimide
Potassium (K+)	To evaluate the kidney function	7.29 mmol/L	High (hyperkalemia) and treated immediately to prevent cardiac arrest and then to reduce the K level in blood to improve renal function

(continues)

Table 12-1 Parameters used in this case study (*continued*)

Parameters	Purpose	In this Study's Patient	Significance/Implications
Arterial blood gas (ABG) analysis	To evaluate the metabolic status and lung ventilation status of the patient	pH: 7.32, P_{CO_2}: 26, P_{O_2}: 95.3, HCO_3: 13.5	Mild metabolic acidosis and treatment of ongoing illness is sufficient for its management
Total carbon-dioxide (tCO_2)	To evaluate the tCO_2 in blood (to know the role of tCO_2 causing respiratory difficulty)	10.6 mmol/L	Low (known as metabolic acidosis) and treatment of ongoing illness is sufficient for its management
Ilius (distension of abdomen with absent bowel sound)	Either due to infection in blood by bacteria or obstruction in abdomen	Ilius probably due to infection in blood by bacteria and hyperkalemia	Deterioration of the ongoing illness and antibiotic was changed for the management
Mechanical ventilation with SIMV/P mode (with 100% FiO_2, PEEP: 5 cm of water, control pressure 25 mm Hg, RR of 25/min, inspiratory time of 0.7 second)	To ensure adequate oxygen and to provide adequate support for proper respiration	Brief period with adequate ventilation followed by rapid deterioration	Deterioration of the ongoing illness even under adequate ventilator support and tried different set of ventilation and nothing worked

At 3:30 p.m. that day, serum electrolytes were remeasured. Creatinine had dropped to 312.9 μmol/L, and potassium (K+) had dropped to 6.87. The patient's abdomen gradually distended and eventually developed **ileus**. The patient remained on nothing per oral (NPO), nasogastric suction, and IV fluids and metronidazol. An abdominal X-ray showed dilated bowel loops. Signs of renal failure led to administration of a single dose of frusimide (1 mg/kg) to increase urine output, which remained stable at 0.5 ml/kg/hr. Physicians adjusted the antibiotic doses because of ARF, adjusted the required fluid volume to manage renal failure, and maintained the intake output chart strictly. Except the renal component, the boy's other measures of circulation were maintained: pulse had good volume, mean arterial pressure was less than 60 mm Hg, capillary refilling time was normal. However, without improvement of the renal condition, the patient would need to be referred to another facility for renal dialysis.

Deteriorating Condition and Death

That evening, the patient's condition further deteriorated. He became drowsy, and SpO2 dropped to 75% despite continued high O_2 flow. He developed severely labored respiration with severe abdominal contraction. The next ABG showed pH of 6.92, P_{CO_2} of 56, P_{O_2} of 40, and HCO_3 of 13 mmol/L, all indicating abnormally high acidity and leading to immediate intubation and normalizing of SpO2, or partial pressure of oxygen. However, peripheral perfusion severely worsened (pulse: 104, low-volume; BP: nonrecordable; CRT: a low 4 seconds; periphery: cold). The antibiotic was changed to meropenum instead of ceftriaxone and levofloxacin, and the boy was kept under mechanical ventilation. However, at 11:15 p.m., saturation was no longer maintained despite mechanical ventilation, spontaneous respiration ceased, and the patient developed bradycardia instead of under ventilation. Cardiopulmonary respiration (CPR) was carried out according to the hospital protocol, with three doses of adrenaline and two doses of atropine. The patient's respiration did not improve, and there was no spontaneous cardiac activity. After 30 minutes of CPR and observation of dilated, nonreacting pupils, the patient did not show any signs of life. At 11:45 p.m., the patient was declared dead.

Final clinical diagnosis: Severe acute malnutrition with very severe pneumonia with ARF

Cause of death: Cardiorespiratory failure due to very severe pneumonia

Antecedent cause: ARF and severe malnutrition

Discussion Questions

- What were the causes of this child's tragic death and hundreds of thousands of similar cases each year?

- What is the best way to diagnose and treat SAM and pneumonia in children to prevent death after presentation at a hospital?

- Which modifiable risk factors can public health interventions target to reduce SAM and pneumonia in children?

- How can public health programs intervene among high-risk populations?

Introduction

Public health measures that could potentially have prevented this tragic death and others like it could aim to initiate early and aggressive management of pneumonia by helping the earlier admission of patients to the hospital. Education of parents and caregivers about the higher risk of developing pneumonia in malnutrition and about the visible simple clinical parameters of pneumonia can help. This chapter examines pneumonia and SAM, and introduces public health perspectives on these major public health threats to millions of children around the globe.

Introduction to Pneumonia and Malnutrition

Pneumonia is the inflammation of lung tissue due to infection by an agent such as a virus, bacterium, or fungus. Worldwide, pneumonia kills 1 child every 15 seconds.[1] Risk factors for childhood pneumonia include younger age, increasing birth order, **low birth weight (LBW)**, young maternal age, limited parental education, day care attendance, exposure to tobacco smoke, industrial pollution, urban residence, congenital heart disease, chronic lung disease, male gender, and asthma.[2] Pneumonia often occurs during preschool years when children are first being exposed to pathogens and their **immunity** is weak. Factors affecting its **etiology** include patient age, vaccination status, relevant exposure, immunologic status, and clinical settings in which the disease was acquired.[3] Clinical features include cough and/or fever plus shallow breathing, splinting, rapid breathing, rales, and lung consolidation.[4]

Pneumonia and malnutrition are the two leading causes of death and morbidity in under-5 children in developing countries.[5,6] Pneumonia accounted for 18% of the estimated 7.6 million global deaths in under-5 children in 2010.[7] Approximately 90–95% of these deaths occur in developing countries, especially in South Asia and sub-Saharan Africa.[8,9]

Malnutrition alone is associated with 56% of deaths worldwide among children under age 5 years.[10,11] A common comorbidity in under-5 children with pneumonia in developing nations, severe acute malnutrition (SAM) is associated with 15 times the risk of death compared with children without SAM.[12] Death is usually due to uncommon bacterial etiology compared with those without severe malnutrition.[13,14,15]

Interaction Between Pneumonia and Malnutrition

The majority of childhood deaths globally are associated with malnutrition,[16,17,18,19,20,21,22,23,24,25] yet few studies evaluate the interaction between pneumonia and malnutrition. Mortality risk increases among severely malnourished children with pneumonia.[26] Factors contributing to variations in the magnitude of risk between studies[27] may include differences in the proportion of children with severe malnutrition, geographical variations, and the prevalence of other comorbidities, such as human immunodeficiency virus (HIV) infection. High mortality risk can be linked to immunodeficiency associated with malnutrition, high rates of comorbidities, delayed health-seeking behavior among families of children with malnutrition, and potential delays in diagnosis due to the insensitivity of clinical signs.[28,29,30]

Malnutrition–Infection Complex

The malnutrition–infection complex is a vicious cycle. The first aspect is malnutrition, which compromises host defense. The second is infection, which either exacerbates an existing nutritional deficiency or causes malnutrition during disease pathogenesis. Malnutrition can assist pathogen invasion and promulgation. It increases the likelihood of a secondary infection and thus alters disease pathogenesis and prognosis.[31] Certain infectious diseases, including pneumonia, can cause malnutrition.

Effects of Infection on Metabolism and Nutritional Status

Interactions between malnutrition, immune inhibition, and infection are complex. The infection can suppress appetite and directly affect nutrient metabolism, causing the poor utilization of nutrients[32] and loss of critical body stores of protein, energy, minerals, and vitamins.

During an immune response, hypermetabolism, or increased energy expenditure, is often simultaneous with reduced nutrient intake.[33] The metabolic response to infection also includes negative **nitrogen balance**, increased **gluconeogenesis**, and increased fat oxidation, which is modulated by hormones, cytokines, and other proinflammatory mediators.[34] Negative nitrogen balance persists for days to weeks after the febrile phase, and it appears correlated with loss of body weight. Both conditions result from reduced food intake and infection-induced increased nitrogen excretion, and they contribute to malnutrition.[35,36]

Malnutrition's Effects on Immunity

Malnutrition is associated with impairment of protective activity of vital organs of the body,[37,38,39] leading to poorer immunity and increased susceptibility to infectious diseases, including pneumonia.[40,41]

Leptin, produced by **adipose tissue** during the **acute phase response**, is part of the antibacterial host defense.[42,43,44] Leptin prevents **lymphoid tissue** atrophy, reconstitutes lymphoid **cellularity**, and restores defense activity during malnutrition.[45] Human leptin may also modulate the activation of **CD4+** and CD8+ T-cells from infected malnourished children.[46] Lower serum leptin level reduces cellularity in the spleen and thymus, and is associated with increased susceptibility to infections, such as pneumonia. Serum leptin levels normally increase acutely during infection and inflammation,[47,48] but are lower in children with SAM and pneumonia.[49,50] Thus, diminished leptin concentrations in malnourished children may contribute to susceptibility to pneumonia.[51]

Etiology of Pneumonia in Children with SAM

Bacterial and viral infections are more common causes of pneumonia, although it can also result from fungal infections.

Types of Pneumonia-Causing Bacteria

A recent systematic review revealed that bacteria caused 42% of cases in 509 children with SAM and pneumonia.[52] Among 11 studies that evaluated the etiology of pneumonia

in children with SAM, six used blood cultures alone to identify the causative organism,[53,54,55,56,57,58] four used lung aspirates alone,[59,60,61,62] and one used both methods. The most commonly isolated organisms in severely malnourished children with pneumonia were, in descending order: *Klebsiella* species, *Staphylococcus aureus, Streptococcus pneumonia* (Pneumococcus), *Escherichia coli, Haemophilus influenzae,* and *Salmonella* species (**Figure 12-1**). Species of *Acinetobacter, Pseudomonas, Moraxella,* and *Enterobacter* were rare. Findings varied considerably between individual studies.

Viral Pneumonia

Three of the studies also investigated viral etiology, but diagnostic yields were low.[63,64,65] Only one detailed study of viral agents in malnourished children with pneumonia was identified.[66] In 55 of 158 (35%) children, a viral agent was identified, comprising adenovirus (17%), respiratory syncytial virus (6%), parainfluenza virus (6%), herpes simplex virus (6%), influenza A virus (5%), measles virus (3%), and influenza B virus (1%).

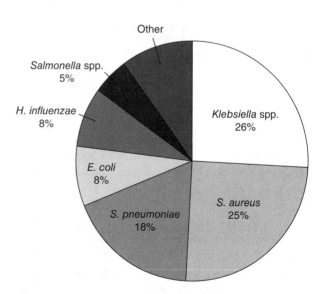

Figure 12-1 Proportion of bacterial isolates in children (n=215) with pneumonia and severe malnutrition from all reports combined

Reproduced from Chisti, M. J., Tebruegge, M., La Vincente, S., Graham, S. M., & Duke, T. (2009). Pneumonia in severely malnourished children in developing countries—mortality risk, etiology and validity of WHO clinical signs: a systematic review. *Tropical Medicine & International Health, 14*(10), 1173-1189.

Studying Pneumonia's Etiology in Malnourished Children: Methods and Challenges

Data on etiology of pneumonia in children with SAM compared with those without SAM are not extensive, in part due to lack of safe and reliable diagnostic procedures. **Percutaneous aspiration** from the consolidated portion of the lung is the gold standard for determining the etiological agent of pneumonia, with isolation rates of 25–79%.[67,68] However, this diagnostic procedure is associated with complications such as **pneumothorax** and mortality,[69,70] especially in children infected with HIV and with pneumonia caused by *Pneumocystis jiroveci*. The use of blood cultures is safer, but yield is below 40%.[71,72,73,74] Improving diagnostic techniques to facilitate case management should be a public health priority.

Some concern over microbiological techniques results from potential underestimation of more fastidious organisms, such as *H. influenzae*.[75,76,77] In addition, the use of antibiotics prior to culture presents a potential bias against isolation of sensitive organisms. Antibiotics are commonly prescribed for acute respiratory infections at peripheral health facilities prior to referral to central hospitals and nutritional rehabilitation units. Furthermore, severely malnourished children who develop pneumonia after admission will usually be receiving a broad-spectrum antibiotic, such as cotrimoxazole, as routine prophylaxis. Also, timing of investigations and interventions vary, and can potentially distort the microbiological data reported. Another factor is whether infections were hospital- rather than community-acquired.

Trends in Etiology

Cases caused by *Pneumococcus* and *H. influenzae* type b are likely to decrease as vaccines against these causative agents become more common in developing nations.[78,79,80,81] *Mycoplasma pneumoniae* is among the common causes of pneumonia in preschool children, as an **opportunistic pathogen**, although it was previously more common in school-aged children.[82]

Differences in Etiology Between Malnourished and Healthy Children

The spectrum and frequency of causative organisms varies between severely malnourished and well-nourished children. *Klebsiella*, *S. aureus* species, and other Gram-negative, enteric organisms, such as *E. coli* and *Salmonella* species, are common in severely malnourished children.[83] In contrast, *S. pneumoniae* is the most common causative bacterial organism of community-acquired pneumonia in children in industrialized countries, while enteric organisms are rare.[84,85,86] Similar observations were made in studies including well-nourished children with pneumonia in developing countries, which reported *S. pneumoniae* and *H. influenzae* as the most common causative agents.[87,88]

Children with malnutrition can be more prone to infections of **Enterobacteriaceae**, including *Klebsiella* species, *E. coli*, *Salmonella* species, and *S. aureus*, because of impaired immune function, including lower leptin levels, and poorer clearance of *S. aureus* from the lungs.[89,90] Increased oropharyngeal colonization with enteric bacilli[91] can facilitate the spread of these pathogens to the lower respiratory tract with or without additional insults, such as viral respiratory tract infections. Breaches of bowel mucosal integrity and translocation of bacteria may lead to Gram-negative **bacteremia** and pneumonia.[92]

Children with SAM have fewer immune cells, such as leukocytes and neutrophils. In addition, leucocytes have reduced ability to kill ingested microorganisms and to replicate, leading to higher morbidity.[93] Defective alveolar macrophage function is another possible explanation for reduced bacterial clearance and increased mortality observed in severely malnourished children with pneumonia.[94] This is a probable reason that despite being uncommon in pneumonic children without SAM, *Klebsiella* species, and *S. aureus* are common in children with pneumonia and SAM; it also necessitates a differential algorithm of antibiotics for the management of this special population.

Future Research Required to Better Address the Problem

Three areas related to the etiology of pneumonia in severely malnourished children remain largely unexplored.[95] First, the role of viral infections is unclear. In particular, data are lacking regarding which viral agents predominate in these children and whether the spectrum of viruses differs from that observed in well-nourished children. Second, the role of *M. tuberculosis* presenting as acute lower respiratory infection in severely malnourished children has not been studied in detail, although this area is likely to be highly important in tuberculosis (TB)-endemic countries. Third, the causes of pneumonia in HIV-infected children with coexisting malnutrition have also not been sufficiently studied,[96,97] despite the great potential relevance to public health in countries with high HIV prevalence.

Pneumonia is closely related to TB and HIV.[98,99] Considering the possibility of TB and HIV in cases of acute pneumonia could help prevent progression of TB infection to TB disease,[100] especially in sub-Saharan Africa.

Pathogenesis of Pneumonia in Children with SAM

This section focuses on the pathogenesis of bacterial pneumonia, which is better defined than that of viral pneumonia in children with SAM. Most cases of pneumonia result from inhalation of contaminated air. Pharyngeal secretions contain saliva with potentially high concentrations of bacteria, and person-to-person transmission through droplets can occur. Even well-nourished children can be infected through inhalation or microaspiration.[101]

Development of pneumonia depends on interactions between bacteria and the host defense and respiratory systems.[102] Most inhaled bacteria are surrounded by moisture, which promotes infection. Smaller droplets are more infectious because they can invade deeper into the lungs, while larger particles do not usually pass through the pharynx.[103]

The respiratory tract below the principal bronchi is usually sterile, but additional host defense mechanisms are recruited when bacteria gain access to the **alveolus**. However, these mechanisms often fail to destroy alveolar bacteria in children with pneumonia and SAM, who are often deficient in certain immune cells. This immunodeficiency leads to inability to efficiently clear bacteria from the lungs[104] and better pathogen survival. This stage is known as the phase of congestion because it is characterized by signs of congestion in the lungs.[105]

In the presence of fluid in the lungs, bacteria can spread quickly among alveoli.[106] The disease can progress with signs including clustering of red blood cells, or red hepatization, and bacterial clumping.[107] Further deterioration leads to the stage known as gray hepatization.[108] This process in children with SAM may be evident without any overt clinical manifestation, a condition often termed occult pneumonia, which often delays the diagnosis as well as management in such children with poor prognosis.[109] In the stage of resolution, white blood cells phagocytocize bacteria and remove cellular debris.[110] If the lung reticular structure remains intact, complete recovery can occur with successful treatment.[111]

Pathogenesis caused by other bacteria varies; complete recovery is often less likely due to rapid bacterial spread throughout the alveolar spaces with a characteristic pneumonia. Rapid spread caused by Gram-negative bacteria and *S. aureus* are responsible for extensive necrosis.[112] Death from bacterial pneumonia is due mainly to respiratory failure due to fluid-filled air spaces complicated by shock and acidosis.[113,114]

Diagnosis and Clinical Manifestations of Pneumonia in Children with SAM

Proper diagnosis of pneumonia and SAM in children and recognition of their clinical manifestations are critical in public health. Rapid, accurate diagnosis allows earlier treatment and better outcomes, while identifying, interpreting, and appropriately treating clinical signs is necessary for optimizing recovery.

Diagnosis of Pneumonia

Diagnosis of pneumonia optimally includes a combination of history, clinical signs, and chest X-ray. An abnormal chest X-ray is considered radiological pneumonia.[115,116] While chest X-rays are generally considered to be a reliable diagnostic tool in all forms of pneumonia, they are prone to interobserver variability in interpretation.[117,118,119] Radiographic changes may be vague, inconclusive, or even absent despite the presence of clinical signs of pneumonia.[120,121,122] Conversely, clinical signs of pneumonia can be absent in the presence of radiological signs of pneumonia.[123,124,125]

Adequate laboratory and radiological services are frequently absent in primary healthcare facilities where malnourished children present with pneumonia, and auscultation has not been sufficiently validated as a diagnostic criterion. WHO therefore recommends basing the diagnosis of pneumonia primarily on visible clinical parameters, including respiratory rate and chest wall in-drawing (**Table 12-2**).[126,127,128]

Among well-nourished children, most of the clinical signs have acceptable sensitivity and specificity.[129,130,131,132,133,134,135,136] Fast breathing and chest in-drawing are usually reported to perform well as clinical predictors of pneumonia. The sensitivity of both parameters appears to be at least 80%; the specificity is above 90%.

In contrast, among children with SAM, the predictive power of most clinical signs is lower. In children with severe malnutrition, the sensitivity of fast breathing as a predictor

Table 12-2 WHO algorithm for the diagnosis of pneumonia (children presenting with cough and/or respiratory difficulty)

Age	Clinical Parameter	Diagnosis
< 2 months of age	• Respiratory rate ≥ 60/min and/or • Lower chest wall in-drawing • (but no signs of very severe pneumonia)	Severe pneumonia
	Any of the below: • Central cyanosis • Not able to drink • Head nodding	Very severe pneumonia
2-60 months of age	• Respiratory rate ≥ 50/min (for 2-11 months of age) • Respiratory rate ≥ 40/min (for 12-60 months of age) • (but no signs of severe or very severe pneumonia)	Pneumonia
	• Lower chest wall in-drawing • (but no signs of very severe pneumonia)	Severe pneumonia
	Any one of the following: • Central cyanosis • Unable to drink • Head nodding	Very severe pneumonia

Reproduced from the World Health Organization (WHO). (2006). *Pocket book of hospital care for children: Guidelines for the management of common illness with limited resources.* Geneva: Author. 69-108.

of radiographically proven pneumonia ranged from 14% to 76%, and specificity from 66% to 100%.[137,138] For chest in-drawing alone, sensitivity was overall poor and widely variable (range: 17–71%), while specificity was high (range: 95–98%). One study reported a sensitivity of 87% for the combination of WHO-defined fast breathing and subcostal retractions (specificity not reported).[139] Another reported 97–100% specificity and sensitivity of 39–60% when fast breathing was defined as at least 50 breaths per minute or at least 40 breaths per minute, respectively.[140]

These studies in children with pneumonia and SAM suggest that 29–86% of pneumonia cases will be missed if fast-breathing and/or chest wall in-drawing are used as the sole diagnostic signs. The wide range may be due to heterogeneity of the study populations, large variation in sample sizes and wide confidence intervals, and bias related to the subjectivity in the assessment of these clinical signs.

Clinical Manifestations

Respiratory muscle weakness is common and may account for the poor predictive power of fast breathing and chest in-drawing in severely malnourished children. Muscle

wasting can result from protein deficiency and depletion of micronutrients and electrolytes, including potassium.[141] Muscle weakness increases mortality risk by delaying diagnosis and treatment, and also because of hypercapnic ventilatory failure. Alternative therapies, such as continuous positive airway pressure (CPAP), may therefore be beneficial.

Children with acute watery diarrhea (AWD) often present with dehydration, which is commonly associated with metabolic acidosis[142,143,144] due to fecal loss of bicarbonate.[145] Clinical features of pneumonia and metabolic acidosis often overlap,[146] making differentiation of pneumonia from metabolic acidosis more difficult.[147] The classic feature of metabolic acidosis in children with dehydrating diarrhea is fast, deep breathing,[148] often misinterpreted as lower chest wall in-drawing by healthcare workers; this sign disappears after the correction of dehydration.[149,150]

When fast breathing and lower chest wall in-drawing are caused by pneumonia, they persist even after full rehydration,[151] thus allowing for diagnosis of pneumonia after full rehydration. However, the slow rate of rehydration[152,153,154] leads to possible delays in initiating appropriate antibiotics, potentially increasing morbidity and deaths. Children with or without SAM and with diarrhea, pneumonia, and metabolic acidosis frequently display clinical dehydration and persistent systolic hypotension even after adequate rehydration.[155] However, because metabolic acidosis has no impact on the diagnostic clinical features of pneumonia in young diarrheal children, early initiation of appropriate antibiotics to combat morbidity and deaths in such populations can occur.[156,157]

Potentially useful clinical diagnostic tools have not been extensively researched. For example, pulse oximetry to detect hypoxemia as an indicator of severe pneumonia has not been sufficiently evaluated in children with SAM.

The laboratory in the Medical Research Council (MRC) in the Gambia achieves relatively high organism yield using lung puncture;[158] currently, this method is being used in the global pneumonia etiology research in child health (PERCH) study.[159] In this context, if facilities are available for careful monitoring and managing complications effectively by trained personnel, percutaneous lung aspiration would be the recommended diagnostic test among certain children with acute pneumonia and SAM and/or HIV. This approach potentially promotes lifesaving early initiation of appropriate antibiotic therapy.

Management of Pneumonia in Children with SAM

Effective management of pneumonia in children with SAM usually involves antibiotics, addressing nutritional deficiencies and respiratory support to avoid or treat hypoxemia. Antibiotic therapy depends on the cause of pneumonia, which often varies if the disease is hospital-acquired. Children should be monitored, and treatment should reflect any changes in condition.

Antibiotics for Pneumonia

Chloramphenicol was formerly recommended as a first-line treatment of pneumonia in severely malnourished children.[160,161,162] However, WHO now recommends a combination of parenteral ampicillin and gentamicin,[163] as they are more effective against enteric Gram-negative bacilli than chloramphenicol.

Guidelines for type and dose of antibiotics and duration of therapy for pneumonia should ideally be based on local patterns, since the extent and spectrum of antibiotic resistance of bacterial organisms vary by region. If treatment fails, *Klebsiella* and *S. aureus* should be considered.[164,165,166,167]

Hospital-acquired pneumonia develops 48 to 72 hours after admission to a hospital. It is the leading cause of death worldwide of nosocomial infections.[168,169] Early-onset hospital-acquired pneumonia appears within five days of admission and is caused by *H. influenza;* methicillin-sensitive *S. aureus* (MSSA); nonresistant enteric Gram-negative organisms, such as *Enterobacter, E. coli, Klebsiella, Proteus,* and *Serratia*; *S. pneumoniae;* and (rarely) *Legionella.* Treatment includes monotherapy with core antibiotics, such as third-generation cephalosporins.

Late-onset hospital-acquired pneumonia occurs five or more days after admission. It is caused by antibiotic-resistant Gram-negatives, such as *Pseudomonas aeruginosa, Acinetobacter,* or, as with early-onset pneumonia, by enteric Gram-negative organisms. Treatment for methicillin-resistant *S. aureus,* or MRSA, involves antipseudomonal cephalosporin plus aminoglycosides, amikacin, or a fluoroquinolone.

In children with SAM, antibiotic therapy should be given for at least seven days in uncomplicated cases of childhood pneumonia. With a comorbidity or complication, such as cystic fibrosis, pulmonary sequestration, bronchiectasis, primary ciliary dyskinesia, immunoglobulin deficiency, HIV, or empyema, treatment should be continued from weeks to months.[170] For suspected *S. aureus* infection, treatment may last 14 to 21 days.[171] Treatment for neonates[172] and for children with hospital-acquired pneumonia[173] should be continued for at least two weeks. Shifting from parenteral therapy to oral therapy is a main objective in the management of childhood pneumonia. It hastens discharge from the hospital and helps prevent subsequent hospital-acquired infections in other hospitalized children. Switching to oral antibiotics takes longer in children with SAM.

Nutritional Management of Pneumonia in Children with SAM

Nutritional therapy should address existing energy and nutrient deficiencies and meet ongoing needs. Routine supplementation of magnesium, potassium chloride, folic acid, and multivitamins for the management of malnutrition, given for at least four weeks, appears to be beneficial.[174]

Calorie Requirements

Adequate energy, or at least 70 to 80 kcal/kg/day, with minimal volume (less than 100 ml/kg/day) is essential. If no diarrhea occurs within 96 hours of admission, fluid volume can be increased to as much as 150 ml/kg/day and calories to 150 kcal/kg/day.[175] To prevent hypoglycemia, children with SAM and pneumonia should not fast for more than four hours.[176,177]

Micronutrient Supplementation

Zinc: Oral daily dose of 20 mg of zinc provided at least until discharge may improve recovery from severe pneumonia by reducing the duration of hypoxemia,[178,179,180] but some research results are conflicting.[181] Thus, zinc should be considered cautiously in each case.

Vitamin A:[182] In children with **xerophthalmia**, vitamin A should be given on each of days 1, 2, and 15 or the day of discharge at doses of 200,000 international units (IU) for children over 1 year of age, 100,000 IU for infants 6 to 12 months, and 50,000 IU for those under 6 months of age. If inflammation is present, eyes are protected with pads and chloramphenicol eyedrops are given every six hours until improvement of signs, such as pus in the eye or redness and watery eyes. For corneal ulceration, atropine eyedrops should be administered once daily in addition to chloramphenicol eyedrops, and the affected eye should be covered with a pad and bandaged. The eyes should be examined very gently, as they easily become damaged in vitamin A deficiency.

Multivitamins:[183] Multivitamin (MV) drops are provided for at least one month, or, for very severely malnourished children, until the end of nutritional rehabilitation. The supplement includes vitamins A, D, C, B1 (thiamine), B2 (riboflavin), B3 (niacin), and B5 (pantothenic acid).

Folic acid:[184] One-quarter of a 5 mg tablet of folic acid is provided daily for at least 15 days or until the end of nutritional rehabilitation.

Potassium:[185] Severely malnourished children have markedly decreased potassium stores. Potassium solution is given by mouth for five days.

Magnesium:[186] Daily intramuscular injection of magnesium sulphate is provided for seven days at a dose dependent on the liquid volume of the diet.

Management of Hypoxemia in Children with SAM

Hypoxemia, a common and the most serious manifestation of childhood pneumonia, is often associated with mortality.[187,188,189] An SpO2 of at least 92% indicates satisfactory oxygenation.[190] Hypoxemia is defined as SpO2 of less than 90% in room air at sea level as measured by pulse oximetry.[191] It can be mild, moderate, or severe.[192]

- Mild hypoxemia: arterial oxygen saturation of 85–89%
- Moderate hypoxemia: arterial oxygen saturation of 80–84%
- Severe hypoxemia: arterial oxygen saturation of less than 80%

In the critical care setting for childhood pneumonia, pulse oximetry is a more common monitoring modality.[193] When pulse oximetry is unavailable, oxygen supplementation should be given when these conditions are present:[194]

1. Central cyanosis
2. Severe lower chest-wall in-drawing
3. Grunting respiration
4. Restlessness (due to hypoxemia)
5. Inability to drink or feed
6. Respiratory rate less than 70 breaths per minute
7. Head nodding

Follow-Up During Management of Pneumonia in SAM

During the acute phase, the patient's condition should be reassessed at least twice daily to evaluate the clinical improvement and discharge. Intravenous therapy should be changed to oral if there is clinical improvement, such as the following:[195]

1. Afebrile for at least 24 hours
2. Normalizing of white blood cell (WBC) count, if data are available
3. No vomiting
4. No other reason for IV therapy

If no improvement occurs, the following possibilities should be considered:[196]

1. Wrong diagnosis
2. Inappropriate antibiotic or route of administration
3. Presence of tuberculosis
4. Host failure, such as immunosuppression or chronic suppurative lung disease (CSLD), with chronic wet cough and lung damage
5. Infection with an unusual pathogen, such as a virus, fungus, or MRSA
6. Complication, such as empyema or effusion

The patient should be discharged if there is clinical improvement with no comorbidities requiring treatment plus the following conditions:[197]

1. CRT less than 3 seconds and RR normal for age
2. Arterial oxygen saturation at least 90%
3. Temperature less than 38 degrees Celsius (100 degrees Fahrenheit) for 24 hours
4. Oral feeding

The subsequent nutritional rehabilitation phase aims to recover lost weight by intensive feeding. The child is stimulated emotionally and physically, and the mother should be trained to continue care at home.[198] Extensive follow-up should be done to prevent nutritional relapse and to ensure the child's proper physical growth and mental development.[199]

Prognosis and Outcome of Pneumonia in Children with SAM

Timely administration of antibiotics improves outcome in bacterial pneumonia. Lung structure and tissue almost always return to normal even in children with complicating empyema and lung abscess.[200] Recurrent pneumonia, defined as at least two episodes in one year or three or more episodes at any age with radiographic cleaning between episodes, should prompt evaluation for other disorders,[201] such as cystic fibrosis, pulmonary sequestration, bronchiectasis, primary ciliary dyskinesia, immunoglobulin deficiency, and HIV.[202]

Complications of Pneumonia in Children with SAM

Data on complications are rare. Most children appear to recover without complications,[203] but some immediate and late complications can occur.

Immediate Complications

Hypoglycemia can indicate infection, and children should be tested on admission and when lethargy, convulsions, or **hypothermia** occur. If blood glucose cannot be measured biochemically, children with SAM suspected to have hypoglycemia should be treated to prevent the chance of death within minutes. A conscious child with blood glucose under 3 mmol/L (54 mg/dl) should receive a 50 ml bolus of 10% glucose or 10% sucrose solution or one rounded teaspoon of sugar in 3.5 tablespoons water orally or by nasogastric tube. The starter diet **F-75** is given every 30 minutes for 2 hours. Thereafter, bi-hourly feeds are continued for 24–48 hours. Children who are unconscious, lethargic, or convulsing should receive sterile 10% glucose (5 ml/kg) by IV, followed by 50 ml of 10% glucose or sucrose by nasogastric tube and, when possible, the starter diet F-75.[204,205]

Septic shock in children with SAM and pneumonia presents with a weak or absent radial pulse, delayed CRT (more than two seconds), cold periphery, or hypoglycemia. Treatment includes isotonic saline of 20 ml/kg over one hour. This rescue therapy should be repeated once if signs of shock remain after the first dose. Broad-spectrum antibiotic coverage includes intravenous daily doses of 100 mg/kg of ceftriaxone and 10 mg/kg levofloxacin. Other supportive measures, including oxygen therapy, and correction of hypoglycemia, hypothermia, or acidosis, should also be taken.[206]

The first step of management of **hypothermia** in children is to wrap them in blankets. An electric lamp may be used, fixing it close to the body for warmth, but the lamp should be kept in a comfortable distance from the body of the child to avoid potential burns. Moreover, to avoid potential hyperthermia, temperature should be measured every 30 minutes during rewarming with a lamp. Feeding should be ensured as soon as possible to prevent the potential development of hypoglycemia, as hypothermia often coexists with hypoglycemia.[207]

Late Complications

Persistent **pleural effusions** and empyema are the most common serious complications of bacterial pneumonia, often with fatal outcome.[208] An **intraparenchymal** cavity containing air that represents a **pneumatocele**, a **cavitation**, an **abscess**, or rarely, a sequel of massive lung **necrosis** is associated with bacterial pneumonia in these children.[209] A pneumatocele typically appears in the convalescent period and may either resolve spontaneously within weeks or linger for months before it gradually diminishes and disappears.[210,211] Sepsis occurs in less than 10% of cases in children with SAM, but it can cause fatal shock. Tension pneumothorax is an uncommon complication and usually associated with *S. aureus* pneumonia.[212]

Prevention of Deaths of Pneumonia in Children with SAM on a Public Health Level

Appropriate management of pneumonia is imperative in reducing childhood deaths.[213] Early diagnosis is critical. A concern in developing nations is that sick children may be taken first to primary healthcare centers that do not have radiological facilities, thus delaying diagnosis and commencement of treatment.[214] In addition, in children with SAM, the use of clinical features to diagnose pneumonia has produced conflicting results due to poor sensitivity and specificity.[215,216]

Role of Public Health in Reducing Effects of Pneumonia

The success of the fourth United Nations Millennium Development Goal (MDG 4) will depend in no small part on a reduction in this enormous burden of child and neonatal mortality related to acute respiratory infection. The first two subsets of this goal specify, respectively, the reduction of the under-5 and infant mortality rates.

> ***Millennium Development Goal 4.A: Reduce by two-thirds, between 1990 and 2015, the under-five mortality rate***
>
> Reproduced from the United Nations. (n.d.). 2015 Millennium Development Goals. Retrieved from http://www.un.org/millenniumgoals/. Accessed August 13, 2013. This source is used for all Millennium Development Goals in this chapter.

Pneumonia is the main disease targeted by the WHO program on acute respiratory infection. Priority interventions to reduce the global burden of deaths of pneumonia include improving nutrition and rates of breastfeeding, reducing indoor air pollution and overcrowded housing, facilitating access to antibiotics, encouraging care-seeking behavior and better referral practices, and improving the quality of case management.[217,218] If the case management of pneumonia is to have a significant impact on global child mortality, the relevant guidelines will need to address those groups of children at highest risk of death. Children with SAM account for a large proportion of this high-risk population, especially in Southeast Asia and sub-Saharan Africa.

Roles of Public Health Professionals in Reducing Effects of Pneumonia

Objectives of public health professionals include:

- Increased awareness of the risk factors of pneumonia in severe malnutrition
- Immediate diagnosis of pneumonia
- Prompt and aggressive treatment
- Reduced cost associated with other unnecessary investigations and complications due to inappropriate treatment
- Prevention of pneumonia through proper nutrition and vaccination
- Prevention of death through appropriate diagnosis and prompt aggressive medical treatment, case monitoring, and maintenance of nutrition with appropriate diet, including micronutrients
- Achieving the best possible care through education of healthcare workers and family members and provision of reassurance to family members

Addressing SAM on a Population Level

Preventing SAM

Public health focuses on prevention, and prevention of SAM is cost-effective as well as likely to lead to better health outcomes. Large-scale malnutrition is typically linked to poverty, and public health programs to prevent malnutrition focus on direct and indirect interventions. Eradication of social injustice is an ambitious but necessary goal to prevent disparities in nutrition status and health outcomes. Governments and other stakeholders must take appropriate measures to minimize the destructive effects of natural disasters and ultimately prevent poverty and hunger.

> ***Public Health Core Competency 1: Analytical /Assessment Skills 1: Identifies the health status of populations and their related determinants of health and illness***
>
> Reproduced from Council on Linkages Between Academia and Public Health Practice. 2010 May. Core Competencies for Public Health Professionals. Washington, DC: Public Health Foundation. http://www.phf.org/resourcestools/Documents/Core_Competencies_for_Public_Health_Professionals_2010May.pdf. Accessed August 13, 2013. This source is used for all Public Health Core Competencies in this chapter.

Community-level and nationwide improvements in **food security** could potentially greatly reduce SAM among children and improve their ability to fight pneumonia-causing pathogens. Food assistance programs can provide increased energy and protein for mothers, leading to healthier children. Adequate provision of micronutrients through supplementation and food fortification can be effective in preventing nutrient deficiencies; these programs require widespread support, often from governments and international organizations. One public health program to reduce pneumonia provided fortified milk with zinc and/or iron supplementation for SAM children. The results included significantly reduced incidence of pneumonia and reduction in deaths of pneumonia in developing countries, including India.[219,220]

Nutrition education to promote exclusive breastfeeding and prevent early and late weaning can not only prevent malnutrition in infants, but also strengthen their immune systems due to factors present only in breastmilk. Prenatal care with adequate micronutrient supplementation during pregnancy is another approach. Finally, public health systems and doctors need to take appropriate measures, such as surveillance, to prevent repeated outbreaks and infections, especially of pneumonia and diarrhea.

These are some examples of recent public health programs to reduce SAM:

- Ready-to-use therapeutic foods (RUTF) are large daily allowances of low-cost, locally available, and culturally acceptable food containing a mixture of milk powder, sugar, vegetable oil, peanut butter, vitamins, and minerals. Programs in Chad and Malawi have shown significant reductions in the severity of malnutrition, and similar programs in other developing nations are likely to be successful.[221]

- Adoption of a public health community-level program for local peanut farmer growers can stimulate the local economy, at the time suffering from 80% unemployment, while increasing the nutrient supply to children.

- Prenatal care with adequate micronutrients supplementation during pregnancy in India showed significant reduction of the rate of low-birth-weight babies that helped to prevent malnutrition.[222]

Treating SAM

Initial treatment needs to avoid providing too much protein, which can lead to refeeding syndrome and the possibility of cardiac or liver failure. Early detection of SAM and prompt and aggressive management of complication in the acute phase (first five to seven days) aims to reduce childhood mortality from SAM. The rehabilitation phase (two to four weeks) aims to attain sufficient growth. Proper evaluation of management during the follow-up phase aims to maintain growth and to prevent potential malnutrition-related mortality at home.

Improving the Environment to Reduce Pneumonia Incidence

Since pneumonia is an infection of the lungs, reducing environmental insults to the lungs can help prevent pneumonia. Indoor air pollution, which the WHO identifies as among the top global risk factors in developing nations, can be reduced with better ventilation and cooking outdoors rather than indoors. Education can be an effective public health approach to reduce indoor air pollution. Reduction of industrial smoke can occur through stricter regulation.

Other measures include reducing housing overcrowding, which is a by-product of poverty. Finally, improving sanitation can reduce the spread of infections. Measures include education to improve handwashing practice among the public and healthcare professionals, as well as the use of safe drinking water.

> *Millennium Development Goal 7: Ensure Environmental Sustainability. Target 7.C: Halve, by 2015, the proportion of people without sustainable access to safe drinking water and basic sanitation*

Policy to Improve Treatment

Policy makers should modify local, national, and WHO guidelines for the management of pneumonia in severely malnourished children. The choice of antibiotics demands special attention, since causes of pneumonia in children with SAM and/or HIV differ from causes in children without severe malnutrition. Evaluation of tuberculosis in children who present with pneumonia and SAM and/or HIV should be an integral part of guidelines for managing pneumonia. Modified policies can improve treatment and reduce morbidity and mortality among children with SAM.

Consistent with WHO recommendations, policy makers should prioritize interventions to reduce the global burden of deaths of pneumonia through improved nutrition, including greater exclusive breastfeeding and appropriate complementary feeding. Other approaches include reducing indoor air pollution and overcrowded housing, facilitating access to antibiotics, encouraging care-seeking behavior and better referral practices, and improving the quality of case management.[223,224] For case management of pneumonia to significantly impact global child mortality, the relevant guidelines need to address those groups of children at highest risk of death.

Policy makers should consider ways to improve education through appropriate media, including the use of mass media, similar to what has been done for management of diarrhea with messages relating to home management and referral to healthcare facilities.[225] Parents and caregivers of children often have poor knowledge about the simple clinical signs of pneumonia.[226] Parents should be educated and cautioned to look for the signs of increasing respiratory distress, danger signs of severe/very severe pneumonia, and clinical signs of hypoxemia and advised to seek medical attention immediately if any of these signs appear.

Health professionals, especially health workers in district hospitals, should receive initial and ongoing training on transmitting knowledge to caregivers and mothers of under-5 children about recognizing the simple clinical signs of pneumonia. Increasing the awareness of signs and risk factors of pneumonia is important to mitigate pneumonia-related deaths.

Future Research

Further research is necessary to better treat pneumonia and SAM in children. Investigators need to know whether the spectrum of viruses differs from that observed in well-nourished children. Another research goal is to evaluate the role of *Mycobacterium tuberculosis* presenting as acute pneumonia in severely malnourished children in TB-endemic countries. Similarly, researchers would like to determine the causes of pneumonia in HIV-infected children with coexisting malnutrition in countries with high HIV prevalence.

Conclusion

Pneumonia and SAM are among the top killers of children under 5 years. Currently available data suggest that the spectrum and frequency of causative agents of pneumonia in severely malnourished children differ from those observed in well-nourished children. Early and appropriate treatment are necessary, but clinical signs are relatively poor predictors of pneumonia in severely malnourished children. Treatment usually consists of injectable antibiotics and nutritional support. To achieve MDG 4, research and improved policy are needed to explore the significance and impact of viral agents and *M. tuberculosis* on acute respiratory disease in malnourished children and ultimately to improve the prevention, early detection, management, and outcome of pneumonia in severely malnourished children in resource-poor settings.

References

1 Liu, L., Johnson, H. L., Cousens, S., Perin, J., Scott, S., Lawn, J. E., . . . Black, R. E.; Child Health Epidemiology Reference Group of WHO and UNICEF. (2012). Global, regional, and national causes of child mortality: An updated systematic analysis for 2010 with time trends since 2000. *Lancet, 379*(9832), 2151-61.

2 Crawford, S. E., & Daum, R. S. (2008). Bacterial pneumonia, lung abscess, and empyema. In L. M. Taussig & L. I. Landau (Eds.), *Pediatric respiratory medicine* (Vol. 2, pp. 501-53). Philadelphia, PA: Mosby Elsevier.

3 Crawford, S. E., & Daum, R. S. (2008). Bacterial pneumonia, lung abscess, and empyema. In L. M. Taussig & L. I. Landau (Eds.), *Pediatric respiratory medicine* (Vol. 2, pp. 501-53). Philadelphia, PA: Mosby Elsevier.

4 Crawford, S. E., & Daum, R. S. (2008). Bacterial pneumonia, lung abscess, and empyema. In L. M. Taussig & L. I. Landau (Eds.), *Pediatric respiratory medicine* (Vol. 2, pp. 501-53). Philadelphia, PA: Mosby Elsevier.

5 Black, R. E., Cousens, S., Johnson, H. L., Lawn, J. E., Rudan, I., Bassani, D. G., . . . Mathers, C., for the Child Health Epidemiology Reference Group of WHO and UNICEF. (2010). Global, regional, and national causes of child mortality in 2008: A systematic analysis. *Lancet, 375*(9730), 1969-87.

6 Chisti, M. J., Tebruegge, M., La Vincente, S., Graham, S. M., & Duke, T. (2009). Pneumonia in severely malnourished children in developing countries: Mortality risk, etiology and validity of WHO clinical signs: A systematic review. *Tropical Medicine & International Health, 14*(10), 1173-89.

7 Liu, L., Johnson, H. L., Cousens, S., Perin, J., Scott, S., Lawn, J. E., . . . Black, R. E.; Child Health Epidemiology Reference Group of WHO and UNICEF. (2012). Global, regional, and national causes of child mortality: An updated systematic analysis for 2010 with time trends since 2000. *Lancet, 379*(9832), 2151-61.

8 Mulholland, K. (2003). Global burden of acute respiratory infections in children: Implications for interventions. *Pediatric Pulmonology, 36*(6), 469-74.

9 Williams, B. G., Gouws, E., Boschi-Pinto, C., Bryce, J., & Dye, C. (2002). Estimates of world-wide distribution of child deaths from acute respiratory infections. *Lancet Infectious Diseases, 2*(1), 25-32.

10 Pelletier, D. L., Frongillo, E. A., Jr., Schroeder, D. G., & Habicht, J. P. (1995). The effects of malnutrition on child mortality in developing countries. *Bulletin of the World Health Organization, 73*(4), 443-48.

11 Rodriguez, L., Cervantes, E., & Ortiz, R. (2011). Malnutrition and gastrointestinal and respiratory infections in children: A public health problem. *International Journal of Environmental Research and Public Health, 8*(4), 1174-1205.

12 Chisti, M. J., Tebruegge, M., La Vincente, S., Graham, S. M., & Duke, T. (2009). Pneumonia in severely malnourished children in developing countries: Mortality risk, etiology and validity of WHO clinical signs: A systematic review. *Tropical Medicine & International Health, 14*(10), 1173-89.

13 Chisti, M. J., Tebruegge, M., La Vincente, S., Graham, S. M., & Duke, T. (2009). Pneumonia in severely malnourished children in developing countries: Mortality risk, etiology and validity of WHO clinical signs: A systematic review. *Tropical Medicine & International Health, 14*(10), 1173-89.

14 Adegbola, R. A., Falade, A. G., Sam, B. E., Aidoo, M., Baldeh, I., Hazlett, D., . . . Mulholland E. K. (1994). The etiology of pneumonia in malnourished and well-nourished Gambian children. *Pediatric Infectious Disease Journal, 13*(11), 975-82.

15 Falade, A. G., Mulholland, E. K., Adegbola, R. A., & Greenwood, B. M. (1997). Bacterial isolates from blood and lung aspirate cultures in Gambian children with lobar pneumonia. *Annals of Tropical Paediatrics, 17*(4), 315-19.

16 Pelletier, D. L., Frongillo, E. A., Jr., Schroeder, D. G., & Habicht, J. P. (1995). The effects of malnutrition on child mortality in developing countries. *Bulletin of the World Health Organization, 73*(4), 443-48.

17 Brown, P. (2003). Malnutrition leading cause of death in postwar Angola. *Bulletin of the World Health Organization, 81*(11), 849-50.

18 Suskind, D. M. K., & Suskind, R. M. (1990). The malnourished child: An overview. In R. M. Suskind & L. Suskind (Eds.), *The malnourished child* (pp. 1-22). New York, NY: Vevey/Raven Press.

19 Spooner, V., Barker, J., Tulloch, S., Lehmann, D., Marshall, T. F., Kajoi, M., & Alpers, M. P. (1989). Clinical signs and risk factors associated with pneumonia in children admitted to Goroka Hospital, Papua New Guinea. *Journal of Tropical Pediatrics, 35*(6), 295-300.

20 De Onis, M., & Blossner, M. (2003). The World Health Organization global database on child growth and malnutrition: Methodology and applications. *International Journal of Epidemiology, 32*(4), 518-26.

21 Puoane, T., Sanders, D., Ashworth, A., Chopra, M., Strasser, S., & McCoy, D. (2004). Improving the hospital management of malnourished children by participatory research. *International Journal for Quality in Health Care, 16*(1), 31-40.

22 Bachou, H., Tumwine, J. K., Mwadime, R. K., & Tylleskar, T. (2006). Risk factors in hospital deaths in severely malnourished children in Kampala, Uganda. *BMC Pediatrics, 6,* 7.

23 Ahmed, T., Ali, M., Ullah, M. M., Choudhury, I. A., Haque, M. E., Salam, M. A., . . . Fuchs, G. J. (1999). Mortality in severely malnourished children with diarrhea and use of a standardised management protocol. *Lancet, 353*(9168), 1919-22.

24 Deivanayagam, N., Nedunchelian, K., Ramasamy, S., Sudhandirakannan, & Ratnam, S. R. (1992). Risk factors for fatal pneumonia: A case control study. *Indian Pediatrics, 29*(12), 1529-32.

25 Tupasi, T. E., Mangubat, N. V., Sunico, M. E., Magdangal, D. M., Navarro, E. E., Leonor, Z. A., . . . Lucero, M. G. (1990). Malnutrition and acute respiratory tract infections in Filipino children. *Reviews of Infectious Diseases, 12*(Suppl. 8), S1047-54.

26 Chisti, M. J., Tebruegge, M., La Vincente, S., Graham, S. M., & Duke, T. (2009). Pneumonia in severely malnourished children in developing countries: Mortality risk, etiology and validity of WHO clinical signs: A systematic review. *Tropical Medicine & International Health, 14*(10), 1173-89.

27 Chisti, M. J., Tebruegge, M., La Vincente, S., Graham, S. M., & Duke, T. (2009). Pneumonia in severely malnourished children in developing countries: Mortality risk, etiology and validity of WHO clinical signs: A systematic review. *Tropical Medicine & International Health, 14*(10), 1173-89.

28 Black, R. E., Cousens, S., Johnson, H. L., Lawn, J. E., Rudan, I., Bassani, D. G., . . . Mathers, C., for the Child Health Epidemiology Reference Group of WHO and UNICEF. (2010). Global, regional, and national causes of child mortality in 2008: A systematic analysis. *Lancet, 375*(9730), 1969-87.

29 Chisti, M. J., Duke, T., Robertson, C. F., Ahmed, T., Faruque, A. S., Bardhan, P. K., . . . Salam, M. A. (2011). Co-morbidity: Exploring the clinical overlap between pneumonia and diarrhea in a hospital in Dhaka, Bangladesh. *Annals of Tropical Paediatrics, 31*(4), 311-19.

30 Chisti, M. J., Ahmed, T., Faruque, A. S., & Abdus Salam, M. (2010). Clinical and laboratory features of radiologic pneumonia in severely malnourished infants attending an urban diarrhea treatment center in Bangladesh. *Pediatric Infectious Disease Journal, 29*(2), 174-77.

31 Borelli, P., Blatt, S. L., Rogero, M. M., & Fock, R. A. (2004). Haematological alterations in protein malnutrition. *Revista Brasileira de Hematologia e Hemoterapia, 26,* 49-56.

32 Bloss, E., Wainaina, F., & Bailey, R. C. (2004). Prevalence and predictors of underweight, stunting, and wasting among children aged 5 and under in western Kenya. *Journal of Tropical Pediatrics, 50*(5), 260-70.

33 Cunningham-Rundles, S., McNeeley, D. F., & Moon, A. (2005). Mechanisms of nutrient modulation of the immune response. *Journal of Allergy and Clinical Immunology, 115*(6), 1119-28; quiz 1129.

34 Rodriguez, L., Cervantes, E., & Ortiz, R. (2011). Malnutrition and gastrointestinal and respiratory infections in children:

A public health problem. *International Journal of Environmental Research and Public Health, 8*(4), 1174-1205.

35 Powanda, M. C., & Beisel, W. R. (2003). Metabolic effects of infection on protein and energy status. *Journal of Nutrition, 133*(1), 322S-327S.

36 Phillips, R. S., Enwonwu, C. O., Okolo, S., & Hassan, A. (2004). Metabolic effects of acute measles in chronically malnourished Nigerian children. *Journal of Nutritional Biochemistry, 15*(5), 281-88.

37 Morgan, G. (1997). What, if any, is the effect of malnutrition on immunological competence? *Lancet, 349*(9066), 1693-95.

38 Stiehm, E. R. (1980). Humoral immunity in malnutrition. *Federation Proceedings, 39*(13), 3093-97.

39 Suskind, D. M. K., & Suskind, R. M. (1990). The malnourished child: An overview. In R. M. Suskind & L. Suskind (Eds.), *The malnourished child* (pp. 1-22). New York, NY: Vevey/Raven Press.

40 Feigin, R. D., & Garg, R. (1987). Interaction of infection and nutrition. In R. D. Feigin & J. D. Cherry (Eds.), *Textbook of pediatric infectious diseases* (2nd ed.) (pp. 17-27). Philadelphia, PA: Saunders.

41 Fulginiti, V. A. (1987). Immunological responses to infection. In R. D. Feigin & J. D. Cherry (Eds.), *Textbook of pediatric infectious diseases* (2nd ed.) (pp. 28-40). Philadelphia, PA: Saunders.

42 Gainsford, T., Willson, T. A., Metcalf, D., Handman, E., McFarlane, C., Ng, A., . . . Hilton, D. J. (1996). Leptin can induce proliferation, differentiation, and functional activation of hematopoietic cells. *Proceedings of the National Academy of Sciences of the United States of America, 93*(25), 14564-68.

43 Loffreda, S., Yang, S. Q., Lin, H. Z., Karp, C. L., Brengman, M. L., Wang, D. J., . . . Diehl, A. M. (1998). Leptin regulates proinflammatory immune responses. *Federation of American Societies for Experimental Biology Journal, 12*(1), 57-65.

44 Lord, G. M., Matarese, G., Howard, J. K., Baker, R. J., Bloom, S. R., & Lechler, R. I. (1998). Leptin modulates the T-cell immune response and reverses starvation-induced immunosuppression. *Nature, 394*(6696), 897-901.

45 Faggioni, R., Jones-Carson, J., Reed, D. A., Dinarello, C. A., Feingold, K. R., Grunfeld, C., & Fantuzzi, G. (2000). Leptin-deficient (ob/ob) mice are protected from T cell-mediated hepatotoxicity: Role of tumor necrosis factor alpha and IL-18. *Proceedings of the National Academy of Sciences of the United States of America, 97*(5), 2367-72.

46 Rodriguez, L., Graniel, J., & Ortiz, R. (2007). Effect of leptin on activation and cytokine synthesis in peripheral blood lymphocytes of malnourished infected children. *Clinical & Experimental Immunology, 148*(3), 478-85.

47 Moshyedi, A. K., Josephs, M. D., Abdalla, E. K., Mackay, S. L., Edwards, C. K., 3rd, Copeland, E. M., 3rd, & Moldawer, L. L. (1998). Increased leptin expression in mice with bacterial peritonitis is partially regulated by tumor necrosis factor alpha. *Infection and Immunity, 66*(4), 1800-02.

48 Faggioni, R., Feingold, K. R., & Grunfeld, C. (2001). Leptin regulation of the immune response and the immunodeficiency of malnutrition. *Federation of American Societies for Experimental Biology Journal, 15*(14), 2565-71.

49 Soliman, A. T., El Zalabany, M. M., Salama, M., & Ansari, B. M. (2000). Serum leptin concentrations during severe protein-energy malnutrition: Correlation with growth parameters and endocrine function. *Metabolism, 49*(7), 819-25.

50 Sanchez-Margalet, V., Martin-Romero, C., Santos-Alvarez, J., Goberna, R., Najib, S., & Gonzalez-Yanes, C. (2003). Role of leptin as an immunomodulator of blood mononuclear cells: Mechanisms of action. *Clinical & Experimental Immunology, 133*(1), 11-19.

51 Palacio, A., Lopez, M., Perez-Bravo, F., Monkeberg, F., & Schlesinger, L. (2002). Leptin levels are associated with immune response in malnourished infants. *Journal of Clinical Endocrinology & Metabolism, 87*(7), 3040-46.

52 Chisti, M. J., Tebruegge, M., La Vincente, S., Graham, S. M., & Duke, T. (2009). Pneumonia in severely malnourished children in developing countries: Mortality risk, etiology and validity of WHO clinical signs: A systematic review. *Tropical Medicine & International Health, 14*(10), 1173-89.

53 Chisti, M. J., Ahmed, T., Faruque, A. S., & Abdus Salam, M. (2010). Clinical and laboratory features of radiologic pneumonia in severely malnourished infants attending an urban diarrhea treatment center in Bangladesh. *Pediatric Infectious Disease Journal, 29*(2), 174-77.

54 Shimeles, D., & Lulseged, S. (1994). Clinical profile and pattern of infection in Ethiopian children with severe protein-energy malnutrition. *East African Medical Journal, 71*(4), 264-67.

55 Johnson, A. W., Osinusi, K., Aderele, W. I., & Adeyemi-Doro, F. A. (1993). Bacterial etiology of acute lower respiratory infections in pre-school Nigerian children and comparative predictive features of bacteraemic and non-bacteraemic illnesses. *Journal of Tropical Pediatrics, 39*(2), 97-106.

56 Johnson, W. B., Aderele, W. I., & Gbadero, D. A. (1992). Host factors and acute lower respiratory infections in pre-school children. *Journal of Tropical Pediatrics, 38*(3), 132-36.

57 Friedland, I. R. (1992). Bacteremia in severely malnourished children. *Annals of Tropical Paediatrics, 12*(4), 433-40.

58 Berkowitz, F. E. (1983). Infections in children with severe protein-energy malnutrition. *Annals of Tropical Paediatrics, 3*(2), 79-83.

59 Fagbule, D. O. (1993). Bacterial pathogens in malnourished children with pneumonia. *Tropical & Geographical Medicine, 45*(6), 294-96.

60 Diallo, A. A., Siverman, M., & Egler, L. J. (1979). Bacteriology of lung puncture aspirates in malnourished children in Zaria. *Nigerian Medical Journal, 9*(4), 421-23.

61 Morehead, C. D., Morehead, M., Allen, D. M., & Olson, R. E. (1974). Bacterial infections in malnourished children. *Journal of Tropical Pediatrics and Environmental Child Health, 20*(3), 141-47.

62 Hughes, J. R., Sinha, D. P., Cooper, M. R., Shah, K. V., & Bose, S. K. (1969). Lung tap in childhood: Bacteria, viruses, and mycoplasmas in acute lower respiratory tract infections. *Pediatrics, 44*(4), 477-85.

63 Johnson, A. W., Osinusi, K., Aderele, W. I., & Adeyemi-Doro, F. A. (1993). Bacterial etiology of acute lower respiratory infections in pre-school Nigerian children and comparative predictive features of bacteraemic and non-bacteraemic illnesses. *Journal of Tropical Pediatrics, 39*(2), 97-106.

64 Berkowitz, F. E. (1983). Infections in children with severe protein-energy malnutrition. *Annals of Tropical Paediatrics, 3*(2), 79-83.

65 Hughes, J. R., Sinha, D. P., Cooper, M. R., Shah, K. V., & Bose, S. K. (1969). Lung tap in childhood: Bacteria, viruses, and mycoplasmas in acute lower respiratory tract infections. *Pediatrics, 44*(4), 477-85.

66 Adegbola, R. A., Falade, A. G., Sam, B. E., Aidoo, M., Baldeh, I., Hazlett, D., . . . Mulholland, E. K. (1994). The etiology of pneumonia in malnourished and well-nourished Gambian children. *Pediatric Infectious Disease Journal, 13*(11), 975-82.

67 Fagbule, D. O. (1993). Bacterial pathogens in malnourished children with pneumonia. *Tropical & Geographical Medicine, 45*(6), 294-96.

68 Morehead, C. D., Morehead, M., Allen, D. M., & Olson, R. E. (1974). Bacterial infections in malnourished children. *Journal of Tropical Pediatrics and Environmental Child Health, 20*(3), 141-47.

69 Escobar, J. A., Dover, A. S., Duenas, A., Leal, E., Medina, P., Arguello, A., . . . Reyes, M. A. (1976). Etiology of respiratory tract infections in children in Cali, Colombia. *Pediatrics, 57*(1), 123-30.

70 Shann, F., Gratten, M., Germer, S., Linnemann, V., Hazlett, D., & Payne, R. (1984). Etiology of pneumonia in children in Goroka Hospital, Papua New Guinea. *Lancet, 2*(8402), 537-41.

71 Shimeles, D., & Lulseged, S. (1994). Clinical profile and pattern of infection in Ethiopian children with severe protein-energy malnutrition. *East African Medical Journal, 71*(4), 264-67.

72 Johnson, A. W., Osinusi, K., Aderele, W. I., & Adeyemi-Doro, F. A. (1993). Bacterial etiology of acute lower respiratory infections in pre-school Nigerian children and comparative predictive features of bacteraemic and non-bacteraemic illnesses. *Journal of Tropical Pediatrics, 39*(2), 97-106.

73 Johnson, W. B., Aderele, W. I., & Gbadero, D. A. (1992). Host factors and acute lower respiratory infections in pre-school children. *Journal of Tropical Pediatrics, 38*(3), 132-36.

74 Berkowitz, F. E. (1983). Infections in children with severe protein-energy malnutrition. *Annals of Tropical Paediatrics, 3*(2), 79-83.

75 Shann, F., Gratten, M., Germer, S., Linnemann, V., Hazlett, D., & Payne, R. (1984). Etiology of pneumonia in children in Goroka Hospital, Papua New Guinea. *Lancet, 2*(8402), 537-41.

76 Shann, F., Gratten, M., Germer, S., Linnemann, V., Hazlett, D., & Payne, R. (1984). Etiology of pneumonia in children in Goroka Hospital, Papua New Guinea. *Lancet, 2*(8402), 537-41.

77 Berman, S. (1991). Epidemiology of acute respiratory infections in children of developing countries. *Reviews of Infectious Diseases, 13*(Suppl. 6), S454-62.

78 Adegbola, R. A., Secka, O., Lahai, G., Lloyd-Evans, N., Njie, A., Usen, S., . . . Milligan, P. J. (2005). Elimination of *Haemophilus influenzae* type b (Hib) disease from The Gambia after the introduction of routine immunisation with a Hib conjugate vaccine: A prospective study. *Lancet, 366*(9480), 144-150.

79 Martin, M., Casellas, J. M., Madhi, S. A., Urquhart, T. J., Delport, S. D., Ferrero, F., . . . Feikin, D. R. (2004). Impact of *Haemophilus influenzae* type b conjugate vaccine in South Africa and Argentina. *Pediatric Infectious Disease Journal, 23*(9), 842-47.

80 Morris, S. K., Moss, W. J., & Halsey, N. (2008). Haemophilus influenzae type b conjugate vaccine use and effectiveness. *Lancet Infectious Diseases, 8*(7), 435-43.

81 Centers for Disease Control and Prevention. (2008). Progress in introduction of pneumococcal conjugate vaccine: Worldwide, 2000-2008. *Morbidity and Mortality Weekly Report, 57*(42), 1148-51.

82 Crawford, S. E., & Daum, R. S. (2008). Bacterial pneumonia, lung abscess, and empyema. In L. M. Taussig & L. I. Landau (Eds.), *Pediatric respiratory medicine* (Vol. 2, pp. 501-53). Philadelphia, PA: Mosby Elsevier.

83 Chisti, M. J., Tebruegge, M., La Vincente, S., Graham, S. M., & Duke, T. (2009). Pneumonia in severely malnourished children in developing countries: Mortality risk, etiology and validity of WHO clinical signs: A systematic review. *Tropical Medicine & International Health, 14*(10), 1173-89.

84 Sinaniotis, C. A., & Sinaniotis, A. C. (2005). Community-acquired pneumonia in children. *Current Opinion in Pulmonary Medicine, 11*(3), 218-25.

85 McCracken, G. H., Jr. (2000). Diagnosis and management of pneumonia in children. *Pediatric Infectious Disease Journal, 19*(9), 924-28.

86 Hale, K. A., & Isaacs, D. (2006). Antibiotics in childhood pneumonia. *Paediatric Respiratory Reviews, 7*(2), 145-51.

87 Shann, F., Gratten, M., Germer, S., Linnemann, V., Hazlett, D., & Payne, R. (1984). Etiology of pneumonia in children in Goroka Hospital, Papua New Guinea. *Lancet, 2*(8402), 537-41.

88 Berman, S. (1991). Epidemiology of acute respiratory infections in children of developing countries. *Reviews of Infectious Diseases, 13*(Suppl. 6), S454-62.

89 Martin, T. R. (1987). The relationship between malnutrition and lung infections. *Clinics in Chest Medicine, 8*(3), 359-72.

90 Rodriguez, L., Cervantes, E., & Ortiz, R. (2011). Malnutrition and gastrointestinal and respiratory infections in children: A public health problem. *International Journal of Environmental Research and Public Health, 8*(4), 1174-1205.

91 Gilman, R. H., Brown, K. H., Gilman, J. B., Gaffar, A., Alamgir, S. M., Kibriya, A. K., & Sack, R. B. (1982). Colonization of the oropharynx with Gram-negative bacilli in children with severe protein-calorie malnutrition. *American Journal of Clinical Nutrition, 36*(2), 284-89.

92 Chisti, M. J., Ahmed, T., Faruque, A. S., & Abdus Salam, M. (2010). Clinical and laboratory features of radiologic pneumonia in

severely malnourished infants attending an urban diarrhea treatment center in Bangladesh. *Pediatric Infectious Disease Journal, 29*(2), 174-77.

93 Deshmukh, P. R., Dongre, A. R., Sinha, N., & Garg, B. S. (2009). Acute childhood morbidities in rural Wardha: Some epidemiological correlates and health care seeking. *Indian Journal of Medical Science, 63*(8), 345-54.

94 Rodriguez, L., Cervantes, E., & Ortiz, R. (2011). Malnutrition and gastrointestinal and respiratory infections in children: A public health problem. *International Journal of Environmental Research & Public Health, 8*(4), 1174-1205.

95 Chisti, M. J., Tebruegge, M., La Vincente, S., Graham, S. M., & Duke, T. (2009). Pneumonia in severely malnourished children in developing countries: Mortality risk, etiology and validity of WHO clinical signs: A systematic review. *Tropical Medicine & International Health, 14*(10), 1173-89.

96 Robertson, M. A., & Molyneux, E. M. (2001). Description of cause of serious illness and outcome in patients identified using ETAT guidelines in urban Malawi. *Archives of Disease in Childhood, 85*(3), 214-17.

97 Bachou, H., Tylleskar, T., Downing, R., & Tumwine, J. K. (2006). Severe malnutrition with and without HIV-1 infection in hospitalised children in Kampala, Uganda: Differences in clinical features, haematological findings and CD4+ cell counts. *Nutrition Journal, 5,* 27.

98 Jeena, P. M., Pillay, P., Pillay, T., & Coovadia, H. M. (2002). Impact of HIV-1 co-infection on presentation and hospital-related mortality in children with culture proven pulmonary tuberculosis in Durban, South Africa. *International Journal of Tuberculosis and Lung Disease, 6*(8), 672-78.

99 Moore, D. P., Klugman, K. P., & Madhi, S. A. (2010). Role of *Streptococcus pneumoniae* in hospitalization for acute community-acquired pneumonia associated with culture-confirmed *Mycobacterium* tuberculosis in children: A pneumococcal conjugate vaccine probe study. *Pediatric Infectious Disease Journal, 29*(12), 1099-1104.

100 Moore, D. P., Klugman, K. P., & Madhi, S. A. (2010). Role of *Streptococcus pneumoniae* in hospitalization for acute community-acquired pneumonia associated with culture-confirmed *Mycobacterium* tuberculosis in children: A pneumococcal conjugate vaccine probe study. *Pediatric Infectious Disease Journal, 29*(12), 1099-1104.

101 Laurenzi, G. A., Potter, R. T., & Kass, E. H. (1961). Bacteriologic flora of the lower respiratory tract. *New England Journal of Medicine, 265,* 1273-78.

102 Crawford, S. E., & Daum, R. S. (2008). Bacterial pneumonia, lung abscess, and empyema. In L. M. Taussig & L. I. Landau (Eds.), *Pediatric respiratory medicine* (Vol. 2, pp. 501-53). Philadelphia, PA: Mosby Elsevier.

103 Crawford, S. E., & Daum, R. S. (2008). Bacterial pneumonia, lung abscess, and empyema. In L. M. Taussig & L. I. Landau (Eds.), *Pediatric respiratory medicine* (Vol. 2, pp. 501-53). Philadelphia, PA: Mosby Elsevier.

104 Martin, T. R. (1987). The relationship between malnutrition and lung infections. *Clinics in Chest Medicine, 8*(3), 359-72.

105 Crawford, S. E., & Daum, R. S. (2008). Bacterial pneumonia, lung abscess, and empyema. In L. M. Taussig & L. I. Landau (Eds.), *Pediatric respiratory medicine* (Vol. 2, pp. 501-53). Philadelphia, PA: Mosby Elsevier.

106 Crawford, S. E., & Daum, R. S. (2008). Bacterial pneumonia, lung abscess, and empyema. In L. M. Taussig & L. I. Landau (Eds.), *Pediatric respiratory medicine* (Vol. 2, pp. 501-53). Philadelphia, PA: Mosby Elsevier.

107 Crawford, S. E., & Daum, R. S. (2008). Bacterial pneumonia, lung abscess, and empyema. In L. M. Taussig & L. I. Landau (Eds.), *Pediatric respiratory medicine* (Vol. 2, pp. 501-53). Philadelphia, PA: Mosby Elsevier.

108 Crawford, S. E., & Daum, R. S. (2008). Bacterial pneumonia, lung abscess, and empyema. In L. M. Taussig & L. I. Landau (Eds.), *Pediatric respiratory medicine* (Vol. 2, pp. 501-53). Philadelphia, PA: Mosby Elsevier.

109 Chisti, M. J., Salam, M. A., Sharifuzzaman, & Pietroni, M. A. (2009). Occult pneumonia: An unusual but perilous entity presenting with severe malnutrition and dehydrating diarrhea. *Journal of Health, Population and Nutrition, 27*(6), 808-12.

110 Crawford, S. E., & Daum, R. S. (2008). Bacterial pneumonia, lung abscess, and empyema. In L. M. Taussig & L. I. Landau (Eds.), *Pediatric respiratory medicine* (Vol. 2, pp. 501-53). Philadelphia, PA: Mosby Elsevier.

111 Tuomanen, E. I., Austrian, R., & Masure, H. R. (1995). Pathogenesis of pneumococcal infection. *New England Journal of Medicine, 332*(19), 1280-84.

112 Crawford, S. E., & Daum, R. S. (2008). Bacterial pneumonia, lung abscess, and empyema. In L. M. Taussig & L. I. Landau (Eds.), *Pediatric respiratory medicine* (Vol. 2, pp. 501-53). Philadelphia, PA: Mosby Elsevier.

113 Crawford, S. E., & Daum, R. S. (2008). Bacterial pneumonia, lung abscess, and empyema. In L. M. Taussig & L. I. Landau (Eds.), *Pediatric respiratory medicine* (Vol. 2, pp. 501-53). Philadelphia, PA: Mosby Elsevier.

114 Anderson, V. M., & Turner, T. (1991). Histopathology of childhood pneumonia in developing countries. *Reviews of Infectious Diseases, 13*(Suppl. 6), S470-76.

115 Chisti, M. J., Ahmed, T., Faruque, A. S., & Abdus Salam, M. (2010). Clinical and laboratory features of radiologic pneumonia in severely malnourished infants attending an urban diarrhea treatment center in Bangladesh. *Pediatric Infectious Disease Journal, 29*(2), 174-77.

116 Chisti, M. J., Salam, M. A., Bardhan, P. K., Ahad, R., La Vincente, S., & Duke, T. (2010). Influences of dehydration on clinical features of radiological pneumonia in children attending an urban diarrhea treatment centre in Bangladesh. *Annals of Tropical Paediatrics, 30*(4), 311-16.

117 Pauls, S., Kruger, S., Richter, K., Muche, R., Marre, R., Welte, T., . . . Suttorp, N. (2007). [Interobserver agreement in the assessment of pulmonary infiltrates on chest radiography in community-acquired pneumonia]. [Article in German]. *RöFo: Fortschritte auf dem Gebiete der Röntgenstrahlen und der Nuklearmedizin, 179*(11), 1152-58.

118 Bada, C., Carreazo, N. Y., Chalco, J. P., & Huicho, L. (2007). Inter-observer agreement in interpreting chest X-rays on children with acute lower respiratory tract infections and concurrent wheezing. *São Paulo Medical Journal, 125*(3), 150-54.

119 Sarria, E., Fischer, G. B., Lima, J. A., Menna Barreto, S. S., Flores, J. A., & Sukiennik, R. (2003). [Interobserver agreement in the radiological diagnosis of lower respiratory tract infections in children]. [Article in Portuguese]. *Jornal de Pediatria Sociedade Brasileira de Pediatria, 79*(6), 497-503.

120 Wafula, E. M., Ngamau, D. W., Onyango, F. E., Mirza, N. M., & Njeru, E. K. (1998). X-ray diagnosable pneumonia in children with severe malnutrition at Kenyatta National Hospital. *East African Medical Journal, 75*(10), 567-71.

121 Hamid, M., Qazi, S. A., & Khan, M. A. (1996). Clinical, nutritional and radiological features of pneumonia. *Journal of the Pakistan Medical Association, 46*(5), 95-99.

122 Doherty, J. (1991). WHO guidelines on detecting pneumonia in children. *Lancet, 338*, 1454.

123 Chisti, M. J., Salam, M. A., Sharifuzzaman, & Pietroni, M. A. (2009). Occult pneumonia: An unusual but perilous entity presenting with severe malnutrition and dehydrating diarrhea. *Journal of Health, Population and Nutrition, 27*(6), 808-12.

124 Bachur, R., Perry, H., & Harper, M. B. (1999). Occult pneumonias: Empiric chest radiographs in febrile children with leukocytosis. *Annals of Emergency Medicine, 33*(2), 166-73.

125 Murphy, C. G., van de Pol, A. C., Harper, M. B., & Bachur, R. G. (2007). Clinical predictors of occult pneumonia in the febrile child. *Academic Emergency Medicine, 14*(3), 243-49.

126 Cashat-Cruz, M., Morales-Aguirre, J. J., & Mendoza-Azpiri, M. (2005). Respiratory tract infections in children in developing countries. *Seminars in Pediatric Infectious Diseases, 16*(2), 84-92.

127 World Health Organization. (1990). *Acute respiratory infections in children: Case management in small hospitals in developing countries: A manual for doctors and other senior health workers.* Geneva, Switzerland: World Health Organization.

128 World Health Organization. (1991). *Technical bases for the WHO recommendations on the management of pneumonia in children at first-level health facilities.* Paper presented at the WHO/ARI/91.20. Geneva, Switzerland: World Health Organization.

129 Gupta, D., Mishra, S., & Chaturvedi, P. (1996). Fast breathing in the diagnosis of pneumonia--a reassessment. *Journal of Tropical Pediatrics, 42*(4), 196-99.

130 Palafox, M., Guiscafre, H., Reyes, H., Munoz, O., & Martinez, H. (2000). Diagnostic value of tachypnoea in pneumonia defined radiologically. *Archives of Disease in Childhood, 82*(1), 41-45.

131 Mulholland, E. K., Simoes, E. A., Costales, M. O., McGrath, E. J., Manalac, E. M., & Gove, S. (1992). Standardized diagnosis of pneumonia in developing countries. *Pediatric Infectious Disease Journal, 11*(2), 77-81.

132 Singhi, S., Dhawan, A., Kataria, S., & Walia, B. N. (1994). Validity of clinical signs for the identification of pneumonia in children. *Annals of Tropical Paediatrics, 14*(1), 53-58.

133 Campbell, H., Byass, P., & Greenwood, B. M. (1988). Simple clinical signs for diagnosis of acute lower respiratory infections. *Lancet, 2*(8613), 742-43.

134 Falade, A. G., Tschappeler, H., Greenwood, B. M., & Mulholland, E. K. (1995). Use of simple clinical signs to predict pneumonia in young Gambian children: The influence of malnutrition. *Bulletin of the World Health Organization, 73*(3), 299-304.

135 Cherian, T., Steinhoff, M. C., Simoes, E. A., & John, T. J. (1997). Clinical signs of acute lower respiratory tract infections in malnourished infants and children. *Pediatric Infectious Disease Journal, 16*(5), 490-94.

136 Shamo'on, H., Hawamdah, A., Haddadin, R., & Jmeian, S. (2004). Detection of pneumonia among children under six years by clinical evaluation. *Eastern Mediterranean Health Journal, 10*(4-5), 482-87.

137 Wafula, E. M., Ngamau, D. W., Onyango, F. E., Mirza, N. M., & Njeru, E. K. (1998). X-ray diagnosable pneumonia in children with severe malnutrition at Kenyatta National Hospital. *East African Medical Journal, 75*(10), 567-71.

138 Falade, A. G., Tschappeler, H., Greenwood, B. M., & Mulholland, E. K. (1995). Use of simple clinical signs to predict pneumonia in young Gambian children: The influence of malnutrition. *Bulletin of the World Health Organization, 73*(3), 299-304.

139 Cherian, T., Steinhoff, M. C., Simoes, E. A., & John, T. J. (1997). Clinical signs of acute lower respiratory tract infections in malnourished infants and children. *Pediatric Infectious Disease Journal, 16*(5), 490-94.

140 Aref, G. H., Osman, M. Z., Zaki, A., Amer, M. A., & Hanna, S. S. (1992). Clinical and radiologic study of the frequency and presentation of chest infection in children with severe protein energy malnutrition. *Journal of the Egyptian Public Health Association, 67*(5-6), 655-73.

141 Suskind, D. M. K., Suskind, R. M. (1990). The malnourished child: An overview. In R. M. Suskind & L. Suskind (Eds.), *The malnourished child* (pp. 1-22). New York, NY: Vevey/Raven Press.

142 Chisti, M. J., Salam, M. A., Bardhan, P. K., Ahad, R., La Vincente, S., & Duke, T. (2010). Influences of dehydration on clinical features of radiological pneumonia in children attending an urban diarrhea treatment centre in Bangladesh. *Annals of Tropical Paediatrics, 30*(4), 311-16.

143 Salam, M. A., Ronan, A., Saha, D., & Khan, W. A. (2002). *Diagnosis of pneumonia in children with dehydrating diarrhea at a diarrheal hospital* [Abstract no. G-146]. Presented at the 42nd Interscience Conference on Antimicrobial Agents and Chemotherapy (ICAAC), San Diego, California.

144 Wang, F., Butler, T., Rabbani, G. H., & Jones, P. K. (1986). The acidosis of cholera: Contributions of hyperproteinemia, lactic acidemia, and hyperphosphatemia to an increased serum anion gap. *New England Journal of Medicine, 315*(25), 1591-95.

145 Richards, L., Claeson, M., & Pierce, N. F. (1993). Management of acute diarrhea in children: Lessons learned. *Pediatric Infectious Disease Journal, 12*(1), 5-9.

146 Salam, M. A., Ronan, A., Saha, D., & Khan, W. A. (2002). *Diagnosis of pneumonia in children with dehydrating diarrhea at a diarrheal hospital* [Abstract no. G-146]. Presented at the 42nd Interscience Conference on Antimicrobial Agents and Chemotherapy (ICAAC), San Diego, California.

147 Chisti, M. J., Salam, M. A., Bardhan, P. K., Ahad, R., La Vincente, S., & Duke, T. (2010). Influences of dehydration on clinical features of radiological pneumonia in children attending an urban diarrhea treatment centre in Bangladesh. *Annals of Tropical Paediatrics, 30*(4), 311-16.

148 Greenbaum, L. A. (2012). Electrolyte and acid-base disorders. In R. M. Kliegman, R. E. Behrman, H. B. Jenson, & B. F. Stanton (Eds.), *Nelson textbook of pediatrics* (19th ed., pp. 267-309). Philadelphia, PA: Saunders.

149 Nathoo, K. J., Glyn-Jones, R., & Nhembe, M. (1987). Serum electrolytes in children admitted with diarrheal dehydration managed with simple salt sugar solution. *Central African Journal of Medicine, 33*(8), 200-204.

150 Ahmed, S. M., Islam, M. R., & Butler, T. (1986). Effective treatment of diarrheal dehydration with an oral rehydration solution containing citrate. *Scandinavian Journal of Infectious Diseases, 18*(1), 65-70.

151 Salam, M. A., Ronan, A., Saha, D., & Khan, W. A. (2002). *Diagnosis of pneumonia in children with dehydrating diarrhea at a diarrheal hospital* [Abstract no. G-146]. Presented at the 42nd Interscience Conference on Antimicrobial Agents and Chemotherapy (ICAAC), San Diego, California.

152 Ahmed, T., Ali, M., Ullah, M. M., Choudhury, I. A., Haque, M. E., Salam, M. A., . . . Fuchs G. J (1999). Mortality in severely malnourished children with diarrhea and use of a standardised management protocol. *Lancet, 353*(9168), 1919-22.

153 Ahmed, S. M., Islam, M. R., & Butler, T. (1986). Effective treatment of diarrheal dehydration with an oral rehydration solution containing citrate. *Scandinavian Journal of Infectious Diseases, 18*(1), 65-70.

154 Alam, N. H., & Ashraf, H. (2003). Treatment of infectious diarrhea in children. *Paediatric Drugs, 5*(3), 151-65.

155 Chisti, M. J., Ahmed, T., Ashraf, H., Faruque, A. S., Bardhan, P. K., Dey, S. K., . . . Salam, M. A. (2012). Clinical predictors and outcome of metabolic acidosis in under-five children admitted to an urban hospital in Bangladesh with diarrhea and pneumonia. *PLOS One, 7*(6), e39164.

156 Chisti, M. J., Ahmed, T., Ashraf, H., Faruque, A. S., Bardhan, P. K., Dey, S. K., . . . Salam, M. A. (2012). Clinical predictors and outcome of metabolic acidosis in under-five children admitted to an urban hospital in Bangladesh with diarrhea and pneumonia. *PLOS One, 7*(6), e39164.

157 World Health Organization. (2006). *Pocket book for hospital care of children: Guidelines for the management of common illness with limited resources* (pp. 173-96). Geneva: World Health Organization.

158 Adegbola, R. A., Falade, A. G., Sam, B. E., Aidoo, M., Baldeh, I., Hazlett, D., . . . Mulholland, E. K. (1994). The etiology of pneumonia in malnourished and well-nourished Gambian children. *Pediatric Infectious Disease Journal, 13*(11), 975-82.

159 Hammitt, L. L., Murdoch, D. R., Scott, J. A., Driscoll, A., Karron, R. A., Levine, O. S., et al. (2012). Specimen collection for the diagnosis of pediatric pneumonia. *Clinical Infectious Diseases, 54*(Suppl. 2), S132-39.

160 Ahmed, T., Ali, M., Ullah, M. M., Choudhury, I. A., Haque, M. E., Salam, M. A., . . . Fuchs, G. J. (1999). Mortality in severely malnourished children with diarrhea and use of a standardised management protocol. *Lancet, 353*(9168), 1919-22.

161 World Health Organization. (1991). *Technical bases for the WHO recommendations on the management of pneumonia in children at first-level health facilities.* Paper presented at the WHO/ARI/91.20. Geneva: World Health Organization.

162 World Health Organization. (1999). *Management of severe malnutrition: A manual for physicians and other senior health workers.* Geneva: World Health Organization.

163 Asghar, R., Banajeh, S., Egas, J., Hibberd, P., Iqbal, I., Katep-Bwalya, M., . . . Qazi, S.; Severe Pneumonia Evaluation Antimicrobial Research Study Group. (2008). Chloramphenicol versus ampicillin plus gentamicin for community acquired very severe pneumonia among children aged 2-59 months in low resource settings: Multicentre randomised controlled trial (SPEAR study). *BMJ, 336*(7635), 80-84.

164 Chisti, M. J., Tebruegge, M., La Vincente, S., Graham, S. M., & Duke, T. (2009). Pneumonia in severely malnourished children in developing countries: Mortality risk, etiology and validity of WHO clinical signs: A systematic review. *Tropical Medicine & International Health, 14*(10), 1173-89.

165 World Health Organization. (2006). *Pocket book for hospital care of children: Guidelines for the management of common illness with limited resources* (pp. 173-96). Geneva: World Health Organization.

166 Shann, F. (2010). *Drug doses* (15th ed.). Melbourne, Australia: Collective P/L.

167 Ashraf, H., Chisti, M. J., & Alam, N. H. (2010). Treatment of childhood pneumonia in developing countries. In K. Śmigórski (Ed.), *Health management* (Vol. 1, pp. 59-88). Rijeka, Croatia: Sciyo.

168 Niederman, M. S. (2003). Bacterial pneumonia. In R. E. Rakel & E. T. Bope (Eds.), *Conn's current therapy.* Philadelphia, PA: Saunders.

169 Deshmukh, C. T., Tullu, M. S., & Parmar, R. C. (2002). Nosocomial Pneumonia. In S. Gupte (Ed.), *Recent advances in pediatrics pulmonology* (special volume 10). New Delhi, India: Jaypee.

170 Wald, E. R. (1990). Recurrent pneumonia in children. *Advances in Pediatric Infectious Diseases, 5,* 183-203.

171 Ashraf, H., Chisti, M. J., & Alam, N. H. (2010). Treatment of childhood pneumonia in developing countries. In K. Śmigórski (Ed.), *Health management* (Vol. 1, pp. 59-88). Rijeka, Croatia: Sciyo.

172 Ashraf, H., Chisti, M. J., & Alam, N. H. (2010). Treatment of child-hood pneumonia in developing countries In K. Śmigórski (Ed.), *Health management* (Vol. 1, pp. 59-88). Rijeka, Croatia: Sciyo.

173 Niederman, M. S. (2003). Bacterial pneumonia. In R. E. Rakel & E. T. Bope (Eds.), *Conn's current therapy*. Philadelphia, PA: Saunders.

174 Ahmed, T., Ali, M., Ullah, M. M., Choudhury, I. A., Haque, M. E., Salam, M. A., . . . Fuchs, G. J. (1999). Mortality in severely mal-nourished children with diarrhea and use of a standardised management protocol. *Lancet, 353*(9168), 1919-22.

175 Ahmed, T., Ali, M., Ullah, M. M., Choudhury, I. A., Haque, M. E., Salam, M. A., . . . Fuchs, G. J. (1999). Mortality in severely mal-nourished children with diarrhea and use of a standardised management protocol. *Lancet, 353*(9168), 1919-22.

176 Chisti, M. J., Ahmed, T., Ashraf, H., Faruque, A. S. G., Huq, S., & Hossain, M. I. (2011). Hypoglycemia in children attending the critical care medicine in developing countries. In E. C. Rigobelo (Ed.), *Diabetes: Damages and treatments* (Vol. 2, pp. 27-46). Rijeka, Croatia: InTech.

177 Chisti, M. J., Ahmed, T., Bardhan, P. K., & Salam, M. A. (2010). Evaluation of simple laboratory investigations to predict fatal outcome in infants with severe malnutrition presenting in an urban diarrhea treatment centre in Bangladesh. *Tropical Medicine & International Health, 15*(11), 1322-25.

178 Brooks, W. A., Yunus, M., Santosham, M., Wahed, M. A., Nahar, K., Yeasmin, S., & Black RE. (2004). Zinc for severe pneumonia in very young children: Double-blind placebo-controlled trial. *Lancet, 363*(9422), 1683-88.

179 Mahalanabis, D., Chowdhury, A., Jana, S., Bhattacharya, M. K., Chakrabarti, M. K., Wahed, M. A., et al. (2002). Zinc supple-mentation as adjunct therapy in children with measles accom-panied by pneumonia: a double-blind, randomized controlled trial. *American Journal of Clinical Nutrition, 76*(3), 604-7.

180 Shakur, M. S., Malek, M. A., Bano, N., & Islam, K. (2004). Zinc sta-tus in well-nourished Bangladeshi children suffering from acute lower respiratory infection. *Indian Pediatrics, 41*(5), 478-81.

181 Bose, A., Coles, C. L., Gunavathi, John, H., Moses, P., Raghupathy, P., et al. (2006). Efficacy of zinc in the treatment of severe pneumonia in hospitalized children <2 y old. *American Journal of Clinical Nutrition, 83*(5), 1089-96; quiz 1207.

182 Ahmed, T., Ali, M., Ullah, M. M., Choudhury, I. A., Haque, M. E., Salam, M. A., . . . Fuchs, G. J. (1999). Mortality in severely mal-nourished children with diarrhea and use of a standardised management protocol. *Lancet, 353*(9168), 1919-22.

183 Ahmed, T., Ali, M., Ullah, M. M., Choudhury, I. A., Haque, M. E., Salam, M. A., . . . Fuchs, G. J. (1999). Mortality in severely mal-nourished children with diarrhea and use of a standardised management protocol. *Lancet, 353*(9168), 1919-22.

184 Ahmed, T., Ali, M., Ullah, M. M., Choudhury, I. A., Haque, M. E., Salam, M. A., . . . Fuchs, G. J. (1999). Mortality in severely mal-nourished children with diarrhea and use of a standardised management protocol. *Lancet, 353*(9168), 1919-22.

185 Ahmed, T., Ali, M., Ullah, M. M., Choudhury, I. A., Haque, M. E., Salam, M. A., . . . Fuchs, G. J. (1999). Mortality in severely

malnourished children with diarrhea and use of a standardised management protocol. *Lancet, 353*(9168), 1919-22.

186 Ahmed, T., Ali, M., Ullah, M. M., Choudhury, I. A., Haque, M. E., Salam, M. A., . . . Fuchs, G. J. (1999). Mortality in severely mal-nourished children with diarrhea and use of a standardised management protocol. *Lancet, 353*(9168), 1919-22.

187 Onyango, F. E., Steinhoff, M. C., Wafula, E. M., Wariua, S., Musia, J., & Kitonyi, J. (1993). Hypoxemia in young Kenyan children with acute lower respiratory infection. *BMJ, 306*(6878), 612-15.

188 Duke, T., Mgone, J., & Frank, D. (2001). Hypoxemia in children with severe pneumonia in Papua New Guinea. *International Journal of Tuberculosis and Lung Disease, 5*(6), 511-19.

189 Chisti, M. J., Duke, T., Robertson, C. F., Ahmed, T., Faruque, A. S., Ashraf, H., et al. (2011). Clinical predictors and outcome of hypoxemia among under-five diarrhoeal children with or without pneumonia in an urban hospital, Dhaka, Bangladesh. *Tropical Medicine & International Health, 17*(1), 106-11.

190 Ashraf, H., Chisti, M. J., & Alam, N. H. (2010). Treatment of childhood pneumonia in developing countries In K. Śmigórski (Ed.), *Health management* (Vol. 1, pp. 59-88). Rijeka, Croatia: Sciyo.

191 World Health Organization. (2006). *Pocket book for hospital care of children: Guidelines for the management of common ill-ness with limited resources* (pp. 173-96). Geneva: World Health Organization.

192 Ashraf, H., Chisti, M. J., & Alam, N. H. (2010). Treatment of childhood pneumonia in developing countries In K. Śmigórski (Ed.), *Health management* (Vol. 1, pp. 59-88). Rijeka, Croatia: Sciyo.

193 World Health Organization. (2006). *Pocket book for hospital care of children: guidelines for the management of common ill-ness with limited resources* (pp. 173-96). Geneva, Switzer-land: World Health Organization.

194 Ashraf, H., Chisti, M. J., & Alam, N. H. (2010). Treatment of childhood pneumonia in developing countries In K. Śmigórski (Ed.), *Health management* (Vol. 1, pp. 59-88). Rijeka, Croatia: Sciyo.

195 Crawford, S. E., & Daum, R. S. (2008). Bacterial pneumonia, lung abscess, and empyema. In L. M. Taussig & L. I. Landau (Eds.), *Pediatric respiratory medicine* (Vol. 2, pp. 501-53). Philadelphia, PA: Mosby Elsevier.

196 Crawford, S. E., & Daum, R. S. (2008). Bacterial pneumonia, lung abscess, and empyema. In L. M. Taussig & L. I. Landau (Eds.), *Pediatric respiratory medicine* (Vol. 2, pp. 501-53). Philadelphia, PA: Mosby Elsevier.

197 Crawford, S. E., & Daum, R. S. (2008). Bacterial pneumonia, lung abscess, and empyema. In L. M. Taussig & L. I. Landau (Eds.), *Pediatric respiratory medicine* (Vol. 2, pp. 501-53). Philadelphia, PA: Mosby Elsevier.

198 Ahmed, T., Ali, M., Ullah, M. M., Choudhury, I. A., Haque, M. E., Salam, M. A., . . . Fuchs, G. J. (1999). Mortality in severely mal-nourished children with diarrhea and use of a standardised management protocol. *Lancet, 353*(9168), 1919-22.

199 Ahmed, T., Ali, M., Ullah, M. M., Choudhury, I. A., Haque, M. E., Salam, M. A., . . . Fuchs, G. J. (1999). Mortality in severely malnourished children with diarrhea and use of a standardised management protocol. *Lancet, 353*(9168), 1919-22.

200 Crawford, S. E., & Daum, R. S. (2008). Bacterial pneumonia, lung abscess, and empyema. In L. M. Taussig & L. I. Landau (Eds.), *Pediatric respiratory medicine* (Vol. 2, pp. 501-53). Philadelphia, PA: Mosby Elsevier.

201 Wald, E. R. (1990). Recurrent pneumonia in children. *Advances in Pediatric Infectious Diseases, 5,* 183-203.

202 Crawford, S. E., & Daum, R. S. (2008). Bacterial pneumonia, lung abscess, and empyema. In L. M. Taussig & L. I. Landau (Eds.), *Pediatric respiratory medicine* (Vol. 2, pp. 501-53). Philadelphia, PA: Mosby Elsevier.

203 Ashraf, H., Chisti, M. J., & Alam, N. H. (2010). Treatment of childhood pneumonia in developing countries In K. Śmigórski (Ed.), *Health management* (Vol. 1, pp. 59-88). Rijeka, Croatia: Sciyo.

204 Ahmed, T., Ali, M., Ullah, M. M., Choudhury, I. A., Haque, M. E., Salam, M. A., . . . Fuchs, G. J. (1999). Mortality in severely malnourished children with diarrhea and use of a standardised management protocol. *Lancet, 353*(9168), 1919-22.

205 Chisti, M. J., Ahmed, T., Ashraf, H., Faruque, A. S. G., Huq, S., & Hossain, M. I. (2011). Hypoglycemia in children attending the critical care medicine in developing countries. In E. C. Rigobelo (Ed.), *Diabetes: Damages and treatments* (Vol. 2, pp. 27-46). Rijeka, Croatia: InTech.

206 Ahmed, T., Ali, M., Ullah, M. M., Choudhury, I. A., Haque, M. E., Salam, M. A., . . . Fuchs, G. J. (1999). Mortality in severely malnourished children with diarrhea and use of a standardised management protocol. *Lancet, 353*(9168), 1919-22.

207 Ahmed, T., Ali, M., Ullah, M. M., Choudhury, I. A., Haque, M. E., Salam, M. A., . . . Fuchs, G. J. (1999). Mortality in severely malnourished children with diarrhea and use of a standardised management protocol. *Lancet, 353*(9168), 1919-22.

208 Crawford, S. E., & Daum, R. S. (2008). Bacterial pneumonia, lung abscess, and empyema. In L. M. Taussig & L. I. Landau (Eds.), *Pediatric respiratory medicine* (Vol. 2, pp. 501-53). Philadelphia, PA: Mosby Elsevier.

209 Crawford, S. E., & Daum, R. S. (2008). Bacterial pneumonia, lung abscess, and empyema. In L. M. Taussig & L. I. Landau (Eds.), *Pediatric respiratory medicine* (Vol. 2, pp. 501-53). Philadelphia, PA: Mosby Elsevier.

210 Boisset, G. F. (1972). Subpleural emphysema complicating staphylococcal and other pneumonias. *Journal of Pediatrics, 81*(2), 259-66.

211 Victoria, M. S., Steiner, P., & Rao, M. (1981). Persistent post-pneumonic pneumatoceles in children. *Chest, 79*(3), 359-61.

212 Crawford, S. E., & Daum, R. S. (2008). Bacterial pneumonia, lung abscess, and empyema. In L. M. Taussig & L. I. Landau (Eds.), *Pediatric respiratory medicine* (Vol. 2, pp. 501-53). Philadelphia, PA: Mosby Elsevier.

213 Graham, S. M., English, M., Hazir, T., Enarson, P., & Duke, T. (2008). Challenges to improving case management of childhood pneumonia at health facilities in resource-limited settings. *Bulletin of the World Health Organization, 86*(5), 349-55.

214 Chisti, M. J., Ahmed, T., Faruque, A. S., & Abdus Salam, M. (2010). Clinical and laboratory features of radiologic pneumonia in severely malnourished infants attending an urban diarrhea treatment center in Bangladesh. *Pediatric Infectious Disease Journal, 29*(2), 174-77.

215 Chisti, M. J., Ahmed, T., Faruque, A. S., & Abdus Salam, M. (2010). Clinical and laboratory features of radiologic pneumonia in severely malnourished infants attending an urban diarrhea treatment center in Bangladesh. *Pediatric Infectious Disease Journal, 29*(2), 174-77.

216 Chisti, M. J., Tebruegge, M., La Vincente, S., Graham, S. M., & Duke, T. (2009). Pneumonia in severely malnourished children in developing countries: Mortality risk, etiology and validity of WHO clinical signs: A systematic review. *Tropical Medicine & International Health, 14*(10), 1173-89.

217 Mulholland, K. (2007). Childhood pneumonia mortality: A permanent global emergency. *Lancet, 370*(9583), 285-89.

218 Sazawal, S., & Black, R. E. (1992). Meta-analysis of intervention trials on case-management of pneumonia in community settings. *Lancet, 340*(8818), 528-33.

219 Sazawal, S., Dhingra, U., Dhingra, P., Hiremath, G., Kumar, J., Sarkar, A., et al. (2007). Effects of fortified milk on morbidity in young children in north India: Community based, randomised, double masked placebo controlled trial. *BMJ, 334*(7585), 140.

220 Aggarwal, R., Sentz, J., & Miller, M. A. (2007). Role of zinc administration in prevention of childhood diarrhea and respiratory illnesses: a meta-analysis. *Pediatrics, 119*(6), 1120-30.

221 Dewey, K. G., & Arimond, M. (2012). Lipid-based nutrient supplements: How can they combat child malnutrition? *PLoS Medicine, 9*(9), e1001314.

222 Shankar, A. H., Jahari, A. B., Sebayang, S. K., Aditiawarman, Apriatni, M., Harefa, B., et al. (2008). Effect of maternal multiple micronutrient supplementation on fetal loss and infant death in Indonesia: A double-blind cluster-randomised trial. *Lancet, 371*(9608), 215-27.

223 Mulholland, K. (2007). Childhood pneumonia mortality: A permanent global emergency. *Lancet, 370*(9583), 285-89.

224 Sazawal, S., & Black, R. E. (1992). Meta-analysis of intervention trials on case-management of pneumonia in community settings. *Lancet, 340*(8818), 528-33.

225 Chisti, M. J., Duke, T., Robertson, C. F., Ahmed, T., Faruque, A. S., Bardhan, P. K., et al. (2011). Co-morbidity: Exploring the clinical overlap between pneumonia and diarrhea in a hospital in Dhaka, Bangladesh. *Annals of Tropical Paediatrics, 31*(4), 311-19.

226 Chisti, M. J., Duke, T., Robertson, C. F., Ahmed, T., Faruque, A. S., Bardhan, P. K., et al. (2011). Co-morbidity: Exploring the clinical overlap between pneumonia and diarrhea in a hospital in Dhaka, Bangladesh. *Annals of Tropical Paediatrics, 31*(4), 311-19.

Chapter 13

Childhood Diarrhea and Severe Malnutrition

Abu Syed Golam Faruque, MBBS, MPH
Sumon Kumar Das, MBBS
Mohammod Jobayer Chisti, MBBS, MMed
Farzana Afroze, MBBS
Hasan Ashraf, MBBS, MCPS, MD
Md. Iqbal Hossain, MBBS, DCH, PhD
Md. Munirul Islam, MBBS, PhD
Tahmeed Ahmed, MBBS, PhD

"Contaminated food is a major cause of diarrhea, substantially contributing to malnutrition and killing about 2.2 million people each year, most of them children."–Gro Harlem Brundtland

Learning Objectives

- Understand the global burden of childhood diarrhea associated with malnutrition and severe acute malnutrition.

- Understand the etiology of childhood diarrhea with malnutrition and its case management.

- Increase awareness about childhood diarrhea with malnutrition.

- Recognize the significance of early diagnosis and management of acute malnutrition.

- Reduce case fatality and prevention of mortality and morbidity due to childhood diarrhea.

- Reduce costs associated with other unnecessary investigations and complications due to inappropriate treatment.

- Understand how public health interventions can improve treatment of diarrhea and severe acute malnutrition in children.

Case Study: Diarrhea in a Malnourished Infant in Bangladesh

A girl aged 6 months and 15 days, third child of non-consanguineous parents, was admitted to the Acute Respiratory Infections (ARI) ward of the Longer Stay Unit in the Dhaka Hospital of International Center for Diarrheal Disease Research (icddr,b) on July 2, 2012, at 1:30 p.m. She had had fever, cough, and breathing difficulty for seven days, passage of loose stool for four days, and low activity for the past six hours. She was immunized as per the **Expanded Program on Immunization (EPI)** schedule, partially breastfed, and from a low-**socioeconomic status (SES)** family. Watery stools passed four to five times per day, but were not mixed with visible blood or mucus. She had low-grade, intermittent fever, but no chills, rigor, or dry cough. Her mother had given her four to five packets of properly diluted **oral rehydration salt (ORS)** solution for four days prior to admission, and received some medical advice from the local unqualified physician. However, the mother could not name the prescribed drugs. The baby had been delivered normally at home at 39 weeks of gestation, and prenatal and postnatal events were normal.

Initial Examination and Diagnosis

On admission to the ARI ward, the girl had sunken eyes and was thirsty. Systemic examination found severe lower chest wall in-drawing and labored breathing but adequate arterial oxygen saturation (SpO2) (**Table 13-1**). Her lungs had bilateral fine crackles at base, both anterior (front) and posterior (back). The abdomen was slightly distended but soft with no rebound tenderness, and bowel sounds were present. Other systemic examination revealed normal findings. So, patient was diagnosed with acute watery diarrhea with some dehydration with **kwashiorkor**, as well as severe **pneumonia**.

Treatment and Disease Progression

Initial treatment included ORS for dehydration, antibiotics for pneumonia, and micronutrients and vitamins as per the protocolized management for **severe acute malnutrition** as well as pneumonia. Laboratory investigations revealed low **hemoglobin** levels. High white blood cell (WBC) and low platelet counts suggested infections. Serum **electrolyte** revealed **hypokalemia** and mild hypernatremia, suggesting dehydration. The chest X-ray was abnormal as well. Oral supplementation of potassium was continued (**Table 13-2**).

The patient's diarrheal condition improved in terms of decreased frequency of diarrhea and rehydration, but the pneumonia remained static for two days. Then, she developed hypoxemia and was transferred to the intensive care unit (ICU). She had shortness of breath and was provided supplemental oxygen. She was maintaining SpO2 (98%), and respiratory distress was improving gradually. In the ICU, the patient was diagnosed with acute diarrhea, very severe pneumonia, **urinary tract infection (UTI)**, **ileus**, **sepsis**, hyperkalemia, and kwashiorkor. The patient's pneumonia deteriorated clinically, WBC increased, and platelet counts fell, so antibiotic treatment was accordingly altered (**Table 13-3**). In addition, the child was provided with salbutamol and calcium gluconate to address hypokalemia. The patient was kept on nothing per oral (NPO) for her ileus, and fluid rations and intravenous (IV) nutrition were started.

On July 5, 2012, the patient was doing well as oxygen treatment was allowing O_2 saturation to be maintained. The girl remained afebrile and had normal urine output. However, hypokalemia and hypernatremia persisted. Upon confirmation of an infection with *Pseudomonas* species, antibiotics were changed. The girl remained almost static throughout the day.

Table 13-1 Initial clinical measures

Temperature	36.5° Celsius
Heart rate	132/minute
Respiratory rate	68/minute (low volume)
Blood pressure	100/50 mm Hg
Edema	Present
Dehydration	Some
Periphery	Cold
Weight	5.6 kg
Height	62 cm
Weight-for-age z score	−2.36
Weight-for-age (% of NCHS median)	74.6%
Weight-for-height z score	−1.47
Weight-for-height (% of NCHS median)	86%

Table 13-2 Results of early bloodwork

Hemoglobin (Hb)	8 gm/l
White blood cell (WBC)	17,650/cmm
Neutrophil (N)	74%
Lymphocyte (L)	21%
Platelet	50,000/cmm
Serum sodium (Na⁺)	153.1 mmol/L
Serum potassium (K⁺)	2.97 mmol/L
Serum chloride (Cl⁻)	126.2 mmol/L
Stool routine microscopic examination (R/M/E)	
Pus cell	21–50
Red blood cell	1–5

Table 13-3 Clinical measures and bloodwork with treatment

Hemoglobin (Hb)	8 gm/l
White blood cell (WBC)	19,710/cmm
Neutrophil (N)	74%
Lymphocyte (L)	22%
Platelet	20,000/mcL
Arterial blood gas (ABG)	
p^H	7.26
Pco_2	38
Base excess (BE)	−9.4
tco_2	18.1
HCO_3	16.9
Serum Na^+	153.1 mmol/L
Serum K^+	5.95 mmol/L
Serum Cl^-	130.5 mmol/L
Serum creatinine	106.3 mmol/L
Serum calcium (Ca^{++})	1.97
Serum magnesium (Mg^{++})	1.47
Urine routine microscopy (R/M)	
Pus cell	Numerous
RBC	15-20
Protein	++

Critical Deterioration and Death

By 2:00 a.m. on the night of July 6, 2012, the patient's respiratory distress gradually increased, with the development of head nodding and nasal flaring. However, by 6:00 a.m., the patient gradually developed bradycardia with gasping respiration and reduced oxygen saturation SpO2. The patient also developed poor peripheral perfusion (peripheral pulses were absent, BP not recordable, periphery was cold). Cardiopulmonary resuscitation (CPR) was given, along with infusion of normal saline (20 ml/kg). After 20 to 30 minutes, cardiac activities became spontaneous, but her breathing pattern was still gasping and irregular, so the baby was intubated and kept under ventilatory support.

Circulation did not improve, and after 1.5 hours, despite adequate ventilator support, patient again developed hypoxemia with bradycardia. CPR was repeated according to the standard Advance Cardiovascular Life Support

(ACLS) protocol, but failed to restore the patient's cardiac activities. At that time, pupils became dilated and nonreactive to light. The patient was declared dead at 7:45 a.m. on July 6, 2012.

The urinary culture report was available after the patient's death, and it showed that there was growth of *E. coli* (1.0×10^4), which was resistant to the antibiotics provided.

> *Cause of death:* Septic shock (due to *Pseudomonas* sepsis)

> *Antecedent cause:* Kwashiorkor with very severe pneumonia with urinary tract infection with ileus

Discussion Questions

- How did malnutrition contribute to this tragic death?
- Could better preventive care and more prudent use of antibiotics have significant public health benefits?
- What is the global impact of nutrition and diarrhea on childhood mortality and morbidity?
- Which public health interventions could have prevented this death from occurring?

Introduction

Diarrhea is the second-leading cause of death and a top cause of malnutrition in children under 5.[1] Public health programs can address diarrheal diseases through preventing malnutrition, reducing ingestion of contaminated food through exclusive breastfeeding or appropriate complementary feeding, and increasing awareness. This chapter will explore causes, consequences, and interventions for childhood diarrhea and malnutrition.

Epidemiology of Childhood Diarrhea and Malnutrition

The World Health Organization (WHO) defines diarrhea as passage of three or more loose or watery stools by an individual in a 24-hour period. Diarrhea lasting 14 days or more is called "persistent diarrhea." Diarrhea is usually due to intestinal infection, mainly from viruses, although it may be caused by bacteria and parasites also. The disease is mainly transmitted through the fecal–oral route as a result of consumption of contaminated food. Water and electrolyte imbalance is the main concern, and children are at greater risk than adults of life-threatening dehydration because water constitutes a greater proportion of their body weight.

Global Epidemiology of Childhood Diarrhea

In 1976, Rohde and Northrup estimated that diarrhea kills up to 5 million children in developing countries annually, and urged the scientific community to "take science where the diarrhea is."[2] Around that time, Snyder and Merson estimated that under-5-year-olds averaged 2.2 episodes of diarrhea per year, resulting in 4.6 million deaths.[3] In 1980 to 1990, annual episodes of diarrhea and deaths were 2.6 per child and 3.3 million, respectively.[4] Annual mortality in 1990 to 2000 further decreased to 2.5 million deaths per year, accounting for 21% of all deaths among children under 5.[5] A different estimate, published in 2000, was 1.4 million deaths per year based on information from national vital registration systems, sample registration systems, population laboratories, and epidemiological studies.[6] By 2010, annual deaths were as much as 751,000, or 10% of total childhood deaths, and diarrhea is the second-leading cause of global childhood mortality.[7]

Global Epidemiology of Childhood Malnutrition

There is no universally accepted definition of **malnutrition** or **protein–energy malnutrition (PEM)**; however, WHO states that malnutrition is the cellular imbalance between supply of nutrients and energy, and the body's demand for them to ensure growth, maintenance, and specific functions.[8] Nutrient needs increase dramatically with illnesses. Suboptimal dietary intake, metabolic stress, malabsorption, and increased nutrient demands put patients with gastrointestinal (GI) diseases at especially high risk for malnutrition.

Severely malnourished children who are hospitalized with severe illnesses have a fatality rate of more than 20%.[9] Cross-sectional data from 241 nationally representative surveys show that prevalence of stunting has fallen in developing countries from 47% in 1980 to 33% in 2000 (that is, a reduction by 40 million). In 2010, stunting decreased to 27%, or 171 million, with 167 million in developing countries, and was projected to decrease to 22%, or 142 million, by 2020.[10] Progress is uneven between regions.[11] Stunting has increased in eastern Africa, but decreased in southeastern Asia, south-central Asia, and South America; northern Africa and the Caribbean observed modest improvement; and western Africa and Central America had little progress.[12] Strikingly, the prevalence of malnutrition in India, Bangladesh, Afghanistan, and Pakistan (38–51%) is much higher than in sub-Saharan Africa (26%).[13]

Relationship Between Childhood Diarrhea and Malnutrition: Global Concern

In children, malnutrition increases the frequency and duration of diarrheal illnesses, doubling the burden of diarrhea measured by days of diarrhea.[14] About 60% of all deaths among under-5 children in developing countries could be attributed to malnutrition. It has been estimated that nearly 50.6 million under-5 children are malnourished, and at least 90% of these children are from developing countries. Globally, 35% of deaths among children under 5 are related to malnutrition.[15] Stunting, severe wasting, and intrauterine growth restriction together were responsible for 2.2 million deaths and 21% of disability-adjusted life-years (DALYs) for children under 5.[16] In addition to growth failure and micronutrient deficiencies,[17] undernutrition can cause cognitive and behavioral impairments even with long-term nutritional rehabilitation.[18]

The presence of diarrhea among hospitalized children with **severe acute malnutrition (SAM)** increases mortality,[19,20] and conversely, children with SAM are at higher risk of life-threatening conditions, such as **hypoglycemia**, **hypothermia**, serious infections, and electrolyte imbalances.[21] **Underweight**, **stunting**, and **wasting** are each associated with synergistic increases in mortality from diarrhea, respiratory diseases, and infections such as measles.[22]

Etiology of Acute and Chronic Diarrhea and Malnutrition

Diarrhea in children in developing nations is usually caused by infection with microorganisms. Identifying causes of diarrhea is difficult because of the broad spectrum of possible microorganisms. *Vibrio cholerae, Shigella* species, *Salmonella* species, enteropathogenic *Escherichia coli* (EPEC), enteroaggregative *E. coli* (EAEC), enterotoxigenic *E. coli* (ETEC), *Aeromonas,* and *Campylobacter jejuni* are the most frequent bacterial enteric pathogens that cause severe acute diarrhea.[23,24,25,26,27,28] Intestinal helminth infections may also impair intestinal function, absorption, and growth.[29,30] Parasites such as *Entamoeba histolytica, Giardia lamblia,* and *Cryptosporidium* are often responsible for growth faltering and childhood diarrhea. Viruses that are responsible for diarrhea can include rotavirus, norovirus, astrovirus, sapovirus, and adenovirus.

Joaquin Cravioto, a prominent Mexican nutritionist, stated, "The basic origin of malnutrition is to be found in the

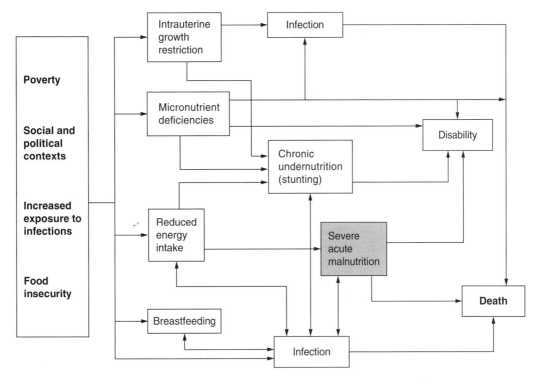

Figure 13-1 Direct and indirect causes of malnutrition and conceptual model of pathway to death and disability

Reproduced from Bhutta, Z. A., Ahmed, T., Black, R. E., Cousens, S., Dewey, K., Giugliani, E., ... Shekar, M. (2008). What works? Interventions for maternal and child undernutrition and survival. *Lancet, 371* (9610), 417-40.

malfunctioning of society as a whole and the accompanying injustices."[31] Examination of direct and indirect causes of malnutrition confirms the role of poverty (**Figure 13-1**). Poverty and food insecurity constrain the accessibility of nutritious diets that have high protein quality, adequate nutrient density, high micronutrient content, and large bioavailability, and are rich in macrominerals and essential fatty acids.[32,33] Inadequate diet is a primary cause of malnutrition, and secondary causes include impaired nutrient absorption in the GI tract and increased nutrient demands and/or nutrient excretion.[34] The severity of malnutrition depends on the cause, intensity, and duration of the deficiency.

Pathophysiology of Childhood Diarrhea and Malnutrition

Bacteria

Shigella flexneri, S. sonnei, Shigella boydii, and *Shigella dysenteriae* are among the most common causes of **dysentery**.[35]

Shigella-induced inflammation occurs partly in response to bacterial products[36] during bacterial translocation across **M cells** within the GI tract, and partly as an inflammatory immune response.[37,38,39] Intracellular invasion and spread in gut epithelium leads to **necrosis** and dysentery.[40,41]

Current *Shigella* Concerns

Emerging variants of *Shigella* have been reported in Vietnam and Bangladesh, implying the potential for antibiotic resistance and increased difficulties in treatment.

Millennium Development Goal 7: Ensure Environmental Sustainability. Target 7.C: Halve, by 2015, the proportion of the population without sustainable access to safe drinking water and basic sanitation

Reproduced from the United Nations. (n.d.). 2015 Millennium Development Goals. Retrieved from http://www.un.org/millenniumgoals/. Accessed August 13, 2013. This source is used for all Millennium Development Goals in this chapter.

Cholera causes severe watery diarrhea and can lead to rapid death without proper treatment. It is caused by water or food contaminated with *V. cholerae*. *V. cholerae* produces several antibodies known as hemagglutinins (HA) that enhance attachment and colonization of the small intestinal epithelium and produces cholera toxin (CT).[42] A series of steps[43,44,45,46] due to CT in the small intestine leads to increased chloride secretion and decreased sodium absorption, producing the massive fluid and electrolyte loss characteristic of cholera.[47,48]

Current Cholera Concerns

Only isolates in the serogroup *Vibrio cholerae* O1 (consisting of two biotypes known as "classical" and "El Tor") and the derivative O139 can cause epidemic cholera.[49] The Haitian Ministry of Public Health and Population (MSPP) reported a cholera outbreak in 2010.[50] Within a month, the outbreak had spread to almost every corner of the country, and four weeks later, the outbreak totaled 121,518 cases, including 63,711 hospitalizations and 2,591 deaths.[51] The National Public Health Laboratory (LNSP) in Haiti and an investigation team from MSPP and the Centers for Disease Control and Prevention's Haiti Office reported that *Vibrio cholera*, serogroup O1, serotype Ogawa, biotype El Tor from stool specimens was responsible for this large-scale outbreak.[52] Prevention and control measures implemented by MSPP with assistance from governmental and nongovernmental partners included (1) increasing access to treated drinking water; (2) providing education on better sanitation, hygiene, and food preparation practices; (3) advising ill persons to use ORS immediately and seek health care at the onset of watery diarrhea; (4) enhancing cholera treatment capacity at existing healthcare institutions; and (5) establishing cholera treatment centers.[53]

> *Public Health Core Competency 1: Analytical /Assessment Skills 1: Identifies the health status of populations and their related determinants of health and illness*
>
> Reproduced from Council on Linkages Between Academia and Public Health Practice. 2010 May. Core Competencies for Public Health Professionals. Washington, DC: Public Health Foundation. http://www.phf.org/resourcestools/Documents/Core_Competencies_for_Public_Health_Professionals_2010May.pdf. Accessed August 13, 2013. This source is used for all Public Health Core Competencies in this chapter.

Diseases caused by *Helicobacter pylori* include chronic gastritis and gastric adenocarcinoma.[54] Infection occurs primarily in early childhood,[55] and it can initiate a vicious cycle of events causing malnutrition, growth retardation, and increased morbidity and mortality.[56,57] Acute *H. pylori* infection causes chloride imbalances[58,59] and diarrhea.[60] Acid concentrations and gastric juice secretion rates are diminished in severely malnourished children,[61] allowing higher levels of bacterial colonization[62,63] and a further decrease in stomach acidity.[64] Hypochlorydia also increases susceptibility to enteric infections such as salmonellosis, cholera, giardiasis, shigellosis, and others due to the reduction of the gastric acid barrier.[65,66]

Enteroaggregative *E. coli* (EAEC) causes disease mainly by inducing host inflammation and changes in function in the epithelial cells lining the gut.[67]

Viruses

Rotavirus causes diarrhea through multiple mechanisms. Malabsorption occurs from destruction of enterocytes, or cells lining the GI tract. A toxic rotavirus protein induces imbalances of the electrolytes potassium and sodium and inhibits reabsorption of water. It also impairs enzyme activity, leading to **lactose intolerance** that can last for weeks.[68,69,70] A recurrence of mild diarrhea often follows the reintroduction of formula milk to the child's diet,[71] but breastfeeding can help prevent rotavirus diarrhea.

Current Rotavirus Concerns

In 2004, rotavirus accounted for 527,000 under-5 deaths, or 29% of all diarrhea-caused deaths. Twenty-three percent of deaths due to rotavirus disease occurred in India, and Nigeria, Congo, Ethiopia, China, and Pakistan together accounted for one-quarter of deaths due to rotavirus.[72] In Bangladesh, 5,600 to 9,400 under-5 deaths annually are attributable to rotavirus diarrhea. The proportion of diarrhea from rotavirus rose from 22% in 1993 to 42% in 2004 in urban Dhaka, and was common among children aged 3 to 24 months.[73]

Current Concerns with Other Viruses

From 2001 to 2003, 73 outbreaks of norovirus occurred in Switzerland and in the United States,[74,75] with additional outbreaks in Brazil,[76] Scotland,[77] the Netherlands,[78] and Germany.[79,80] In Japan, an outbreak of saporovirus occurred in 2004.[81] Also in Japan, an outbreak of acute gastroenteritis adenovirus occurred in infants and children.[82]

Parasites

Amebiasis, caused by the invasion of the intestinal wall by the protozoan parasite *Entamoeba histolytica,* is strongly associated with a high incidence of diarrhea in malnourished children. *E. histolytica* infection results from ingestion of the parasite through fecally contaminated food or water. In developing countries, *E. histolytica* causes 2–10% of diarrheal episodes in children, and *E. histolytica*–induced amebiasis leads to 50 million infections and 100,000 deaths worldwide annually.[83] The increased incidence of *E. histolytica* in malnourished children may result from an impaired immune system and reductions in protective IgA antibodies.[84,85,86] *Cryptosporidium* species is another parasite that can cause diarrheal disease.

Interaction Between Diarrhea and Malnutrition

The epithelium of the GI tract is a single layer of cells acting as a barrier to the rest of the body and regulates nutrient digestion, secretion, and absorption.[87] Epithelial damage can lead to GI infections and diarrhea. Anorexia and malabsorption of carbohydrates, lipids, proteins, and micronutrients can lead to malnutrition,[88,89] impaired weight and height gain, and delayed physical and cognitive development.[90,91,92,93] Conversely, malnutrition causes abnormalities in the GI epithelium.[94]

The GI-associated lymphoid tissues, such as Peyer's patches, contain immune cells and effect immune responses against GI pathogens.[95] Antigens in the gut are transported to Peyer's patches, where they can be neutralized through IgA-mediated responses.[96] Malnutrition compromises this gut mucosal immunity through decreases in T-cell function, **cytokine** production, and the ability of lymphocytes to respond appropriately to cytokines.[97,98,99,100] Malnourished children have altered production of cytokines, including IL-2, IL-4, IL-6, and IL-10. Altered physiology of lymphocytes may be the predominant cause of the immune impairment observed in malnourished children.[101] Loss of protein with anorexia during *Shigella* is another important factor.

Malnutrition is a major predictor for prolonged and persistent diarrhea,[102,103,104,105] which lasts for at least 14 days.[106] A review investigating morbidity and mortality caused by persistent diarrhea over the past three decades included data from Bangladesh, Brazil, Ethiopia, India, Indonesia, and Peru. An estimated 3 to 5 billion diarrheal illness cases and 5 to 10 million diarrhea-related deaths occurred annually during those three decades among 3 billion people in Africa, Asia, and Latin America.[107]

Clinical Assessment of Dehydration and Malnutrition

Diarrhea manifests as dehydration due to loss of water and **electrolytes**, or sodium, chloride, potassium, and bicarbonate, which are lost during diarrheal episodes. Dehydration can be assessed using clinical signs (**Table 13-4**).[108]

Table 13-4 Clinical assessment of dehydration

Parameters	Clinical Findings		
Condition*	Normal	Irritable/less active*	Lethargic/comatose*
Eyes	Normal	Sunken	
Mucosa	Normal	Dry	
Thirst*	Normal	Thirsty*	Inability to drink*
Skin turgor*	Normal	Reduced*	
Radial pulse*	Normal		Uncountable/absent*
Diagnosis	No dehydration	If at least two signs, including one key sign (*) are present, diagnose: Some dehydration	If some dehydration plus one of the above key signs (*) are present, diagnose: Severe dehydration
Estimated body weight loss	0-4%	5-10%	>10%

Reproduced from Chisti, M. J., Salam, M. A., Bardhan, P. K., Ahad, R., La Vincente, S., & Duke, T. (2010). Influences of dehydration on clinical features of radiological pneumonia in children attending an urban diarrhoea treatment centre in Bangladesh. *Annals of Tropical Paediatrics*, 30(4), 311-16.

Table 13-5 Classification of malnutrition according to the National Center for Health Statistics (NCHS)

	Well Nourished	First Degree (Mild)	Second Degree (Moderate)	Third Degree (Severe)
Weight-for-age (WA)	90-120%	75-89%	60-74%	< 60% (Severe undernutrition)
Weight-for-height (WH)	90-120%	80-89%	70-79%	< 70% (Severe wasting)
Height-for-age (HA)	95-110%	90-94%	85-89%	< 85% (Severe stunting)

Data from World Health Organization and United Nations Children's Fund. (2009). WHO child growth standards and the identification of severe acute malnutrition in infants and children. Accessed August 26, 2013 from http://www.who.int/nutrition/publications/severemalnutrition/9789241598163_eng.pdf.

Several anthropometric approaches can be used to assess malnutrition. Comparison with median weights and heights of healthy children using reference values from the National Center for Health Statistics (NCHS) is an example of a quantitative method useful in community and clinical settings for estimating prevalence and severity of malnutrition (**Table 13-5**).[109,110,111] The Wellcome classification is used in clinical settings. It is based upon weight-for-age (W/A) and the presence or absence of nutritional edema (**Table 13-6**).[112]

The mid-upper arm circumference (MUAC) is useful for rapid assessment of nutritional status of children in a field setting or in an emergency situation, such as famine. However, it is appropriate only for children between 1 and 5 years of age (**Table 13-7**).

Nutritional status may also be expressed in terms of standard deviation (SD) score of an anthropometric index such as weight-for-height (W/H). This score, also known as the z score, indicates deviation of a child's nutritional status from NCHS reference values (**Table 13-8**).[113]

Table 13-6 Wellcome classification for assessing malnutrition

W/A (% of NCHS median)	Edema	
	Present	Absent
80-60	Kwashiorkor	Undernutrition
< 60	Marasmic kwashiorkor	Marasmus

Reproduced from Food and Agriculture Organization of the United Nations (1997). Food and Nutrition Series. No. 29. Available at: http://www.fao.org/docrep/w0073e/w0073e05.htm

Table 13-7 Classification of malnutrition by MUAC

MUAC	Nutritional Status
> 13.5 cm	Not malnourished
11.5-13.5 cm	Moderately malnourished
< 11.5 cm	Severely malnourished

Data from World Health Organization and United Nations Children's Fund. (2009). WHO child growth standards and the identification of severe acute malnutrition in infants and children. Accessed August 26, 2013, from http://www.who.int/nutrition/publications/severemalnutrition/9789241598163_eng.pdf

Table 13-8 Classification of malnutrition by Standard Deviation Score

	Well nourished	Moderate	Severe
Weight-for-age z score	$\geq$ –2 z score	– 3 to < –2 z score	< – 3 z score (Severe undernutrition)
Weight-for-height z score	$\geq$ –2 z score	– 3 to < –2 z score	< – 3 z score (Severe wasting)
Height-for-age z score	$\geq$ –2 z score	– 3 to < –2 z score	< – 3 z score (Severe stunting)

Data from World Health Organization and United Nations Children's Fund. (2009). WHO child growth standards and the identification of severe acute malnutrition in infants and children. Accessed August 26, 2013 from http://www.who.int/nutrition/publications/severemalnutrition/9789241598163_eng.pdf

Treatment of Diarrhea with Severe Malnutrition Including Dehydration

Management of children with severe malnutrition has three phases: acute, nutrition rehabilitation, and follow-up. Treatment is based on severe wasting or severe undernutrition or nutritional edema.

Phase 1: Acute Phase

Hypoglycemia, hypothermia, water–electrolyte imbalance, and infection are four life-threatening conditions during the acute phase, and management of this stage must begin as soon as possible. Antimicrobial treatment, appropriate feeding, and correction of micronutrient deficiencies are initiated.[114]

Antimicrobial Treatment and Nutritional Support

WHO guidelines recommend broad-spectrum antimicrobials for children with SAM due to increased vulnerability to pneumonia, diarrhea, and urinary tract infections due to bacterial infections.[115,116] Broad-spectrum antimicrobial treatment immediately after admission improves the outcome of feeding, prevents shock, and reduces death rate.[117] Local sensitivity patterns of common bacteria, availability and cost-effectiveness of antimicrobials should be considered. Appropriate antimicrobials are required to treat specific infections, with specific recommendations for shigellosis, salmonellosis, cholera, and amebiasis, for example. Ampicillin, gentamicin, and ceftriaxone are likely options for treatment of diarrheal disease. Dose, frequency, and mode of administration— that is, intramuscular (IM) or IV, must be considered. All children aged 1 year and above should be dewormed. Deworming treatment should be done every six months during the follow-up phase.

The course of treatment must be reevaluated if the child: has no clinical improvement of fever or respiratory rate within 48 hours; develops a weak pulse; has a deterioration of condition after 24 hours of treatment; has suspected septicemia with presence of weak pulse, hypothermia, hypoglycemia, or shock; or is dehydrated.

Oral Rehydration Therapy and Energy and Macronutrient Support

Diarrhea with dehydration is common among children with SAM. Although serum sodium is reduced in malnourished children, total body sodium is normal or increased.[118] To prevent fluid overload and heart failure, the provision of ORS for rehydrating children with SAM occurs over 10 to 12 hours, compared with 3 to 6 hours for well-nourished patients. ORS may need to be administered through a nasogastric (NG) tube drip for children who are unable to drink due to extreme weakness or severe vomiting.

The use of IV fluids is delayed as long as possible, but it is needed in the following conditions:

1. Severe dehydration
2. Septic shock
3. Severe abdominal distension with absent bowel sounds
4. Severe vomiting
5. High purging

The total fluid required is calculated and the prescription is given in terms of drops per minute (1 ml = 60 drops, by a microdrip or soluset). If the child is unable to drink due to extreme weakness or severe vomiting, ORS is administered through NG tube drip. Reassessment should be done every 30 minutes to prevent the relapse of severe dehydration.

Treatment should include adherence to a specific feeding schedule from the beginning of treatment or within two hours of starting rehydration. Breastfeeding must be continued if the child is able to suck. Feeding is started with a liquid diet at a volume of 10 ml/kg at each feeding. Feedings should be every two hours, or 12 times per day, and provide 80 kcal/kg per day. As the child's appetite improves shortly after admission, quantity should increase to 100 kcal/kg per day. Protein intake should be 1 to 1.5 g/kg per day.

Vitamin and Mineral Supplementation

Vitamin A: If **xerophthalmia** is not present, vitamin A is given. Doses are 200,000 international units (IU) (8 drops) for children over 1 year old, 100,000 IU (4 drops) for infants 6 to 12 months, and 50,000 IU (2 drops) for those below 6 months.[119,120] If the child has xerophthalmia, higher doses of vitamin A should be provided, taking care to prevent irritation of any inflammation that is present.

Zinc: WHO and UNICEF recommend zinc supplementation during acute diarrhea.[121] The amount of 2 mg/kg/day of elemental zinc is given for at least one month and continued through nutritional rehabilitation for very severely malnourished children (W/A less than 50%, or W/H less than 70%, or with edema).[122,123]

Multivitamins: A multivitamin containing 5,000 IU vitamin A (as palmitate), 1,000 IU vitamin D, 1.6 mg thiamine hydrochloride, 1 mg riboflavin, 1 mg pyridoxine hydrochloride, 10 mg nicotinamide, 5 mg calcium D-pantothenate, and 50 mg ascorbic acid[124,125,126,127] should be provided for at least one month in a dose of 1 ml twice daily for children more than 1 year of age, and 0.5 ml twice daily for infants (less than 1 year of age), and should be continued until nutritional rehabilitation is complete.

Folic acid: Folic acid, one-quarter tablet (5 mg/tablet), is given once daily for at least 15 days, and continued through nutritional rehabilitation for very severely malnourished children.[128,129]

Potassium: Depletion of potassium, an electrolyte, is common among children with SAM. Oral potassium solution is provided at the dose of 4 mmol/kg per day, three times daily for five days.[130]

Magnesium: Magnesium sulfate (50%), 0.1 ml/kg (0.4 mmol/kg), is injected daily for seven days.[131,132]

Early Recognition of Complications and Their Proper Management

Hypoglycemia: Blood glucose levels can be measured by dextrostix. If it occurs within the first two days of treatment, hypoglycemia, or blood glucose less than 3.0 mmol (54 mg/dl), can lead to death. It can result from severe systemic infection or improper feeding. Signs of hypoglycemia include low body temperature, clouding of consciousness, lethargy, and convulsions.

Treatment should begin immediately on suspicion, before confirmation of hypoglycemia. Children who are able to drink should receive 25–50 ml of 10% glucose (or 5 g sugar in 50 ml water). If the child is unconscious or has convulsions, 2 ml/kg of 25% glucose is administered intravenously followed by 25–50 ml of 10% glucose or table sugar in water (25 ml for a very small infant) through NG tube to prevent recurrence. If the dose of IV glucose cannot be given quickly, NG treatment is given first.

Hypothermia: Children with temperature under 35.5 degrees Celsius (less than 96 degrees Fahrenheit) (rectal) or temperature under 35 degrees Celsius (less than 95 degrees Fahrenheit) (axillary/underarm) should be wrapped in blankets. A warm electric lamp can be used, but must be placed far enough from the patient to avoid burns. Rectal temperature should be measured every 30 minutes during rewarming with a lamp, as the child may rapidly become hyperthermic. Hypoglycemia should be suspected.

Septic shock: Signs of septic shock include weak or absent radial pulse, signs of dehydration without a history of watery diarrhea, hypothermia, and hypoglycemia. It should be corrected with isotonic infusion of 20 ml/kg with 5% dextrose over one hour. Cholera saline is preferred over normal saline if there is a history of watery diarrhea. This therapy can be repeated once if septic shock persists. Additional treatment includes broad-spectrum antibiotics, oxygen therapy, and correction of hypoglycemia, hypothermia, and acidosis as necessary.

Acidosis: Common in cases of diarrhea with dehydration, **acidosis** usually requires no treatment other than appropriate correction of dehydration. If symptoms such as rapid and deep breathing and low total serum CO_2 (< 6 mmol/L) persist, 1 mg/kg of 8.4% sodium bicarbonate can be infused slowly.

Hypokalemia: Oral rather than IV-administered potassium should be sufficient for **hypokalemia** in children with SAM and without significant diarrhea, vomiting, or the need for IV rehydration. The risk of fluid overload with IV fluids is of great concern. For all children with hypokalemia, oral potassium should be administered at 4 mmol/kg per day in three divided doses for five days. Children requiring IV fluids for severe dehydration or with a large stool output that cannot be managed with ORS can receive potassium via IV, with dose based on blood potassium levels.

Abdominal distension: If there is increasing abdominal distension, food is offered at three- to four-hour intervals. If the problem does not resolve, a single intramuscular injection of magnesium sulfate 50%, 0.3 ml/kg, may be given, to a maximum of 2 ml. This bolus dose is in addition to the daily maintenance dose of injection magnesium sulfate. If the problem does not resolve even with this treatment, then feeding may be discontinued and IV fluids given as half-strength cholera saline with 5% dextrose, 75 ml/kg per

24 hours (3 ml/kg per hour). If possible, 13 mmol of injection potassium chloride is added to one liter of the infusion.

Very severe anemia: 10 ml/kg of packed red cells or whole blood transfused over a period of three hours should be given in cases of very severe anemia (hemoglobin of less than 5 g/100 ml or hematocrit of less than 15%). Iron tablets or syrup are not given during the acute phase due to a risk of increase in the infection's severity.

Congestive heart failure (CHF): CHF can result from overhydration, very severe anemia, overly large or rapid blood transfusion, or high-sodium diets. Heart failure must be distinguished from pneumonia or septic shock. Heart failure from fluid overload requires cessation of IV fluid and administration of IV furosemide of 1 mg/kg. Digoxin can be provided only if the diagnosis of heart failure is confirmed, such as by raised jugular venous pressure, and blood potassium is normal.

Widespread weeping skin lesions: Weeping skin lesions are commonly seen in and around the buttocks of children with **kwashiorkor**. Affected areas are bathed in 1% potassium permanganate solution for 15 minutes daily. This dries the lesions, helps to prevent loss of serum, and inhibits infection.

Phase 2: Nutritional Rehabilitation Phase

The aim of this phase is to recover lost weight through intensive feeding. The child is stimulated emotionally and physically, and the mother is trained to continue care at home.

Once diarrhea has resolved, other infections are controlled, and appetite has improved, severely malnourished children (W/H < 70%, W/A < 50%, or with nutritional edema) need nutritional rehabilitation. Children requiring NG tube feeding are not yet ready for this phase. Infants less than 49 cm in length, which is less than the lowest reference length in the NCHS chart, should be admitted if weight-for-age is less than 60. In the nutritional rehabilitation phase, calories and protein are gradually increased in a programmed manner over a period of time to achieve rapid growth. A weight gain of more than 10 g/kg (1% of body weight) per day should be the goal of this phase. A key point is that the diet's proteins should mainly be from vegetable-derived foods. Animal-source foods (ASF), such as milk, eggs,

meat, and fish, are expensive and typically unaffordable for mothers when continuing children's nutritional rehabilitation at home.[133,134]

Phase 3: Follow-Up Phase

Goals of follow-up are to prevent relapse of severe malnutrition and to ensure proper physical growth and mental development of the child.

Prevention of Diarrhea

The World Health Organization has recommended the use of rotavirus vaccines in childhood immunization schedules.[135] The vaccines RV1 and RV5 have been approved in more than 100 countries in both developed as well as developing countries, including Bangladesh.[136,137,138,139,140,141,142,143,144,145,146,147,148,149,150] This vaccine is cost effective, and many experts support its immediate inclusion in the National Immunization Programme.[151,152,153,154,155]

Nonvaccine interventions for the prevention of childhood diarrhea in developing countries are: proper breastfeeding, appropriate complementary feeding, improvements of water and sanitation, promotion of personal and domestic hygiene, weaning education/food hygiene, vitamin A supplementation, and the prevention of low birth weight.[156,157,158,159,160]

Public Health Implications: Prevention of Malnutrition

Nearly one-third of children in developing countries suffer from chronic malnutrition.[161] Reducing malnutrition through prevention and treatment can reduce incidence of diarrhea as well as other diseases like pneumonia by preventing infections. Possible public health interventions to improve maternal and child nutrition include promotion of breastfeeding and proper complementary feeding, with or without provision of food supplements; micronutrient interventions; general supportive strategies to improve family and community nutrition; and reduction of the disease burden through the promotion of handwashing and strategies to reduce malaria in pregnancy.[162]

> *Millennium Development Goal 1: Eradicate Extreme Poverty and Hunger. Target 1.C: Halve, between 1990 and 2015, the proportion of people who suffer from hunger*

Progress toward Millennium Development Goal (MDG) 1 has been slow, however.[163] Initiation of breastfeeding within one hour of birth occurred among fewer than half of infants. Prevalence of exclusive breastfeeding among infants younger than 6 months is only 36%. Only about 60% of children receive age-appropriate breastfeeding, defined as exclusive breastfeeding before 6 months and continuing to receive breastmilk while being given complementary foods from 6 to 23 months.[164]

Approaches to Improving Dietary Adequacy

Dietary improvements by processing (dehulling, germinating, fermenting), fortification, and adding animal-source foods (for example, milk) or other specific nutrients are highly prioritized. Formulated foods to reduce malnutrition include fortified blended foods, commercial infant cereals, and ready-to-use foods (RUFs), such as pastes, compressed bars, and biscuits. Complementary food supplements containing milk powder, high-quality vegetable oil, peanut paste, sugar, and micronutrients include micronutrient powders or powdered complementary food supplements. Their protein, amino acids, and/or enzymes or lipid-based nutrient supplements can supply an additional 120–250 kcal/day.[165]

Multiple food fortification programs have seen some success. In India, a randomized control trial investigated the effects of supplemental nutrition among children 1 to 3 years old. The yearlong intervention included milk fortified with iron; zinc; vitamins A, C, and E; selenium; and copper. Children receiving the milk had 15% fewer days with severe illnesses, 18% lower incidence of diarrhea, and 26% lower incidence of acute lower respiratory illness.[166] Anemia was also reduced.[167,168] Vitamin A fortification of commodities, including sugar, cooking oils, and monosodium glutamate (MSG), is a promising strategy; mortality among children aged 6 to 49 months was reduced by 30% in the study in India.[169,170,171,172] In resource-poor settings, vitamin A supplementation can reduce diarrhea and all-cause childhood mortality.[173,174]

In Kenya, provision of maize fortified with high-dose sodium iron edetic acid reduced iron-deficiency anemia among children aged 3 to 8 years in Kenya.[175] In addition, distribution of micronutrients, including iron, through sachets that can be added to prepared food as a form of home fortification among young children under 2 years has led to increased hemoglobin concentrations and reduced iron-deficiency anemia.[176,177,178,179,180] However, iron supplementation also appears to increase incidence of diarrhea without significantly impacting growth.[181]

Zinc supplementation has a protective effect on child growth and development.[182] Zinc supplementation in children showed a weighted average effect size for change in height and weight[183] and led to fewer episodes of diarrhea, severe diarrhea or dysentery, persistent diarrhea, and lower respiratory infections,[184,185] and 9% lower child mortality.[186,187,188,189]

Thus, interventions that provide micronutrients are potentially effective in reducing stunting, micronutrient deficiencies, and childhood morbidity and mortality. Food assistance, breastfeeding counseling, micronutrient supplementation, and food fortification are also essential in food-insecure areas.

Increased Energy and Protein

Lipid-based nutrient supplements (LNS) can help prevent stunting (chronic malnutrition), wasting (acute malnutrition), recurring diarrheal diseases, and growth faltering after contracting diarrhea.[190] These fortified, lipid-based products range from energy-dense, ready-to-use therapeutic foods (RUTF), with several hundred kcal and relatively low micronutrient concentrations, to point-of-use supplements, with daily doses of 1 to 4 teaspoons, under 100 kcal and higher micronutrient concentrations.[191,192]

Prenatal Care and Sanitation and Hygiene Interventions

Multiple micronutrient supplementation is recommended during pregnancy.[193,194] It reduces maternal anemia and decreases the risk of low birth weight (LBW)[195,196,197] and small-for-gestational-age (SGA) babies. Recent systematic reviews found that hygiene interventions, such as handwashing, water treatment, sanitation, and health education, can reduce malnutrition and comorbidities of malnutrition, diarrhea, and dysentery.[198,199,200]

Dietary Diversification and Food Security

Agricultural interventions promoting home gardening, livestock, cash crops, and irrigation are promising and culturally relevant.[201] These can potentially reduce food insecurity, increase dietary diversity, and improve nutritional outcomes. While they are culturally relevant, they have generally been implemented only at a small scale, and have not been adequately assessed.[202,203,204] Dietary modification techniques, such as germination, fermentation, and malting, can improve children's micronutrient intakes and status,[205,206] but again, these techniques have not been proven effective on a large scale. Food security is necessary for acute and long-term prevention and control.[207,208,209,210,211]

In community-based dietary diversification/modification intervention in rural southern Malawi, the aim was to introduce and enhance the content and bioavailability of micronutrients in maize-based diets of stunted children aged 30 to 90 months. Two villages received the dietary intervention, which included more animal-source foods, especially soft-boned fish, more vitamin A–rich fruits, such as mangoes, and treatment of maize and legumes to lower content of phytates, which inhibit absorption of non-heme iron, zinc, and calcium. Median intakes of energy, protein, calcium, available zinc, heme iron, and vitamin B12 were greater in the intervention villages.[212]

Influence of Social Determinants

WHO identifies 10 categories of **social determinants** of health: social gradient, stress, early life, social exclusion, work, unemployment, social support, addiction, food, and transport.[213] Social determinants have significant impact on health status,[214] and public health interventions from both government and nongovernmental organizations (NGOs) must consider social determinants of health when developing programs to prevent and treat malnutrition and diarrheal diseases. Social awareness campaigns emphasizing health education programs led by efficient and experienced healthcare workers with adequate and simple training kits are essential.[215,216] Improving interpersonal communication can also be effective.[217] Benefits of prenatal education can include improving weight gain during pregnancy, reducing LBW, and improving breastfeeding practices.[218,219] To be more effective, education programs should be administered in conjunction with aid programs such as conditional cash transfer.[220,221]

Mexico's PROGRESA program, for example, includes cash transfer contingent on children's regular school attendance and health clinic visits. The program, which started in 1997 and covered 40% of all rural Mexican families by 2000, is now known as Oportunidades. Its aim is to reduce poverty. This program substantially increased caloric acquisition by increasing income and nutritional knowledge.[222] The program includes nutritional supplementation and education, and has improved the nutritional status among children 12 to 36 months in poor rural communities.[223,224] Average growth increased by one-sixth per year among these children, with greater increases among the poorest children.[225]

Conclusion

Malnutrition adversely affects the immune system and is therefore considered the most common cause of immunodeficiency throughout the world. Malnutrition increases the risk for diarrhea, which is among the most important causes of high morbidity and mortality in malnourished children. Conversely, children with diarrhea are at increased risk of developing malnutrition. Severely malnourished patients have higher mortality rates and more frequent hospital admissions than their well-nourished counterparts. Public health nutrition programs can reduce deaths due to diarrhea and malnutrition, with strategies including nutritional supplementation and education and policies to alleviate poverty.

References

1 World Health Organization. (2013, April). *Diarrhoeal disease.* Fact Sheet No. 330. Retrieved from http://www.who.int/mediacentre/factsheets/fs330/en/index.html

2 Gill, D. M. (1976). The arrangement of subunits in cholera toxin. *Biochemistry* 15(6), 1242-48.

3 Snyder, J. D., & Merson, M. H. (1982). The magnitude of the global problem of acute diarrheal disease: A review of active surveillance data. *Bulletin of the World Health Organization, 60*(4), 605-13.

4 Bern, C., Martines, J., de Zoysa, I., & Glass, R. I. (1992). The magnitude of the global problem of diarrhoeal disease: A ten-year update. *Bulletin of the World Health Organization, 70*(6), 705-14.

5 Kosek, M., Bern, C., & Guerrant, R. L. (2003). The global burden of diarrhoeal disease, as estimated from studies published between 1992 and 2000. *Bulletin of the World Health Organization, 81*(3), 197-204.

6 Murray, C. J. L., Lopez, A. D., Mathers, C. D., & Stein, C. (2001). *The Global Burden of Disease 2000 Project: Aims, methods, and data sources.* Geneva: World Health Organization.

7 Liu, L., Johnson, H. L., Cousens, S., Perin, J., Scott, S., Lawn, J. E., Rudan, I., . . . Black, R. E. (2012). Global, regional, and national causes of child mortality: An updated systematic analysis for 2010 with time trends since 2000. *Lancet, 379*(9832), 2151-61.

8 World Health Organization. (n.d.). *Malnutrition—the global picture, 2000.* Retrieved from http://www.who.int/home-page

9 Ahmed, T., Ali, M., Ullah, M. M., Choudhury, I. A., Haque, M. E., Salam, M. A., Rabbani, G. H., Suskind, R. M., & Fuchs, G. J. (1999). Mortality in severely malnourished children with diarrhoea and use of a standardised management protocol. *Lancet, 353*(9168), 1919-22.

10 de Onis, M., Blössner, M., & Borghi, E. (2012). Prevalence and trends of stunting among pre-school children, 1990-2020. *Public Health Nutrition, 15*(1), 142-48.

11 de Onis, M., Frongillo, E. A., & Blössner, M. (2000). Is malnutrition declining? An analysis of changes in levels of child malnutrition since 1980. *Bulletin of the World Health Organization, 78*(10), 1222-33.

12 de Onis, M., Frongillo E. A., & Blössner, M. (2000). Is malnutrition declining? An analysis of changes in levels of child malnutrition since 1980. *Bulletin of the World Health Organization, 78*(10), 1222-33.

13 Ahmed, T., Haque, R., Shamsir Ahmed, A. M., Petri, W. A., Jr., & Cravioto, A. (2009). Use of metagenomics to understand the genetic basis of malnutrition. *Nutrition Review, 67*(Suppl. 2), S201-6.

14 Guerrant, R. L., Schorling, J. B., McAuliffe, J. F., & de Souza, M. A. (1992). Diarrhea as a cause and an effect of malnutrition: Diarrhea prevents catch-up growth and malnutrition increases diarrhea frequency and duration. *American Journal of Tropical Medicine and Hygiene, 47*(1, Pt. 2), 28-35.

15 World Health Organization. (2004). *Severe acute malnutrition*. Geneva: World Health Organization.

16 Black, R. E., Allen, L. H., Bhutta, Z. A., Caulfield, L. E., de Onis, M., Ezzati, M., Mathers, C., & Rivera, J. (2008). Maternal and child undernutrition: Global and regional exposures and health consequences. *Lancet 371*(9608), 243-60.

17 Pasricha, S. R., & Biggs, B. A. (2010). Undernutrition among children in South and South-East Asia. *Journal of Paediatrics & Child Health, 46*(9), 497-503.

18 Galler, J. R., Bryce, C. P., Zichlin, M. L., Fitzmaurice, G., Eaglesfield, G. D., & Waber, D. P. (2012). Infant malnutrition is associated with persisting attention deficits in middle adulthood. *Journal of Nutrition, 142*(4), 788-94.

19 Talbert, A., Thuo, N., Karisa, J., Chesaro, C., Ohuma, E., Ignas, J., . . . Maitland, K. (2012). Diarrhoea complicating severe acute malnutrition in Kenyan children: A prospective descriptive study of risk factors and outcome. *PLOS One, 7*(6), e38321.

20 Irena, A. H., Mwambazi, M., & Mulenga, V. (2011). Diarrhea is a major killer of children with severe acute malnutrition admitted to inpatient set-up in Lusaka, Zambia. *Nutrition Journal, 10*, 110.

21 World Health Organization. (2004). *Maternal, newborn, child and adolescent health: Serious childhood problems in countries with limited resources*. Geneva: World Health Organization.

22 Black, R. E., Allen, L. H., Bhutta, Z. A., Caulfield, L. E., de Onis, M., Ezzati, M., Mathers, C., & Rivera, J. (2008). Maternal and child undernutrition: Global and regional exposures and health consequences. *Lancet 371*(9608), 243-60.

23 Mondal, D., Petri, W. A., Jr., Sack, R. B., Kirkpatrick, B. D., & Haque, R. (2006). *Entamoeba histolytica*-associated diarrheal illness is negatively associated with the growth of preschool children: Evidence from a prospective study. *Transactions of the Royal Society of Tropical Medicine and Hygiene, 100*(11), 1032-38.

24 Checkley, W., Epstein, L. D., Gilman, R. H., Black, R. E., Cabrera, L., & Sterling, C. R. (1998). Effects of *Cryptosporidium parvum* infection in Peruvian children: Growth faltering and subsequent catch-up growth. *American Journal of Epidemiology, 148*(5), 497-506.

25 Steiner, T. S., Lima, A. A., Nataro, J. P., & Guerrant, R. L. (1998). Enteroaggregative *Escherichia coli* produce intestinal inflammation and growth impairment and cause interleukin-8 release from intestinal epithelial cells. *Journal of Infectious Diseases, 177*(1), 88-96.

26 Tarleton, J. L., Haque, R., Mondal, D., Shu J., Farr, B. M., & Petri, W. A., Jr. (2006). Cognitive effects of diarrhea, malnutrition, and *Entamoeba histolytica* infection on school age children in Dhaka, Bangladesh. *American Journal of Tropical Medicine and Hygiene, 74*(3), 475-81.

27 Qadri, F., Saha, A., Ahmed, T., Al Tarique, A., Begum, Y. A., & Svennerholm, A. M. (2007). Disease burden due to enterotoxigenic *Escherichia coli* in the first 2 years of life in an urban community in Bangladesh. *Infection and Immunity, 75*(8), 3961-68.

28 Denno, D. M., Shaikh, N., Stapp, J. R., Qin, X., Hutter, C. M., Hoffman, V., . . . Klein, E. J. (2012). Diarrhea etiology in a pediatric emergency department: A case control study. *Clinical Infectious Diseases, 55*(7), 897-904.

29 Raj, S. M., Sein, K. T., Anuar, A. K., & Mustaffa, B. E. (1996). Effect of intestinal helminthiasis on intestinal permeability of early primary schoolchildren. *Transcriptions of the Royal Society of Tropical Medicine and Hygiene, 90*(6), 666-69.

30 Muniz, P. T., Ferreira, M. U., Ferreira, C. S., Conde, W. L., & Monteiro, C. A. (2002). Intestinal parasitic infections in young children in Sao Paulo, Brazil: Prevalences, temporal trends and associations with physical growth. *Annals of Tropical Medicine & Parasitology, 96*(5), 503-12.

31 Arroyo, P., & Mandujano, M. (2000). Joaquin Cravioto (1922-1998). *Journal of Nutrition, 130*(12), 2867-69.

32 De Pee, S., & Bloem, M. W. (2009). Current and potential role of specially formulated foods and food supplements for preventing malnutrition among 6- to 23-month-old children and for treating moderate malnutrition among 6- to 59-month-old children. *Food and Nutrition Bulletin, 30*(3 Suppl.), S434-63.

33 Müller, O., & Krawinkel, M. (2005). Malnutrition and health in developing countries. *CMAJ, 173*(3), 279-86.

34 Gomez, F., Ramos Galvan, R., Frenk, S., Cravioto Munoz, J., Chavez, R., & Vazquez, J. (2000). Mortality in second and third degree malnutrition, 1956. *Bulletin of the World Health Organization, 78*(10), 1275-80.

35 Hale, T. L., & Keusch, G. T. (1996). *Shigella*. In S. E. Baron (Ed.), *Medical microbiology*. Galveston, TX: University of Texas Medical Branch at Galveston.

36 Phalipon, A., & Sansonetti, P. J. (2003). Shigellosis: Innate mechanisms of inflammatory destruction of the intestinal epithelium, adaptive immune response, and vaccine development. *Critical Reviews in Immunology, 23*(5-6), 371-401.

37 Zychlinsky, A., Fitting, C., Cavaillon, J. M., & Sansonetti, P. J. (1994). Interleukin 1 is released by murine macrophages during apoptosis induced by *Shigella flexneri. Journal of Clinical Investigation, 94*(3), 1328-32.

38 Zychlinsky, A., Prevost, M. C., & Sansonetti, P. J. (1992). *Shigella flexneri* induces apoptosis in infected macrophages. *Nature, 358*(6382), 167-69.

39 Sansonetti, P. J. (1991). Genetic and molecular basis of epithelial cell invasion by *Shigella* species. *Reviews of Infectious Diseases, 13*(Suppl. 4), S285-92.

40 Perdomo, J. J., Gounon, P., & Sansonetti, P. J. (1994). Polymorphonuclear leukocyte transmigration promotes invasion of colonic epithelial monolayer by *Shigella flexneri. Journal of Clinical Investigation, 93*(2), 633-43.

41 Perdomo, O. J., Cavaillon, J. M., Huerre, M., Ohayon, H., Gounon, P., & Sansonetti, P. J. (1994). Acute inflammation causes epithelial invasion and mucosal destruction in experimental shigellosis. *Journal of Experimental Medicine, 180*(4), 1307-19.

42 Gill, D. M. (1976). The arrangement of subunits in cholera toxin. *Biochemistry, 15*(6), 1242-48.

43 Mekalanos, J. J., Collier, R. J., & Romig, W. R. (1979). Enzymic activity of cholera toxin. II. Relationships to proteolytic processing, disulfide bond reduction, and subunit composition. *Journal of Biological Chemistry, 254*(13), 5855-61.

44 Yamamoto, S., Takeda, Y., Yamamoto, M., et al. (1997). Mutants in the ADP-ribosyltransferase cleft of cholera toxin lack diarrheagenicity but retain adjuvanticity. *Journal of Experimental Medicine. 185*(7), 1203-10.

45 Cassel, D., & Pfeuffer, T. (1978). Mechanism of cholera toxin action: Covalent modification of the guanyl nucleotide-binding protein of the adenylate cyclase system. *Proceedings of the National Academies of Science of the United States of America, 75*(6), 2669-73.

46 Gill, D. M., & Meren, R. (1978). ADP-ribosylation of membrane proteins catalyzed by cholera toxin: basis of the activation of adenylate cyclase. *Proceedings of the National Academies of Science of the United States of America, 75*(7), 3050-54.

47 Holmgren, J. (1981). Actions of cholera toxin and the prevention and treatment of cholera. *Nature, 292*(5822), 413-17.

48 Gilman, A. G. (1984). G proteins and dual control of adenylate cyclase. *Cell, 36*(3), 577-79.

49 Mutreja, A., Kim, D. W., Thomson, N. R., Connor, T. R., Lee, J. H., . . . Dougan G. (2011). Evidence for several waves of global transmission in the seventh cholera pandemic. *Nature, 477*(7365), 462-65.

50 Centers for Disease Control and Prevention. (2010). Update: Cholera outbreak–Haiti, 2010. *Morbidity and Mortality Weekly Report, 59*(45), 1473-79.

51 Centers for Disease Control and Prevention. (2010). Update on cholera–Haiti, Dominican Republic, and Florida, 2010. *Morbidity and Mortality Weekly Report, 59*(50), 1637-41.

52 Centers for Disease Control and Prevention. (2010). Update: Cholera outbreak–Haiti, 2010. *Morbidity and Mortality Weekly Report, 59*(45), 1473-79.

53 Centers for Disease Control and Prevention. (2010). Update: cholera outbreak–Haiti, 2010. *Morbidity and Mortality Weekly Report, 59*(45), 1473-79.

54 Furuta, T., El-Omar, E. M., Xiao, F., Shirai, N., Takashima, M., & Sugimura, H. (2002). Interleukin 1 beta polymorphisms increase risk of hypochlorhydria and atrophic gastritis and reduce risk of duodenal ulcer recurrence in Japan. *Gastroenterology, 123*(1), 92-105.

55 Windle, H. J., Kelleher, D., & Crabtree, J. E. (2007). Childhood *Helicobacter pylori* infection and growth impairment in developing countries: A vicious cycle? *Pediatrics, 119*(3), e754-59.

56 Windle, H. J., Kelleher, D., & Crabtree, J. E. (2007). Childhood *Helicobacter pylori* infection and growth impairment in developing countries: A vicious cycle? *Pediatrics, 119,* (3), e754-59.

57 Bravo, L. E., Mera, R., Reina, J. C., Pradilla, A., Alzate, A., Fontham, E., & Correa, P. (2003). Impact of *Helicobacter pylori* infection on growth of children: A prospective cohort study. *Journal of Pediatric Gastroenterology and Nutrition, 37*(5), 614-19.

58 Dale, A., Thomas, J. E., Darboe, M. K., Coward, W. A., Harding, M., & Weaver, L. T. (1998). *Helicobacter pylori* infection, gastric acid secretion, and infant growth. *Journal of Pediatric Gastroenterology and Nutrition, 26*(4), 393-97.

59 Weaver, L. T. (1995). Royal Society of Tropical Medicine and Hygiene Meeting at Manson House, London, February 16, 1995. Aspects of *Helicobacter pylori* infection in the developing and developed world. *Helicobacter pylori* infection, nutrition and growth of West African infants. *Transactions of the Royal Society of Tropical Medicine and Hygiene, 89*(4), 347-50.

60 Windle, H. J., Kelleher, D., & Crabtree, J. E. (2007). Childhood *Helicobacter pylori* infection and growth impairment in developing countries: A vicious cycle? *Pediatrics, 119*(3), e754-59.

61 Mata, L. (1992). Diarrheal disease as a cause of malnutrition. *American Journal of Tropical Medicine and Hygiene, 47*(1, Pt. 2), 16-27.

62 Gilman, R. H., Partanen, R., Brown, K. H., Spira, W. M., Khanam, S., Greenberg, B., Bloom, S. R., & Ali, A. (1988). Decreased gastric acid secretion and bacterial colonization of the stomach in severely malnourished Bangladeshi children. *Gastroenterology, 94*(6), 1308-14.

63 Stockbruegger, R. W. (1985). Bacterial overgrowth as a consequence of reduced gastric acidity. *Scandinavian Journal of Gastroenterology,* (Suppl. 111), 7-16.

64 Cook, G. C. (1985). Infective gastroenteritis and its relationship to reduced gastric acidity. *Scandinavian Journal of Gastroenterology,* (Suppl. 111), 17-23.

65 Windle, H. J., Kelleher, D., & Crabtree, J. E. (2007). Childhood *Helicobacter pylori* infection and growth impairment in developing countries: A vicious cycle? *Pediatrics, 119*(3), e754-59.

66 Torres, J., Perez, G. P., Ximenez, C., Munoz, L., Camorlinga-Ponce, M., Ramos, F., Gomez, A., & Munoz, O. (2003). The association of intestinal parasitosis and *H. pylori* infection in children and adults from a Mexican community with high prevalence of parasitosis. *Helicobacter, 8*(3),179-85.

67 Petri, W. A., Jr., Miller, M., Binder, H. J., Levine, M. M., Dillingham, R., & Guerrant, R. L. (2008). Enteric infections, diarrhea, and their impact on function and development. *Journal of Clinical Investigation, 118*(4), 1277-90.

68 Hyser, J. M., & Estes, M. K. (2009). Rotavirus vaccines and pathogenesis: 2008. *Current Opinion in Gastroenterology, 25*(1), 36-43.

69 Farnworth, E. R. (2008). The evidence to support health claims for probiotics. *Journal of Nutrition, 138*(6), 1250S-1254S.

70 Ouwehand, A., & Vesterlund, S. (2003). Health aspects of probiotics. *IDrugs, 6*(6), 573-80.

71 Arya, S. C. (1984). Rotaviral infection and intestinal lactase level. *Journal of Infectious Diseases, 150*(5), 791.

72 Parashar, U. D., Burton, A., Lanata, C., Boschi-Pinto, C., Shibuya, K., Steele, D., Birmingham, M., & Glass, R. I. (2009). Global mortality associated with rotavirus disease among children in 2004. *Journal of Infectious Diseases, 200*(Suppl. 1), S9-S15.

73 Tanaka, G., Faruque, A. S., Luby, S. P., Malek, M. A., Glass, R. I., & Parashar, U. D. (2007). Deaths from rotavirus disease in Bangladeshi children: Estimates from hospital-based surveillance. *Pediatric Infectious Disease Journal, 26*(11), 1014-18.

74 Fretz, R., Svoboda, P., Luthi, T. M., Tanner, M., & Baumgartner, A. (2005). Outbreaks of gastroenteritis due to infections with Norovirus in Switzerland, 2001-2003. *Epidemiology and Infection, 133*(3), 429-37.

75 Widdowson, M. A., Sulka, A., Bulens, S. N., Beard, R. S., Chaves, S. S., Hammond, R., . . . Glass, R. I. (2005). Norovirus and food-borne disease, United States, 1991-2000. *Emerging Infectious Diseases, 11*(1), 95-102.

76 Fioretti, J. M., Ferreira, M. S., Victoria, M., Vieira, C. B., Xavier Mda, P., Leite, J. P., & Miagostovich, M. P. (2011). Genetic diversity of noroviruses in Brazil. *Memórias do Instituto Oswaldo Cruz, 106*(8), 942-47.

77 McAllister, G., Holmes, A., Garcia, L., Cameron, F., Cloy, K., Danial, J., . . . Templeton, K. E. (2012). Molecular epidemiology of norovirus in Edinburgh healthcare facilities, Scotland 2007-2011. *Epidemiology and Infection, 140*(12), 2273-81.

78 Svraka, S., Duizer, E., Vennema, H., de Bruin, E., van der Veer, B., Dorresteijn, B., & Koopmans, M. (2007). Etiological role of viruses in outbreaks of acute gastroenteritis in The Netherlands from 1994 through 2005. *Journal of Clinical Microbiology, 45*(5), 1389-94.

79 Koch, J., Schneider, T., Stark, K., & Schreier, E. (2006). [Norovirus infections in Germany]. *Bundesgesundheitsblatt Gesundheitsforschung Gesundheitsschutz, 49*(3), 296-309.

80 Matthews, J. E., Dickey, B. W., Miller, R. D., Felzer, J. R., Dawson, B. P., Lee, A. S., . . . Leon, J. S. (2012). The epidemiology of published norovirus outbreaks: a review of risk factors associated with attack rate and genogroup. *Epidemiology and Infection, 140*(7), 1161-72.

81 Phan, T. G., Trinh, Q. D., Yagyu, F., Sugita, K., Okitsu, S., Muller, W. E., & Ushijima, H. (2006). Outbreak of sapovirus infection among infants and children with acute gastroenteritis in Osaka City, Japan, during 2004-2005. *Journal of Medical Virology, 78*(6), 839-46.

82 Shimizu, H., Phan, T. G., Nishimura, S., Okitsu, S., Maneekarn, N., & Ushijima, H. (2007). An outbreak of adenovirus serotype 41 infection in infants and children with acute gastroenteritis in Maizuru City, Japan. *Infection, Genetics and Evolution, 7*(2), 279-84.

83 Stanley, S. L., Jr. (2003). Amoebiasis. *Lancet, 361*(9362), 1025-34.

84 Villena, J., Barbieri, N., Salva, S., Herrera, M., & Alvarez, S. (2009). Enhanced immune response to pneumococcal infection in malnourished mice nasally treated with heat-killed *Lactobacillus casei*. *Microbiology and Immunology, 53*(11), 636-46.

85 Holmgren, J., & Czerkinsky, C. (2005). Mucosal immunity and vaccines. *Nature Medicine, 11*(4 Suppl.), S45-53.

86 Haque, R., Mondal, D., Duggal, P., Kabir, M., Roy, S., Farr, B. M., Sack, R. B., & Petri W. A., Jr. (2006). *Entamoeba histolytica* infection in children and protection from subsequent amebiasis. *Infection and Immunity, 74*(2), 904-9.

87 Bjerknes, M., & Cheng, H. (2005). Gastrointestinal stem cells. II. Intestinal stem cells. *American Journal of Physiology. Gastrointestinal and Liver Physiology, 289*(3), G381-87.

88 Jambunathan, L. R., Neuhoff, D., & Younoszai, M. K. (1981). Intestinal disaccharidases in malnourished infant rats. *American Journal of Clinical Nutrition, 34*(9), 1879-84.

89 Akuyam, S. A. (2007). A review of some metabolic changes in protein-energy malnutrition. *Nigerian Postgraduate Medical Journal, 14*(2), 155-62.

90 Mata, L. (1992). Diarrheal disease as a cause of malnutrition. *American Journal of Tropical Medicine and Hygiene, 47*(1, Pt. 2), 16-27.

91 Lima, A. A., Brito, L. F., Ribeiro, H. B., Martins, M. C., Lustosa, A. P., Rocha, E. M., . . . Guerrant, R. L. (2005). Intestinal barrier function and weight gain in malnourished children taking glutamine supplemented enteral formula. *Journal of Pediatric Gastroenterology Nutrition, 40*(1), 28-35.

92 Islam, S., Mitra, A. K., Chowdhury, A. K., & Alam, N. H. (2006). Intestinal enzymes during malnutrition & infection in rabbits. *Indian Journal of Medical Research, 124*(3), 313-18.

93 Martorell, R., Yarbrough, C., Yarbrough, S., & Klein, R. E. (1980). The impact of ordinary illnesses on the dietary intakes of malnourished children. *American Journal of Clinical Nutrition, 33*(2), 345-50.

94 Martorell, R., Yarbrough, C., Yarbrough, S., & Klein, R. E. (1980). The impact of ordinary illnesses on the dietary intakes of malnourished children. *American Journal of Clinical Nutrition, 33*(2), 345-50.

95 Erickson, K. L., & Hubbard, N. E. (2009). Assessing mucosal immunity with new concepts and innovative, time-honored strategies. *Nutrition Review, 67*(Suppl. 2), S172-82.

96 Erickson, K. L., & Hubbard, N. E. (2009). Assessing mucosal immunity with new concepts and innovative, time-honored strategies. *Nutrition Review, 67*(Suppl. 2), S172-82.

97 Ing, R., Su, Z., Scott, M. E., & Koski, K. G. (2000). Suppressed T helper 2 immunity and prolonged survival of a nematode parasite in protein-malnourished mice. *Proceedings of the National Academy of Sciences of the United States, 97*(13), 7078-83.

98 Rodriguez, L., Gonzalez, C., Flores, L., Jimenez-Zamudio, L., Graniel, J., & Ortiz, R. (2005). Assessment by flow cytometry of cytokine production in malnourished children. *Clinical and Diagnostic Laboratory Immunology, 12*(4), 502-7.

99 Chandra, R. K. (1992). Protein-energy malnutrition and immunological responses. *Journal of Nutrition, 122*(3 Suppl.), 597-600.

100 Pelletier, L., Frongillo. A., & Habicht. P. (1993). Nutrition and immunology. *American Journal of Public Health, 83,* 1130-33.

101 González, C., Rodriguez, L., Bonilla, E., Betancourt, M., Siller, N., Zumano, E., & Ortiz, R. (1997). Electrophoretic analysis of plasmatic and lymphocytes secreted proteins in malnourished children. *Medical Science Research, 25,* 643-46.

102 Bhandari, N., Bhan, M. K., Sazawal, S., Clemens, J. D. C., Bhatnagar, S., & Khoshoo, V. (1989). Association of antecedent malnutrition with persistent diarrhoea: A case-control study. *BMJ, 298,* 1284-87.

103 Moore, S. R., Lima, N. L., Soares, A. M., Oria, R. B., Pinkerton, R. C., & Barrett, L. J. (2010). Prolonged episodes of acute diarrhea reduce growth and increase risk of persistent diarrhea in children. *Gastroenterology, 139,* 1156-64.

104 Sodeinde, O., Adeyemo, A. A., Gbadegesin, R. A., & Ademowo, O. G. (1997). Persistent diarrhoea in Nigerian children aged less than five years: A hospital-based study. *Journal of Diarrhoeal Diseases Research, 15,* 155-60.

105 Mahalanabis, D., Alam, A. N., Rahman, N., & Hasnat, A. (1991). Prognostic indicators and risk factors for increased duration of acute diarrhoea and for persistent diarrhoea in children. *International Journal of Epidemiology, 20,* 1064-72.

106 Dialogue on Diarrhoea and the Applied Diarrhoeal Disease Research Project. (1992). *Clinical update: Persistent diarrhoea.* Retrieved from http://rehydrate.org/dd/pdf/su48.pdf

107 Lima, A. A., & Guerrant, R. L. (1992). Persistent diarrhea in children: Epidemiology, risk factors, pathophysiology, nutritional impact, and management. *Epidemiology Review, 14,* 222-42.

108 Chisti, M.. J., Salam, M. A., Bardhan, P. K., Ahad, R., La Vincente, S., & Duke, T. (2010). Influences of dehydration on clinical features of radiological pneumonia in children attending an urban diarrhoea treatment centre in Bangladesh. *Annals of Tropical Paediatrics, 30*(4), 311-16.

109 de Onis, M., Frongillo, E. A., & Blössner, M. (2000). Is malnutrition declining? An analysis of changes in levels of child malnutrition since 1980. *Bulletin of the World Health Organization 78*(10), 1222-33.

110 Gomez, F., Galvan, R. R., Cravioto, J., & Frenk, S. (1955). Malnutrition in infancy and childhood, with special reference to kwashiorkor. *Advances in Pediatrics, 7,* 131-69.

111 Waterlow, J. C., Buzina, R., Keller, W., Lane, J. M., Nichaman, M. Z., & Tanner, J. M. (1977). The presentation and use of height and weight data for comparing the nutritional status of groups of children under the age of 10 years. *Bulletin of the World Health Organization, 55*(4), 489-98.

112 Waterlow, J. C. (1996). *Malnutrición proteico-energética* (pp. 261-62). Washington, DC: Organización Panamericana de la Salud.

113 Pinstrup-Andersen, P., Burger, S., Habicht, J. P., & Peterson, K. (1993). Protein-energy malnutrition. In D. T. Jamison, W. H. Mosley, A. R. Measham, & J. L. Bobadilla (Eds.), *Disease control priorities in developing countries* (2nd ed.) (pp. 391-420). Oxford: Oxford University Press.

114 Picot, J., Hartwell, D., Harris, P., Mendes, D., Clegg, A. J., & Takeda, A. (2012). The effectiveness of interventions to treat severe acute malnutrition in young children: A systematic review. *Health Technology Assessment, 16*(19), 1-316.

115 Frenk, S. (1985). Protein-energy malnutrition (pp. 153-93). In Arneil, G. C., Metcoff, J. (Eds.), *Pediatric nutrition.* London: Butterworths.

116 Lazzerini, M., & Tickell, D. (2011). Antibiotics in severely malnourished children: Systematic review of efficacy, safety and pharmacokinetics. *Bulletin of the World Health Organization, 89*(8), 594-607.

117 World Health Organization. (1999). *Management of severe malnutrition: A manual for physicians and other senior health workers.* Geneva: World Health Organization.

118 Ahmed, T., Begum, B., Badiuzzaman, A. M., & Fuchs, G. (2001). Management of severe malnutrition and diarrhea. *Indian Journal of Pediatrics, 68*(1), 45-51.

119 Picot, J., Hartwell, D., Harris, P., Mendes, D., Clegg, A. J., & Takeda, A. (2012). The effectiveness of interventions to treat severe acute malnutrition in young children: A systematic review. *Health Technology Assessment, 16*(19), 1-316.

120 Sattar, S., Ahmed, T., Rasul, C. H., Saha, D., Salam, M. A., & Hossain, M. I. (2012). Efficacy of a high-dose in addition to daily low-dose vitamin A in children suffering from severe acute malnutrition with other illnesses. *PLOS One, 7*(3), e33112.

121 Lazzerini, M., & Ronfani, L. (2012). Oral zinc for treating diarrhoea in children. *Cochrane Database of Systematic Reviews, 6,* CD005436.

122 Lazzerini, M., & Ronfani, L. (2012). Oral zinc for treating diarrhoea in children. *Cochrane Database of Systematic Reviews, 6,* CD005436.

123 Imdad, A., Sadiq, K., & Bhutta, Z. A. (2011). Evidence-based prevention of childhood malnutrition. *Current Opinion in Clinical Nutrition and Metabolic Care, 14*(3), 276-85.

124 Mtvarelidze, Z. G., Kvezereli-Kopadze, A. N., & Kvezereli-Kopadze, M. A. (2009). [Megaloblastic-vitamin B12 deficiency anemia in childhood]. *Georgian Medical News,* (170), 57-60.

125 Reinken, L., Stolley, H., & Droese, W. (1979). Biochemical assessment of thiamine nutrition in childhood. *European Journal of Pediatrics, 131*(4), 229-35.

126 Mathew, L., Lobel, S. A., & Miale, T. D. (1984). The clinical diagnosis of megaloblastic anemias in infancy and childhood. *Indian Journal of Pediatrics, 51*(411), 429-42.

127 Viteri, F. E., & Gonzalez, H. (2002). Adverse outcomes of poor micronutrient status in childhood and adolescence. *Nutrition Reviews, 60*(5, Pt. 2), S77-83.

128 Mtvarelidze, Z. G., Kvezereli-Kopadze, A. N., & Kvezereli-Kopadze, M. A. (2009). [Megaloblastic-vitamin B12 deficiency anemia in childhood]. *Georgian Medical News,* (170), 57-60.

129 Marshall, K. G., Howell, S., Badaloo, A. V., Reid, M., Farrall, M., Forrester, T., & McKenzie, C. A. (2006). Polymorphisms in genes involved in folate metabolism as risk factors for oedematous severe childhood malnutrition: A hypothesis-generating study. *Annals of Tropical Paediatrics, 26*(2), 107-14.

130 Nutzenadel, W. (2011). Failure to thrive in childhood. *Deutsches Ärzteblatt International, 108*(38), 642-49.

131 Nutzenadel, W. (2011). Failure to thrive in childhood. *Deutsches Ärzteblatt International, 108*(38), 642-49.

132 Brewster, D. R. (2011). Inpatient management of severe malnutrition: Time for a change in protocol and practice. *Annals of Tropical Paediatrics, 31*(2), 97-107.

133 Nutzenadel, W. (2011). Failure to thrive in childhood. *Deutsches Ärzteblatt International, 108*(38), 642-49.

134 Brewster, D. R. (2011). Inpatient management of severe malnutrition: Time for a change in protocol and practice. *Annals of Tropical Paediatrics, 31*(2), 97-107.

135 Soares-Weiser K., Maclehose H., Ben-Aharon I., Goldberg E., Pitan F., & Cunliffe N. (2010). Vaccines for preventing rotavirus diarrhoea: Vaccines in use. *Cochrane Database of Systematic Reviews,* (5), CD008521.

136 Soares-Weiser, K., Maclehose, H., Bergman, H., Ben-Aharon, I., Nagpal, S., Goldberg, E., . . . & Cunliffe, N. (2012). Vaccines for preventing rotavirus diarrhoea: Vaccines in use. *Cochrane Database of Systematic Reviews, 2,* CD008521.

137 De Zoysa, I., & Feachem, R. G. (1985). Interventions for the control of diarrhoeal diseases among young children: Rotavirus and cholera immunization. *Bulletin of the World Health Organization, 63*(3), 569-83.

138 Taniguchi, K. (2012). [Human rotavirus vaccine]. *Uirusu, 62*(1), 87-96.

139 Soares-Weiser, K., Maclehose, H., Bergman, H., Ben-Aharon, I., Nagpal, S., Goldberg, E., . . . Cunliffe, N. (2012). Vaccines for preventing rotavirus diarrhoea: Vaccines in use. *Cochrane Database of Systematic Reviews, 11,* CD008521.

140 Bellido-Blasco, J. B., Sabater-Vidal, S., Salvador-Ribera, M. D., Arnedo-Pena, A., Tirado-Balaguer, M. D., Meseguer-Ferrer, N., . . . Moreno-Munoz, M. R. (2012). Rotavirus vaccination effectiveness: A case-case study in the EDICS project, Castellón (Spain). *Vaccine, 30*(52), 7536-40.

141 Dey, A., Wang, H., Menzies, R., & Macartney, K. (2012). Changes in hospitalisations for acute gastroenteritis in Australia after the national rotavirus vaccination program. *Medical Journal of Australia, 197*(8), 453-57.

142 Lee, W. S., Lim, B. T., Chai, P. F., Kirkwood, C. D., & Lee, J. K. (2012). Rotavirus genotypes in Malaysia and Universal rotavirus vaccination. *Human Vaccines and Immunotherapeutics, 8*(10), 1401-6.

143 Wang, F. T., Mast, T. C., Glass, R. J., Loughlin, J., & Seeger, J. D. (2012). Effectiveness of an incomplete RotaTeq (RV5) vaccination regimen in preventing rotavirus gastroenteritis in the United States. *Pediatric Infectious Disease Journal, 32*(3), 278-83.

144 Dudareva-Vizule, S., Koch, J., An der Heiden, M., Oberle, D., Keller-Stanislawski, B., & Wichmann, O. (2012). Impact of rotavirus vaccination in regions with low and moderate vaccine uptake in Germany. *Human Vaccines and Immunotherapeutics, 8*(10), 1407-15.

145 Braeckman, T., Van Herck, K., Meyer, N., Pircon, J.Y., Soriano-Gabarro, M., Heylen, E., . . . Van Damme, P. (2012). Effectiveness of rotavirus vaccination in prevention of hospital admissions for rotavirus gastroenteritis among young children in Belgium: Case-control study. *BMJ, 345,* e4752.

146 Breiman, R. F., Zaman, K., Armah, G., Sow, S. O., Anh, D. D., Victor, J. C., . . . K.M. (2012). Analyses of health outcomes from the 5 sites participating in the Africa and Asia clinical efficacy trials of the oral pentavalent rotavirus vaccine. *Vaccine, 30*(Suppl. 1), A24-29.

147 Feller, A. J., Zaman, K., Lewis, K. D., Hossain, I., Yunus, M., & Sack, D. A. (2012). Malnutrition levels among vaccinated and unvaccinated children between 2 and 3 years of age following enrollment in a randomized clinical trial with the pentavalent rotavirus vaccine (PRV) in Bangladesh. *Vaccine, 30*(Suppl. 1), A101-5.

148 Shin, S., Anh, D. D., Zaman, K., Yunus, M., Mai le, T.P., Thiem, V. D., . . . Ciarlet M. (2012). Immunogenicity of the pentavalent rotavirus vaccine among infants in two developing countries in Asia, Bangladesh and Vietnam. *Vaccine, 30*(Suppl. 1), A106-13.

149 Sow, S. O., Tapia, M., Haidara, F. C., Ciarlet, M., Diallo, F., Kodio, M., . . . Levine M.M. (2012). Efficacy of the oral pentavalent rotavirus vaccine in Mali. *Vaccine, 30*(Suppl. 1), A71-78.

150 Zaman, K., Sack, D. A., Yunus, M., Arifeen, S. E., Podder, G., Azim, T., . . . Bock, H. L. (2009). Successful co-administration of a human rotavirus and oral poliovirus vaccines in Bangladeshi infants in a 2-dose schedule at 12 and 16 weeks of age. *Vaccine, 27*(9), 1333-39.

151 Van Hoek, A. J., Ngama, M., Ismail, A., Chuma, J., Cheburet, S., Mutonga, D., . . . Nokes, D. J. (2012). A cost effectiveness and capacity analysis for the introduction of universal rotavirus vaccination in Kenya: Comparison between Rotarix and RotaTeq vaccines. *PLOS One, 7*(10), e47511.

152 Fisman, D. N., Chan, C. H., Lowcock, E., Naus, M., & Lee, V. (2012). Effectiveness and cost-effectiveness of pediatric rotavirus vaccination in British Columbia: A model-based evaluation. *Vaccine, 30*(52), 7601-7.

153 Kumar, A., Goel, M. K., Jain, R. B., Khanna, P., & Vibha, V. (2012). Rotavirus vaccine: A cost effective control measure for India. *Human Vaccines and Immunotherapeutics, 8*(4), 501-4.

154 Atkins, K. E., Shim, E., Carroll, S., Quilici, S., & Galvani, A. P. (2012). The cost-effectiveness of pentavalent rotavirus vaccination in England and Wales. *Vaccine, 30*(48), 6766-76.

155 Seheri, L. M., Page, N. A., Mawela, M. P., Mphahlele, M. J., & Steele, A. D. (2012). Rotavirus vaccination within the South African Expanded Programme on Immunisation. *Vaccine, 30*(Suppl. 3), C14-20.

156 Huttly, S. R., Morris, S. S., & Pisani, V. (1997). Prevention of diarrhoea in young children in developing countries. *Bulletin of the World Health Organization, 75*(2), 163-74.

157 Aung Myo, H., & Thein, H. (1989). Prevention of diarrhoea and dysentery by hand washing. *Transactions of the Royal Society of Tropical Medicine and Hygiene, 83*(1), 128-31.

158 Ejemot, R. I., Ehiri, J. E., Meremikwu, M. M., & Critchley, J. A. (2008). Hand washing for preventing diarrhoea. *Cochrane Database of Systematic Reviews,* (1), CD004265.

159 Clasen, T. F., Bostoen, K., Schmidt, W. P., Boisson, S., Fung, I. C., Jenkins, M. W., . . . Cairncross, S. (2010). Interventions to improve disposal of human excreta for preventing diarrhoea. *Cochrane Database of Systematic Reviews,* (6), CD007180.

160 Clasen, T., Roberts, I., Rabie, T., Schmidt, W., & Cairncross, S. (2006). Interventions to improve water quality for preventing diarrhoea. *Cochrane Database of Systematic Reviews,* (3), CD004794.

161 Ahmed, T., Haque, R., Shamsir Ahmed, A. M., Petri, W. A., Jr., & Cravioto, A. (2009). Use of metagenomics to understand the genetic basis of malnutrition. *Nutrition Reviews, 67*(Suppl. 2), S201-06.

162 Bhutta, Z. A., Ahmed, T., Black, R.,E., Cousens, S., Dewey, K., Giugliani, E., . . . Shekar, M. (2008). What works? Interventions for maternal and child undernutrition and survival. *Lancet, 371*(9610), 417-40.

163 Lutter, C. K., Daelmans, B. M., de Onis, M., Kothari, M. T., Ruel, M. T., . . . Borghi, E. (2011). Undernutrition, poor feeding practices, and low coverage of key nutrition interventions. *Pediatrics, 128*(6), e1418-27.

164 Lutter, C. K., Daelmans, B. M., de Onis, M., Kothari, M. T., Ruel, M. T., . . . Borghi, E. (2011). Undernutrition, poor feeding practices, and low coverage of key nutrition interventions. *Pediatrics, 128*(6), e1418-27.

165 De Pee, S., & Bloem, M. W. (2009). Current and potential role of specially formulated foods and food supplements for preventing malnutrition among 6- to 23-month-old children and for treating moderate malnutrition among 6- to 59-month-old children. *Food Nutrition Bulletin, 30*(3 Suppl.), S434-63.

166 Sazawal, S., Dhingra, U., Dhingra, P., Hiremath, G., Kumar, J., Sarkar, A., . . . Black, R. E. (2007). Effects of fortified milk on morbidity in young children in north India: Community based, randomised, double masked placebo controlled trial. *BMJ, 334*(7585), 140.

167 Sazawal, S., Dhingra, U., Dhingra, P., Hiremath, G., Sarkar, A., Dutta, A., . . . Black R.E. (2010). Micronutrient fortified milk improves iron status, anemia and growth among children 1-4 years: a double masked, randomized, controlled trial. *PLOS One, 5*(8), e12167.

168 Sazawal, S., Dhingra, U., Hiremath, G., Sarkar, A., Dhingra, P., Dutta, A., . . . Black, R. E. (2010). Prebiotic and probiotic fortified milk in prevention of morbidities among children: community-based, randomized, double-blind, controlled trial. *PLoS One, 5*(8), e12164.

169 Muhilal, Permeisih D., Idjradinata Y. R., Muherdiyantiningsih, & Karyadi, D. (1988). Vitamin A-fortified monosodium glutamate and health, growth, and survival of children: a controlled field trial. *American Journal of Clinical Nutrition, 48*(5), 1271-76.

170 Beaton, G. H., Martorell, R., Aronson, K. J., Edmonston, B., McCabe, G., Ross, A. C., & Harvey, B. (1993). *Effectiveness of vitamin A supplementation in the control of young child morbidity and mortality in developing countries.* Nutrition Policy Discussion Paper No. 13. United Nations Administrative Committee on Coordination/Sub-Committee on Nutrition, Geneva, Switzerland. Toronto: International Nutrition Program, University of Toronto. Retrieved from http://www.unscn.org/layout/modules/resources/files/Policy_paper_No_13.pdf

171 Krause, V. M., Delisle, H., & Solomons, N. W. (1998). Fortified foods contribute one half of recommended vitamin A intake in poor urban Guatemalan toddlers. *Journal of Nutrition, 128*(5), 860-64.

172 Dary, O., & Mora, J. O. (2002). Food fortification to reduce vitamin A deficiency: International Vitamin A Consultative Group recommendations. *Journal of Nutrition, 132*(9 Suppl.), 2927S-2933S.

173 Grotto, I., Mimouni, M., Gdalevich, M., & Mimouni, D. (2003). Vitamin A supplementation and childhood morbidity from diarrhea and respiratory infections: A meta-analysis. *Journal of Pediatrics, 142*(3), 297-304.

174 Long, K. Z., Montoya, Y., Hertzmark, E., Santos, J. I., & Rosado, J. L. (2006). A double-blind, randomized, clinical trial of the effect of vitamin A and zinc supplementation on diarrheal disease and respiratory tract infections in children in Mexico City, Mexico. *American Journal of Clinical Nutrition, 83*(3), 693-700.

175 Andang'o, P. E., Osendarp, S. J., Ayah, R., West, C. E., Mwaniki, D. L., De Wolf, C. A., . . . Verhoef, H. (2007). Efficacy of iron-fortified whole maize flour on iron status of schoolchildren in Kenya: A randomised controlled trial. *Lancet, 369*(9575), 1799-1806.

176 Hirve, S., Bhave, S., Bavdekar, A., Naik, S., Pandit, A., Schauer, C., . . . Zlotkin S. (2007). Low dose "Sprinkles"–an innovative approach to treat iron deficiency anemia in infants and young children. *Indian Pediatrics, 44*(2), 91-100.

177 Christofides, A., Asante, K. P., Schauer, C., Sharieff, W., Owusu-Agyei, S., & Zlotkin, S. (2006). Multi-micronutrient Sprinkles including a low dose of iron provided as microencapsulated ferrous fumarate improves haematologic indices in anaemic children: A randomized clinical trial. *Maternal and Child Nutrition, 2*(3), 169-80.

178 Menon, P., Ruel, M. T., Loechl, C. U., Arimond, M., Habicht, J. P., Pelto, G., & Michaud, L. (2007). Micronutrient Sprinkles reduce anemia among 9- to 24-mo-old children when delivered through an integrated health and nutrition program in rural Haiti. *Journal of Nutrition, 137*(4), 1023-30.

179 Giovannini, M., Sala, D., Usuelli, M., Livio, L., Francescato, G., Braga, M., . . . Riva E. (2006). Double-blind, placebo-controlled trial comparing effects of supplementation with two different combinations of micronutrients delivered as sprinkles on growth, anemia, and iron deficiency in Cambodian infants. *Journal of Pediatric Gastroenterology and Nutrition, 42*(3), 306-12.

180 Sharieff, W., Yin, S. A., Wu, M., Yang, Q., Schauer, C., Tomlinson, G., & Zlotkin S. (2006). Short-term daily or weekly administration of micronutrient Sprinkles has high compliance and does not cause iron overload in Chinese schoolchildren: A cluster-randomised trial. *Public Health Nutrition, 9*(3), 336-44.

181 Gera, T., Sachdev, H. P., Nestel, P., & Sachdev, S. S. (2007). Effect of iron supplementation on haemoglobin response in children: Systematic review of randomised controlled trials. *Journal of Pediatric Gastroenterology and Nutrition, 44*(4), 468-86.

182 Brown, K. H., Peerson, J. M., Rivera, J., & Allen, L. H. (2002). Effect of supplemental zinc on the growth and serum zinc concentrations of prepubertal children: A meta-analysis of randomized controlled trials. *American Journal of Clinical Nutrition, 75*(6), 1062-71.

183 Bhutta, Z. A., Black, R. E., Brown, K. H., Gardner, J. M., Gore, S., Hidayat, A., . . . Shankar A. (1999). Prevention of diarrhea and pneumonia by zinc supplementation in children in developing countries: Pooled analysis of randomized controlled trials. Zinc Investigators' Collaborative Group. *Journal of Pediatrics, 135*(6), 689-97.

184 Bhutta, Z. A., Black, R. E., Brown, K. H., Gardner, J. M., Gore, S., Hidayat, A., . . . Shankar A. (1999). Prevention of diarrhea and pneumonia by zinc supplementation in children in developing countries: pooled analysis of randomized controlled trials. Zinc Investigators' Collaborative Group. *Journal of Pediatrics, 135*(6), 689-97.

185 Aggarwal, R., Sentz, J., & Miller, M. A. (2007). Role of zinc administration in prevention of childhood diarrhea and respiratory illnesses: A meta-analysis. *Pediatrics, 119*(6), 1120-30.

186 Tielsch, J. M., Khatry, S. K., Stoltzfus, R. J., Katz, J., LeClerq, S. C., Adhikari, R., . . . Shresta, S. (2007). Effect of daily zinc supplementation on child mortality in southern Nepal: A community-based, cluster randomised, placebo-controlled trial. *Lancet, 370*(9594), 1230-39.

187 Sazawal, S., Black, R. E., Ramsan, M., Chwaya, H. M., Dutta, A., Dhingra, U., . . . Kabole, F. M. (2007). Effect of zinc supplementation on mortality in children aged 1-48 months: A community-based randomised placebo-controlled trial. *Lancet, 369*(9565), 927-34.

188 Sazawal, S., Black, R. E., Ramsan, M., Chwaya, H. M., Stoltzfus, R. J., Dutta, A., Dhingra, U., . . . Kabole, F. M. (2006). Effects of routine prophylactic supplementation with iron and folic acid on admission to hospital and mortality in preschool children in a high malaria transmission setting: Community-based, randomised, placebo-controlled trial. *Lancet 367*(9505), 133-43.

189 Tielsch, J. M., Khatry, S. K., Stoltzfus, R. J., Katz, J., LeClerq, S. C., Adhikari, R., . . . Black, R. E. (2006). Effect of routine prophylactic supplementation with iron and folic acid on preschool child mortality in southern Nepal: Community-based, cluster-randomised, placebo-controlled trial. *Lancet, 367*(9505), 144-52.

190 Dewey, K. G., & Arimond, M. (2012). Lipid-based nutrient supplements: How can they combat child malnutrition? *PLOS Medicine, 9*(9), e1001314.

191 Chaparro, C. M., & Dewey, K. G. (2010). Use of lipid-based nutrient supplements (LNS). to improve the nutrient adequacy of general food distribution rations for vulnerable sub-groups in emergency settings. *Maternal and Child Nutrition, 6*(Suppl. 1), 1-69.

192 Dewey, K. G., & Arimond, M. (2012). Lipid-based nutrient supplements: How can they combat child malnutrition? *PLOS Medicine, 9*(9), e1001314.

193 Haider, B. A., & Bhutta, Z. A. (2012). Multiple-micronutrient supplementation for women during pregnancy. *Cochrane Database of Systematic Reviews, 11,* CD004905.

194 Haider, B. A., & Bhutta, Z. A. (2006). Multiple-micronutrient supplementation for women during pregnancy. *Cochrane Database of Systematic Reviews,* (4), CD004905.

195 Shankar, A. H., Jahari, A. B., Sebayang, S. K., Aditiawarman, Apriatni, M., Harefa, B., . . . Sofia, G. (2008). Effect of maternal multiple micronutrient supplementation on fetal loss and infant death in Indonesia: A double-blind cluster-randomised trial. *Lancet, 371*(9608), 215-27.

196 Gupta, P., Ray, M., Dua, T., Radhakrishnan, G., Kumar, R., & Sachdev, H. P. (2007). Multimicronutrient supplementation for undernourished pregnant women and the birth size of their offspring: A double-blind, randomized, placebo-controlled trial. *Archives of Pediatric and Adolescent Medicine, 161*(1), 58-64.

197 Fawzi, W. W., Msamanga, G. I., Urassa, W., Hertzmark, E., Petraro, P., Willett, W. C., & Spiegelman, D. (2007). Vitamins and perinatal outcomes among HIV-negative women in Tanzania. *New England Journal of Medicine, 356*(14), 1423-31.

198 Curtis, V., & Cairncross, S. (2003). Effect of washing hands with soap on diarrhoea risk in the community: A systematic review. *Lancet Infect Dis 3 (5),* 275-281.

199 Fewtrell, L., Kaufmann R.B., Kay D., Enanoria W., Haller L., & Colford J.M., Jr. (2005). Water, sanitation, and hygiene interventions to reduce diarrhoea in less developed countries: A systematic review and meta-analysis. *Lancet Infectious Diseases, 5*(1), 42-52.

200 Zwane, A. P., & Kremer, M. (2007). *What works in fighting diarrheal diseases in developing countries? A critical review.* CID Working Paper, 140.

201 Hoddinott, J., & Skoufias, E. (2003, May). The impact of PROGRESA on food consumption. International Food Policy Research Institute (IFPRI), FCND Discussion Paper No. 150. *Food and Nutrition Bulletin, 24*(4), 379-80.

202 Berti, P. R., Krasevec, J., & FitzGerald, S. (2004). A review of the effectiveness of agriculture interventions in improving nutrition outcomes. *Public Health Nutrition, 7*(5), 599-609.

203 Faber, M., Phungula, M. A., Venter, S. L., Dhansay, M. A., & Benade, A. J. (2002). Home gardens focusing on the production of yellow and dark-green leafy vegetables increase the serum retinol concentrations of 2-5-y-old children in South Africa. *American Journal of Clinical Nutrition, 76*(5), 1048-54.

204 Leroy, J. L., & Frongillo, E. A. (2007). Can interventions to promote animal production ameliorate undernutrition? *Journal of Nutrition, 137*(10), 2311-16.

205 Gibson, R. S., Yeudall, F., Drost, N., Mtitimuni, B. M., & Cullinan, T. R. (2003). Experiences of a community-based dietary intervention to enhance micronutrient adequacy of diets low in animal source foods and high in phytate: A case study in rural Malawian children. *Journal of Nutrition, 133*(11 Suppl. 2), 3992S-3999S.

206 Yeudall, F., Gibson, R. S., Cullinan, T. R., & Mtimuni, B. (2005). Efficacy of a community-based dietary intervention to enhance micronutrient adequacy of high-phytate maize-based diets of rural Malawian children. *Public Health Nutrition, 8*(7), 826-36.

207 Parikh, K., Marein-Efron, G., Huang, S., O'Hare, G., Finalle, R., & Shah, S. S. (2010). Nutritional status of children after a food-supplementation program integrated with routine health care through mobile clinics in migrant communities in the Dominican Republic. *American Journal of Tropical Medicine and Hygiene, 83*(3), 559-64.

208 Park, K., Kersey, M., Geppert, J., Story, M., Cutts, D., & Himes, J. H. (2009). Household food insecurity is a risk factor for iron-deficiency anaemia in a multi-ethnic, low-income sample of infants and toddlers. *Public Health Nutrition, 12*(11), 2120-28.

209 Skalicky, A., Meyers, A. F., Adams, W. G., Yang, Z., Cook, J. T., & Frank, D. A. (2006). Child food insecurity and iron deficiency anemia in low-income infants and toddlers in the United States. *Maternal and Child Health Journal, 10*(2), 177-85.

210 Mason, J. B., White, J. M., Heron, L., Carter, J., Wilkinson, C., & Spiegel, P. (2012). Child acute malnutrition and mortality in populations affected by displacement in the Horn of Africa, 1997-2009. *International Journal of Environmental Research and Public Health, 9*(3), 791-806.

211 Da Fonseca, M. A. (2012). The effects of poverty on children's development and oral health. *Pediatric Dentistry, 34*(1), 32-38.

212 Gibson, R. S., Yeudall, F., Drost, N., Mtitimuni, B. M., & Cullinan, T. R. (2003). Experiences of a community-based dietary intervention to enhance micronutrient adequacy of diets low in animal source foods and high in phytate: A case study in rural Malawian children. *Journal of Nutrition, 133*(11 Suppl. 2), 3992S-3999S.

213 Bambra, C., Gibson, M., Sowden, A., Wright, K., Whitehead, M., & Petticrew, M. (2010). Tackling the wider social determinants of health and health inequalities: Evidence from systematic reviews. *Journal of Epidemiology and Community Health, 64*(4), 284-91.

214 Evci Kiraz, E. D., Ergin, F., Okur, O., Saruhan, G., & Beser, E. (2012). Local decision makers' awareness of the social determinants of health in Turkey: A cross-sectional study. *BMC Public Health, 12,* 437.

215 Ritte, S. A., & Kessy, A. T. (2012). Social factors and lifestyle attributes associated with nutritional status of people living with HIV/AIDS attending care and treatment clinics in Ilala District, Dar Es Salaam. *East African Journal of Public Health, 9*(1), 33-38.

216 Schmitz, B. A., Moreira, E. A., de Freitas, M. B., Fiates, G. M., Gabriel, C. G., & Fagundes, R. L. (2011). Public intervention in food and nutrition in Brazil. *Archivos Latinoamericanos de Nutrición, 61*(4), 361-66.

217 Shahrawat, R., & Joon, V. (2012). Role of interpersonal communication in infant and young child feeding practices in an urban slum: An overview based on case studies. Advance online publication. *Indian Journal of Pediatrics.*

218 Akter, S. M., Roy, S. K., Thakur, S. K., Sultana, M., Khatun, W., Rahman, R., . . . Alam N. (2012). Effects of third trimester counseling on pregnancy weight gain, birthweight, and breastfeeding among urban poor women in Bangladesh. *Food Nutrition Bulletin, 33*(3), 194-201.

219 Thakur, S. K., Roy, S. K., Paul, K., Khanam, M., Khatun, W., & Sarker, D. (2012). Effect of nutrition education on exclusive breastfeeding for nutritional outcome of low birth weight babies. *European Journal of Clinical Nutrition, 66*(3), 376-81.

220 Lagarde, M., Haines, A., & Palmer, N. (2007). Conditional cash transfers for improving uptake of health interventions in low- and middle-income countries: A systematic review. *JAMA, 298*(16), 1900-1910.

221 Hoddinott, J., & Skoufias, E. (2003, May). The impact of PROGRESA on food consumption. International Food Policy Research Institute (IFPRI), FCND Discussion Paper No. 150. *Food and Nutrition Bulletin, 24*(4), 379-80.

222 Hoddinott, J., & Skoufias, E. (2003, May). The impact of PROGRESA on food consumption. International Food Policy Research Institute (IFPRI), FCND Discussion Paper No. 150. *Food and Nutrition Bulletin, 24*(4), 379-80.

223 Behrman, J., & Hoddinott, J. (2001). *An evaluation of the impact of PROGRESA on pre-school child height.* International Food Policy Research Institute (IFPRI), FCND Discussion Paper No. 104. Washington, DC: Food Consumption and Nutrition Division, International Food Policy Research Institute.

224 Villalpando, S., Shamah, T., Rivera, J. A., Lara, Y., & Monterrubio, E. (2006). Fortifying milk with ferrous gluconate and zinc oxide in a public nutrition program reduced the prevalence of anemia in toddlers. *Journal of Nutrition, 136*(10), 2633-37.

225 Behrman, J., & Hoddinott, J. (2001). *An evaluation of the impact of PROGRESA on pre-school child height.* International Food Policy Research Institute (IFPRI), FCND Discussion Paper No 104. Washington, DC: Food Consumption and Nutrition Division, International Food Policy Research Institute.

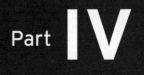

Part **IV**

Public Health Nutrition for Children and Adults

Food Security and Special Diets: Meeting Children's Nutrient Needs in Industrialized Nations

Natalie Stein, MS, MPH
Juliana F. W. Cohen, ScD, ScM

"Food security is defined as access by all people at all times to enough food for an active, healthy life. . . . Food insecurity exists whenever the ability of nutritionally adequate and safe foods or the ability to acquire acceptable food in socially acceptable ways is limited or uncertain. Hunger . . . [is] the uneasy or painful sensation caused by lack of food."–Food and Agriculture Organization

Food and Agriculture Organization. (2002). The State of Food Insecurity in the World 2001. Rome, Italy.

Learning Objectives

- Define food security and describe the scope of children's food insecurity in industrialized nations.

- Identify risk factors for food insecurity.

- Describe the effects of food insecurity on food choices and nutrient intake.

- Link children's food insecurity to educational challenges and disparities in health outcomes.

- Define a rights-based approach to food and explain how cultural differences can affect the likelihood of a nation embracing it.

- Explain different public health strategies for addressing children's food insecurity and the reasoning behind each. Include supplemental food programs, cash assistance programs, and fortification programs.

- Describe nutritional implications of vegetarian diets.

- Understand dietary considerations for individuals with lactose intolerance, gluten intolerance, and food allergies, and discuss the role of public health programs in meeting these needs.

Case Study: Project Bread

In many low-income middle schools in Boston, where most students were eligible for free or reduced-price meals, principals observed students throwing away unappetizing foods from their school meals before sitting down to eat lunch. Project Bread, a nonprofit organization in Boston, partnered with the Harvard School of Public Health (HSPH), the Boston Public Health Commission, Boston Public Schools, and a professional chef to provide students with more appealing meals that surpassed the United States Department of Agriculture's (USDA) nutritional requirements for school meals.

> *Public Health Core Competency 5: Community Dimensions of Practice Skills 2: Demonstrates the capacity to work in community-based participatory research efforts*
>
> Reproduced from Council on Linkages Between Academia and Public Health Practice. 2010 May. Core Competencies for Public Health Professionals. Washington, DC: Public Health Foundation. http://www.phf.org/resourcestools/Documents/Core_Competencies_for_Public_Health_Professionals_2010May.pdf. Accessed August 13, 2013. This source is used for all Public Health Core Competencies in this chapter.

In the fall of 2007, the "Chef Initiative" launched. Trans fats were no longer used, and saturated fats were reduced by using low-fat cheese, eliminating whole and 2% milk, and cooking with unsaturated oils instead of butter. Sugar was reduced by removing pastries, limiting chocolate milk to less than three times per week, and by replacing fruits canned in syrup with fresh or frozen fruit. To reduce sodium, cafeteria staff used fewer high-sodium sauces and dressings, and served fresh or frozen vegetables instead of canned. Student taste tests assessed the palatability of new recipes. More whole-grain products were served, and each lunch provided at least five grams of fiber (**Figure 14-1**). Chef Conrad created new recipes and trained the staff in culinary skills to make the changes sustainable.

After the Chef Initiative had been in the schools for two years, HSPH conducted a **plate waste study (Figure 14-2 and Box 14-1)** to compare students' consumption in the Chef Initiative schools and two matched control schools. Students in Chef Initiative schools chose more whole grains and ate more vegetables than students in control schools. Furthermore, these students consumed the same amount of their low-sugar, low-sodium entrees as did students receiving standard meals. Also promising was that

Menu items	
Chef Initiative Schools	**Boston Public Schools**
Entrées Whole-wheat pasta and meatballs with homemade lower-sodium sauce Low-fat grilled cheese on whole-wheat bread Baked, seasoned chicken Tuna salad on whole wheat-bread with lettuce, tomato, and onion	**Entrées** Meatball sandwich on refined-wheat roll Prepackaged grilled cheese with refined wheat Chicken nuggets Tuna salad on white bread
Milk Nonfat and 1% milk (flavored milk served twice per week)	**Milk** Milk variety offered daily (e.g., whole milk, chocolate milk, 1% plain)
Vegetables Salad with homemade dressing Homemade soup with fresh and frozen vegetables Seasoned frozen broccoli sautéed in oil and garlic Corn (canned) and black bean salsa	**Vegetables** Canned peas and carrots Canned green beans Frozen broccoli (plain) Canned corn
Fruit Fresh apples Fresh oranges	**Fruit** Canned applesauce Canned mixed fruit in syrup
Sides Seasoned brown rice Whole-wheat rolls	**Sides** White rice Refined-wheat rolls

Figure 14-1 Menu items offered in the Chef Initiative plate waste study

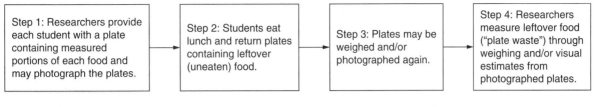

Figure 14-2 Plate waste study

Data from USDA. Chapter 7: Plate waste data collection and analysis. Accessed September 5, 2013 at http://naldc.nal.usda.gov/download/55286/PDF_007.

when access to chocolate milk was limited, it was replaced with consumption of white milk, allowing total milk consumption to remain high.

This success led to the hiring of more chefs and program expansion in Boston and other low-income school districts in Massachusetts, with the support of private donations. Other programs throughout the nation are now using chefs to train school staff. One such program is First Lady Michelle Obama's "Chefs Move to Schools" initiative, which connects local chefs with schools.

Discussion Questions

- Why do low-income, food-insecure children face malnutrition and obesity?
- How does the Chef Initiative serve as an example of a community-wide effort to improve nutrition?

- Which public health nutrition programs are available in the United States and other industrialized nations to reduce childhood food insecurity?
- How can public health nutrition programs consider other cultural factors to increase success?

Introduction to Childhood Food Security

Among school-aged children, desired outcomes that require good nutrition include normal physical growth, development, emotional, social and cognitive gains, and preparation for the pubertal growth spurt.[1] Proper nutrition during childhood also helps prevent obesity and lowers the risk of developing obesity-related diseases, such as cardiovascular disease, type 2 diabetes, and fatty liver disease.[2]

Box 14-1 Plate Waste Study: A method to assess consumption

A plate waste study is often considered a gold standard because it does not rely on study participants' memory to determine foods consumed. The steps necessary to conduct a plate waste study in a school setting are:

1. Weigh foods on a food scale before study participants begin the meal.

2. Label each tray with a unique identifying number.

3. Record the foods selected by study participants along with the tray number (e.g., at cash registers as students pay for their meals).

4. When feasible, observe students during the meal to record any food trading,

5. At the end of the meal, collect all of the study participants' trays,

6. Weigh each item remaining on each tray.

7. The preweight and postweight values can be used to determine the servings, weight, and percent consumed. Foods that were recorded as selected by students and are not on the tray at the end of collection are considered entirely consumed.*

*An exception is for foods that are served in a container (e.g., milk) or typically leave food remnants behind (e.g., bananas with peels); these food items should be recorded as missing.

The Universal Declaration of Human Rights (UDHR) states that "everyone has the right to a standard of living adequate for the health and well-being of himself and of his family, including food, clothing, housing and medical care and necessary social services."[3] Further, all children have the right to extra aid. More than six decades after the United Nations (UN) General Assembly adopted the UDHR, inadequate and unhealthy diets remain threats to children worldwide, including in wealthy industrialized nations. This is the focus of much of this chapter. Also discussed are children who follow special diets for medical or cultural reasons, who can be at higher risk for impaired nutritional status.

> *Public Health Core Competency 6: Basic Public Health Sciences Skills 3: Relates public health science skills to the Core Public Health Functions and Ten Essential Services of Public Health*

Definitions, Assessment, and Prevalence of Food Security and Insecurity

Public health interventions can address children's food insecurity and improve nutritional status through each of the **core functions** of public health.[4] Assessment of children's food insecurity demonstrates the scope of the problem. Policy development supports a healthier food environment. Finally, assurance ideally allows all children to get consistent and socially acceptable access to the food and nutrients they need.[5]

Public health has a natural role in improving nutrition among disadvantaged children, but addressing food insecurity first requires clear definitions of food security and insecurity.[6] Many industrialized nations facing children's food insecurity in the 1980s were slow to recognize and address it because of inadequate definitions. The **Food and Agriculture Organization (FAO)** adopted a standardized definition in 2001, and many nations since then have used that definition or similar ones.[7]

Definitions of Food Security and Food Insecurity

According to FAO, "Food security is defined as access by all people at all times to enough food for an active, healthy life and includes at a minimum: (a) the ready availability of nutritionally adequate and safe foods, and (b) the assured ability to acquire acceptable food in socially acceptable ways (e.g., without resorting to emergency food supplies, scavenging, stealing and other coping strategies)."[8] In contrast, "food insecurity exists whenever the ability of nutritionally adequate and safe foods or the ability to acquire acceptable food in socially acceptable ways is limited or uncertain."[9] FAO defines hunger, a more extreme condition, as "the uneasy or painful sensation caused by lack of food."[10]

The USDA previously stated that food secure "households had access, at all times, to enough food for an active, healthy life for all household members."[11] In 2006, the USDA further divided food security into **high food security**, in which "households had no problems, or anxiety about, consistently accessing adequate food," and **marginal food security**, in which "households had problems at times, or anxiety about, accessing adequate food, but the quality, variety, and quantity of their food intake were not substantially reduced." The USDA uses the terms low and very low food security instead of food insecurity. With **low food security**, "households reduced the quality, variety, and desirability of their diets, but the quantity of food intake and normal eating patterns were not substantially disrupted," and with **very low food security**, "eating patterns of one or more household members were disrupted and food intake reduced because the household lacked money and other resources for food."[12] **Table 14-1** summarizes characteristics of food security.

Assessment of Food Insecurity

Assessment of food insecurity, often through surveys, considers quantity and quality of food and psychological and social acceptability (see Table 14-1). Methods must have **validity**, or be appropriate for achieving identified objectives, such as estimating prevalence of and monitoring food insecurity, investigating causes and risk factors, and evaluating programs to reduce food insecurity.[13] A valid survey should have high sensitivity, or ability to correctly identify food insecurity, and specificity, or ability to accurately assess food security.[14]

> *Public Health Core Competency 1: Analytical/ Assessment Skills 5: Identifies sources of public health data and information*

The **National Health and Nutrition Examination Survey (NHANES)** is a well-established survey in the United States with a range of dietary and additional methods to assess health and nutrition. However, it underestimated

Table 14-1 The four dimensions of food security at the individual and household levels

Dimension	Individual Level	Household Level
Quantity	Adequacy of dietary intake	Repleteness of household stores
Quality	Adequacy of nutrient intake	Quality and safety of available food
Psychological acceptability	Feelings of deprivation of restricted choice	Anxiety about food supplies
Social acceptability	Normal meal patterns	Sources of food

Data from: Kendall, A., Olson, C., & Frongillo, E. A. (2002). Validation of the Radimer/Cornell measures of hunger and food insecurity in a general population survey. *The Journal of Nutrition, 125*, 2793-2801.

food insecurity, and a more sensitive survey was necessary. The 10-item Radimer/Cornell Scale and the Community Childhood Hunger Identification Project, or CCHIP, achieved acceptable sensitivity of 84–89% and specificity of 63–71%.[15] The 10-item Radimer/Cornell Scale includes a food anxiety component with four questions to assess food insecurity at the household level. Qualitative components include three questions to assess adult-level food insecurity and three questions to assess child-level food insecurity.[16]

The 10-Year Comprehensive Plan set forth in the National Nutrition Monitoring and Related Research Act of 1990 (NNMRR), required the USDA to develop a "standardized mechanism and instrument(s) for obtaining data on the prevalence of 'food security' and 'food insecurity.'"[17] The USDA and collaborators defined food security and food insecurity and developed and tested an 18-question Food Security Survey Module, in which seven questions are focused on identifying children's food insecurity (**Box 14-2**). The USDA's

---

Box 14-2 Food Insecurity Assessment survey

The Economic Research Service of the USDA uses the 18-question U.S. Food Security Survey Module to assess food security. Seven questions pertain to children's food security. The presence of two to four conditions of food insecurity is an indicator of "low food insecurity among children," while the presence of five or more conditions indicates "very low food security among children." Adults with one or more children answer the following questions to determine children's food security.

11. "We relied on only a few kinds of low-cost food to feed our children because we were running out of money to buy food." Was that often, sometimes, or never true for you in the last 12 months?

12. "We couldn't feed our children a balanced meal because we couldn't afford that." Was that often, sometimes, or never true for you in the last 12 months?

13. "The children were not eating enough because we just couldn't afford food." Was that often, sometimes, or never true for you in the last 12 months?

14. In the last 12 months, did you ever cut the size of any of the children's meals because there wasn't enough money for food? (Yes/No)

15. "In the last 12 months, were the children ever hungry but you couldn't afford food?" (Yes/No)

16. In the last 12 months, did any of the children ever skip meals because there wasn't enough money for food?" (Yes/No)

17. (If yes to question 16) How often did this happen—almost every month, some months but not every month, or in only 1 or 2 months?"

18. In the last 12 months, did any of the children ever not eat for a whole day because there wasn't enough money for food? (Yes/No)

Reproduced from Bickel, G., Nord, M., Price, C., Hamilton, W., & Cook, J. (2000). Guide to measuring household food security revised 2000. (Office of Analysis, Nutrition and Evaluation, Food and Nutrition Service, United States Department of Agriculture).

Economic Research Service (ERS) publishes survey results annually.

The European Union Statistics on Income and Living Conditions (EU-SILC) survey has collected cross-sectional and longitudinal data since 2003.[18] By 2011, all EU member states and Switzerland used the EU-SILC, which includes data from national surveys. France, for example, adapted the EU-SILC by combining it with national census data to generate a tool for measuring subjective poverty.[19] The resulting European Depression Index has potential for future use in distinct European nations because of its consideration of national characteristics. Census-based deprivation indices have also been used in the United Kingdom and other European nations.[20,21] Statistics Canada has used the Survey of Household Spending to analyze household food expenditures and assess food insecurity.[22] The Serbia Multiple Indicator Cluster Survey is another example of a national survey for measuring risk factors for food insecurity.[23]

> *Healthy People 2020: NWS-12: Eliminate very low food security among children*
>
> *Healthy People 2020: NWS-13: Reduce household food security and in doing so reduce hunger*
>
> Reproduced from the U.S. Department of Health and Human Services. Healthypeople.gov. Retrieved from http://www.healthypeople.gov/2020/default.aspx. Last updated July 30, 2013. Accessed August 13, 2013. All *Healthy People 2020* in this chapter is from this source.

Global Prevalence of Food Security and Food Insecurity

The United States has the highest national **gross domestic product (GDP)** in the world, but only 85.5% of U.S. households were food secure in 2010.[24] In the remaining households, 9.1%, or 10.9 million, had low food security; the remaining 5.4%, or 6.4 million households, had very low food security.[25] Prevalence of food insecurity (low or very low food secure) in households with children is 20.2%, nearly double the 11.2% among households without children.

Childhood food insecurity is also substantial in other industrialized nations. More than 10% of Canadian children were food insecure in 1998–1999,[26] and 16–21% of households from low-income neighborhoods in Sydney, Australia, were food insecure.[27] South Korea has a per

capita GDP among the top 30 in the world, but a sample of low-income urban areas found a prevalence of low or very low food security, also known as "child hunger," of 62.7%, based on the 10-item Radimer/Cornell Scale.[28,29] The United Kingdom and other western European nations have similar levels of food insecurity.

Children's food insecurity is even more evident in central and eastern Europe and is likely related to lower income and other socioeconomic factors. Serbia, for example, received a ranking of only 59 ("high human development") on the **Human Development Index (HDI)** in 2011.[30] In contrast, most western European nations were ranked as "very high human development," and with global rankings ranging from first (Norway) to 41st (Portugal). Malnutrition is evident among high-risk children in Serbia.[31]

Various surveys identified children's food insecurity and poverty in the United Kingdom. Children's poverty, defined as household income less than one-half of the median, had a prevalence of 33% in the United Kingdom in 1998–1999.[32] The Low Income Diet and Nutrition Survey, developed specifically to assess diet and nutritional status in low-income populations, sampled from the 15% of the population with the lowest socioeconomic indicators from 2003 to 2005.[33] The survey found that 29% of respondents were food insecure, and that the insecurity was caused by lack of money or other factors, such as transportation or limited access to food. Thirty-nine percent of participants worried that food would run out before they were able to purchase more, 22% skipped or reduced their meal size occasionally, and 1 out of 20 had fasted an entire day because they could not afford to purchase food.

Risk Factors for Children's Food Insecurity

Children are at risk for food insecurity because they depend on parents or others for food and money. They rely on household food distribution patterns, and may not receive an equal or adequate amount of food during times of scarcity. Many socioeconomic risk factors for children's food insecurity have been identified.

Income

Lower income is linked to higher risk of food insecurity. In the United States, 40.2% of households with household income below the **poverty threshold** had food insecurity in 2009, compared with the aforementioned national average of 14.5%.[34] Similarly, low-income Canadian families had a prevalence of food insecurity of 35% in comparison to the national average of 10%; 14% of middle-income families were also food insecure.[35] Nations in Europe,[36,37] Asia,[38] and Australia[39] also have these patterns.

Lower household income is linked to children's food insecurity; limited money is available for food and other essentials, such as housing, heating, medicine, and clothing.[40] Spending over 30% of the household budget on housing is a risk factor for food insecurity,[41] although household income is not a perfect predictor of children's food insecurity.[42] Children from low-income households may receive food aid to prevent insecurity, while children from higher-income households might be food insecure due to inequality in distribution of household resources. Nevertheless, assessing poverty helps identify food security risk because it is quantitative and often regularly monitored.

Household Composition

Living in a single-parent household is a risk factor for food insecurity.[43,44,45] In 2010, children in households headed by single women and single men had a prevalence of food insecurity of 35.1% and 25.4%, respectively. In the United Kingdom, single-mother households had more than five times the relative risk of being poor.[46] Other risk factors are being in households with more than two children[47] and being left in the care of another child.[48]

Minority Groups

Racial or ethnic minority groups can be at higher risk for food insecurity. Black and Hispanic children are at higher risk for food insecurity than white children and other non-Hispanic minorities in the United States.[49] Aboriginal people living off-reservation in Canada have double the risk of food insecurity,[50] and recent immigrants to the United Kingdom have more than five times the relative risk of being poor as nonminorities.[51] Children in the Roma population, the largest ethnic minority in central and eastern Europe, are likely not only to be living in poverty, but also to display signs of malnutrition.[52] In Serbia, 20% of Roma children were stunted, compared with a national average of 7.7%, and 7.7% were underweight, compared with the 1.4% average overall. Similar patterns of malnutrition among Roma children are seen in Macedonia and the Czech Republic.[53]

Additional Risk Factors

Living in low-income urban neighborhoods is a risk factor for food insecurity. Rural dwellers can also be at high risk for inadequate nutritious food if they depend mainly on home-grown crops. In the United States, suburban dwellers have lower rates of children's food insecurity than inhabitants of **Metropolitan Statistical Areas (MSA)** and rural regions.[54] Among low-income Roma minorities in Serbia, those who live in crowded urban settlements are more likely to have signs of malnutrition.[55] Refugees are particularly vulnerable, and one study found food insecurity to be 100% prevalent among children of low-income refugees, based on the 10-item Radimer/Cornell Scale.[56] In East London, refugees were found to have a 60% rate of very low food security.[57]

Effects of Food Insecurity Among Children

Children's food insecurity can compromise dietary intake and nutritional status, harm physical and psychological health, and impair growth and development. Children with food insecurity may face higher rates of infections and chronic diseases, such as asthma, because their families cannot afford both food and other essentials, such as heat, medicine, and health care.[58] Food insecurity in childhood is also associated with obesity.

Dietary Effects of Food Insecurity

Compared with diets of food-secure individuals, diets of food-insecure individuals tend to be less healthy, consisting of more **energy-dense** and fewer **nutrient-dense** foods. Such patterns have been observed in the United States, Canada, Europe, Asia, and Australia.[59,60]

Less Healthy Food Choices

Food insecurity is associated with increased consumption of unhealthy choices, such as whole milk and fatty meats, which are high in **saturated fat**, deli meats,[61] which are high in **sodium**, rapidly digestible carbohydrates,[62] such as white bread and potatoes,[63] foods with solid fats, or saturated and trans fats, and more **added sugars**, such as sweets, sugar-sweetened beverages, and ice cream.[64,65,66] These dietary patterns can increase the risk for obesity and chronic diseases such as heart disease, hypertension, and diabetes.[67]

Low-income children drink less low-fat and fat-free milk than children from higher-income households.[68,69] They may also consume less oily fish, which provides **omega-3 fatty acids**, and **whole grains** than food-secure individuals.[70,71]

Fruit and vegetable intake in low-income and food-insecure populations is consistently below recommendations in studies in the United States, Europe, South Korea, and Australia.[72,73,74] Households below the poverty threshold were twice as likely to report not having purchased fruits or vegetables in the past week as higher-income households. On average, low-income individuals spent $3.59 per week on fruits and vegetables, compared with $5.02 for high-income individuals.[75] The World Health Organization lists a low intake of fruit and vegetables as among the top 10 actual causes of death worldwide,[76] and fruit and vegetable consumption is associated with a lower risk of heart disease, hypertension, cancer, and diabetes.[77] These foods have low energy density, thus reducing the risk of obesity. Lower consumption in low-income households is a source of health disparities.

Nutrient Intake Patterns and Food Insecurity

Children's food insecurity is associated with inadequate **calcium** intake, which can lead to lower peak bone mineral density and a higher risk for **osteoporosis** later in life.[78,79] **Iron** is another nutrient of concern, with low intakes prevalent and likely to cause anemia. **Vitamin D,**[80] **riboflavin**, **vitamin C**, and **folate** have also been identified as nutrients that are often inadequate among low food-secure individuals.

Food Insecurity and Obesity

Food insecurity is associated with obesity and overweight.[81] This observation seems ironic because food insecurity is the lack of certainty about procuring sufficient nutrition, while obesity results from the overconsumption of calories. However, the relationship between poverty or food insecurity and obesity holds true around the world. The low cost of energy-dense, low-nutrient foods likely contributes to this relationship.[82] In one example in Australia, a head of lettuce cost $9, while a candy bar cost $2, making higher-calorie candy bars far more accessible than lettuce.[83]

Childhood obesity is a growing public health concern worldwide. Recent rates of childhood overweight and obesity are 35% in Spain, 14% in France, 12% in Greece, 30% in Australia, and 17% in the United States.[84,85,86] Risk factors for childhood obesity parallel those of food insecurity and include having racial or ethnic minority status,[87] having low socioeconomic statues (SES),[88,89] and living in low-income urban areas.[90] Crime, fear of dogs, and fewer facilities for exercise can be barriers to physical activity and raise obesity risk.[91]

Physiological effects of obesity include a higher risk for heart disease, type 2 diabetes, metabolic syndrome, hypertension, and fatty liver disease.[92,93] Obese children are more likely to become obese adults and maintain their increased risk of chronic diseases,[94] and suffer social stigma and low self-esteem.

Additional Effects of Food Insecurity

Psychosocial consequences of childhood food insecurity include behavior problems, depression, and stress. On average, children from food-insecure households have impaired cognitive development, as measured by lower scores on math and reading tests and slower rates of improvement than same-age peers.[95]

Consequences of Food Insecurity at the Community Level

Malnourished children can increase strain on the healthcare system due to infections and psychological trouble.[96] Children may be embarrassed to invite their peers home. Skipping meals or consuming less undesirable foods at school can further isolate children. Universal school meal programs can prevent this stigma by providing the same food for all students. In the United States, low-income students who receive free or reduced-price school meals receive the same food as students who pay the full price.

Impaired Growth from Severe Food Insecurity

Malnutrition from severe food insecurity can interfere with normal growth and development in children. The minority Roma people, in central and eastern Europe, provide an example. Some research indicates that children living in extreme poverty in Roma communities had a prevalence of as high as 20% **stunting**, 4.3% **wasting**, and 8.0% **underweight**.[97] Each of these values was at least twice the national average, demonstrating the effect of poverty on anthropometric indicators of nutritional status.

Examples of Interventions for Reducing Children's Food Security

Strategies for increasing food security among children include school meal programs and providing supplemental groceries or vouchers for food. These strategies are used in the United States. Another approach is to provide parents or guardians with funds to purchase food or nonfood goods. Better household finances can increase food expenditures and thus improve children's nutrition.

Organizations that can play a role in reducing food insecurity include government agencies at the federal, state, or regional and local levels. Nonprofit organizations, faith-based groups, and other community groups often run food pantries. University extension or outreach programs can direct food assistance programs or community garden programs, conduct research to assess need and evaluate program effectiveness, and supply educational materials and classes on topics such as stretching the food budget and making healthy recipes. This section of the chapter focuses on national, government-run strategies to improve children's health.

Public Health Initiatives in the United States: Food Assistance Programs

The **National School Lunch Program (NSLP)** is one of several USDA programs to reduce food insecurity among children and families. Others include the **Supplemental Nutrition Assistance Program (SNAP)**, formerly known as the Food Stamp Program, the **National School Breakfast Program**, the Summer Food Service Program, and the Special Supplemental Nutrition Assistance Program for Women, Infants, and Children (WIC).

Background on USDA Programs

The first Food Stamp Program in the United States lasted from 1939 to 1943 and served low-income individuals.[98] Food assistance via these stamps targeted nutritionally at-risk populations in the United States. Over the next several decades, the program grew, received more funding, and developed structure through legislation, including the Food Stamp Act of 1964. The Women, Infants, and Children (WIC) program was established in 1972 to serve nutritionally at-risk and low-income pregnant women, mothers, and children up to age 5.[99] Participants receive vouchers for nutritious foods, such as milk, cereal, and eggs; nutrition education; and breastfeeding support. The National Nutrition Monitoring and Related Research Act of 1990 called for a 10-year plan to measure food insecurity in the United States.[100]

The Child and Adult Care Food Program, or CACFP, provides reimbursement for healthy meals for low-income child care centers and after-school programs, and for meals for children who are homeless or displaced because of emergencies. The Special Milk Program subsidizes milk for low-income children without access to school meals, which can occur if schools do not participate in NSLP or children attend half-day kindergarten programs. The Fresh Fruit and Vegetable Program, a collaborative effort of the USDA and the Department of Defense (DoD), provides students in low-income elementary schools with free fresh fruits and vegetables throughout the day outside of school meals.[101]

National School Lunch Program

Ninety-five percent of schools in the United States participate in the National School Lunch Program. Of the 32 million meals served daily in the NSLP,[102] 63% are provided for free or reduced cost.[103] Students can receive free meals if their household incomes are no more than 130% of the poverty line, or $29,965 for a family of four during the 2012–2013 school year.[104] Household income under 185% of the poverty line, or $42,643 for a family of four, qualifies students for reduced-price meals[105] at a maximum cost of $0.40.[106] Local school districts determine the price of full-cost meals, but must operate as nonprofit programs.

To be eligible for federal reimbursement, participating schools must serve lunches that meet nutritional standards as required in the Healthy, Hunger Free Kids Act of 2010. Intended to comply with the Dietary Guidelines for Americans, lunches must on average provide one-third of the Recommended Dietary Allowances (RDA) for nutrients of concern, including protein, calories, calcium, iron, vitamin A, and vitamin C. Students who received school lunches consumed twice as many servings of vegetables at lunch compared with students not participating in the NSLP.[107] However, among low-income children, evidence does not show that students who participate in the NSLP have healthier diets overall than nonparticipants.[108]

School lunch participants consume more calories and fiber. Middle and high school student participants consumed more calcium, potassium, vitamin A, vitamin B6, vitamin C, folate, thiamin, magnesium, and phosphorous. Among high school students, NSLP participants also had high sodium intakes.[109]

Public Health Core Competency 2: Policy Development/ Program Planning Skills 7: Identifies mechanisms to monitor and evaluate programs for their effectiveness and quality

Healthy People 2020: NWS-14: Increase the contribution of fruits to the diets of the population aged 2 years and older

Healthy People 2020: NWS-15: Increase the variety and contribution of fruits and vegetables to the diets of the population aged 2 years and older

Healthy People 2020: NWS-16: Increase the contribution of whole grains to the diets of the population aged 2 years and older

Public Health Initiatives in Europe and Australia: Cash Assistance Programs

As described, the United States tends to use nutrition assistance programs to address children's food insecurity. Some programs in many other industrialized nations instead provide parents with cash benefits[110] in the form of one-time grants to new parents or regular stipends that last until the child reaches a certain age. Eligibility for some programs is based on income, while other programs include all parents.

As with food assistance programs for low-income families in the United States, the objective of these cash assistance programs is to enable families to spend more money on children's other needs, such as health care, clothing, and school supplies. Evidence supports the benefits of nonfood assistance, such as cash assistance or subsidized housing, for reducing children's food insecurity.[111] For example, in an evaluation of a housing subsidy program for families in a low-income urban area, the Canadian Survey of Household Spending found an inverse relationship between the proportion of income spent on housing and positive dietary factors, such as amount of money spent on food and adequacy of diet.[112]

The different approaches to assistance for children may reflect different attitudes toward social welfare between the United States compared with other industrialized nations. Universal assistance is more characteristic of social welfare states, such as many nations in Europe, than of the United States, which values individualism. Providing special foods, visible coupons, special debit cards, or vouchers to low-income families, as done in the United States, can be seen as demeaning or a form of social stigma in other nations.[113]

Paid Maternity or Paternity Leave

A number of programs in Europe and Australia require employers to provide paid leave during pregnancy and for some time after birth. For example, Australia's Department of Health Services allows parents to choose between the Baby Bonus, which is a 26-week stipend, and the Paid Parental Leave program, which allows parents to receive pay while staying home to care for infants.[114] An additional component of Paid Parental Leave is Dad and Partner Pay, which began in 2013 with two weeks of paid leave. Benefit amounts are based on family income. Every nation in the European Union has a maternity leave program, and many have paternity leave provisions.[115]

Ireland's Health and Safety Benefit is an example of an initiative to support **breastfeeding**. The program allows mothers to stay home to breastfeed and receive weekly payments from their employers or the government.[116] Women are eligible if they wish to breastfeed but are unable to safely do so while working because of unsafe conditions, such as exposure to chemicals, or if they work night shifts.

Cash Assistance for Children in Australia

The Australian Department of Health Services runs the Parental Payment program to help with the costs of raising children. The stipend, consisting of biweekly payments from the Australian government, is for lower-income single parents of children up to 8 years old and couples with children up to 6 years old. Stipend amounts are inversely related to income, and in 2012, parents were eligible for participation if annual household income was under $43,278, or approximately 82% of the per capita GDP of Australia in 2011.[117,118] Parents under 19 years old who participate in Parental Payment may receive additional aid, such as counseling to increase the chances of finishing high school.[119]

Managed Income and the Centrelink BasicsCard

Another Australian program to aid families with limited budgets is a managed income program, whose objective is to assist with household budgeting.[120] The program is mandatory for parents and other individuals who receive other government assistance, and for parents who are referred by a social service worker because of perceived benefits of participation. Voluntary participation is incentivized for other individuals in Australia.[121] The goal is for parents to be able to take better care of their children with less money, and it includes financial counseling.[122]

The program includes a Centrelink BasicsCard, which is funded with money from the family's personal accounts within the managed income program. This money can be used only in approved stores for "essential goods and services," such as food, clothes, health necessities, appliances, fuel, and furniture in approved stores. It cannot be used for alcohol, tobacco, pornography, or cash withdrawals.

Assistance for Children in the United Kingdom

The United Kingdom provides free school lunches for low-income families and offers other cash assistance programs for families with children.[123] Sure Start Maternity Grants are tax-free, one-time payments for low-income, first-time parents.[124] In households in which the new parent is under 20 years old and living as a dependent of the head of household, the head of household may be eligible for a grant. Recipients must be on government aid such as unemployment benefits or pension credit.

The Child Benefit is a payment to parents for each child in the household until the age of 16 years. The stipend is paid every four weeks, or every two weeks for parents who are low-income and receiving other government services. Similar programs in Europe may include one-time grants or repeating stipends, and are often related to income.[125]

Assistance for Children in Ireland

Pregnant women and new mothers may request Maternity Benefits to receive payment without working for the last four weeks of pregnancy and eight weeks after giving birth. Unemployed mothers seeking work may receive benefits for longer.[126] Parents who have paid into the Irish Social Insurance System can receive monthly payments until their children reach the age of 16 years, or 18 years for children with disabilities. The goal of increasing the household budget is to allow more money to be spent on food and thereby improve children's nutritional status and health. In Ireland, the perception of poverty is closely tied to food insecurity.[127]

Food Fortification to Reduce Disparities and Improve Nutritional Status

Children's food insecurity is related to poorer diet quality, often characterized by more energy-dense foods and higher intakes of saturated fat, sodium, and added sugars compared with food-secure children.[128] Children with low or very low food security are also likely to have lower or inadequate intakes of certain essential **micronutrients**, such as calcium, iron, vitamin D, and/or riboflavin. Consumption of fruits, vegetables, and whole-grain products is lower, and

these nutrient-dense foods are natural sources of **dietary fiber**, vitamin C, **beta-carotene**, and **vitamin E**.[129]

Food fortification programs are public health nutrition interventions that can effectively improve nutritional status in susceptible populations, including children with food insecurity. Universal food fortification, such as grain fortification with thiamin, riboflavin, and niacin, can benefit hard-to-reach populations without specifically targeting them or requiring conscious behavior change.[130] This can be beneficial for low food-secure families that may reside in remote rural areas, have inadequate money to purchase additional nutritious foods, and be unlikely to change behaviors based on educational materials or media campaigns. Another benefit of appropriate food fortification programs is their affordability; purchasing fortified foods may remain a more affordable option than purchasing naturally nutrient-dense foods that are less common among food-insecure children. Mandatory iodization of salt is a program that has virtually eliminated **endemic** iodine deficiency in regions that have adopted it.

Examples of Food Fortification Programs

Vitamin D is naturally present only in limited foods, such as fish oil, and adequate exposure to radiation from the sun is necessary for endogenous production. Deficiency is common among children in industrialized nations, increasing the risk for bone disorders, such as **rickets** and **osteomalacia**, and a higher risk for osteoporosis later in life. The World Health Organization recommends fortifying milk with vitamin D.[131]

Folic Acid and Vitamin B12 Fortification of Grains

Some public health nutritionists argue for universal fortification of flour with folic acid,[132] which is commonly deficient in children's food insecurity and is essential for proper growth and the prevention of **neural tube birth defects**. The United States implemented mandatory folic acid fortification of flour in 1996.

Much remains to be done, however; folic acid deficiency is still widespread worldwide. Only about 10% of potentially preventable neural tube birth defects are actually being prevented.[133] Few European nations require folic acid fortification because of the fear of toxicity symptoms, such as masking vitamin B12 deficiency in vulnerable populations, such as older adults and children who eat plant-based diets. However, vitamin B12 fortification can prevent the possibility of high folic acid intake masking a vitamin B12 deficiency. Hungary adopted the strategy of fortifying bread with folic acid, **vitamin B12**, and **vitamin B6**.

Food Fortification: Successes and Critiques

Since implementing mandatory folic acid fortification at the rate of 140 micrograms per 100 grams of flour in the United States, NTDs have decreased and serum folate levels have increased. In the United Kingdom, food-insecure individuals who consumed breakfast cereals had higher intakes of thiamin, riboflavin, niacin, biotin, folate, vitamin B6, vitamin B12, iron, and zinc. Their calcium intake was also higher, probably due to higher milk consumption.[134]

To be sustainable, food fortification programs need to be affordable and easy for consumers to participate in. The cost of fortification needs to be low enough so that low-income families, who are at highest risk for food insecurity and micronutrient deficiencies, are able and willing to purchase fortified foods. Governments can support programs by providing guidelines, initial or ongoing funds, technical support, and enforcement of mandatory programs. In addition, governments can implement policies to include fortified foods, such as vitamin D–fortified milk, in food assistance programs to ensure that food-insecure children receive them. Voluntary fortification programs lacking government and popular support risk failure.[135] Consumer perceptions of natural foods being superior to fortified foods can interfere with national fortification programs.[136]

Lessons Learned in Addressing Children's Food Insecurity

Public health actions to reduce children's food insecurity include assessment and monitoring of prevalence and effects, development, and implementation of policies to alleviate and prevent food insecurity and underlying causes, and implementation and outcome evaluation of programs designed to reduce children's food insecurity.

Objectives Related to Children's Food Insecurity

Objectives are targets or specific goals based on careful assessment of the problem, such as prevalence, causes, and consequences of food insecurity. They are important because they acknowledge problems, increase awareness, guide public health interventions, and enable evaluation of progress.

The United States and the European Union are currently working toward a variety of objectives related to children's food insecurity. *Healthy People 2020* objectives include eliminating "very low food security among children" from a baseline of 1.3% prevalence in 2008 to a goal of 0.2% by 2020. Another objective is to "reduce household food insecurity" from a baseline of 14.6% to a goal of 6%.[137] Among the United States Department of Agriculture's Strategic Goals is to allow all children "access to safe, nutritious and affordable meals," including subgoals to "increase access to nutritious food" and "promote healthy diet and physical activity behaviors."[138] Europe 2020 Targets, within the European Union, include reducing social exclusion and poverty by 20 million people.[139] Many nations have set individual targets as well.

Establishing these objectives and monitoring progress indicates recognition of the importance of children's food insecurity. Some programs have demonstrated reductions in food insecurity or higher nutrient intake. However, much remains to be done. The prevalence of children's food insecurity in the United States has not changed markedly since 1995, when the first food insecurity poll was taken.[140] In the European Union, the prevalence of poverty remains at 8.1%, which is down from 10.7% in 2005 but far from desirable.[141]

Considerations for Programs to Reduce Children's Food Insecurity

Observations from previously implemented programs can guide more successful ones in the future.

Components to Include: Lessons from the Farm Bill and Food Stamp Program

Every public health program must be carefully crafted based on the particular situation at the community, national, or regional level, but examination of previous and current programs for reducing children's food insecurity suggests that certain components should be carefully considered when designing a program.

One lesson from the **Farm Bill**[142] in the United States is that programs should be distinct from each other but coordinated to facilitate administration and reduce cost. Programs should serve current needs based on careful assessment, and be affordable based on current economic conditions. Each program must have clear methods of demonstrating effectiveness and have oversight methods in place to monitor compliance and avoid waste.

Based on SNAP, formerly known as the Food Stamp Program,[143] the U.S. Government Accountability Office (GAO) suggests that assistance programs include only some foods to encourage the purchase of nutritious foods among individuals whose food budget is limited. Planners should recognize that the amount of aid affects participation and costs of the program. Finally, including families can increase effectiveness of food aid programs.

Program Accessibility

A measure of a program's success is accessibility to the majority of its target population, including awareness of the program among eligible populations. Food assistance programs, such as NSLP and cash benefit programs, such as the Australian Parenting Payment, can be publicized via other government assistance programs, such as WIC clinics or physician offices. Community organizations and volunteers can help raise awareness and provide registration assistance.

Public Health Core Competency 3: Communication Skills 4: Conveys public health information using a variety of approaches

Accessibility also requires the ability to sign up for the program without trouble. Fast registration online or over the telephone can remove time,[144] transportation, and social stigma barriers associated with requiring in-person attendance at a specified office or clinic. Another potential benefit of using electronic systems to sign up is the reduced occurrence of fraud[145] and procedural denials resulting from delays in paperwork.[146]

Promoting Nutrition Through Accessibility

A sufficient and nutritious diet may be inaccessible to food-insecure children because of the food environment.[147] Children's food insecurity may result from residency in low-income neighborhoods, which can often be defined as food deserts without large supermarkets. Policies to require the stocking of healthy foods in all neighborhoods can be a solution.[148]

The cost of high-nutrient, low-energy-dense food is another major barrier to a nutritious diet for children with food insecurity. Policies that promote healthy choices and discourage less healthy options include subsidies for healthy foods,[149] inclusion of fresh produce from farmers' markets in programs, and prohibiting the use of electronic banking cards for purchasing junk food, since many nutritionists are concerned that energy-dense foods purchased with electronic banking cards may increase risk for obesity among SNAP participants.[150] School-based policies to improve dietary choices include the current policy of requiring reduced-fat milk, fruits, and vegetables to be served in the National School Lunch Program. Another strategy, which is currently enforced only on district or statewide levels, is banning the sale of junk foods, such as soft drinks and candy, from vending machines. School-based programs that focus on the palatability of the healthier foods can also lead to improvements in children's diets, as was seen with the Chef Initiative.

Rights-Based Approach to Food Security

The Universal Declaration of Human Rights recognizes that all people have a right to food, and that children should receive extra aid. Furthermore, the statement that "all children, whether born in or out of wedlock, shall receive the same social protection" implies a mandate to eliminate children's food insecurity.[151] The rights-based approach to food is evident in Europe, especially states known as welfare states, such as the United Kingdom and Ireland.[152] The Irish, for example, associate poverty with food poverty.

A rights-based approach is less likely in the United States.[153] Such an approach would address underlying social and economic disparities and focus on public awareness, oversight, transparency, and protection of vulnerable groups. Barriers to a rights-based approach in the United States include widespread belief that government would be meddling and interfere with social, economic, and cultural rights by directly providing them. Rights-based approach proponents might argue that this position demonstrates lack of understanding of the need for a long-term plan to reduce poverty and disparities.

Evidence suggests that "safety nets," or ongoing programs to alleviate food insecurity, do not encourage laziness and are not necessarily an economic drain.[154] Food-based safety nets are more difficult than cash to provide because of perishability and distribution, but they may have greater immediate benefits.

Public Health Core Competency 4: Cultural Competency Skills 1: Incorporates strategies for interacting with persons from diverse backgrounds

Role of Nutrition Education

Nutrition education, focusing on choosing and preparing healthy foods, can improve diet quality among food-insecure families.[155] Education can take place in classes or through media campaigns to targeted audiences.[156] Free online resources are easily accessible. The Food and Nutrition Service within the USDA provides materials, including interactive games for children and recipes.[157] Many materials are available in Spanish, the language spoken at home in 12% of U.S. households in 2007.[158] In addition, the USDA and the Department of Health and Human Services (DHHS) publish *Dietary Guidelines for Americans* to help guide food choices. The Food Safety Authority of Ireland and the Food Standards Agency in the United Kingdom have similar resources.[159,160]

Education from university outreach programs can include lessons on healthy choices, shopping for healthy foods on a budget, and preparing foods provided in food assistance programs.[161] Classes on home economics in schools have also been proposed.[162]

Special Diets and Children's Nutrition

Children may alter their diets because of health conditions, such as allergies or intolerances, or because of their or their caregivers' beliefs or values. Special diets can place children at higher risk of nutritional concerns when they involve avoiding certain foods or food groups. Usually, well-planned diets can meet children's physiological nutritional needs and allow them to enjoy meals with their peers. Fortified foods or dietary supplements can help meet nutrient requirements.

Lactose Intolerance

Lactose, or "milk sugar," is the carbohydrate in milk. In lactose intolerance, inadequate levels of the enzyme lactase in the small intestine cause incomplete digestion of lactose. Symptoms may include stomach cramps, diarrhea, nausea, and bloating. More than two-thirds of the world's population is lactose intolerant.[163] Primary lactose intolerance, the most common type, often develops as children grow up, diversify their diets, and have less need for lactase. Nearly all Asian and American Indian populations and 50–80% of Hispanic, black, and Ashkenazi Jewish adults are lactose intolerant.

Most lactose-intolerant individuals can have small amounts of lactose. Small servings of yogurt, aged cheese, milk

chocolate, ice cream, and reduced-lactose milk are often tolerated. Dairy products are important sources of calcium for children, contributing an average of 70% of total calcium intake in the United States.[164] A cup of milk or yogurt or one and a half ounces of cheese provides about 300 milligrams of calcium, or 23% of the adequate intake of 1,300 milligrams per day for children 9 to 18 years old. Sufficient calcium during childhood is necessary for achieving peak bone mass.

If they are careful, lactose-intolerant individuals can meet calcium and other nutritional needs without consuming dairy products. Canned bony fish and calcium-fortified orange juice, soy milk, and rice milk are good sources. **Table 14-2** summarizes nutrients in dairy products and alternative sources for individuals with lactose intolerance.

Celiac Disease or Gluten Intolerance

Celiac disease is an autoimmune disorder that leads to reactions to gluten, a protein in wheat, rye, and barley.[165] Nearly 1% of Americans have celiac disease. Symptoms include diarrhea, fatigue, and irritability. Children may have poor weight gain, slowed growth, and discolored tooth enamel due to nutrient malabsorption.

Avoiding gluten prevents symptoms. A gluten-free diet excludes wheat, barley, and rye, along with products that may contain them, such as beer, broth, soy sauce, products made with wheat flour, wheat starch, and many sauces and other processed foods. Fruits, vegetables, beans, corn, oatmeal, meat, eggs, dairy products, nuts, rice, and amaranth are naturally gluten-free, although some products can become contaminated with gluten during storage or processing if silos or processing equipment has residues of gluten. Children on gluten-free diets and their parents must choose foods whose labels state "gluten free." Regulations for the "gluten-free" designation on food products are similar in the United Kingdom and other European nations.[166,167]

Carefully planned gluten-free diets can be nutritionally adequate. Fortified grains in the United States provide iron, thiamin, niacin, riboflavin, and folic acid. Children with gluten intolerance can avoid wheat and instead choose fortified gluten-free grains.

Strict Vegetarian, or Vegan, Diets

Semi-vegetarians eat meat, poultry, and seafood less than once per week.[168] Pesco-vegetarians exclude meat and poultry but include seafood. Lacto-ovo vegetarians, or vegetarians, exclude meat, poultry, and seafood and include eggs and dairy products. Vegan diets include only plant-based

Table 14-2 Affected nutrients in special diets

Affected Nutrients in Special Diets	Alternative Sources
Lactose intolerance: nutrients found in milk and dairy products	
Calcium	Canned bony fish, leafy green vegetables
Vitamin D	Fatty fish, fortified juices and cereals
	Exposure to sunlight
Riboflavin	Fortified grains
Magnesium	Nuts, legumes, whole grains, leafy green vegetables
Phosphorus	Meat, poultry, fish, eggs,
Potassium	Fruits, vegetables, potatoes, legumes, eggs
Vegan diet: nutrients in dairy, eggs, meat, poultry, and seafood	
Nutrients from dairy products (see lactose intolerance), plus the following:	Same sources as lactose intolerance, but excluding all animal products
Calories	If necessary, choose more nutrient-dense foods to reduce necessary bulk to achieve energy needs
Protein	Soy-based foods, legumes, nuts, grains, peanuts, seeds, vegetables
Vitamin B12	Fortified soy milk, nutritional yeast and other dietary supplements
Iron	Fortified grains, nuts, legumes, dried fruits, leafy green vegetables
Zinc	Wheat germ, whole grains, legumes, vegetables
Long-chain omega-3 fatty acids DHA and EPA	Flaxseed, flax, canola oil and walnuts (ALA), DHA and EPA or fish oil supplements
Celiac disease: nutrients in wheat, barley, and rye products	
Thiamin	Fortified rice, fortified gluten-free breakfast cereals, yeast, pork, seeds, soy milk, legumes
Riboflavin	Milk, fortified rice, fortified gluten-free breakfast cereals and breads, leafy green vegetables, eggs, fish, meat
Niacin	Fortified rice, fortified gluten-free breakfast cereals, fish, meat, eggs, legumes, coffee, tea
Folic acid	Fortified rice, fortified gluten-free breakfast cereals, green vegetables, mushrooms, legumes, fruit, liver
Iron	Fortified rice, fortified gluten-free breakfast cereals and breads, meat, liver, seafood, nuts, legumes, seafood, dried fruits, leafy green vegetables

Data from Gropper, S. S., Smith, J. L., & Groff, J. L. (2009). *Advanced nutrition and human metabolism* (5th ed.). Belmont, CA: Wadsworth Publishing.

foods and exclude all meat, poultry, seafood, dairy products, and eggs. Vegan diets require supplementation or fortified foods for nutritional adequacy.

In 2006, 3% of U.S. children reported following vegetarian diets, and 1% followed vegan diets.[169] Reasons include religious beliefs, ethical principles, concern for the environment, and the belief that vegetarian diets are healthier.[170] Younger children and preadolescents are likely to follow the habits in their households; older adolescents might independently decide to follow vegetarian diets.

Varied lacto-ovo vegetarian diets emphasizing nutrient-dense foods can be sufficient for normal growth and development. Children on vegan diets emphasizing filling, low-calorie-dense foods, such as fruits and vegetables, can have difficulty eating enough calories.[171] More calorie-dense foods that can increase total energy intake without providing much extra bulk include nuts and nut butters, seeds, grains, and soy-based products.

Legumes, or beans, split peas and lentils, soy-based products, nuts, peanuts, and whole grains are plant-based sources of protein that can meet children's needs for quantity and quality of protein. Soy protein is a **complete protein**, but most plant-based proteins are incomplete. Still, **protein combining**, or using **complementary proteins**, can help children meet their amino acid requirements on vegan diets. Eating incomplete proteins from two different food groups supplies a complete protein. A peanut butter sandwich (peanuts and grains), beans and rice (legumes and grains), and a bean burrito (legumes with grains) are examples of complementary proteins.

Fortified foods or supplements are necessary to supply vitamin B12, which is found naturally only in animal-derived foods. Children who do not eat fish are likely to have low intakes of the omega-3 fatty acids, docohexaenoic acid (DHA), and eicosapentaenoic acid (EPA). Plant-based diets can be low in calcium and vitamin D due to avoidance of dairy products. Lacto-ovo vegetarians have higher-than-average calcium intake, while vegans have a higher risk of bone fractures later in life, likely indicating low calcium and vitamin D intake.[172]

Vegetarian diets may be protective against coronary heart disease and lower total and low-density lipoprotein (LDL) cholesterol levels.[173] Individuals on vegetarian diets tend to have higher intakes of some beneficial nutrients, such as dietary fiber, vitamin C, and vitamin E, and lower consumption of saturated fat.[174] The potential benefits for children are not certain. Vegetarian diets have not been shown to be protective against childhood obesity.[175] In addition, the former American Dietetic Association, now the Academy of Nutrition and Dietetics, states that children on vegetarian diets have slower growth rates. The lower consumption of vitamin D associated with vegetarian diets can lead to reduced calcium absorption and bone disorders.

Allergies

An allergy is an immune response to a specific protein after eating a food.[176] Food allergies are more prevalent among children, with prevalence of 4–8%, than among adults,

with prevalence of 2% in the United States. Symptoms of an allergic reaction may include hives, itching, wheezing, a runny nose, and dizziness. Symptoms of potentially fatal anaphylactic reactions include trouble breathing and low blood pressure. Children with allergies must avoid the food, and very severe allergies may require avoidance of smelling or touching the food.

The eight most commonly allergenic foods are peanuts, tree nuts, wheat, shellfish, fish, soybeans, eggs, and milk.[177] The Food Allergen Labeling and Consumer Protection Act requires listing of these foods on food labels. In the United Kingdom, the Food Standards Agency recognizes 14 allergens: gluten, crustaceans, mollusks, eggs, fish, peanuts, nuts, soybeans, milk, celery, lupin, mustard, sesame, and sulfur dioxide above a threshold level.[178]

Allergies do not usually affect nutritional status unless multiple allergies force children to consume overly restrictive diets. In addition to carefully reading labels to avoid ingesting an allergen, children or their parents may need to request that group-prepared meals, such as in school cafeterias, be prepared without a specific allergen. Food preparers may need to be educated about reading labels and avoiding the implicated ingredient.

Children may need to bring their own food to school. The NSLP requires schools to provide a "safe meal, non-allergenic meal to the child if the condition is disabling,"[179] but not if the condition is not serious. To receive reimbursement for accommodating food substitutions that are not (i.e., minor allergy or intolerance), schools must provide a student's medical statement with descriptions of the diet or condition, prohibited foods, and included food substitutions.

Improving Nutrition Among Children with Special Diets

As seen above, legislation and enforcement of accurate food labeling is an important step in allowing children to avoid foods that can trigger adverse health effects. Widespread food fortification and targeted dietary supplements can help compensate for missed nutrients. Education for parents, children, and food handlers on choosing nutritious, safe foods can also prevent nutritional problems related to special diets.

A healthy diet for children with special needs goes beyond simply writing down a nutritionally adequate meal and supplement plan.[180] Children need to enjoy their food and feel equal to their peers. This has become easier with the increase in vegetarian, gluten-free, and lactose-free menu items in restaurants and substitute products, such as soy milk, meat substitutes, and gluten-free bread, in supermarkets.[181] Vegan children can, for example, enjoy veggie burgers while peers are eating hamburgers.

Conclusion

Although industrialized nations are wealthier and have generally stable food supplies, many children in industrialized nations are still at risk for poor nutritional status and health outcomes. Children with food insecurity may be low in key micronutrients while simultaneously facing obesity and chronic diseases; children with dietary restrictions due to chronic conditions or cultural reasons may also be at risk for nutrient deficiencies. Public health interventions can support better nutrition using a variety of strategies, such as nutrition assistance and economic support for parents to indirectly improve household food availability. Food labeling, promotion of a balanced diet, and support for nutrition education and fortification programs can improve childhood nutritional status.

References

1 Woolridge, N. H. (2011). Child and preadolescent nutrition. In J. Brown (Ed.), *Nutrition through the life cycle* (pp. 311-37). Belmont, CA: Wadsworth.

2 Berenson, G. S., & Bogalusa Heart Study Group. (2012). Health consequences of obesity. *Pediatric Blood & Cancer, 58*, 117-21.

3 Food and Agriculture Organization. (2002). *The state of food insecurity in the world, 2001*. Rome, Italy: Food and Agriculture Organization.

4 Centers for Disease Control and Prevention. (2010, December 9). *Core functions of public health and how they relate to the 10 essential public health services*. Retrieved from http://www.cdc.gov/nceh/ehs/EPHLI/core_ess.htm

5 Committee on Assuring the Health of the Public in the 21st Century. (2002). *The future of public health in the 21st century*. Washington, DC: National Academies Press.

6 Radimer, K. L., & Radimer, K. L. (2002). Measurement of household food security in the USA and other industrialized countries. *Public Health Nutrition, 5*, 859-64.

7 Food and Agriculture Organization. (2002). *The state of food insecurity in the world, 2001*. Rome, Italy: Food and Agriculture Organization.

8 Anderson, S. A. (Ed.). (1990). Core indicators of nutritional state for difficult-to-sample populations. *Journal of Nutrition, 120*, 1559-99.

9 Anderson, S. A. (Ed.). (1990). Core indicators of nutritional state for difficult-to-sample populations. *Journal of Nutrition, 120*, 1559-99.

10 Anderson, S. A. (Ed.). (1990). Core indicators of nutritional state for difficult-to-sample populations. *Journal of Nutrition, 120*, 1559-99.

11 Nord, M., & Coleman-Jensen, A. (2012, August 15). *Food security in the U.S.: Measurement of food security*. Retrieved from http://www.ers.usda.gov/topics/food-nutrition-assistance/food-security-in-the-us/definitions-of-food-security.aspx

12 Nord, M., & Coleman-Jensen, A. (2012, June 4). *Food security in the U.S.: Definitions of food security*. Retrieved from http://www.ers.usda.gov/topics/food-nutrition-assistance/food-security-in-the-us/definitions-of-food-security.aspx

13 Frongillo, E. A. (1999). Validation of measures of food insecurity and hunger. *Journal of Nutrition, 129*, 506S-509S.

14 Frongillo, E. A., Rauschenbach, B. S., Olson, C. M., Kendall, A., & Colmenares, A. G. (1997). Questionnaire-based measures are valid for the identification of rural households with hunger and food insecurity. *Journal of Nutrition, 127*, 699-705.

15 Frongillo, E. A., Rauschenbach, B. S., Olson, C. M., Kendall, A., & Colmenares, A. G. (1997). Questionnaire-based measures are valid for the identification of rural households with hunger and food insecurity. *Journal of Nutrition, 127*, 699-705.

16 Kendall, A., Olson, C. M., & Frongillo, E. A. (1996). Relationship of hunger and food insecurity to food availability and consumption. *Journal of the American Dietetic Association, 96*, 1019-24.

17 Nord, M., & Coleman-Jensen, A. (2012, June 4). Food security in the U.S: History and background. Retrieved from http://www.ers.usda.gov/topics/food-nutrition-assistance/food-security-in-the-us/history-background.aspx

18 Eurostat, European Union Commission. (2010, April 4). *European Union statistics on income and living conditions (EU-SILC)*. Retrieved from http://epp.eurostat.ec.europa.eu/portal/page/portal/microdata/eu_silc.

19 Pornet, C., Delpierre, C., Dejardin, O., Grosclaude, P., Launay, L., Guittet, L., . . . Launoy, G. (2012). Construction of an adaptable European transnational ecological deprivation index: The French version. *Journal of Epidemiology and Community Health, 66*(11), 982-89.

20 Gordon, D. (1995). Census based deprivation indices: Their weight and validation. *Journal of Epidemiology and Community Health, 49*, S39-S44.

21 Bradshaw, J., & Mayhew, E., for the European Commission. (2011). *The measurement of extreme poverty in the European Union*. Brussels: European Commission, DG Employment, Social Affairs and Inclusion.

22 Kirkpatrick, S. I., & Tarasuk, V. (2007). Adequacy of food spending is related to housing expenditures among lower-income Canadian households. *Public Health Nutrition, 10*, 1464-73.

23 Janevic, T., Petrovic, O., Bjelic, I., & Kubera, A. (2010). Risk factors for childhood malnutrition in Roma settlements in Serbia. *BMC Public Health, 10,* 509.

24 Nord, M. (2009, September). *Food insecurity in households with children: Prevalence, severity and household characteristics.* Economic Information Bulletin No. EIB-56. Retrieved from http://www.ers.usda.gov/publications/eib-economic-information-bulletin/eib56.aspx#.Umq0HxXD8y8

25 Nord, M. (2009, September). *Food insecurity in households with children: Prevalence, severity and household characteristics.* Economic Information Bulletin No. EIB-56. Retrieved from http://www.ers.usda.gov/publications/eib-economic-information-bulletin/eib56.aspx#.Umq0HxXD8y8

26 Che, J., & Chen, J. (2001). Food insecurity in Canadian households. *Health Reports, 12*(4), 11-22.

27 Nolan, M., Williams, M., Rikard-Bell, G., & Mohsin, M. (2006). Food insecurity in three socially disadvantaged localities in Sydney, Australia. *Health Promotion Journal of Australia, 17*(3), 247-54.

28 International Monetary Fund. (2012, April). *World economic outlook.* Retrieved from http://www.imf.org/external/pubs/ft/weo/2012/01/weodata/index.aspx

29 Oh, S. Y., & Hong, M. J. (2003). Food insecurity is associated with dietary intake and body size of Korean children from low-income families in urban areas. *European Journal of Clinical Nutrition, 57,* 1598-1604.

30 United Nations Development Program. (2011). *Human development report 2011: sustainability and equity: A better future for all.* New York, NY: Human Development Report Team.

31 Janevic, T., Petrovic, O., Bjelic, I., & Kubera, A. (2010). Risk factors for childhood malnutrition in Roma settlements in Serbia. *BMC Public Health, 10,* 509.

32 Nelson, M., Erens, B., Bates, B., Church, S., & Boshier, T. (2007). *Low income diet and nutrition survey: Summary of key findings.* Food Standards Agency. Norwich, UK: The Stationary Office. Retrieved from http://www.food.gov.uk/multimedia/pdfs/lidnssummary.pdf

33 Nelson, M., Erens, B., Bates, B., Church, S., & Boshier, T. (2007). *Low income diet and nutrition survey: Summary of key findings.* Food Standards Agency. Norwich, UK: The Stationary Office. Retrieved from http://www.food.gov.uk/multimedia/pdfs/lidnssummary.pdf

34 Nord, M., & Coleman-Jensen, A. (2012, July 13). *Food security in the U.S: Key statistics and graphics.* Retrieved from http://www.ers.usda.gov/topics/food-nutrition-assistance/food-security-in-the-us/key-statistics-graphics.aspx

35 Che, J., & Chen, J. (2001). Food insecurity in Canadian households. *Health Reports, 12*(4), 11-22.

36 Nelson, M., Erens, B., Bates, B., Church, S., & Boshier, T. (2007). *Low income diet and nutrition survey: Summary of key findings.* Food Standards Agency. Norwich, UK: The Stationary Office. Retrieved from http://www.food.gov.uk/multimedia/pdfs/lidnssummary.pdf

37 Janevic, T., Petrovic, O., Bjelic, I., & Kubera, A. (2010). Risk factors for childhood malnutrition in Roma settlements in Serbia. *BMC Public Health, 10,* 509.

38 Oh, S. Y., & Hong, M. J. (2003). Food insecurity is associated with dietary intake and body size of Korean children from low-income families in urban areas. *European Journal of Clinical Nutrition, 57,* 1598-1604.

39 Nolan, M., Williams, M., Rikard-Bell, G., & Mohsin, M. (2006). Food insecurity in three socially disadvantaged localities in Sydney, Australia. *Health Promotion Journal of Australia, 17*(3), 247-54.

40 Nord, M. (2009, September). *Food insecurity in households with children: prevalence, severity and household characteristics.* Economic Information Bulletin No. EIB-56. Retrieved from http://www.ers.usda.gov/publications/eib-economic-information-bulletin/eib56.aspx#.Umq0HxXD8y8

41 Kirkpatrick, S. I., & Tarasuk, V. (2011). Housing circumstances are associated with food access among low-income urban families. *Journal of Urban Health, 88,* 284-96.

42 Gordon, D., Levitas, R., Pantazis, C., Patsios, D., Payne, S., & Townsend, P. (1990). *Poverty and social exclusion in Britain.* York, United Kingdom: Joseph Rowntree Foundation. Retrieved from http://www.bris.ac.uk/poverty/pse/Poverty%20and%20Social%20Exclusion%20in%20Britain%20JRF%20Report.pdf

43 Nord, M., & Coleman-Jensen, A. Economic Research Service, U.S. Department of Agriculture. (2012, July 13). *Food security in the U.S: Key statistics and graphics.* Retrieved from http://www.ers.usda.gov/topics/food-nutrition-assistance/food-security-in-the-us/key-statistics-graphics.aspx

44 Che, J., & Chen, J. (2001). Food insecurity in Canadian households. *Health Reports, 12*(4), 11-22.

45 Che, J., & Chen, J. (2001). Food insecurity in Canadian households. *Health Reports, 12*(4), 11-22.

46 Gordon, D., Levitas, R., Pantazis, C., Patsios, D., Payne, S., & Townsend, P. (1990). *Poverty and social exclusion in Britain.* York, United Kingdom: Joseph Rowntree Foundation. Retrieved from http://www.bris.ac.uk/poverty/pse/Poverty%20and%20Social%20Exclusion%20in%20Britain%20JRF%20Report.pdf

47 Nord, M. (2009, September). *Food insecurity in households with children: Prevalence, severity and household characteristics.* Economic Information Bulletin No. EIB-56. Retrieved from http://www.ers.usda.gov/publications/eib-economic-information-bulletin/eib56.aspx#.Umq0HxXD8y8

48 Janevic, T., Petrovic, O., Bjelic, I., & Kubera, A. (2010). Risk factors for childhood malnutrition in Roma settlements in Serbia. *BMC Public Health, 10,* 509.

49 Nord, M. (2009, September). *Food insecurity in households with children: Prevalence, severity and household characteristics.* Economic Information Bulletin No. EIB-56. Retrieved from http://www.ers.usda.gov/publications/eib-economic-information-bulletin/eib56.aspx#.Umq0HxXD8y8

50 Che, J., & Chen, J. (2001). Food insecurity in Canadian households. *Health Reports, 12*(4), 11-22.

51 Gordon, D., Levitas, R., Pantazis, C., Patsios, D., Payne, S., & Townsend, P. (1990). *Poverty and social exclusion in Britain.* York, United Kingdom: Joseph Rowntree Foundation. Retrieved from http://www.bris.ac.uk/poverty/pse/Poverty%20and%20Social%20Exclusion%20in%20Britain%20JRF%20Report.pdf

52 Janevic, T., Petrovic, O., Bjelic, I., & Kubera, A. (2010). Risk factors for childhood malnutrition in Roma settlements in Serbia. *BMC Public Health, 10,* 509.

53 Janevic, T., Petrovic, O., Bjelic, I., & Kubera, A. (2010). Risk factors for childhood malnutrition in Roma settlements in Serbia. *BMC Public Health, 10,* 509.

54 Nord, M. (2009, September). *Food insecurity in households with children: Prevalence, severity and household characteristics.* Economic Information Bulletin No. EIB-56. Retrieved from http://www.ers.usda.gov/publications/eib-economic-information-bulletin/eib56.aspx#.Umq0HxXD8y8

55 Janevic, T., Petrovic, O., Bjelic, I., & Kubera, A. (2010). Risk factors for childhood malnutrition in Roma settlements in Serbia. *BMC Public Health, 10,* 509.

56 Gordon, D., Levitas, R., Pantazis, C., Patsios, D., Payne, S., & Townsend, P. (1990). *Poverty and social exclusion in Britain.* York, United Kingdom: Joseph Rowntree Foundation. Retrieved from http://www.bris.ac.uk/poverty/pse/Poverty%20and%20Social%20Exclusion%20in%20Britain%20JRF%20Report.pdf

57 Selen, D. W., Tedstone, A. E., & Frize, J. (2002). Food insecurity among refugee families in East London: Results of a pilot assessment. *Public Health Nutrition, 5,* 637-44

58 Chilton, M., & Rose, D. (2009). A rights-based approach to food insecurity in the United States. *American Journal of Public Health, 99,* 1203-11.

59 Darmon, N., & Drewnowski, A. (2008). Does social class predict diet quality? *American Journal of Clinical Nutrition, 87,* 1107-17.

60 Oh, S. Y., & Hong, M. J. (2003). Food insecurity is associated with dietary intake and body size of Korean children from low-income families in urban areas. *European Journal of Clinical Nutrition, 57,* 1598-1604.

61 Rolland-Cachera, M. F., & Bellisle, F. (1986). No correlation between adiposity and food intake: why are working class children fatter? *American Journal of Clinical Nutrition, 44,* 779-87.

62 Darmon, N., & Drewnowski, A. (2008). Does social class predict diet quality? *American Journal of Clinical Nutrition, 87,* 1107-17.

63 Rolland-Cachera, M. F., & Bellisle, F. (1986). No correlation between adiposity and food intake: Why are working class children fatter? *American Journal of Clinical Nutrition, 44,* 779-87.

64 Rolland-Cachera, M. F., & Bellisle, F. (1986). No correlation between adiposity and food intake: why are working class children fatter? *American Journal of Clinical Nutrition, 44,* 779-87.

65 Xie, B., Gilliland, F. D., Li, Y. F., & Rockett, H. R. (2003). Effects of ethnicity, family income, and education on dietary intake among adolescents. *Preventive Medicine, 36,* 30-40.

66 Oh, S. Y., & Hong, M. J. (2003). Food insecurity is associated with dietary intake and body size of Korean children from low-income families in urban areas. *European Journal of Clinical Nutrition, 57,* 1598-1604.

67 World Health Organization. (2003). *Diet, nutrition and the prevention of chronic diseases: report of a WHO study group.* Geneva: World Health Organization.

68 Xie, B., Gilliland, F. D., Li, Y. F., & Rockett, H. R. (2003). Effects of ethnicity, family income, and education on dietary intake among adolescents. *Preventive Medicine, 36,* 30-40.

69 Darmon, N., & Drewnowski, A. (2008). Does social class predict diet quality? *American Journal of Clinical Nutrition, 87,* 1107-17.

70 Briefel, R. R. (2007). The changing consumption patterns and health and nutritional status in the United States: Evidence from national surveys. In E. Kennedy and R. Deckelbaum (Eds.), *The nation's nutrition* (pp. 11-27). Washington, DC: International Life Sciences Institute Press.

71 Nelson, M., Erens, B., Bates, B., Church, S., & Boshier, T. (2007). *Low income diet and nutrition survey: Summary of key findings.* Food Standards Agency. Norwich, United Kingdom: The Stationary Office. Retrieved from http://www.food.gov.uk/multimedia/pdfs/lidnssummary.pdf

72 Irala, J. D., Groth, M., Johansson, L., Oltersdorf, U., Prattala, R., & Martinez-Gonzalez, M. A. (2000). A systematic review of socio-economic differences in food habits in Europe: Consumption of fruits and vegetables. *Nature, 54,* 706-14.

73 Oh, S. Y., & Hong, M. J. (2003). Food insecurity is associated with dietary intake and body size of Korean children from low-income families in urban areas. *European Journal of Clinical Nutrition, 57,* 1598-1604.

74 Darmon, N., & Drewnowski, A. (2008). Does social class predict diet quality? *American Journal of Clinical Nutrition, 87,* 1107-17.

75 Office of Research and Analysis, Food and Nutrition Service, U.S. Department of Agriculture. (2009, December 18). *Healthy Incentives pilot evaluation: Public summary.* Retrieved from http://www.fns.usda.gov/SNAP/HIP/docs/eval.pdf

76 World Health Organization. (2003, August 25-27). *Fruit and vegetable promotion initiative: A meeting report.* Geneva: World Health Organization. Retrieved from http://www.who.int/dietphysicalactivity/publications/f&v_promotion_initiative_report.pdf

77 Office of Research and Analysis, Food and Nutrition Service, U.S. Department of Agriculture. (2009, December 18). *Healthy Incentives pilot evaluation: Public summary.* Retrieved from http://www.fns.usda.gov/SNAP/HIP/docs/eval.pdf

78 Oh, S. Y., & Hong, M. J. (2003). Food insecurity is associated with dietary intake and body size of Korean children

from low-income families in urban areas. *European Journal of Clinical Nutrition, 57,* 1598-1604.

79 Darmon, N., & Drewnowski, A. (2008). Does social class predict diet quality? *American Journal of Clinical Nutrition, 87,* 1107-17.

80 Darmon, N., & Drewnowski, A. (2008). Does social class predict diet quality? *American Journal of Clinical Nutrition, 87,* 1107-17.

81 Oh, S. Y., & Hong, M. J. (2003). Food insecurity is associated with dietary intake and body size of Korean children from low-income families in urban areas. *European Journal of Clinical Nutrition, 57,* 1598-1604.

82 Darmon, N., & Drewnowski, A. (2008). Does social class predict diet quality? *American Journal of Clinical Nutrition, 87,* 1107-17.

83 Australian Red Cross. (n.d.). *High food price hurdle.* Retrieved from http://www.obesityaction.org/wp-content/uploads/OAC-Insurance-Piece.pdf

84 Dehgan, M., Akhtar-Danesh, N., & Merchant, A. T. (2005). Childhood obesity, prevalence and prevention. *Nutrition Journal, 4,* 24.

85 Cretikos, M. A., Valenti, L., Britt, H. C., & Baur, L. A. (2008). General practice management of overweight and obesity in children and adolescents in Australia. *Medical Care, 46,* 1163-69.

86 Ogden, C. L., Flegal, K. M., Carroll, M. D., & Johnson, C. L. (2010). Prevalence of high body mass index in U.S. children and adolescents, 1999-2000. *Journal of the American Medical Association, 303,* 242-49.

87 DeNavas-Walt, C., Proctor, B. D., & Smith, J. C. (2010, September). *Income, poverty, and health insurance coverage in the United States, 2009* (pp. 60-238, and Detailed Tables—Table HINC-06). Current Population Reports, P60-238. Washington, DC: U.S. Government Printing Office.

88 Rolland-Cachera, M. F., & Bellisle, F. (1986). No correlation between adiposity and food intake: Why are working class children fatter? *American Journal of Clinical Nutrition, 44,* 779-87.

89 Office of Research and Analysis, Food and Nutrition Service, U.S. Department of Agriculture. (2008). *Healthy Incentives pilot evaluation: Public summary.* Retrieved from http://www.fns.usda.gov/snap/hip/docs/eval.pdf.

90 Linz, P., Bell, L., & Lee, M. *Obesity, poverty and participation in nutrition assistance programs, February 2005.* Family Programs Report No. FSP-04-PO. Washington, DC: The Office of Analysis, Nutrition and Evaluation, Food and Nutrition Services, United States Department of Agriculture.

91 Linz, P., Bell, L., & Lee, M. *Obesity, poverty and participation in nutrition assistance programs, February 2005.* Family Programs Report No. FSP-04-PO. Washington, DC: The Office of Analysis, Nutrition and Evaluation, Food and Nutrition Services, United States Department of Agriculture.

92 Caprio, S., Daniels, S. R., Drewnowski, A., Kaufman, F. R., Palinkas, L. A., Rosenbloom, A. L., & Schwimmer, J. B. (2008). Influence of race, ethnicity and culture on childhood obesity: Implications for prevention and treatment: A consensus statement of Shaping America's Health and the Obesity Society. *Diabetes Care, 31,* 2211-21.

93 Berenson, G. S., & Bogalusa Heart Study Group. (2012). Health consequences of obesity. *Pediatric Blood & Cancer, 58,* 117-21.

94 Barton, M. (2012). Childhood obesity: A life-long health risk. *Acta Pharmacologica Sinica, 33,* 189-93.

95 Nord, M. (2009, September). *Food insecurity in households with children: prevalence, severity and household characteristics.* Economic Information Bulletin No. EIB-56. Retrieved from http://www.ers.usda.gov/publications/eib-economic-information-bulletin/eib56.aspx#.Umq0HxXD8y8

96 Hamelin, A. M., Habicht, J. P., & Beaudry, M. (1999). Food insecurity: Consequences for the household and broader social implications. *Journal of Nutrition, 129,* 525.

97 Janevic, T., Petrovic, O., Bjelic, I., & Kubera, A. (2010). Risk factors for childhood malnutrition in Roma settlements in Serbia. *BMC Public Health, 10,* 509.

98 Food and Nutrition Service, U.S. Department of Agriculture (2012). *Supplemental Nutrition Assistance Program: A short history of SNAP.* Retrieved from http://www.fns.usda.gov/snap/rules/Legislation/about.htm

99 Oliveira, V., Racine, E., Olmsted, J., & Ghelfi, L. M. (2002). *The WIC program: Background, trends, and issues.* Food Assistance and Nutrition Research Report No. 27 (FANRR-27). Retrieved from http://www.ers.usda.gov/media/327957/fanrr27_1_.pdf

100 Nord, M., & Coleman-Jensen, A. (2012, June 4). *Food security in the U.S.: History and background.* Retrieved from http://www.ers.usda.gov/topics/food-nutrition-assistance/food-security-in-the-us/history-background.aspx

101 Food and Nutrition Service. U.S. Department of Agriculture. (2010, December). *Fresh Fruit and Vegetable Program: A handbook for schools.* Retrieved from http://www.fns.usda.gov/cnd/FFVP/handbook.pdf

102 Food and Nutrition Service, U.S. Department of Agriculture. (2007, April). *USDA school meals: Healthy meals, healthy schools, healthy kids.* Retrieved from http://www.fns.usda.gov/cga/factsheets/school_meals.pdf

103 Food and Nutrition Service, U.S. Department of Agriculture. (2007, April). *USDA school meals: Healthy meals, healthy schools, healthy kids.* Retrieved from http://www.fns.usda.gov/cga/factsheets/school_meals.pdf

104 Food and Nutrition Service, U.S. Department of Agriculture. (2012, August). *National School Lunch Program.* Retrieved from http://www.fns.usda.gov/cnd/lunch/AboutLunch/NSLPFactSheet.pdf

105 Food and Nutrition Service, U.S. Department of Agriculture. (2012, August). *National School Lunch Program.* Retrieved from http://www.fns.usda.gov/cnd/lunch/AboutLunch/NSLPFactSheet.pdf

106 Food and Nutrition Service, U.S. Department of Agriculture. (2012, August). *National School Lunch Program.* Retrieved

from http://www.fns.usda.gov/cnd/lunch/AboutLunch/NSLP FactSheet.pdf

107 Food and Nutrition Service, United States Department of Agriculture. (2007, April). *USDA Healthy meals, healthy schools, healthy kids*. Retrieved from http://www.fns.usda.gov/cga/factsheets/school_meals.pdf

108 Ben-Shalom, Y., Fox, M. K. & Newby, P. K.; U.S. Department of Agriculture, Food and Nutrition Service, Office of Research and Analysis. (2012). *Characteristics and dietary patterns of healthy and less-healthy eaters in the low-income population*. Retrieved from http://www.fns.usda.gov/ORA/menu/Published/SNAP/FILES/Participation/HEI.pdf

109 Gordon, A. R., Crepinsek, M. K., Briefel, R. R., Clark, M. A., & Fox, M. K. (2009) The third school nutrition dietary assessment study: Summary and implications. *Journal of the American Dietetic Association, 109*, S129-35.

110 Mutual Information System on Social Protection in the EU Member States and the EEA. (2012). *Comparative tables on social protection: Results* [data file]. Retrieved from http://ec.europa.eu/employment_social/missoc/db/public/compareTables.do

111 Kirkpatrick, S. I., & Tarasuk, V. (2011). Housing circumstances are associated with food access among low-income urban families. *Journal of Urban Health, 88*, 284-96.

112 Kirkpatrick, S. I., & Tarasuk, V. (2007). Adequacy of food spending is related to housing expenditures among lower-income Canadian households. *Public Health Nutrition, 10*, 1464-73.

113 Government Accountability Office. (1988). *Practices of the European community and selected member nations*. GAO Publication No. RCED 88-102. Washington, DC: U.S. Government Printing Office. Retrieved from http://www.gao.gov/assets/150/146151.pdf

114 Australia Government Department of Health Services. (2012, August 10). *Payments to help you raise children*. Retrieved from http://www.humanservices.gov.au/customer/subjects/payments-to-help-you-raise-children

115 Mutual Information System on Social Protection in the EU Member States and the EEA. (2012). *Comparative tables on social protection: Results* [data file]. Retrieved from http://ec.europa.eu/employment_social/missoc/db/public/compareTables.do

116 Citizens Information Board. (2012, February 7). *Pregnancy and social welfare benefits*. Retrieved from http://www.citizensinformation.ie/en/social_welfare/social_welfare_payments/social_welfare_payments_to_families_and_children/pregnancy_and_social_welfare_payments.html

117 Australian Government Department of Health Services. (2012, August 7). *Income and assets tests for parenting payment*. Retrieved from   http://www.humanservices.gov.au/customer/enablers/centrelink/parenting-payment/income-and-assets-test

118 World Bank. (2012). *World development indicators and global development finance*. Retrieved from http://databank.

worldbank.org/Data/Views/Reports/TableView.aspx?IsShared=true&IsPopular=series

119 Australian Government Department of Health Services. (2012, June 29). *Helping young parents*. Retrieved from http://www.humanservices.gov.au/customer/services/centrelink/helping-young-parents

120 Australia Government Department of Human Services. (n.d.). *CentreLink: BasicsCard: Making purchases easy for you*. Retrieved from http://www.humanservices.gov.au/spw/customer/publications/resources/9240/9240-1205.pdf

121 Australia Department of Health Services. (n.d.). *About income management*. Retrieved from http://www.humanservices.gov.au/customer/enablers/centrelink/income-management/about-income-management

122 Australia Department of Health Services. (n.d.). *Income management*. Retrieved from http://www.humanservices.gov.au/customer/services/centrelink/income-management

123 Gov.uk. (n.d.). *Nutrition and school lunches*. Retrieved from http://www.direct.gov.uk/en/Parents/Schoolslearninganddevelopment/SchoolLife/DG_4016089

124 Gov.uk. (n.d.). *Sure Start Maternity Grant*. Retrieved from http://www.direct.gov.uk/en/MoneyTaxAndBenefits/BenefitsTaxCreditsAndOtherSupport/Expectingorbringingupchildren/DG_10018854

125 Mutual Information System on Social Protection in the EU Member States and the EEA. (2012). *Comparative tables on social protection: Results* [data file]. Retrieved from http://ec.europa.eu/employment_social/missoc/db/public/compareTables.do

126 Citizens Information Board. (2012, February 7). *Pregnancy and social welfare benefits*. Retrieved from http://www.citizensinformation.ie/en/social_welfare/social_welfare_payments/social_welfare_payments_to_families_and_children/pregnancy_and_social_welfare_payments.html

127 Dowler, E. A., O'Connor, D. (2012). Rights-based approaches to addressing food poverty and food insecurity in Ireland and UK. *Social Science and Medicine, 74*, 44-51.

128 Rolland-Cachera, M. F., & Bellisle, F. (1986). No correlation between adiposity and food intake: Why are working class children fatter? *American Journal of Clinical Nutrition, 44*, 779-87.

129 Darmon, N., & Drewnowski, A. (2008). Does social class predict diet quality? *American Journal of Clinical Nutrition, 87*, 1107-17.

130 Harrison, G. (2010). Public health interventions to combat micronutrient deficiencies. *Public Health Reviews, 32*, 243-55.

131 Harrison, G. (2010). Public health interventions to combat micronutrient deficiencies. *Public Health Reviews, 32*, 243-55.

132 Oakley, G. P., & Tulchinsky, T. H. (2010). Folic acid and vitamin B12 fortification of flour: A global basic food security requirement. *Public Health Reviews, 32*, 256-66.

133 Oakley, G. P., & Tulchinsky, T. H. (2010). Folic acid and vitamin B12 fortification of flour: A global basic food security requirement. *Public Health Reviews, 32,* 256-66.

134 Holmes, B. A., Kaffa, N., Campbell, K., & Sanders, T. A. (2012). The contribution of fortified cereals to the nutritional intake of the materially deprived British population. *European Journal of Clinical Nutrition, 66,* 10-11.

135 Czeizel, A. E., & Merhala, Z. (1998). Bread fortification with folic acid, vitamin B12 and vitamin B6 in Hungary. *Lancet, 352,* 1225.

136 Ionescu, C. (2005). Improving nutrition in Romania. *Lancet, 365, 561-62.*

137 HealthyPeople.gov (2012, July 26). *2020 nutrition and weight status: Objectives.* Retrieved from http://www.healthy-people.gov/2020/topicsobjectives2020/objectiveslist.aspx?topicId=29

138 Food and Nutrition Service, United States Department of Agriculture. (2012, March 8). *USDA strategic plan and the FNS.* Retrieved from http://www.fns.usda.gov/ora/MENU/gpra/StrategicPlan.htm

139 European Commission. (2011, August 17). *Europe 2020 targets.* Retrieved from http://ec.europa.eu/europe2020/targets/eu-targets/index_en.htm

140 Nord, M. (2009, September). *Food insecurity in households with children: Prevalence, severity and household characteristics.* Economic Information Bulletin No. EIB-56. Retrieved from http://www.ers.usda.gov/publications/eib-economic-information-bulletin/eib56.aspx#.Umq0HxXD8y8

141 European Commission. (2012, August 20). *Headline indicators.* Retrieved from http://epp.eurostat.ec.europa.eu/portal/page/portal/europe_2020_indicators/headline_indicators.

142 U.S. Government Accountability Office. (2012). *Farm Bill: Issues to reconsider for reauthorization.* GAO Publication No. GAO-12-338SP. Washington, DC: Government Printing Office.

143 U.S. Government Accountability Office. (2008). *Food stamp program: Options for delivering financial incentives to participants for purchasing targeted foods.* GAO Publication No. GAO-08-415. Washington, DC: Government Printing Office.

144 Caprio, S., Daniels, S. R., Drewnowski, A., Kaufman, F. R., Palinkas, L. A., Rosenbloom, A. L., & Schwimmer, J. B. (2008). Influence of race, ethnicity and culture on childhood obesity: Implications for prevention and treatment: A consensus statement of Shaping America's Health and the Obesity Society. *Diabetes Care, 31,* 2211-21.

145 U.S. Government Accountability Office. (2007). *Food stamp program: FS could improve guidance and monitoring to help ensure appropriate use of noncash categorical eligibility.* GAO Publication No. GAO-07-465. Washington, DC: Government Printing Office.

146 U.S. Government Accountability Office. (2007). *Food stamp program: Use of alternative methods to apply for and maintain benefits could be enhanced by additional evaluation and information on promising practices.* GAO Publication No. GAO-07-573. Washington, DC: Government Printing Office.

147 Darmon, N., & Drewnowski, A. (2008). Does social class predict diet quality? *American Journal of Clinical Nutrition, 87,* 1107-17.

148 Darmon, N., & Drewnowski, A. (2008). Does social class predict diet quality? *American Journal of Clinical Nutrition, 87,* 1107-17.

149 Darmon, N., & Drewnowski, A. (2008). Does social class predict diet quality? *American Journal of Clinical Nutrition, 87,* 1107-17.

150 Briefel, R. R. (2007). The changing consumption patterns and health and nutritional status in the United States: Evidence from national surveys. In *The Nation's Nutrition.* Washington, DC: International Life Sciences Institute.

151 United Nations General Assembly. (1948). *The universal declaration of human rights.* Retrieved from http://daccess-dds-ny.un.org/doc/RESOLUTION/GEN/NR0/043/88/IMG/NR004388.pdf?OpenElement

152 Dowler, E. A., O'Connor, D. (2012). Rights-based approaches to addressing food poverty and food insecurity in Ireland and UK. *Social Science and Medicine, 74,* 44-51.

153 Chilton, M., & Rose, D. (2009). A rights-based approach to food insecurity in the United States. *American Journal of Public Health, 99,* 1203-11.

154 Brown, L., & Gentilini, U. (2006). *On the edge: The role of food-based safety nets in helping vulnerable households manage food insecurity.* World Institute for Development Economics Research of the United Nations University, Research Paper No. 2006/11.

155 Oh, S. Y., & Hong, M. J. (2003). Food insecurity is associated with dietary intake and body size of Korean children from low-income families in urban areas. *European Journal of Clinical Nutrition, 57,* 1598-1604.

156 Office of Research and Analysis, Food and Nutrition Service, U.S. Department of Agriculture. (2009, December 18). *Healthy Incentives pilot evaluation: Public summary.* Retrieved from http://www.fns.usda.gov/SNAP/HIP/docs/eval.pdf

157 Food and Nutrition Service, U.S. Department of Agriculture. (2012, February 2). *Nutrition education.* Retrieved from http://www.fns.usda.gov/fns/nutrition.htm

158 Census Bureau. (2010, April 27). *New Census Bureau report analyzes nation's linguistic diversity: Population speaking a language other than English at home increases by 140 percent in past three decades* [press release]. Retrieved from http://www.census.gov/newsroom/releases/archives/american_community_survey_acs/cb10-cn58.html

159 Food Safety Authority of Ireland. (n.d.). Retrieved from http://www.fsai.ie/home.html

160 Food Standards Agency. (n.d.). Website, http://food.gov.uk/.

161 Briefel, R. R. (2007). The changing consumption patterns and health and nutritional status in the United States: Evidence from national surveys. In *The Nation's Nutrition.* Washington, DC: International Life Sciences Institute.

162 Grant, D. K., & Maxwell, S. (1999) Food coping strategies: A century on from Rowntree. *Nutrition and Health, 13,* 45-60.

163 Heymann, M. B. (2006). Lactose intolerance in infants, children and adolescents. *Pediatrics, 118,* 1279-86.

164 Fulgoni, V. L., 3rd, Keast, D. R., Auestad, N., & Quann, E. E. (2011). Nutrients from dairy foods are difficult to replace in diets of Americans: Food pattern modeling and an analysis of the National Health and Nutrition Examination Survey, 2003-2006. *Nutrition Research, 31,* 759-65.

165 Niewinski, M. M. (2008). Advances in celiac disease and gluten-free diets. *Journal of the American Dietetic Association, 96,* 661-72.

166 *Food Standards Agency. (n.d.). Labelling of "gluten-free" foods.* Retrieved from http://www.food.gov.uk/policy-advice /allergyintol/guide/gluten/

167 European Parliament. (2011, October 25). Regulation (EU) No. 1169/2011 of the European Parliament and the Council of 25 October 2011. *Official Journal of the European Union.* Retrieved from http://eur-lex.europa.eu/LexUriServ /LexUriServ.do?uri=OJ:L:2011:304:0018:0063:EN:PDF

168 Fraser, G. E. (2009). Vegetarian diets: What do we know of their effects on common chronic diseases? *American Journal of Clinical Nutrition, 89,* 1607S-1612S.

169 Craig, W. J., & Mangels, A. R. (2009). Position of the American Dietetic Association: vegetarian diets. *Journal of the American Dietetic Association, 109,* 1266-82.

170 Haverstock, K., & Forgays, D. K. (2012). To eat or not to eat: A comparison of current and former animal product limiters. *Appetite, 58,* 1030-36.

171 Messina, V., & Mangels, A. (2001). Considerations in planning vegan diets: Children. *Journal of the American Dietetic Association, 101,* 661-69.

172 Craig, W. J., & Mangels, A. R. (2009). Position of the American Dietetic Association: Vegetarian diets. *Journal of the American Dietetic Association, 109,* 1266-82.

173 Fraser, G. E. (2009). Vegetarian diets: What do we know of their effects on common chronic diseases? *American Journal of Clinical Nutrition, 89,* 1607S-1612S.

174 Craig, W. J., & Mangels, A. R. (2009). Position of the American Dietetic Association: Vegetarian diets. *Journal of the American Dietetic Association, 109,* 1266-82.

175 Newby, P. K. (2009). Plant foods and plant-based diets: protective against obesity? *American Journal of Clinical Nutrition, 10,* 1572S-1587S.

176 Food Safety and Inspection Service, United States Department of Agriculture. (2011, July 26). *Allergies and food safety.* Retrieved from http://www.fsis.usda.gov/Fact _Sheets/Allergies_and_Food_Safety/index.asp

177 U.S. Food and Drug Administration. (2012, May 14). *Food allergies: What you need to know.* Retrieved from http://www.fda .gov/Food/ResourcesForYou/Consumers/ucm079311.htm

178 Food Standards Agency. (n.d.) *Food allergen labelling.* Retrieved from http://www.food.gov.uk/policy-advice/allergyintol/label

179 Food and Nutrition Service, U.S. Department of Agriculture. (2001). *Accommodating children with special dietary needs in the school nutrition programs: Guidance for school food service staff.* Washington, DC. Retrieved from http://www.fns.usda .gov/cnd/Guidance/special_dietary_needs.pdf

180 Peregrin, T. (2001). A successful diet for children nourishes the child. *Journal of the American Dietetic Association, 101,* 669.

181 Craig, W. J., & Mangels, A. R. (2009). Position of the American Dietetic Association: Vegetarian diets. *Journal of the American Dietetic Association, 109,* 1266-82.

Chapter 15

Children's Dietary Needs and the Role of School Meals

Natalie Stein, MS, MPH
Juliana F. W. Cohen, ScD, ScM

"The State shall, in particular, direct its policy toward securing . . . that children are given opportunities and facilities to develop in a healthy manner and conditions of freedom and dignity and that children and youth are protected against exploitation and against moral and material abandonment."–Article 39(f), Part IV ["Directives Principles of State Policy"] of the Constitution of India
"The State shall regard the raising of the level of nutrition and the standard of living of its people and the improvement of public health as among its primary duties."–Article 47, Part IV ["Directives Principles of State Policy"] of the Constitution of India

Article 39(f) and 47, Part IV ["Directives Principles of State Policy"] of the Constitution of India.

Learning Objectives

- Justify schools as settings for public health nutrition interventions for children worldwide, and recognize potential benefits of school meal programs for children and communities.

- Relate malnutrition to disparities in health outcomes, socioeconomic status, and education.

- Identify goal nutrition outcomes during childhood. Explain the functions, sources, deficiency symptoms, and prevalence of deficiency for energy and key nutrients of concern.

- Use anthropometric methods to assess nutritional status during childhood.

- Identify Millennium Development Goals related to childhood hunger, poverty, equality, and education.

- Explain why development of school meal and other public health nutrition programs must be based on specific community needs and resources. Provide examples and point out differences in cultural factors, nutrient content, and integration with other programs.

- Describe school meal programs in India, the United States, Japan, and Uganda and explain their regulation, implementation, and progress toward meeting goals.

- Explain the significance of collaboration between schools, government, community members, families, and other stakeholders in developing, implementing, and sustaining school-based meal programs.

- Identify components of successful school-based programs.

Case Study: National School Lunch Program in Uttar Pradesh, India

India's national school lunch program, the Mid-Day Meal Scheme, aims to improve nutritional status among Indian schoolchildren. The federal government provides some funding, food, and advisory support, and India's 28 states and 7 union territories administer regional programs. Many states have long histories of school meals, and the Mid-Day Meal Scheme builds on these traditions.

Particular Challenges in the Uttar Pradesh State of India

Uttar Pradesh is a southern state with some of the poorest socioeconomic indicators in India. Its infant mortality rate and female life expectancy are 160 per 1,000 and 55 years, respectively, rates that are similar to those of sub-Saharan Africa; the respective averages in India are 66 deaths and 63 years. Maternal death rates in childbirth are high, and per capita income, the proportion of households with electricity, and literacy rates are low. Two out of five individuals over age 7, including only one-quarter of females, are literate. Regional differences exist, and the urbanized western area is wealthier than rural areas. Forty-six percent of children under age 5 are underweight in India; prevalence in parts of Uttar Pradesh is 72%.[1]

Malnutrition in Uttar Pradesh

In a study published in 2010, in the Mathura District of Uttar Pradesh, more than 90% of schoolchildren aged 5 to 12 had protein–energy malnutrition (PEM).[2] Sixty-three percent of girls and 54% of women had moderate to severe PEM as categorized using the **Gomez classification (Box 15-1)**.[3] Two-fifths of study participants had **conjunctival xerosis**, a sign of vitamin A deficiency. The prevalence of deficiency of vitamin D, vitamin B complex, or vitamin C was about 10–15% for each. Iodine deficiency and goiter were found to affect 87% of schoolchildren in this state.[4] School-based public health nutrition interventions can potentially improve these figures.

Implementation of the Mid-Day Meal Scheme in Uttar Pradesh

The history of school meals in Uttar Pradesh dates back to 1953 with the initiation of a voluntary school meal program. The original program provided boiled chickpeas, nuts, rice, and fruits. The Mid-Day Meal Scheme was implemented in 1995, and all government schools in India were required to have it by 2002. By 2012, the state program in Uttar Pradesh had expanded to serve school meals to 1.4 million children each day under the Mid-Day Meal Scheme. States and villages administer their own programs and are encouraged to partner with community members.

Box 15-1 The Gomez Classification for assessing malnutrition

A Mexican pediatrician developed the Gomez Classification in 1956 by examining relationships between degree of malnourishment in child patients and their hospital mortality rates. He defined a healthy child as having a weight over 90% of the ideal. First-degree malnutrition, with "mild clinical" effects, was defined as 76–90% of desirable weight. Second-degree malnutrition with this scale is 61-75%. Gomez reported that children with third-degree malnutrition had much greater risk of mortality within two days of admittance to the hospital.

Assessment with the Gomez Classification is relatively easy because it considers only a child's weight and age. However, critics say that the system is out of date and has other limitations. Neglecting to measure height to assess stunting, a measure of chronic malnutrition, prevents distinction from wasting, or acute malnutrition. Another criticism is that the cut-points are not based on sufficient evidence. Finally, the system does not consider obesity, which is a growing problem in industrialized and developing nations. Suggested modifications to the Gomez classification include using standard weight-for-age reference values, such as those of the World Health Organization; using normative values, such as standard deviations from the mean, as indicators for concern; and using weight-for-age on a population level while using weight-for-height for individual patients.

Source: Gueri, M., Gurney, J. M., & Jutsum, P. (1980). The Gomez classification: Time for a change? *Bulletin of the World Health Organization, 58,* 773-777.

Innovative Mid-Day Meal Scheme for Addressing Malnutrition in Uttar Pradesh

In many villages, panchayats, or local governments, take responsibility for providing a hot meal each day to each student. In some villages, the Akshay Patra Foundation, a nongovernmental agency, delivers meals that were cooked in centralized or localized kitchens. The Akshay Patra Foundation set up its first kitchen in the Matthura District of Uttar Pradesh in 2003. The foundation's mission is to reduce hunger and promote education with the objective of reducing poverty.[5] In 2012, the foundation served hot meals to 1.3 million children per day.

Neither panchayat-administered school meal programs nor programs with Akshay Patra Foundation involvement were found to significantly reduce prevalence or degree of underweight, although both interventions led to increased growth rates. Evidence that school-based programs can be effective includes findings that the prevalence of anemia in girls aged 10 to 19 years in Uttar Pradesh decreased from 73% to 25% after implementation of a four-year school-based program that included weekly iron and folic acid supplements, family education twice a month, and semiannual distribution of deworming tablets. The intervention cost $0.36 per child per year.[6] Deworming helps rid the body of intestinal parasites that can be prevalent among Indian schoolchildren[7] and impair health, nutritional status, and academic performance.[8]

Despite nationwide efforts, malnutrition, low literacy rates, and poverty remain prevalent in many parts of Uttar Pradesh and elsewhere in India. By serving 140 million children throughout India, the Mid-Day Meal Scheme is an example of a large-scale, cost-effective public health intervention to address a deep-rooted problem in India. It has the potential to address these problems by improving nutritional status and student retention, and reducing gender and caste discrimination.

Discussion Questions

- What are the objectives of the Mid-Day Meal Scheme? How do they compare to the objectives of school lunch programs in other nations?
- Why is India's Mid-Day Meal Scheme an example of a multilevel public health intervention? Which features help integrate it into the community and make it sustainable?
- Which elements of the program are successful? Which modifications should be made?

Introduction

Appropriate nutrition during childhood supports healthy growth and development. Children with adequate nutrient intake have better attendance, academic performance, and behavior than children who skip breakfast, are hungry, or have nutrient deficiencies.[9] Proper nutrition can improve health, school attendance, academic performance, and retention rates, and it can help break poverty cycles linked to poor health and low academic achievement.[10] School-based programs can address widespread local nutrition concerns and encourage school achievement. This chapter introduces nutritional needs and common concerns during childhood.

Energy and Nutrient Concerns During Childhood

Public Health Core Competency 6: Basic Public Health Sciences Skills 5: Describes the scientific evidence related to a public health issue, concern, or intervention

Reproduced from Council on Linkages Between Academia and Public Health Practice. 2010 May. Core Competencies for Public Health Professionals. Washington, DC: Public Health Foundation. http://www.phf.org/resourcestools/Documents/Core_Competencies_for_Public_Health_Professionals_2010May.pdf. Accessed August 13, 2013. This source is used for all Public Health Core Competencies in this chapter.

Hunger, food insecurity, seasonal variability, and monotonous diets can cause malnutrition in the United States and worldwide. Effects may include obesity, undernutrition, and infectious diseases, such as malaria, pneumonia, diarrheal diseases, and measles, which are public health threats, especially in low-income developing nations. These diseases are more likely to occur in children with micronutrient deficiencies.[11]

Energy

Sufficient energy is necessary for children to support growth and physical activity. Energy needs, expressed as **calories** per day, are based on children's height, weight, age, gender, needs for growth, and physical activity level.[12] Protein and carbohydrates each provide 4 calories per gram, and fat provides 9 calories per gram. Alcohol, a nonessential nutrient, provides 7 calories per gram.

Energy balance, when energy consumption matches energy expenditure, allows maintenance of a healthy weight. Overconsumption of calories relative to need leads to obesity, which is a growing problem among children worldwide. Obesity increases the risk for chronic diseases, such as type 2 diabetes, heart disease, and asthma. Chronic energy deficiency can cause impaired growth, or **stunting**, and **underweight**. Chronic and widespread inadequate energy intake is rare in industrialized nations, but is evident in many developing nations. School meal programs should be designed to promote a healthy weight, with menus tailored to community needs.

Protein

Protein is a source of energy. In the body, proteins are also enzymes, structural components of body tissues, major components of the immune system, hormones, and regulators of acid–base and fluid balance.[13] The U.S. **Recommended Daily Allowance (RDA)** for children aged 4 to 13 is 0.95 grams of protein per kilogram of body weight, compared with 0.8 grams per kilogram for adults. All proteins are made up of amino acids. Of the 20 dietary amino acids, nine are indispensable, or **essential**. Adequate protein intake requires not only total quantity, but also consumption of adequate amounts of each of the essential amino acids. **Complete**, or high-quality, **proteins** include those from animal-derived foods, including meat, poultry, fish, eggs, and dairy products, as well as soy protein. **Incomplete proteins** include most vegetables, grains, legumes, nuts, and seeds. Incomplete proteins can complement each other to create complete proteins and meet protein requirements on plant-based diets.

Protein deficiency is rare in the United States.[14] In 2007–2008, average daily intake was 61.9 grams for 6- to 11-year-old girls and 70.8 grams for boys. In developing nations, however, protein deficiency is more prevalent, with 31% of children underweight and 31% with stunted growth.[15] Other consequences include fatty liver, coarse hair, and frequent infections, with effects such as diarrheal diseases and helminth worm infections. Two types of severe protein–energy deficiency are **marasmus** and **kwashiorkor**.

Iron

Iron is a component of **hemoglobin** and **myoglobin**. Iron is also involved in aerobic metabolism, antioxidant and healthful pro-oxidant functions, and DNA synthesis. Iron deficiency, which can lead to **anemia**, is the most common

nutritional deficiency worldwide, affecting more than two billion individuals, or more than 30% of the world's population. Children have higher iron requirements because of growth and expanding blood, and approximately 40% of children have iron deficiency. In 1999–2000, 4% of children in the United States were iron deficient.[16] Dietary sources include liver, beef, other meats, dark meat poultry, shellfish, and fish. Beans, broccoli, spinach, and other leafy greens, such as collards and kale, also provide iron. In the United States, enriched grains have been fortified since 1941.[17] Worldwide, 27% of wheat flour was fortified with iron in 2007.[18]

Iodine

Iodine is a mineral required for the synthesis of the thyroid hormones thyroxine, which contains four iodine molecules, and triiodothyronine, which has three. The thyroid hormones affect nearly every cell, regulating energy production, basal metabolic rate, growth, neurotransmitter synthesis, and body temperature. Iodine deficiency is the leading preventable cause of cognitive impairment worldwide. Iodine deficiency disorders in children also lead to **goiter**, juvenile hypothyroidism, impaired physical development, and increased susceptibility to nuclear radiation.[19,20] More than 30% of children worldwide had inadequate iodine intake in 2007. Intake is adequate in the United States and other nations with comprehensive fortification programs.[21] India's Mid-Day Meal Scheme has seen success with annual administration of iodine supplements as part of a health package. In contrast, iodine deficiency in Europe remains a public health concern. This region has the lowest rate of iodized salt among all of the World Health Organization (WHO) regions, with 27% of households consuming iodine-fortified salt in 1999. Seafood is rich in iodine; iodine content of plant-based and animal products depends on soil content. For this reason, iodine deficiency is typically endemic by region. Universal fortification and regular administration of supplements are options that can virtually eliminate iodine deficiency. In Europe in 2004, the prevalence of iodine deficiency among schoolchildren aged 6 to 12 years was 47.8%.[22]

Calcium

Calcium is the most abundant mineral in the body, with most stored in bone mineral. In addition to helping prevent **osteoporosis** and an increased risk for fractures later in life, some, but not all, data suggest an association between calcium and reduced adiposity.[23] Dairy products, such as milk, yogurt, and cheese, provide up to 80% of dietary calcium in

Box 15-2 Milk Matters and Special Milk Program

In the United States, children consume less than 900 milligrams of calcium per day on average, compared with an adequate intake (AI) of 1,000 to 1,200 milligrams of calcium. Milk Matters and the Special Milk Program are two initiatives for increasing calcium intake among children in the United States.

The Milk Matters campaign encourages children from 11 to 15 years old to increase consumption of calcium from dairy products. The campaign is run by the Eunice Kennedy Shriver National Institute of Child Health and Human Development (NICHD), within the National Institutes of Health, in partnership with physicians, other government agencies, and nongovernmental organizations. The program provides educational materials and activities in English and Spanish for healthcare providers, parents, and children age 11 to 15. The school-based component includes lesson plans and other educational materials for teachers to use in classrooms.

The Special Milk Program is for children who do not participate in national school meal programs. The U.S. Department of Agriculture reimburses schools for fat-free and 1% reduced-fat milk fortified with vitamins A and D. Schools that participate in the National School Breakfast and National School Lunch Programs also receive federal reimbursement for eligible milk served at school meals. The Special Milk Program helps ensure children's access to milk, an important source of calcium and vitamin D.

Data from the Agricultural Research Service, United States Department of Agriculture. (2012, July 16). What We Eat in America. Retrieved from http://www.ars.usda.gov/Services/docs.htm?docid=13793; Data also from the Institute of Medicine (U.S.) Committee to Review Dietary Reference Intakes for Vitamin D and Calcium. (2011). Dietary reference intakes for calcium and vitamin D. Washington, DC: National Academies Press; and Data from the Food and Nutrition Service, United States Department of Agriculture. (2012 August). Special Milk Program. Retrieved from http://www.fns.usda.gov/cnd/milk/AboutMilk/SMPFactSheet.pdf

industrialized nations (**Box 15-2**).[24] Other natural sources are canned bony fish and leafy green vegetables, although some vegetables contain oxalates, which are compounds that can inhibit calcium absorption. Foods in the United States that are often fortified with calcium include orange juice, breakfast cereals, soy milk, and tofu; the United Kingdom mandates fortification of refined flour; and calcium fortification of soy beverages is common in Asian nations. Meeting calcium requirements is possible, but less likely, without consuming dairy products.[25]

Vitamin D

Low-serum vitamin D can lead to bone disorders such as rickets or osteomalacia and is a risk factor for developing osteoporosis in older adulthood and in younger children. Vitamin D is naturally found in few foods, such as fish oils, fatty fish, and butter. In the United States, fortified milk and some other fortified products contain vitamin D. Healthy individuals can synthesize vitamin D upon exposure to radiation from the sun, but low vitamin D is a risk among populations who live in northern climates, with low levels of sun radiation; among dark-skinned individuals, whose conversion of vitamin D is limited; and among children who routinely use sunscreen. One study found that 45% of adolescent girls in Beijing, China, had low serum levels of vitamin D during the winter months.[26]

Zinc

Zinc is necessary for zinc-dependent enzymes, for regulation of gene expression, and as a component of cell membranes and some proteins.[27] Average intake among children in the United States is 9 to 11 milligrams, compared with the RDA of 5 to 8 milligrams. As much as 20% of the world's population may be deficient, with south Asia, Africa, and nations in the Pacific at greatest risk.[28] Effects include stunting, from impaired protein synthesis, cell division, and growth, and frequent infections, such as from malaria. Zinc deficiency is associated with diarrheal diseases and vitamin A and protein deficiencies. Shellfish, meat, poultry, and dairy products are good sources of zinc. Nuts and legumes provide less absorbable forms of zinc. Vegetarians and children on grain-based diets are more likely to experience zinc deficiency.

Anthropometric Assessment of Nutritional Status in Childhood

Anthropometric measurements are useful for assessing recent and longer-term nutritional status during childhood. Childhood is a period of growth, and normal growth requires proper nutrition. Anthropometric measurements, such as height and weight, are practical for public health applications because they are relatively inexpensive, simple, and fast.

Recommended Growth Charts

Growth charts allow comparisons of children's heights and weights to established norms. The Centers for Disease Control and Prevention (CDC) recommends using its **growth references** for children. These charts, which are used to determine appropriate **body mass index (BMI)**, height, and weight by age, are based on data collected from 1963 to 1994 during the **National Health and Nutrition Examination Survey (NHANES)** I, II, and III.[29]

Globally based growth charts are also available for anthropometric assessment around the world. Growth standards are used up through 59 months of age from data collected in various nations: Davis, California, United States; Accra, Ghana; Pelota, Brazil; Delhi, India; Oslo, Norway; and Muscat, Oman. Data are from WHO's Multicentre Growth Reference Study (MGRS), and the National Center for Health Statistics (NCHS).[30] WHO provides height-for-age and weight-for-age charts for boys and girls 5 to 10 years old, and BMI-for-age charts for children ages 5 to 19 years.[31]

Interpretation of Growth Charts

Interpretation of anthropometric data using growth charts is based on norms, such as standard deviations above or below the mean, or above or below a given percentile.[32] Stunting is low height-for-age, and it indicates chronic nutrient deficiency. Wasting, or low weight-for-height, indicates acute malnutrition, possibly due to famine or illness. Underweight is a low weight-for-age. High BMI-for-age indicates overweight and obesity.

Millennium Development Goals

In an effort to eradicate poverty by 2015, the United Nations created the Millennium Development Goals (MDGs) in 1990.[33] The MDGs are based on values of peace, increasing equality, and improving living conditions worldwide through international cooperation.[34] In 2000, 189 United Nations (UN) member states signed the Millennium Resolution, and the values and targets were reaffirmed in 2005.[35,36] The first three of the eight main targets are of particular relevance to this chapter.

Millennium Development Goal 1: Eradicate Extreme Poverty and Hunger

Reproduced from the United Nations. (n.d.). 2015 Millennium Development Goals. Retrieved from http://www.un.org/millenniumgoals/. Accessed August 13, 2013. This source is used for all Millennium Development Goals in this chapter.

The first target is to end poverty and hunger worldwide, with the first specific objectives being to "halve the proportion of people who suffer from hunger." The objective recognizes the fact that 25% of children in the developing world are underweight, with higher rates among children who live in rural areas or whose families live in poverty.[37] A specific indicator for tracking improvements is a reduction in the proportion of individuals who are unable to meet their daily energy requirements. As evidence of progress, by 2012, the UN development regions of Northern Africa, Eastern and Southeastern Asia, Latin America, the Caribbean, Caucasus, and Central America had already met the goal or were on pace to achieve it by 2015.[38] Southeastern Asia still had hunger rates of 14%, significantly down from 24% in 1990–1992. Southern Asia had hunger rates of 20% in 2006–2008, down from 22% in 1990–1992, and the prevalence of hunger in sub-Saharan Africa was 27%, compared with a baseline of 31%.[39]

Millennium Development Goal 2: Achieve Universal Primary Education

The second MDG is to achieve universal education, with subgoals of enrolling all children in school and having all children who enroll in first grade complete their primary education. Primary education enrollment and completion is lowest in sub-Saharan Africa, where nearly 25% children are not in school. In southern Asia 7% of children are not in school.

Millennium Development Goal 3: Promote Gender Equality and Empower Women

The third MDG is to achieve gender equality, with a subgoal of equal education for boys and girls. The World Bank's position is that gender equality, including equal education opportunities, is essential for a nation's development and prosperity.[40] As of 2012, this MDG had been achieved, or was on pace to be achieved by 2015, in most UN regions. Sub-Saharan Africa, a region with among the greatest gender gaps, had a regional ratio of 91 girls to every 100 boys in primary school; the number decreases to 64 girls by tertiary school.[41] Individual nations may have different trends than their average regional trend.[42]

> *Public Health Core Competency 8: Leadership and Systems Thinking Skills 2: Describes how public health operates within a larger system*

The MDGs are interrelated with the common overarching goals of peacefully reducing poverty and improving health. For example, a reciprocal relationship between attending school and income is evident. Higher socioeconomic status, often defined as higher income or education, is linked to better health outcomes and nutritional status.[43] Higher SES leads to higher food security, increased likelihood of choosing healthy foods, better nutritional status, and lower risk for hunger or chronic disease.[44]

Improving Nutrition in Childhood Worldwide with School-Based Interventions

Schools are potentially ideal settings for effective nutrition interventions, with possible programs including school meals, nutrition education, physical activity programs, and outreach to parents and communities. Each program must reflect the most pressing community needs, whether related to protein or energy malnutrition, micronutrient deficiencies, overnutrition, sedentary lifestyles, and/or nutritional knowledge.

School Lunch Program: United States

As a "measure of national security," President Truman signed the National School Lunch Act in 1946[45] after large numbers of men were rejected from military service in World War II because of malnutrition.[46] All students whose schools participate in the program can purchase National School Lunch Program (NSLP) meals, which are offered for free or at reduced cost to low-income students. Schools participating in the NSLP receive federal reimbursement for all school lunches served that meet the NSLP nutrient requirements (**Table 15-1**). In 2012–2013, schools received $2.86 for each meal provided free, $2.46 for meals provided at reduced cost, and $0.27 for each meal sold at full cost. The cost of food accounts for 46% of spending;[47] the

remainder pays for operating the food service program, including labor costs.[48]

The U.S. Department of Agriculture (USDA) also offers schools discounted **commodity foods**, also known as entitlement foods, such as meat/meat alternatives like beef, pork, poultry, and cheese; grain products, such as flour, rice, and pasta; canned, frozen, or dried fruits and vegetables; and oils. "Bonus" foods are occasionally donated to states due to agricultural surpluses.[49] Recent examples are fruits, beans, and low-fat cheese. Each state receives a list of available entitlement foods and prepares a list of offerings. Each school district can then select which entitlement foods to purchase from the list. School food service programs must ensure their meals meet the nutrition requirements, but have the freedom to decide which specific foods to serve and how to prepare them. While 20% of foods served are from USDA entitlement foods, the remaining 80% are purchased from outside vendors.[50]

NSLP Nutrient Standards

NSLP nutrition standards for school meals are based on the USDA's **Dietary Guidelines for Americans** and must meet specific requirements daily or over the course of one week. These guidelines were created to provide students with roughly one-third of the Recommended Dietary Allowances (RDA) for nutrients of concern, including protein, calories, calcium, iron, vitamin A, and vitamin C. After years of adherence to the 1995 *Dietary Guidelines*, the Healthy, Hunger-Free Kids Act of 2010 updated NSLP nutrition standards to reflect the most recent *Dietary Guidelines for Americans*. Each lunch must include a meat or meat alternative, a grain, low-fat or fat free milk, a fruit, and a vegetable. Current standards include whole grain requirements, limits on sodium and saturated fats, restrictions on *trans* fats, and acceptable calorie ranges.

The NSLP must address the growing problem of overweight and obesity among school-aged children.[51] Since nearly 70% of children report consuming school meals at least three times per week, with the majority from low-income households, the NSLP can play a particularly important role in addressing this epidemic.[52] Research examining NSLP participation and overweight has found mixed results, with some studies reporting that participants were more likely to be overweight or obese.[53] This may be due to schools providing meals with too many calories or the use of inexpensive commodity foods that are energy dense and high in saturated fats, like meats and cheese.[54] To help address this, many schools have opted to implement "Offer versus

Table 15-1 National School Lunch guidelines

Meal Pattern	Lunch Meal Pattern		
	Grades K-5	Grades 6-8	Grades 9-12
	Amount of Food Per Week (Minimum Per Day)		
Fruit (cups)[a,b]	$2\frac{1}{2}$ ($\frac{1}{2}$)	$2\frac{1}{2}$ ($\frac{1}{2}$)	5 (1)
Vegetables (cups)[a,b]	$3\frac{3}{4}$ ($\frac{3}{4}$)	$3\frac{3}{4}$ ($\frac{3}{4}$)	5 (1)
Dark green[c]	$\frac{1}{2}$	$\frac{1}{2}$	$\frac{1}{2}$
Red/orange[c]	$\frac{3}{4}$	$\frac{3}{4}$	$1\frac{3}{4}$
Beans/peas (legumes)[c]	$\frac{1}{2}$	$\frac{1}{2}$	$\frac{1}{2}$
Starchy[c]	$\frac{1}{2}$	$\frac{1}{2}$	$\frac{1}{2}$
Other[c,d]	$\frac{1}{2}$	$\frac{1}{2}$	$\frac{1}{2}$
Additional vegetables to reach total[e]	1	1	$1\frac{1}{2}$
Grains (oz. eq.)[f]	8-9 (1)	8-10 (1)	10-12 (2)
Meat/meat alternatives (oz. eq.)	8-10 (1)	9-10 (1)	10-12 (2)
Fluid milk (cups)[g]	5 (1)	5 (1)	5 (1)
Other specifications: Daily amount based on the average for a five-day week			
Min-max calories (kcal)[h,i]	550-650	600-700	750-850
Saturated fat (% of total calories)	<10	<10	<10
Sodium (mg)[j]	<640	<710	<740
Trans fat	Nutrition label or manufacturer specifications must indicate 0 grams of trans fat per serving		

[a]One-quarter cup of dried fruit counts as $\frac{1}{2}$ cup of fruit; 1 cup of leafy greens counts as $\frac{1}{2}$ cup of vegetables. No more than half of the fruit or vegetable offerings may be in the form of juice. All juice must be 100% full strength.

[b]For breakfast, vegetables may be substituted for fruits, but the first two cups per week of any such substitution must be from the dark green, red/orange, beans/peas (legumes), or "other vegetables" subgroups.

[c]Larger amounts of these vegetables may be served.

[d]The "other vegetables" requirement may be met with any additional amounts from the dark green, red/orange, and beans/peas (legumes) vegetable subgroups.

[e]Any vegetable subgroup may be offered to meet the total weekly vegetable requirement.

[f]At least half of the grains offered must be whole grain-rich in the NSLP beginning July 1, 2012 (SY 2012-2013). All grains must be whole grain-rich in the NSLP beginning July 1, 2014 (SY 2014-15).

[g]Fluid milk must be low-fat (1% milk fat or less, unflavored) or fat-free (unflavored or flavored).

[h]The average daily amount of calories for a five-day school week must be within the range (at least the minimum and no more than the maximum values).

[i]Discretionary sources of calories (solid fats and added sugars) may be added to the meal pattern if within the specifications for calories, saturated fat, trans fat, and sodium. Foods of minimal nutritional value and fluid milk with fat content greater than 1% milk fat are not allowed.

[j]Final sodium specifications are to be reached by SY 2022-2023 or July 1, 2022. Intermediate sodium specifications are established for SY 2014-2015 and 2017-2018.

Modified from: the Food and Nutrition Service. U.S. Department of Agriculture. (2012). Nutrition Standards in the National School Lunch and School Breakfast Programs; Final Rule. *Federal Register, 77*, 17.

Serve," where students may decline up to two of the five food components offered.[55] Additionally, new requirements for school meals limit calories.[56] The goal is to help schools achieve the ***Healthy People 2020*** objective of providing students with "access to safe, nutritious and affordable meals."[57]

Public Health Core Competency 2: Policy Development/ Program Planning Skills 7: Identifies mechanisms to monitor and evaluate programs for their effectiveness and quality

Studies Examining the National School Lunch Program

The main source of information examining the NSLP is the USDA-funded School Nutrition Dietary Assessment Study (SNDA), conducted about every six years. This nationally representative data set collects information from school food service directors, school food service managers, principals, students, and their parents. SNDA-III, conducted before implementation of the Healthy Hunger-Free Kids Act, examined the nutrients and foods offered at lunch, the impact of the school meal program on students' intakes, including "empty calories" from low-nutrient, energy-dense competitive foods and beverages, and prevalence of overweight and obesity among students.[58]

Evaluating NSLP

SNDA-III data showed that while 88% of school lunches provided the required nutrients, 72% of meals exceeded the limit on energy from saturated fats. Meals tended to be very high in sodium and low in fiber. Almost all schools offered a vegetable option daily, but often in the form of french fries or other fried potato products. Fruit was also offered daily, with a canned option served roughly two-thirds of the time. Whole grains or legumes were rarely offered to students. Half of schools offered desserts, and 99% offered flavored milk. SNDA-III data also showed that school lunch participants were about four times more likely than students who did not consume school lunches to drink milk at lunch. School lunch participants also consumed more fruits and vegetables (including french fries) at lunch. Students who received a school lunch were less likely to purchase competitive foods. SNDA-III data also found that while school lunch participation was not associated with a higher prevalence of overweight or obesity, offering french fries or desserts more than once a week was associated with higher rates of obesity among elementary school students.[59] Based on these observations, NSLP appears to be effective at increasing nutrient intake, but less effective at reducing obesity.

Healthy People 2020: NWS-14: Increase the contribution of fruits to the diets of the population aged 2 years and older

Reproduced from the U.S. Department of Health and Human Services. Healthypeople.gov. Retrieved from http://www.healthypeople.gov/2020 /default.aspx. Last updated July 30, 2013. Accessed August 13, 2013. All Healthy People 2020 in this chapter is from this source.

Healthy People 2020: NWS-15: Increase the variety and contribution of fruits and vegetables to the diets of the population aged 2 years and older

Healthy People 2020: NWS-16: Increase the contribution of whole grains to the diets of the population aged 2 years and older

Effectiveness of School-Based Intervention with School Meal Components: CATCH, TEENS, and Shape Up Somerville

Several notable studies related to the school food environment have been met with mixed success. The **Child and Adolescent Trial for Cardiovascular Health (CATCH)** was a 2.5-year, multicomponent intervention in elementary schools that included health education, physical education, and a cafeteria component to decrease the total fat, saturated fat, and sodium content of school meals. Percentages of calories from total fat and saturated fat in the school meals were reduced, but sodium content increased, although less than in control schools.[60] From 24-hour recalls, the CATCH study also found significant reductions in the proportion of energy from total and saturated fats in students attending intervention schools compared with students at control schools.[61] Sodium consumption increased similarly among both groups.

The Teens Eating for Energy and Nutrition at School (TEENS) study was another multifaceted intervention that included classroom, cafeteria, and family components in middle schools and focused on students' intakes of fruits, vegetables, and lower-fat foods.[62] However, the TEENS study found no impact on student's diets at the end of two years. A third intervention, Shape Up Somerville, was a community-based study in Somerville, Massachusetts, that included classroom and cafeteria components for elementary school students. After two years, participants had decreased BMI *z-scores*.

School Lunch Program: India

In 2011, the Global Hunger Index (GHI) (**Box 15-3**) from the International Food Policy Research Institute ranked India as the 67th least food-secure country in the world.[63] India's score of 23.7, categorized as "alarming," was improved from its 1990 mark of 30.4, or "extremely alarming." India's proportion of 20% undernourishment remained stable, while the other two marks improved.

Box 15-3 The Global Hunger Index (GHI)

The International Food Policy Research Institute developed the Global Hunger Index (GHI) to assess and track hunger worldwide. The Welthungerhilfe, a German nonprofit organization, copublishes an annual GHI report that includes national and regional GHI scores. Each report focuses on a major theme; the 2011 report discussed spikes in food costs and price volatility, and the 2010 report emphasized childhood undernutrition.

The GHI is the average of the proportion of the population that is undernourished children, plus the proportion of underweight children under 5 years, plus childhood mortality under 2 years. In theory, the GHI can range from 0 to 100. The following GHI categories are used to describe hunger:

0 to 4.9: low hunger

5 to 9.9: moderate hunger

10 to 19.9: serious

20 to 29.0: alarming

30 and above: extremely alarming

Since its inception in 1990, the world's GHI decreased from 19.7 to 14.6. Eastern Europe, Latin America, and Southeast Asia have made considerable progress. South Asia's barriers include gender and other social inequality. Political conflict and economic trouble hinder sub-Saharan Africa's progress.

Data from International Food Policy Research Institute (IFPRI), Concern Worldwide, & Welthungerhilfe. (2012). *Global Hunger Index: The challenge of hunger: Ensuring sustainable food security under land, water, and energy stresses.* Washington, DC; Dublin; Bonn: Authors. Available at http://www.ifpri.org/sites/default/files/publications/ghi12.pdf. Accessed September 5, 2013.

Public Health Core Competency 1: Analytical/Assessment Skills 2: Describes the characteristics of a population-based health problem

In 2007, 51.4% of Indian women had a BMI under 18.5, classified as underweight, including 15.8% of women with a BMI under 17.[64] More than two-fifths of the population is food insecure, defined as having an income below the absolute poverty line of $1 per person per day.[65] This line is an indicator of risk for malnutrition and infectious diseases. Decreased productivity leads to less ability to earn income and exacerbation of the cycle. Poorer nutrition in Indian schoolchildren is associated with impaired cognition.[66]

Overview of India's Mid-Day Meal Program

The India School Lunch Program, formerly the National Program for Nutrition Support to Primary Education, is also called the Mid-Day Meal Scheme.[67] With more than 140 million children participating, it is the largest school meal program in the world. The Mid-Day Meal Scheme was established in 1995 and made mandatory in 2002 in all government-run primary schools and at rural Education Guarantee Scheme (EGS) sites. Meals must be provided during the summer drought season, when the risk for malnutrition is higher. Objectives are to reduce malnutrition, increase enrollment and attendance, reduce dropouts, and improve learning.[68]

Millennium Development Goal 1: Eradicate Extreme Poverty and Hunger. Target 1.C: Between 1990 and 2015, halve the proportion of people who suffer from hunger.

The federal government regulates the program. Daily, it provides to each student 100 grams of rice or wheat flour, or the cooked equivalent, such as 200 to 300 grams of unleavened flat bread called chappatis.[69] The government reimburses the cost of transporting the grains from local federal depots to schools and cooking the meals; an extra Hill Transport Subsidy is provided to transport grains from local federal depots to schools. These hard-to-reach regions are often the poorest and most in need of nutrition assistance.

Public Health Core Competency 6: Basic Public Health Sciences Skills 1: Describes the scientific evidence related to a public health issue, concern or intervention

State or territorial governments designate a department to oversee the program, a program head in each district, and a school-based entity, such as a parent–teacher association, to take responsibility for local operations. States are responsible for ensuring uninterrupted provision of meals to students, and must have plans in place for possibilities such as delays in grain delivery and cook absence.[70] Schools are encouraged to collaborate with community members and the public and private sectors for assistance such as funding, technical support, and food aid and other supplies. The partnership of the government with the nonprofit organization Akshaya Patra Foundation in Vrindavan, India, is an example. The government subsidizes costs and provides grain, while the nonprofit provides technical and logistical assistance.

Program Designed to Address Nutritional Deficiencies

School lunches in primary schools in India were required in 2004 to provide at least 300 calories and 8 to 12 grams of protein; in 2007, the minimum was raised to 450 calories and 12 grams of protein for younger children and 700 calories and 20 grams of protein for older children. Vitamin A, folic acid, and iron are also required. A typical meal includes pulses (legumes) or soybeans, seasonal vegetables, cooking oil, and a condiment, and drinking water should be available at meal times. Children bring their own cups and eating utensils.

Prevalence of malnutrition among Indian schoolchildren depends on factors such as urban versus rural residency and household income. In the state of Goa, one-third of children aged 10 to 19 were underweight, and 59% reported hunger.[71] Up to 99% of schoolchildren might be folic acid–deficient, two-thirds have low vitamin B12 and vitamin B6 levels, and 44% are low in vitamin A.[72] One in four children has goiter, despite 93% of households having access to iodized salt as mandated in India. Incorrect home storage and chemical changes to the iodine can cause this, implying a potential benefit of using iodized salt in school meals.[73]

The Mid-Day Meal Scheme has been effective when combined with fortification and other interventions. After a **deworming** treatment and eight months of school meals prepared with a multiple micronutrient premix powder, children had improved vitamin A, iron, and folate levels.[74] Similar results and improved physical performance occurred

after using NutriRice, a multiple micronutrient-fortified extruded rice product, for six months.[75] In Bangalore, deworming plus the use of NutriRice was associated with a decrease in iron deficiency from 79% to 49%; prevalence was reduced to 25% among students who received an additional 20-mg iron supplement.[76] Provision of a health package along with the school meal program reduced prevalence of night blindness and vitamin A deficiency from 67% to 39%.[77]

Integration into Existing Programs and Improving Sustainability

Many schools have integrated the Mid-Day Meal Scheme into the School Health Program, a multifaceted approach for helping Indian schoolchildren.[78] Components include screening, health care, and referrals; immunizations; provision of micronutrients; deworming; teacher and staff development; and plans for monitoring. Amenities at Health Promoting Schools may include counselors, peer educators, yoga, physical education programs, and a first aid room.

Uttar Pradesh promotes a School Health Week with the objective to "conduct medical examination of schoolchildren for early detection of anemia, nutrition disorders and worm infestations, eye screenings, dental caries on-site treatment for vital illness."[79] Children in higher grades serve as Health Guides, and physicians from the community partner with schools to provide screening services.

Promoting Equality

The Mid-Day Meal Scheme has a nondiscrimination policy with the objective of reducing socioeconomic disparities by allowing low-income children, especially low-income girls, who are traditionally most likely to stop attending school when food is scarce, to continue attending school. School programs may not discriminate based on student caste or gender. Furthermore, the Mid-Day Meal Scheme promotes women's employment through policies encouraging the employment of women to cook meals.[80]

Millennium Development Goal 3: Promote Gender Equality and Empower Women. Target 3.A: Eliminate gender disparity in primary and secondary education, preferably by 2005, and in all levels of education no later than 2015

School Lunch Program: The Shokuiku Program in Japan

Japan's school lunch program has evolved to meet the nation's changing needs. The program was reinstated in 1946 in response to the need to reduce widespread malnutrition in children after World War II.[81] The United States sent flour and skim milk powder, and dietitians trained students to focus on eating a more Westernized diet—that is, less rice and more meat, dairy products, and eggs. The program was universal in elementary schools by 1952 and expanded to secondary schools in 1954 with the passage of the School Lunch Law with oversight by the Ministry of Education, Culture, Sports, Science, and Technology, or MEXT.

The prevalence of underweight has decreased, and nearly one in four Japanese adults is overweight. More than two-thirds of deaths in Japan are caused by cardiovascular disease, cancer, and other noncommunicable diseases largely related to diet; more than 40% of the population have high blood pressure; and the average fasting blood glucose and cholesterol levels have increased noticeably since 1980.[82] The roles of dietitians and the school lunch program are evolving to address these emerging health concerns. The lunch program is consistent with **Health Japan 21**,[83] similar to the Healthy People 2020 plan in the United States.[84]

In Japan virtually all children complete primary school, so schools provide ideal settings for nutrition and health promotion programs.[85] The 2005 "Basic Law on Shokuiku" established a school lunch program that addresses the nutritional concerns of Japanese children while including features that reflect the nation's culture.[86] In addition to providing supplementary food, the program includes nutrition and health education, with an emphasis on adapting healthy behaviors such as serving appropriate quantities of food, eating breakfast, increasing physical activity, and reducing sedentary time.[87] Another goal of the program is to promote regional produce and rice consumption.[88]

Diet and Nutrition Teachers

Under the Diet and Nutrition Teacher System, established in 2007, Diet and Nutrition Teachers are responsible for menu planning and health promotion. They counsel nutritionally at-risk individuals, such as students with obesity or allergies. They no longer promote Westernized diets, but they do develop educational materials for students, train teachers on nutrition and health, and communicate with parents.[89] MEXT encourages schools to make a Diet and Nutrition Teacher available nearly every day.

The Lunch Environment

Students are engaged in their lunch environments, from setting up for meals to cleaning up later. Students learn about appropriate portion sizes by serving themselves and having the option to return for second helpings. They learn about food safety from Diet and Nutrition Teachers. An objective of the Diet and Nutrition Teacher System is to increase "interest in dietary education" to 90% from a baseline of 70%.

School-Based Programs in Developing Nations: The World Food Programme's School Meals in Africa

The Global Hunger Index (GHI) in many developing nations in Southeast Asia and Latin America has decreased notably since 1990, but much of Africa, particularly sub-Saharan Africa, lags behind. More than half of hungry children in the world live in sub-Saharan Africa. Sub-Saharan Africa made only minor progress from 1990, with a GHI of 25, to 2011, when the score was 20.5. Furthermore, Burundi, Chad, Democratic Republic of Congo, and Eritrea, all in sub-Saharan Africa, have GHI scores greater than 30, which puts them in the "extremely alarming" category in terms of hunger.

The World Food Programme and School Meals

The 2008–2013 Strategic Plan of the **World Food Programme (WFP)** states that the organization's objectives are to save lives and protect livelihoods in emergencies, prepare for emergencies, restore and build lives after emergencies, reduce chronic hunger and undernutrition everywhere, and strengthen the capacity of countries to reduce hunger.[90]

In pursuit of these objectives, WFP and partners served school meals in 62 nations in 2011.[91] Goal outcomes are consistent with the MDGs and include:[92]

1. Nutrition: Improving macronutrient and micronutrient status

2. Education: Improving attendance and reducing dropout rates

3. Gender: Promoting gender equity and reducing barriers for refugees, orphans, low-income students, and individuals with HIV or disabilities

4. Value transfer: Being careful to supply households with enough resources to allow children to attend school without interfering with family livelihood

5. Local development: Linking school meals to local food suppliers

WFP is evolving from being a **food aid** to a **food assistance** program in which school meal and other programs are integrated into society and administered by governments while WFP provides necessary technical assistance. Quality standards that help guide the development of programs include strategies for sustainability, funding, integration into national policy, needs-based and cost-effective design, monitoring and assessment, local food production, and collaboration between sectors and community involvement.[93]

WFP School Meals in Africa

More than half of the 99 million people assisted by WFP nutrition programs in 2011 were in Africa.[94] Recipients included 5.7 million boys and 5.4 million girls in school meal programs. WFP's 2010[95] and 2011[96] annual evaluation reports describe effects and challenges of school feeding programs in various African nations.

Evaluation of School Feeding in Kenya and Côte d'Ivoire: Contrasting Examples

An outcomes evaluation in Kenya investigated effects of school meals on education, nutrition, and value transfer to households.[97] Enrollment, attendance, and student performance increased with the advent of school feeding, although dropout rates between grades 7 and 8 remained at 30%. School meals contributed substantially to daily intake of energy, protein, and micronutrients, but many children still did not meet recommended intakes. Some students received less food at home when they were in school feeding programs. Value transfer to households, resulting from the cost of meals that households did not have to pay for their school children, was 9% of total household income.

Millennium Development Goal 1: Eradicate Extreme Poverty and Hunger. Target 1.C: Halve, between 1990 and 2015, the proportion of people who suffer from hunger.

An accompanying impact analysis acknowledged that low-income children are less likely to attend school. Attendance may also be decreased because of a widespread belief in Kenya that education is a deterrent from cultural traditions. Additional barriers include lack of quality teachers and lack of adequate classrooms and supplies. School feeding cannot directly improve those factors, but they can help reduce community poverty and increase sustainability by increasing local food production through implementation of **Home-Grown School Feeding** (HGSF) programs.[98]

Public Health Core Competency 4: Cultural Competency Skills 2: Recognizes the role of cultural, social, and behavioral factors in the accessibility, availability, acceptability, and delivery of public health services

Similar multiyear outcome and impact evaluations concluded that school feeding was less effective in Côte d'Ivoire. While Kenya's GHI from 1990 to 2011 decreased from 20.6, "alarming," to 18.6, "serious," Côte d'Ivoire's GHI increased from 16.6 to 18.0. The nation is one of only six worldwide to have an increase in GHI since 1990. The others are North Korea, Burundi, Democratic Republic of Congo, Swaziland, and Comoros. Côte d'Ivoire is low on the **Human Development Index**, ranked 170 out of 187 nations.[99]

Millennium Development Goal 2: Achieve Universal Primary Education. Target 2.A: Ensure that, by 2015, children everywhere, boys and girls alike, will be able to complete a full course of primary schooling

School meals in Côte d'Ivoire did not affect enrollment. This may be because school meals were not delivered consistently due to barriers such as lack of infrastructure, high transportation costs, and sociopolitical instability,[100] with civil wars beginning in 2002 and 2010. Objectives of a newly implemented school meal program in Côte d'Ivoire are to provide school meals to 580,000 students and increase return to school of students and teachers after the political turmoil.

School Feeding to Reduce Chronic Hunger in Uganda

Uganda has a history of political turmoil, food insecurity, poverty, and a culture in which girls tend to marry early.[101] Food insecurity is more severe in the drought-susceptible northern region of Karamoja, which has only one growing season, compared with two elsewhere in Uganda. One-third of young children are stunted. Between 2000 and 2006, the prevalence of underweight women increased from 10% to 12%, overweight increased from 13% to 16%, and obesity increased from 0% to 4%. Anemia, vitamin A deficiency, and iodine deficiency are also present. Nevertheless, the GHI improved from 19.0 in 1990 to 16.7 in 2011.

> *Public Health Core Competency 2: Policy Development/ Program Planning Skills 9: Applies strategies for continuous quality improvement*

Education is mandatory starting at age 6 years, but only 25% of students complete their education. School lunch is not universal. Parents are legally required to provide their children with food, shelter, medicine, and transport to school, and many believe that universal education should include school meals. Poor children in Uganda may not be able to eat breakfast and lunch, and skipping these meals is associated with lower achievement.[102]

In Uganda, 266,000 people receive food assistance from WFP. Strategies for reducing chronic hunger include the Agriculture and Market System, which supports infrastructure to support small farmers. Programs to increase food and nutrition security are the Karamoja Productive Assets Program (KPAP), which includes cash-for-work programs in the community, and school meals starting in 2007 as a partnership with World Vision Uganda. The first phase served 32,000 students, and 1.2 million children participated in 2012.

Program evaluation allowed WFP and World Vision Uganda to identify best practices for school feeding in Uganda.[103] A "home-based" feeding program to support local production was effective in improving children's nutritional status and supporting local economies. The program transferred administration and implementation to government and local communities through gradual "sensitization." World Vision Uganda cites "complementary actions" as a positive factor; the organization collaborated with WFP to provide the **Essential Package**,[104] which in this case included building of latrines, developing woodlots and school gardens, providing stoves and food storage pantries, and increasing HIV/AIDS awareness (**Box 15-4**). Other best practices were collaboration with other programs, such as government programs for HIV/AIDS education, and the provision of take-home rations of at least 1,000 calories per day for each child whose attendance was at least 80%. Foods included

grains, pulses, sugar, oil, and a corn–soya blend. Shortfalls in Ministry of Education and community involvement left Parent Teacher Associations as stakeholders without much decision-making power.

> *Millennium Development Goal 3: Promote Gender Equality and Empower Women. Target 3.A: Eliminate gender disparity in primary and secondary education, preferably by 2005, and in all levels of education no later than 2015.*

School Feeding and Gender Equity in Africa

As intended, WFP school feeding programs promoted gender equity in many African nations, with an increase in female enrollment in Chad, Mali, Egypt, and Ghana. In Guinea Bissau women's farming associations receive technical assistance from WFP and the assurance that local schools will purchase their food. Women can also participate in work for food programs, in which work might consist of building latrines or other facilities in exchange for food allowances.

Future Directions for Improving Childhood Nutrition in Africa

Sub-Saharan Africa contains many of the world's most malnourished nations. Sub-Saharan Africa's decrease in malnutrition from 1990 to 2011 was smaller than the drop in South Asia.[105] Barriers to reducing hunger in sub-Saharan Africa include poverty, political turmoil, disease, such as HIV/AIDS, and gender and other inequalities.[106] Experience in Africa demonstrates that school meals are effective and sustainable interventions only when planners consider underlying causes of hunger and consider local circumstances.

A recurring theme in successful school meal programs is that feeding alone is not sufficient. Policies to promote health, increase rural development, and improve education, for example, are responsible for Ghana's better-than-expected GHI score, considering the nation's average income. Ghana's school meal program, fueled by locally produced food, led to improvements in attendance and the economy. Programs require the backing, trust, and sense of ownership of the government, nongovernmental agencies, community members, and other stakeholders. Use and development of infrastructure, such as roads and distribution centers, is also critical.

Box 15-4 FRESH and the Essential Package

The Focusing Resources on Effective School Health, or FRESH, framework is a set of interventions that the WFP proposes to improve child health and nutrition. The assumption is that multifaceted approaches are more likely to provide long-term solutions to underlying causes of malnutrition. The Essential Package is cost-effective, synergizes with other child development initiatives, improves educational outcomes, and increases social equity by allowing girls and disadvantaged children to attend school. These are the 12 interventions in the FRESH framework:

  basic education

  food for education

  promotion of girls' education

  potable water and sanitary latrines

  health, nutrition, and hygiene education

  systematic deworming

  micronutrient supplementation

  HIV and AIDS education

  psychosocial support

  malaria prevention

  school gardens

  improved stores

Data from: the World Food Programme and UNICEF (n.d.). The essential package: Twelve interventions to improve the health and nutrition of school-age children. Retrieved from http://documents.wfp.org/stellent/groups/public/documents/newsroom/wfp212806.pdf

---

Lessons Learned from School Lunch Programs

Lessons learned from school lunch programs have global applications and can be most effective when adapted for specific communities or local circumstances.[107,108]

Stakeholders Should Be Included in the Planning and Design of the Program

For an intervention to be both successfully implemented and maintained, it is essential for people familiar with the school to be involved in the process of developing and approving the intervention. Stakeholders such as teachers, food service directors, principals, students, and/or parents can help identify the problems that need to be addressed in the school, think through implementation challenges, and ensure the program is successfully carried out and sustained. Buy-in and a sense of responsibility for outcomes encourage program success. School staff, parents, and other community members can provide valuable guidance in program development via means such as focus groups.

Public Health Core Competency 5: Community Dimension of Practice Skills 4: Collaborates with community partners to improve the health of the population

The USDA's **Farm to School** initiative involves the community in school meals.[109] School gardens, the purchase of locally grown foods for school meals, and nutrition education can be part of the program.[110] The USDA provides grants and educational materials, such as examples of model programs and suggestions for starting and maintaining a local program.

Inclusion of stakeholders contributed to the success of the school feeding programs in Kenya and Uganda. WFP and World Vision Uganda concluded that similar programs in Ugandan refugee camps were less effective because the government and locals did not feel a sense of ownership.

The Intervention Should Have Clear Benefits and Have No More Than Minimal Burdens

Interventions should be evidence-based and provide obvious health benefits to students, such as increased knowledge, better access to healthy food, and improved physical outcomes, such as lower blood pressure or BMI, or improved growth. Interventions that can be integrated into existing curriculums or food service programs are less burdensome to staff and are easier to implement and maintain.

Stakeholders and decision makers involved in school lunch programs should be aware of how the programs can address specific concerns in their nations or communities. In the United States, the NSLP provides low-income children with nutrients that are of greatest concern. Limiting calories is a strategy to reduce childhood obesity, another public health concern in the United States.

India's Mid-Day Meal Scheme addresses established nutritional concerns, such as protein–energy malnutrition and micronutrient deficiency. Other benefits are that it boosts local economies and reduces gender and caste disparities. Excessive household burden is a potential barrier to successful school feeding and improvements in attendance and retention in developing nations. School meal programs in Kenya and Uganda avoided this by providing a value transfer to households in the form of school meals and take-home rations.

Training Is a Key to Success

For an intervention to be initiated and maintained, staff must be trained. Teachers might be trained to teach a new curriculum, cafeteria staff might learn new cooking techniques or recipes, and administrators might learn how to keep records and conduct periodic evaluations. The USDA provides free training and other informational materials online.[111] The *Coordinated Review Effort* procedures manual, for example, describes acceptable procedures for evaluating implementation of the NSLP at schools.[112] Topics in other resources include updates on laws and regulations regarding food safety, eligibility guidelines, and compliance regulations.

In Japan, Diet and Nutrition Teachers in the Shokuiku program develop curricula to be used in classrooms. In Africa, WFP often provides technical assistance to local producers. In India, the Akshay Patra Foundation teaches women how to cook meals and comply with food safety laws.

Pilot Test and Allow for Flexibility to Make Necessary Changes to the Program

Pilot testing in a small but representative target group allows unforeseen issues to be identified and resolved before implementing the program on a larger scale. During the pilot, communication with stakeholders and any research assistants or supporting agencies that are on site helps determine necessary modifications. Potential hurdles that may occur when it is time to scale up the program should be identified.

Many pilot tests and research studies have been conducted to improve the NSLP. In one example, researchers investigated the effects of offering more milk options by varying containers, temperatures, and locations. Milk consumption increased by 9% to 22% in elementary and secondary schools, and participation in the NSLP increased by 4.8% in secondary schools.[113] These results suggest benefits of providing more milk options.

In Uganda, the World Food Programme and World Vision Uganda began the first phase of a school meal program pilot in early 2007 with 32,000 students; the second phase served 48,000 students in school. Program growth continues to be smooth. Similarly in India, the Akshay Patra Foundation began with a single kitchen and grew to multiple locations.

Maintain a Relationship with the Schools

Results of pilot programs or research studies, changes in policies or procedures, and notifications or reminders of available resources, such as educational tools or additional benefits, should be communicated. Notifications should be easily understood by school staff, administrators, parents, and/or students.

> *Public Health Core Competency 7: Financial Planning and Management Skills 7A: Reports program performance*

The USDA makes National School Lunch Program updates, such as changes in eligibility, available online. To receive benefits as part of India's Mid-Day Meal Scheme, schools must adhere to strict government policies for assessment and evaluation. State agencies or local or school-level officials may carry out the assessments and report results to the state; the state is responsible for communicating with the federal government. Diet and Nutrition Teachers within Japan's Shokuiku program communicate with food service workers, teachers, students, and parents, and provide examples of ongoing communication.

Conclusion

Children need proper nutrition for normal physical and psychosocial growth and development, but millions of children worldwide face overnutrition, hunger, and/or micronutrient deficiencies. School meals can improve children's nutritional status and health, as well as reduce gender disparities and help break the cycle of poverty. Successful programs must address local nutritional concerns and include community stakeholders.

References

1 Monika, M., Arora, S., & Veenu, N. (2011). Nutritional health status of primary school children: A study in Bareilly district. *Indian Educational Review, 48*, 18-29.

2 Sharma, A. K., Singh, S., Meena, S., & Kanna, A. T. (2010). Impact of NGO run midday meal program on nutrition status and growth of primary school children. *Indian Journal of Pediatrics, 77*, 763-69.

3 Gueri, M., Gurney, J. M., & Jutsum, P. (1980). The Gomez classification: Time for a change? *Bulletin of the World Health Organization, 58*, 773-77.

4 Chandra, A. K., Bhattacharjee, A., Malik, T., & Ghosh, S. (2008). Goiter prevalence and iodine nutritional status of school children in a sub-Himalayan Tarai region of eastern Uttar Pradesh. *Indian Pediatrics, 45*, 469-74.

5 Akshaya Patra. (n.d.). Retrieved from http://www.akshaya patra.org

6 Vir, S. C., Singh, N., Nigam, A. K., & Jain, R. (2008). Weekly iron and folic acid supplementation with counseling reduces anemia in adolescent girls: A large-scale effectiveness study in Uttar Pradesh, India. *Food and Nutrition Bulletin, 29*, 186-94.

7 Wani, S. A., Ahmad, F., Zargar, S. A., Dar, P. A., Dar, Z. A., & Jan, T. R. (2008). Intestinal helminthes in a population of children from the Kashmir valley, India. *Journal of Helminthology, 82*(4), 313-17.

8 Osei, A., Houser, R., Bulusu, S., Joshi, T., & Hamer, D. (2010). Nutritional status of primary schoolchildren in Garhwali Himalayan villages of India. *Food and Nutrition Bulletin, 31*(2), 221-33.

9 Taras, H. (2005). Nutrition and student performance at school. *Journal of School Health, 75*(6), 199-213.

10 Kleinman, R. E., Hall, S., Green, H., Korzec-Ramirez, D., Patton, K., Pagano, M. E., & Murphy, J. M. (2002). Diet, breakfast and academic performance in children. *Annals of Nutrition & Metabolism, 42*(Suppl. 1), 24-30.

11 Caulfield, L. E., de Onis, M., Blössner, M., & Black, R. E. (2004). Undernutrition as an underlying cause of child deaths associated with diarrhea, pneumonia, malaria and measles. *American Journal of Clinical Nutrition, 80*, 193-98.

12 Gropper, S. S., Smith, J. L., & Groff, J. L. (2009). *Advanced nutrition and human metabolism* (5th ed.). Belmont, CA: Wadsworth Cengage Learning.

13 Gropper, S. S., Smith, J. L., & Groff, J. L. (2009). *Advanced nutrition and human metabolism* (5th ed.). Belmont, CA: Wadsworth Cengage Learning.

14 Agricultural Research Service, U.S. Department of Agriculture. (2012, July 16). What we eat in America. Retrieved from http://www.ars.usda.gov/Services/docs.htm?docid=13793

15 Muller, O., & Krawinkel, M. (2005). Malnutrition and health in developing countries. *Canadian Medical Association Journal, 173*, 279-86.

16 Looker, A. C., Cogswell, M. E., & Gunter, E. W. (2002). Iron deficiency—United States, 1999-2000. *Morbidity and Mortality Weekly Report, 51*, 897-99.

17 Whittaker, P., Tufaro, P., & Rader, J. I. (2001). Iron and folate in fortified cereals. *Journal of the American College of Nutrition, 20*, 247-54.

18 Maberly, G., Grummer-Strawn, L., Jefferds, M. E., Pena-Rosas, J. P., Serdula, M. K., Tyler, V. Q., . . . , Aburto, N. J. (2008). Trends in wheat flour fortification with folic acid and iron, worldwide, 2004 and 2007. *Morbidity and Mortality Weekly Report, 57*, 8-10.

19 Gembicki, M., Stozharov, A. N., Arinchin, A. N., Moschik, K. V., Petrenko, S., Khmara, I. M., & Baverstock, K. (1997). Iodine deficiency in Belarusian children as a possible factor stimulating the irradiation of the thyroid gland during the Chernobyl catastrophe. *Environmental Health Perspectives, 105*, 1487-90.

20 Hatch, M., Polyanskaya, O., McConnell, R., Gong, Z., Drozdovitch, V., Rozhko, A., . . . Zablotska, L. (2011). Urinary iodine and goiter prevalence in Belarus: Experience of the Belarus-American cohort study of thyroid cancer and other thyroid diseases following the Chernobyl nuclear accident. *Thyroid, 21*, 429-37.

21 De Benoist, B., McLean, E., Andersson, M., & Rogers, L. (2008). Iodine deficiency in 2007: Global progress since 2003. *Food and Nutrition Bulletin, 29*, 195-202.

22 Andersson, M., de Benoist, B., Darnton-Hill, I., & Delange, F. (2007). *Iodine deficiency in Europe: A continuing public health problem.* Geneva: World Health Organization & UNICEF.

23 Davies, K. M., Heaney, R. P., Recker, R. R., Lappe, J. M., Barger-Lux, M. J., Rafferty, K., & Hinders, S. (2000). Calcium intake and body weight. *Journal of Clinical Endocrinology and Metabolism, 85*, 4635-38.

24 Allen, L., de Benoist, B., Dary, O., & Hurrell, R. (2006). *Guidelines on food fortification with micronutrients.* Geneva: World Health Organization & Food and Agricultural Organization.

25 Fulgoni, V. L., 3rd, Keast, D. R., Auestad, N., & Quann, E. E. (2011). Nutrients from dairy foods are difficult to replace in the diets of Americans: Food pattern modeling and an analysis of the National Health and Nutrition Examination Survey, 2003-2006. *Nutrition Research, 31*, 759-65.

26 Du, X., Greenfield, H., Fraser, D. R., Ge, K., Trube, A., & Wang, Y. (2001). Vitamin D deficiency and associated factors in adolescent girls in Beijing. *American Journal of Clinical Nutrition, 74*, 494-500.

27 Gropper, S. S., Smith, J. L., & Groff, J. L. (2009). *Advanced nutrition and human metabolism* (5th edition). Belmont, CA: Wadsworth Cengage Learning.

28 Allen, L., de Benoist, B., Dary, O., & Hurrell, R. (2006). *Guidelines on food fortification with micronutrients.* Geneva: World Health Organization & Food and Agricultural Organization of the United Nations.

29 Grummer-Strawn, L. M., Reinold, C., & Krebs, N. F. (2010). Use of World Health Organization and CDC growth charts for children aged 0-59 months in the United States. *Morbidity and Mortality Weekly Report, 59*, 1-15.

30 De Onis, M., Garza, C., Victora, C. G., Onyango, A. W., Frongillo, E. A., & Martines, J. (2004). Multicentre Growth Reference Study: Planning, study design and methodology. *Food and Nutrition Bulletin, 25,* S15-26.

31 De Onis, M., Onyango, A. W., Borghi, E., Siyam, A., & Nishida, C. (2007). Development of a WHO growth reference for school-aged children and adolescents. *Bulletin of the World Health Organization, 85,* 60-67.

32 Department of Nutrition for Health and Development, World Health Organization. (2008). *Training course on child growth assessment.* Retrieved from http://www.who.int/childgrowth/training/en

33 United Nations. (2012). *Millennium Development Goals: We can end poverty 2015.* Retrieved from http://www.un.org/millennium goals/index.shtml

34 General Assembly of the United Nations. (2000). *United Nations Millennium Declaration.* Retrieved from http://www .un.org/millennium/declaration/ares552e.pdf

35 United Nations. (2008, January 15). *Millennium Development Goals indicators.* Retrieved from http://mdgs.un.org/unsd /mdg/Host.aspx?Content=Indicators/OfficialList.htm

36 General Assembly of the United Nations. (2005). *World summit outcome.* Retrieved from the United Nations website, http://www.un.org/womenwatch/ods/A-RES-60-1-E.pdf

37 United Nations. (2010). *Goal 1: Eradicate extreme poverty and hunger.* Fact sheet. Retrieved from http://www.un.org /millenniumgoals/2008highlevel/pdf/newsroom/Goal%20 1%20FINAL.pdf

38 United Nations. (2012). *Millennium Development Goals: 2012 progress chart.* Retrieved from http://www.un.org/millennium goals/pdf/2012_Progress_E.pdf

39 United Nations. (2012). *The Millennium Development Goals report, 2012.* Retrieved from http://www.un.org/millennium goals/pdf/MDG%20Report%202012.pdf

40 World Bank. (2012). *World development report 2012: Gender equality and development outline.* Washington, DC: World Bank. Retrieved from http://econ.worldbank.org /external/default/main?pagePK=64165259&theSitePK =544849&piPK=64165421&menuPK=64166093&entit yID=000334955_20101103062028

41 United Nations Development Programme. (2011). *Human development report 2011: Sustainability and equity: A better future for all.* New York, NY: United Nations Development Programme.

42 Filmer, D., King, E. M., & Pritchett, L. (1997). *Gender disparity in South Asia: Comparisons between and within countries.* World Bank Policy Research Working Paper No. 1867.

43 Finnegan, J. R., Jr., & Viswanath, K. (2002). Communication theory and health behavior change. In K. Glanz, B. K. Rimer, & F. M. Lewis (Eds.), *Health behavior and health education* (3rd ed.) (pp. 361-38). San Francisco, CA: Jossey-Bass.

44 Wilkinson, R., & Marmot, M. (Eds.). (2003). *Social determinants of health: The solid facts* (2nd ed.). Copenhagen, Denmark: World Health Organization.

45 Food and Nutrition service, U.S. Department of Agriculture. (n.d.). National school Lunch Program (NSLP). Retrieved from http://www.fns.usda.gov/nslp/national-school-lunch-program

46 Food and Nutrition Service, U.S. Department of Agriculture. (n.d.). Food distribution: History and background. Retrieved from http://www.fns.usda.gov/fdd/fdd-history-and-background

47 Food and Nutrition Service, U.S. Department of Agriculture. (2008, April). *School lunch and breakfast cost study. II: Summary of findings.* Retrieved from http://www.fns.usda.gov/ora /menu/published/CNP/FILES/MealCostStudySummary.pdf

48 Food and Nutrition Service, U.S. Department of Agriculture. (2008, April). *School lunch and breakfast cost study. II: Summary of findings.* Retrieved from http://www.fns.usda.gov/ora /menu/published/CNP/FILES/MealCostStudySummary.pdf

49 Food and Nutrition Service. U.S. Department of Agriculture. (2012). *National School Lunch Program.* Retrieved from http:// www.fns.usda.gov/cnd/lunch/AboutLunch/NSLPFactSheet .pdf

50 Food and Nutrition Service, U.S. Department of Agriculture. (2007, April). *USDA school meals: Healthy meals, healthy schools, healthy kids.* Retrieved from http://www.fns.usda .gov/cga/factsheets/school_meals.pdf

51 Ralston, K., Newman, C., Clauson, A., Guthrie, J., & Buzby, J. (2008). *The National School Lunch Program: Background, trends, and issues.* Retrieved from http://www.ers.usda.gov /media/205594/err61_1_.pdf

52 Gordon, A., Crepinsek, M. K., Nogales, R., & Condon, R. (2007). *School nutrition dietary assessment study–III,* Vol. 2: *Student participation and dietary intakes.* Washington, DC: Food and Nutrition Service, U.S. Department of Agriculture. Retrieved from http://www.fns.usda.gov/oane/MENU/Published/CNP/FILES /SNDAIII-Vol2.pdf

53 Ralston, K., Newman, C., Clauson, A., Guthrie, J., & Buzby, J. (2008). *The National School Lunch Program: Background, trends, and issues.* Retrieved from http://www.ers.usda.gov /media/205594/err61_1_.pdf

54 Ralston, K., Newman, C., Clauson, A., Guthrie, J., & Buzby, J. (2008). *The National School Lunch Program: Background, trends, and issues.* Retrieved from http://www.ers.usda.gov /media/205594/err61_1_.pdf

55 Food and Nutrition Service, U. S. Department of Agriculture. (2004). *Resource guide: Offer versus serve in the school nutrition programs.* Retrieved from http://www.fns.usda.gov/tn /Resources/OVS%20Resource%20Guide.pdf

56 Food and Nutrition Service, U.S. Department of Agriculture. (2012). Nutrition standards in the National School Lunch and School Breakfast Programs; Final rule. *Federal Register, 77,* 17.

57 HealthyPeople.gov. (2012, July 26). 2020 nutrition and weight status: Objectives. Retrieved from http://www.healthypeople .gov/2020/topicsobjectives2020/objectiveslist.aspx? topicId=29

58 Gordon, A. R., Crepinsek, M. K., Briefel, R. R., Clark, M. A., & Fox, M. K. (2009). The Third School Nutrition Dietary Assessment Study: Summary and implications. *Journal of the American Dietetic Association, 109,* S129-35.

59 Gordon, A. R., Crepinsek, M. K., Briefel, R. R., Clark, M. A., & Fox, M. K. (2009) The Third School Nutrition Dietary Assessment Study: Summary and implications. *Journal of the American Dietetic Association, 109,* S129-35.

60 Osganian, S. K., Ebzery, M. K., Montgomery, D. H., Nicklas, T. A., Evans, M. A., . . . Parcel, G. S. (1996). Changes in the nutrient content of school lunches: Results from the CATCH Eat Smart food service intervention. *Preventive Medicine, 25,* 400-412.

61 Lytle, L. A., Stone, E. J., Nichaman, M. Z., Perry, C. L., Montgomery, D. H., . . . Galati, T. P. (1996). Changes in nutrient intakes of elementary school children following a school-based intervention: Results from the CATCH study. *Preventive Medicine, 25,* 465-77.

62 Lytle, L. A., Murray, D. M., Perry, C. L., Story, M., Birnbaum, A. S., . . . Varnell, S. (2004). School-based approaches to affect adolescents' diets: Results from the TEENS study. *Health Education & Behavior, 31,* 270.

63 Von Grebmer, K., Torero, M., Olofinbiyi, T., Fritschel, H., Wiesmann, D., & Yohannes, Y. (2011). *Global hunger index: The challenge of hunger: Taming price spikes and excessive food price volatility*. Washington, DC: International Food Policy Research Institute & Concern Worldwide and Welthungerhilfe. Retrieved from http://www.ifpri.org/sites/default/files/publications/ghi11.pdf

64 World Health Organization. (2007*). Country profile: India*. Nutritional Landscape Information System. Retrieved from http://apps.who.int/nutrition/landscape/report.aspx?iso=ind

65 *Help topic: Population below $1 per day*. (n.d.). Retrieved from World Health Organization website, http://apps.who.int/nutrition/landscape/help.aspx?menu=0&helpid=375

66 Eilander, A., Muthayya, S., van der Knaap, H., Srinivasan, K., Thomas, T., Kok, F. J., . . . Osendarp, S. J. (2010). Undernutrition, fatty acid and micronutrient status in relation to cognitive performance in Indian school-children: A cross-sectional study. *British Journal of Nutrition, 103,* 1056-64.

67 Chutani, A. M. (2012). School lunch program in India: Background, objectives and components. *Asia Pacific Journal of Clinical Nutrition, 21,* 151-54.

68 Department of School Education and Literacy. (2004). *Guidelines of revised National Programme of Nutrition Support to Primary Education, 2004*. Retrieved from www.education.nic.in/mdm/mdm2004.asp

69 Department of School Education and Literacy. (2004). *Guidelines of revised National Programme of Nutrition Support to Primary Education, 2004*. Retrieved from www.education.nic.in/mdm/mdm2004.asp

70 Department of School Education and Literacy. (2004). *Guidelines of revised National Programme of Nutrition Support to Primary Education, 2004*. Retrieved from http://www.upmdm.org/docs/MDM2004.pdf

71 Banerjee, S., Dias, A., Shinkre, R., Patel, V. (2011). Under-nutrition among adolescents: A survey in five secondary schools in rural India. *National Medical Journal of India, 24,* 8-11.

72 Sivakumar, B., Nair, K. M., Sreeramulu, D., Suryanarayana, P., Ravinder, P., Shatrugna, V., . . . Raghuramulu, N. (2006). Effect of micronutrient supplement on health and nutritional status of schoolchildren: Biochemical status. *Nutrition, 22,* S15-25.

73 Chandwani, H. R., &Shroff, B. D. (2012). Prevalence of goiter and urinary iodine status in 6-12-year-old rural primary school children of Bharuch District, Gujarat, India. *International Journal of Preventive Medicine, 3,* 54-59.

74 Osei, A. K., Rosenberg, I. H., Houser, R. F., Bulusu, S., Mathews, M., & Hamer, D. H. (2010). Community-level micronutrient fortification of school lunch meals improved vitamin A, folate and iron status of schoolchildren in Himalayan villages of India. *Journal of Nutrition, 140,* 1146-54.

75 Thankachan, P., Rah, J. H., Thomas, T., Selvam, S., Amalrajan, V., Srinivasan, K., Steiger, G., & Kurpad, A. V. (2012). Multiple micronutrient-fortified rice affects physical performance and plasma vitamin B12 and homocysteine concentrations of Indian school children. *Journal of Nutrition, 142,* 846-52.

76 Moretti, D., Zimmermann, M. B., Muthayya, S., Thankachan, P., Lee, T. C., Kurpad, A. V., & Hurrell, R. F. (2006). Extruded rice fortified with micronized ground ferric phosphate reduces iron deficiency in India schoolchildren: A double-blind randomized controlled trial. *American Journal of Clinical Nutrition, 84,* 822-29.

77 Gopaldas, T. (2005). Improved effect of school meals with micronutrient supplementation and deworming. *Food and Nutrition Bulletin, 26,* S220-29.

78 Ministry of Health and Family Welfare, Government of India. (n.d.). *School Health Programme*. Retrieved from http://mdm.nic.in/Files/School%20Health%20Programme/Guidelines_SHP_29TH_JAN_09-FINAL_FINAL.pdf

79 Ministry of Health and Family Welfare, Government of India. (n.d.). *School Health Programme*. Retrieved from http://mdm.nic.in/Files/School%20Health%20Programme/Guidelines_SHP_29TH_JAN_09-FINAL_FINAL.pdf

80 Department of School Education and Literacy. (2004). *Guidelines of revised National Programme of Nutrition Support to Primary Education, 2004*. Retrieved from www.education.nic.in/mdm/mdm2004.asp

81 Nozue, M., Yoshita, K., Jun, K., Ishihara, Y., Taketa, Y., Akiko, N., . . . Ishida, H. (2010). Amounts served and consumed of school lunch differed by gender in Japanese elementary schools. *Nutrition Research and Practice, 4,* 400-404.

82 World Health Organization. (2011). *NCD country profiles: Japan*. Retrieved from http://www.who.int/nmh/countries/jpn_en.pdf

83 Matsuda, R. (2007, April). Midcourse review of "Health Japan 21." *Health Policy Monitor*. Retrieved from http://www.hpm.org/survey/jp/a9/1

84 Fujikura, J., Muto, S., Takemi, Y., Okubo, H., Tanaka, H., Kagawa, A., & Sasaki, S. (2008). The Sakado school-based "shokuiko" food and nutrition education project. *Asia Pacific Journal of Clinical Nutrition, 20,* 57-63.

85 Nakamura, T. (2008).The integration of school nutrition program into health promotion and prevention of lifestyle-related diseases in Japan. *Asia Pacific Journal of Clinical Nutrition, 17,* 349-51.

86 Miyoshi, M., Tsuboyama-Kasaoka, N., & Nishi, N. (2012). School-based "Shokuiku" program in Japan. *Asia Pacific Journal of Clinical Nutrition, 21,* 159-62.

87 Tanaka, N., & Miyoshi, M. (2012). School lunch program for health promotion among children in Japan. *Asia Pacific Journal of Clinical Nutrition, 21,* 155-58.

88 Ministry of Education, Culture, Sports, Science and Technology, Government of Japan. (2008, July 1). Measures to be implemented comprehensively and systematically for the next five years. Chapter 3 in *Basic Plan for the Promotion of Education (provisional translation)*. Retrieved from http://www.mext.go.jp /english/lawandplan/1303463.htm

89 Ministry of Education, Culture, Sports, Science and Technology, Government of Japan. (2004). Sound development of children's minds and bodies. Chapter 1 in *FY2004 White Paper on Education, Culture, Sports, Science and Technology*. Retrieved from http://www.mext.go.jp/english /whitepaper/1302288.htm

90 World Food Programme. (2008). *WFP strategic plan: 2008-2013*. Retrieved from http://one.wfp.org/policies/strategies /documents/WFP_Strategic_Plan_lr.pdf

91 World Food Programme. (2008). *WFP strategic plan: 2008-2013*. Retrieved from http://one.wfp.org/policies/strategies /documents/WFP_Strategic_Plan_lr.pdf

92 World Food Programme. (2012). *School meals—in depth*. Retrieved from http://www.wfp.org/school-meals/in-depth

93 World Food Programme. (n.d.). *Our work: New approach and quality standards*. Retrieved from http://www.wfp.org /our-work/preventing-hunger/school-meals/new-approach -quality-standards

94 World Food Programme. (2012). *WFP in Africa: 2011 facts and figures*. Retrieved from http://www.wfp.org/content /wfp-africa-2011-facts-and-figures

95 World Food Programme. (2011, May). *Annual evaluation report 2010*. Rome, Italy: World Food Programme. Retrieved from http://home.wfp.org/stellent/groups/public/documents /resources/wfp235485.pdf

96 World Food Programme. (2012, May). *Annual evaluation report 2011*. Rome, Italy: World Food Programme.

97 World Food Programme. (2011, May). *Annual evaluation report 2010*. Rome, Italy: World Food Programme. Retrieved from http:// home.wfp.org/stellent/groups/public/documents/resources /wfp235485.pdf

98 World Food Programme. (n.d.). *Home grown school feeding: A framework to link school feeding with local agricultural production*. Retrieved from http://www.wfp.org/content/home -grown-school-feeding

99 United Nations Development Program. (2011). *Human development report 2011: Sustainability and equity: A better future for all*. New York, NY: Human Development Report Team.

100 World Health Organization. (2012). *Côte d'Ivoire: WFP activities*. Retrieved from http://www.wfp.org/countries/c--te-d-ivoire /operations

101 Acham, H., Kikafunda, J. K., Malde, M. K, Oldewage-Theron, W. H., & Egal, A. A. (2012). Breakfast, midday meals and academic achievement in rural primary schools in Uganda: Implications for education and school health policy. *Food and Nutrition Research, 56.*

102 Acham, H., Kikafunda, J. K., Malde, M. K, Oldewage-Theron, W. H., & Egal, A. A. (2012). Breakfast, midday meals and academic achievement in rural primary schools in Uganda: Implications for education and school health policy. *Food and Nutrition Research, 56.*

103 World Health Organization. (n.d.). *Learning from experience: Uganda case study*. Retrieved from http://documents.wfp.org /stellent/groups/public/documents/newsroom/wfp207494 .pdf

104 World Food Programme & United Nations Children's Fund. (2008). *The essential package: Twelve interventions to improve the health and nutrition of school-age children*. Retrieved from http://www.un.org/esa/socdev/poverty/PovertyForum /Documents/The%20Essential%20Package.pdf

105 Von Grebmer, K., Torero, M., Olofinbiyi, T., Fritschel, H., Wiesmann, D., & Yohannes, Y. (2011). *Global hunger index: The challenge of hunger: Taming price spikes and excessive food price volatility*. Washington, DC: International Food Policy Research Institute & Concern Worldwide and Welthungerhilfe. Retrieved from http://www.ifpri.org/sites/ default/files/publications/ghi11.pdf

106 Von Grebmer, K., Ruel, M. T., Menon, P., Nestorova, B., Olofinbiyi, T., Fritschel, H., & Yohannes, Y. (2010). Global hunger index: The challenge of hunger: Focus on the crisis of child undernutrition. Washington, DC: International Food Policy Research Institute & Concern Worldwide and Welthungerhilfe. Retrieved from http://www.ifpri.org/sites/ default/files/publications/ghi10.pdf

107 Franks, A., Kelder, S. H., Dino, G. A., Horn, K. A., Gortmaker, S. L., Wiecha, J. L., & Simoes, E. J. (2007). School-based programs: Lessons learned from CATCH, Planet Health, and Not-On-Tobacco. *Preventing Chronic Disease, 4*(2), A33.

108 Franks, A., Kelder, S. H., Dino, G. A., Horn, K. A., Gortmaker, S. L., Wiecha, J. L., & Simoes, E. J. (2007). School-based programs: Lessons learned from CATCH, Planet Health, and Not-On-Tobacco. *Preventing Chronic Disease, 4*(2), A33.

109 Food and Nutrition Service, United States Department of Agriculture. (2012, April 17). *Farm to school*. Retrieved from http://www.fns.usda.gov/cnd/f2s/about.htm

110 Food and Nutrition Service, United States Department of Agriculture. (2005, December). *Eat smart—farm fresh!* Working draft. Retrieved from http://www.ams.usda.gov/AMSv1.0/ getfile?dDocName=STELDEV3101426

111 Food and Nutrition Service, United States Department of Agriculture. (2012). *Guidance and resources*. Retrieved from http://www.fns.usda.gov/cnd/guidance/default.htm

112 Food and Nutrition Service, United States Department of Agriculture. (2012). *Coordinated review effort procedures manual*. Retrieved from http://www.fns.usda.gov/cnd/guidance /CREmanual.pdf

113 Rafferty, K., Zipay, D., Patey, C., & Meyer, J. (2009). Milk enhancements improve milk consumption and increase meal participation in the NSLP: The School Milk Pilot Test. *Journal of Children Nutrition and Management, 33*(2).

Chapter 16

Prevention of Osteoporosis in Children and Adolescents

May C. Wang, MA, DrPH
Aenor J. Sawyer, MD, MS
Tabashir Z. Nobari, MPH

Osteoporosis is a "pediatric disease with geriatric consequences."–L. Hightower, 2000

Learning Objectives

- Define osteoporosis and discuss its epidemiology and impact on public health.

- Describe bone physiology.

- Describe the pattern of bone mineral acquisition over the life course and explain its contribution to osteoporosis risk in later life.

- Identify nonmodifiable and modifiable factors that affect bone mass, including the roles of nutrition and physical activity.

- Discuss considerations when developing a successful osteoporosis prevention program targeting children and young adults.

Case Study: Reports of Increasing Rates of Bone Fractures in Young Adults

Rates of atraumatic bone fractures in children and adolescents are increasing around the world. For example, a 2010 study reported a 13% increase in fractures among children and adolescents from 1998 to 2007 in Sweden.[1] In 2003, a population-based study of residents of Rochester, Minneosta, found significant increases in age-adjusted incidence rates of distal forearm fractures of 32% and 56% in males and females younger than 35 years of age, respectively, between 1969 and 1971, and 1999 and 2001.[2] The researchers concluded that more research was needed to determine if this increase was due to decreased bone acquisition caused by low physical activity levels, poor calcium intake, or both. Studies in New Zealand have suggested that suboptimal acquistion of bone mass is a risk factor for fractures in children and adolescents.[3]

Numerous public health interventions have been developed in response to increased incidence of bone fractures among children and adolescents, as well as increased recognition of the importance of proper nutrition and physical activity for children and adolescents to achieve optimum bone density. For example, the Milk Matters campaign in the United States encourages pre-teens to consume more calcium-rich foods.[4] The Special Milk Program is another American program aimed at increasing calcium intake; this federal program reimburses eligible schools and institutions for the milk they serve to children.[5] These and other public health nutrition programs can promote better nutrition and more physical activity among children and adolescents, resulting in fewer bone fractures.

Discussion Questions

- Why is the prevalence of low bone mineral density increasing among children and young adults?

- Which factors affect bone mineral density?

- How can public health nutrition programs lead to environments that promote healthier bone mineral density to reduce fracture risk? In which settings should programs be implemented to target children and young adults?

Introduction

Osteoporosis is a condition in which bones become fragile and break more easily. It is the result of the body not making enough bone, losing too much bone, or both. Osteoporotic bones can break from a minor fall, or even from a simple action involving no trauma, such as bumping into furniture or coughing. This condition is usually seen in older adults, particularly in women after menopause, when rapid bone loss naturally occurs. Osteoporosis leads to hip and other fractures, which can be debilitating and increase the risk of premature mortality.[6] Medical expenditures associated with osteoporosis were estimated at $17 billion in 2005.[7] Despite major advances in the treatment of osteoporosis, costs related to annual osteoporosis-related fractures are predicted to be more than $25 billion by 2025.[8]

Prevalence of Osteoporosis in the United States and the World

Osteoporosis is a major global public health problem. More than 200 million people worldwide have osteoporosis,[9] with 75 million in Europe, Japan, and the United States.[10] Because the definition of osteoporosis may vary by country and diagnosis may be difficult, fracture rates among older adults are used to compare osteoporosis rates between countries.[11] An estimated 1.7 million hip fractures occur annually. Rates are higher, although stabilizing, in wealthy industrialized countries.[12] In countries experiencing economic transition, hip fracture rates are generally increasing.[13]

Who Is at Risk for Osteoporosis?

About a quarter of men and half of women aged over 50 years will break or fracture a bone due to osteoporosis. Women have higher osteoporosis rates, with three or four times more fractures than men.[14] In countries where fracture rates are high, two-thirds of hip fractures are experienced by women.[15] In countries with low fracture rates, men and women have similar rates.[16] Among women, hip-fracture rates are the highest among white women in temperate climates, followed by women living in Mediterranean and Asian countries, and lowest among women living in African countries.[17]

Over 10 million Americans have osteoporosis; approximately 34 million have low bone mass and are at higher risk for osteoporosis.[18] Whites, Native Americans, Hispanics, and Asians were about twice as likely to have osteoporosis as blacks, but fracture risk is highest among whites and Hispanics, followed by Native Americans, blacks, and Asians.[19]

Public Health Core Competency 1: Analytical/ Assessment Skills 2: Describes the characteristics of a population-based health problem

Reproduced from Council on Linkages Between Academia and Public Health Practice. 2010 May. Core Competencies for Public Health Professionals. Washington, DC: Public Health Foundation. http:// www.phf.org/resourcestools/Documents/Core_Competencies_for_ Public_Health_Professionals_2010May.pdf. Accessed August 13, 2013. This source is used for all Public Health Core Competencies in this chapter.

Bone Mass and Osteoporosis Risk

Osteoporosis has been referred to as a "pediatric disease with geriatric consequences,"[20] because major risk factors develop during childhood and adolescence and consequences tend to appear in older adulthood. However, consequences can also be evident in childhood. Improving bone acquisition and skeletal development in childhood is therefore important both to reduce incidence of childhood fractures[21,22] and to achieve optimal **peak bone mass (PBM)** and reduce development of osteoprosis and fractures later in life.

Bone strength is partially determined by bone size and geometry;[23] larger bones tend to be more resistant to fracture than smaller ones if both have the same bone mineral density, while individuals with longer **hip axis length** are more likely to suffer a hip fracture.[24] Bone strength is also determined by bone mass, which can be optimized with appropriate nutrition and physical activity.[25] Bone mass acquired by young adulthood is an important determinant of fracture risk in later life. Premenopausal skeletal status explains an estimated 66% of the **variance** in fracture risk in women; later bone loss accounts for the remaining 33%.[26,27]

Before discussing the roles of nutrition and physical activity in bone health and how they can be addressed, it is important to understand some basic facts about bone biology.

> *Public Health Core Competency 1: Analytical/ Assessment Skills 1: Identifies the health status of populations and their related determinants of health and illness (e.g., factors contributing to health promotion and disease prevention, the quality, availability, and use of health services)*

Bone is living, growing tissue, composed mainly of **collagen**. Collagen provides a soft framework for deposition of **calcium phosphate**, a mineral that strengthens and hardens bone. Together, collagen and calcium make bone strong and flexible. The two types of bone are **cortical** bone, which is compact and dense, and forms the outer shell of bone, and **trabecular** bone, which is honeycomb-like and forms the inner core.

Calcium is the most common mineral in the human body and a critical component of bone. More than 99% of the body's calcium is stored in bones and teeth. At birth, the human body has only 2–3% of total adult body calcium. Therefore, skeletal growth is the primary determinant of calcium needs during the first 20 to 30 years of life, when bone mass is increasing. In healthy children and young adults, bone mineral increases steadily throughout childhood, accelerates during puberty, and plateaus as sexual maturity is attained.[28,29,30,31,32,33,34] Bone gains appear to be most rapid between 11 and 14 years in females and between 14 and 17 years in males;[35,36,37] nearly half of adult bone mass is acquired during the teen years.[38]

The age at which PBM is achieved varies by population. Most studies have been among females, and several studies of populations of European origin have concluded that significant gains in bone mass cease in females by the late teens;[39,40,41,42] in girls, 86% of PBM is reached by age 14 or two years after menarche.[43] Slow gains in bone mineral continue into the third decade.[44,45,46,47,48]

> *Public Health Core Competency 6: Public Health Sciences Skills 5: Describes the scientific evidence related to a public health issue, concern, or intervention*

PBM determines about two-thirds of osteoporosis risk and should be optimized to prevent osteoporosis. Genetics, diet, physical activity, and sex hormones affect PBM.[49,50,51,52]

Diet and physical activity are the two primary modifiable determinants of bone mass, accounting for 20–40% of its **variance**.[53] Body size, which is determined by both genetic and environmental factors, also affects bone mass.[54,55,56,57]

Diet and Bone Health

A balanced diet is necessary for bone health. An Institute of Medicine (IOM) committee, appointed to review the evidence on calcium and vitamin D for the purposes of updating the Dietary Reference Intakes (DRI), concluded that these two nutrients are critical for bone health, but that overconsumption may be harmful. This committee established **Recommended Dietary Allowances** (RDAs) and **Tolerable Upper Intake Levels** (UL) for calcium and vitamin D for all age groups except infants (**Table 16-1**).[58] It is inportant to understand that RDAs are established to meet the needs of nearly 98% of the population, and that there are factors affecting individual needs, including genetics and calcium absorption rates. Calcium absorption rates can vary based on type of food consumed and age; highest absorption occurs in infancy. Furthermore, these recommendations are for healthy individuals. Needs can change during illness or while fractures are healing.

Dietary Calcium

On average, about 30% of dietary calcium is absorbed and the rest is excreted. Calcium from dairy products, such as milk, cheese, and yogurt, is relatively well absorbed. Many other foods contain components, such as phytic acid and oxalic acid, that may interfere with the absorption of calcium; examples of foods high in either of these acids are spinach, rhubarb, collard greens, beans, and nuts. Some foods, such as those high in sodium and protein, may reduce calcium available for bones by increasing calcium excretion from urine, feces, and sweat.[59,60,61]

Vitamin D

Vitamin D increases calcium absorption and helps regulate its use in the body. Healthy individuals living in warm climates may get adequate exposure to sunlight for **endogenous** production of vitamin D. However, endogenous production is often inadequate in older adults, dark-skinned adults, and individuals living in northern regions without sufficient exposure to ultraviolet radiation from the sun. Dietary sources of vitamin D include fortified milk, fish oil, and fatty fish, such as salmon and tuna. The DRIs for vitamin D assume minimal endogenous production.

Table 16-1 Dietary Reference Intakes (DRI) for calcium and vitamin D

Age Group	Calcium		Vitamin D	
	Recommended Dietary Allowance (RDA) Per Day	Tolerable Upper Intake Level (UL) Per Day	Recommended Dietary Allowance (RDA) Per Day	Tolerable Upper Intake Level (UL) Per Day
Infants 0-6 months	200 mg*	1000 mg	400 IU (10 mcg)*	1000 IU (25 mcg)
Infants 7-12 months	260 mg*	1500 mg	400 IU (10 mcg)*	1500 IU (38 mcg)
Children 1-3 years	700 mg	2500 mg	600 IU (15 mcg)	2500 IU (63 mcg)
Children 4-8 years	1000 mg	2500 mg	600 IU (15 mcg)	3000 IU (75 mcg)
Children 9-18 years	1300 mg	3000 mg	600 IU (15 mcg)	4000 IU (100 mcg)
Adults 19-50 years	1000 mg	2500 mg	600 IU (15 mcg)	4000 IU (100 mcg)
Adults 51-70 years Men Women	 1000 mg 1200 mg	 2000 mg 2000 mg	 600 IU (15 mcg) 600 IU (15 mcg)	 4000 IU (100 mcg) 4000 IU (100 mcg)
Adults > 70 years	1200 mg	2000 mg	800 IU (20 mcg)	4000 IU (100 mcg)
Pregnancy and lactation 14-18 years 19-50 years	 1300 mg 1000 mg	 3000 mg 2500 mg	 600 IU (15 mcg) 600 IU (15 mcg)	 4000 IU (100 mcg) 4000 IU (100 mcg)

*Only estimates of adequate intakes are available.
Data from the Institute of Medicine. (2011). *Dietary Reference Intakes for Calcium and Vitamin D.* Washington, DC: The National Academies Press.

Considerations for Determining Recommended Intakes

Discussions of dietary recommendations for promoting bone health should consider reviewing the current DRIs as well as health benefits of dairy products, which are considered a primary source of calcium.[62] Some researchers question whether the DRIs for calcium are set too high, especially if vitamin D intake is adequate.[63] With heightened population-wide awareness of the need for calcium and vitamin D, more Americans are taking supplements and eating fortified foods,[64] but excessive intakes of calcium and vitamin D can cause kidney and tissue damage.[65] The UL for calcium and vitamin D for adults over 50 years should not exceed 2000 mg and 4,000 IUs, respectively.[66]

Associations between milk intake and cardiovascular disease (CVD) and some types of cancer have varied.[67,68,69] What is established is that calcium is necessary for bone health, and current recommendations should focus on promoting a balanced diet that includes a variety of sources of calcium, including dairy products, green leafy vegetables, and bean products. Moderate consumption of dairy products is likely to have additional health benefits, such as decreasing the risk of obesity, high blood pressure, and colon cancer,[70,71,72] although there is concern over the potential health effects of bovine feeding practices in the United States.[73] The fatty acids in milk vary according to the feeding practices, with pasture-fed cows producing milk that has higher quality dairy fat than cows that are fed grain.[74] Protein, magnesium, and phosphorus are other nutrients in milk that are important for bone metabolism.[75]

Retrospective and prospective studies demonstrate positive correlations between calcium intake and bone mass in adults,[76,77] and calcium supplementation has led to increased rates of bone mineral acquisition in healthy youth.[78,79,80] Magnitude and duration of calcium's effect on the skeleton appear to be influenced by age and pubertal stage. One study found that calcium intake in **mid-puberty** was associated with increased PBM.[81] In a separate study, prepubertal children given calcium supplements gained more bone mass than controls; however, pubertal subjects did not show similar significant benefits from added calcium.[82] In two follow-up studies, gains in bone mineral were found to disappear once calcium supplementation is discontinued,[83,84] but another study found that girls supplemented before puberty maintained greater bone mass two years after discontinuing the calcium.[85] These findings suggest that calcium intake before pubertal maturity is important for bone modeling and may result in sustained effects on bone mass.[86] However, it is not established that calcium supplementation early in life leads to increased PBM.[87]

Vitamin D has a complex relationship with PBM. Vitamin D increases calcium absorption through mechanisms involving vitamin D–dependent calcium-transport proteins. A dose–response relationship between dietary vitamin D and bone health has not been reported, and results of randomized controlled trials have been inconsistent.[88] One study among 11-year-old girls reported a positive effect on bone mass of vitamin D supplementation at 400 IU for one year;[89] another study found that a considerably higher dose (2000 IU) is needed.[90] However, serum 25-hydroxyvitamin D has been positively correlated with calcium absorption in adults.[91] Dietary needs for vitamin D are affected by endogenous vitamin D synthesis, but vitamin D intake can be linked to bone health using serum 25-hydroxyvitamin D and making assumptions about sunlight exposure.[92]

Individuals who are lactose intolerant or allergic to cow's milk may be more likely to have low calcium and vitamin D intakes because of their avoidance of dairy products. Estimated prevalence of lactose intolerance varies, with a range of 15–80% of American adults suffering from it.[93,94] Lactose-intolerant individuals can often tolerate small amounts of lactose, or the amount in 4 to 8 ounces of milk, throughout the day, especially if consumed with other foods.[95] Low-lactose dairy products, such as aged cheeses, cultured yogurt, and lactose-free milk, may also be tolerated.[96] Nondairy food sources of calcium include some green leafy vegetables, such as kale, bok choy, Chinese cabbage, and broccoli,[97] and calcium-fortified foods.

Physical Activity and Bone Health

Weight-bearing physical activities, such as walking, jogging, dancing, and weightlifting, promote bone strength and increases bone mass gains in young women.[98,99,100,101]

However, intensive exercise, accompanied by weight loss and menstrual irregularities, can have adverse effects on the skeleton.[102] Exercise-induced amenorrhea is associated with bone loss and is a risk factor for spine compression fractures and stress fractures in young women athletes.[103] This is predominately due to low estrogen levels and body weight;

however, higher amounts of calcium lost through sweat may contribute to the problem.[104] The effects of exercise may vary by the skeletal site studied and, as with calcium, with the pubertal stage of the individual.[105,106,107] For example, women who started playing tennis before menarche had a greater increase in bone density in their dominant arm compared with the nondominant one than women who began the sport after menarche.[108] Another study[109] found that physical activity was a significant predictor of bone density at all skeletal sites in prepubertal but not in peripubertal children. Additionally, physical inactivity in prepuberty, but not later stages of puberty, is associated with lower young adult bone mass.[110] The influence of physical activity on bone mineral acquisition is further complicated by the influence of diet.[111,112] Meta-analysis of several studies indicates that physical activity benefits bone mineral only when calcium intake exceeds 1,000 milligrams per day.[113]

Additional Factors Affecting PBM

Pregnancy and contraception may influence PBM. The effects of pregnancy and contraceptive use on PBM are disputed. Several studies have shown that teen pregnancy increases the risk of lower bone density, but did not examine the influence of nutrition.[114,115] The demands of the fetus may have more deleterious effects on the skeleton of teen mothers who typically consume little calcium and have not yet achieved PBM; whether pregnancy ultimately compromises PBM remains undetermined.[116] The effects of oral contraceptive use on bone mass are not clear. In one estimate, each year of contraceptive use contributes to a 1% increase in spinal bone mineral density in 25- to 35-year-old women.[117] However, another study reported higher bone mineral density in physically active women with lower oral contraceptive usage.[118] Given the widespread use of oral contraceptives and the high incidence of teen pregnancy, the effects of these events on PBM must be examined in relation to previous diet and physical activity. Further studies are necessary before making generalized public health recommendations regarding the use of oral contraceptives in relation to bone health.

Body composition can affect PBM. Obesity in adults is associated with increased bone density.[119,120] However, disagreement remains over whether this association is specific to fat mass, **lean mass**, or total body weight, all of which are increased in obesity.[121,122] In adolescents, lean mass has been shown to correlate with bone mineral density,[123] perhaps by directly stimulating bone mineral gains or, alternatively, reflecting the influence of physical activity on both measures. In one study among young adult women, lean and fat mass were both associated with bone mass, with lean mass having a greater effect.[124]

> *Public Health Core Competency 6: Public Health Sciences Skills 5: Describes the scientific evidence related to a public health issue, concern, or intervention*

Public Health Approaches for Optimizing PBM on a Population Level

Given that association between suboptimal acquisition of PBM and osteoporosis, the occurrence of critical stages of physical development during childhood and adolescence when bone is accrued rapidly, and the role of diet and physical activity in achieving PBM, public health efforts to lower osteoporosis risk must focus on improving nutrition and increasing physical activity early in life. Such efforts are consistent with the Healthy People 2010 goal to "promote health and reduce chronic disease risk through the consumption of healthful diets and achievement and maintenance of healthy body weights." Objectives relevant to bone health include reducing sodium intake and increasing calcium intake and physical activity.

Public health focuses on prevention, including preventing risk factors, such as low bone mineral density associated with osteoporosis. Current treatments of osteoporosis can improve but not fully restore deficits in bone mass and microarchitecture once they have developed. Therefore, prevention efforts have focused on optimizing early gains in bone mass during the "acquisition" phase, which is in childhood and adolescence. Following are two examples of public health programs to prevent osteoporosis.

Sample Public Health Program to Reduce Disparities: The California Bone Health Campaign

In 2001, California Project LEAN (Leaders Encouraging Activity and Nutrition) conducted an osteoporosis prevention campaign targeting low-income, Spanish-speaking premenopausal Latina women and their children in San Bernardino County and Monterey County. The California Bone Health Campaign was a social marketing campaign that promoted the consumption of one extra daily serving of 1% low-fat milk through grocery-store taste tests of 1% milk, Spanish-language radio commercials, and community events. The program also included *promotoras,* or trained

community health workers, conducting educational sessions on osteoporosis risk factors and prevention, including the importance of calcium and calcium-rich foods and physical activity. The program was developed based on **formative research** that included focus groups, key informant interviews, and telephone and consumer intercept surveys. An evaluation of the program found that knowledge, attitude, and milk consumption behavior improved in the community that received both the social marketing intervention and *promotora* intervention. Furthermore, grocery-store sales of 1% milk increased in the communities that received the intervention, with the largest increase in the community that had both components of the intervention.

Sample Public Health Program: Best Bones Forever!

In 2009, the National Osteoporosis Foundation and the U.S. Department of Health and Human Services launched a campaign, Best Bones Forever!, with the support of Girl Scouts; Girls Inc.; Action for Healthy Kids; the American Academy of Pediatrics; the American Alliance for Health, Physical Education, Recreation, and Dance; the National Association of School Nurses; the Women's Sports Foundation; and other groups. The goal was to improve bone health and lower osteoporosis risk in the American population. This campaign revamped an earlier campaign, Powerful Bones, Powerful Girls, which was launched in 2001. Based on empirical evidence that early and mid-puberty provide windows of opportunity for accruing bone mineral, and that girls are at greater risk for compromised bone health than boys, it targeted girls 9 to 14 years old. Using a social marketing approach, the campaign considered the influences of peers during this life stage, and also of parents. Therefore, messages were developed for both the girls and their parents, and aimed to empower the girls to act immediately to ensure adequate intakes of calcium and engagement in weight-bearing activities.

Conclusion

Efforts are being made throughout the nation, in schools, work sites, and neighborhoods, to address obesity by promoting healthy eating. It is important to keep in mind that obese individuals are often "malnourished" in the categories of essential micronutrients. These nutrition interventions, while not aiming to address bone health specifically, may lead to improved diets that include adequate intake of calcium- and vitamin D–rich foods and appropriate physical activity. Because dietary recommendations to address all chronic illnesses are quite similar, public health researchers of various chronic health conditions need to convene and learn from one another.

Healthy People 2020: Objectives AOCBC–10: Reduce the proportion of adults with osteoporosis; NWS-20: Increase consumption of calcium in the population aged 2 years and older

Reproduced from the U.S. Department of Health and Human Services. Healthypeople.gov. Retrieved from http://www.healthypeople.gov/2020/default.aspx. Last updated July 30, 2013. Accessed August 13, 2013.

Public Health Core Competency 6: Public Health Sciences Skills 5: Integrates a review of the scientific evidence related to a public health issue, concern, or intervention into the practice of public health

Acknowledgments

Many thanks to Jennifer Arias and M. Pia Chaparro for assistance with word processing and the literature review.

References

1 Hedström, E. M., Svensson, O., Bergström, U., & Michno, P. (2010). Epidemiology of fractures in children and adolescents. *Acta Orthopaedica, 81*(1), 148-53. doi:10.3109/17453671003628780

2 Khosla, S., Melton, L. J., 3rd, Dekutoski, M. B., Achenbach, S. J., Oberg, A. L., & Riggs, B. L. (2003). Incidence of childhood distal forearm fractures over 30 years: A population-based study. *Journal of the American Medical Association, 290*(11), 1479-85.

3 Goulding, A. (2007). Risk factors for fractures in normally active children and adolescents. In R. Daly & M. Petit (Eds.), *Optimizing bone mass and strength: The role of physical activity and nutrition during growth* (Medicine and Sports Science, Vol. 51, pp. 102-20). Basel: Karger.

4 National Institutes of Health. (Updated January 16, 2008). Milk Matters. Retrieved from http://www.nichd.nih.gov/milk/Pages/milk.aspx

5 Food and Nutrition Service, United States Department of Agriculture. (2012, August). *Special Milk Program.* Retrieved from http://www.fns.usda.gov/cnd/milk/AboutMilk/SMPFactSheet.pdf

6 Joint WHO/FAO Expert Consultation. (2003). Recommendations for preventing osteoporosis. In *Population nutrient intake goals for preventing diet-related chronic diseases.* WHO Technical Report Series, no. 916 (pp. 129-33). Geneva: World Health Organization. Retrieved from http://whqlibdoc.who.int/trs/WHO_TRS_916.pdf

7 Burge, R., Dawson-Hughes, B., Solomon, D.H., Wong, J.B., King, A., & Tosteson, A. (2007). Incidence and economic burden of osteoporosis-related fractures in the United States, 2005-2025. *Journal of Bone and Mineral Research, 22*(3), 465-75.

8 Burge, R., Dawson-Hughes, B., Solomon, D. H., Wong, J. B., King, A., & Tosteson, A. (2007). Incidence and economic burden of osteoporosis-related fractures in the United States, 2005-2025. *Journal of Bone and Mineral Research, 22*(3), 465-75.

9 Reginster, J-Y., & Burlet, N. (2006) Osteoporosis: A still increasing prevalence. *Bone, 38,* S4-S9.

10 World Health Organization. (2003). *Prevention and management of osteoporosis.* WHO Technical Report Series 921. Geneva: World Health Organization. Retrieved from http://whqlibdoc.who.int/trs/WHO_TRS_921.pdf

11 Joint WHO/FAO Expert Consultation. (2003). Recommendations for preventing osteoporosis. In *Population nutrient intake goals for preventing diet-related chronic diseases.* WHO Technical Report Series, no. 916 (pp. 129-33). Geneva: World Health Organization. Retrieved from http://whqlibdoc.who.int/trs/WHO_TRS_916.pdf

12 Joint WHO/FAO Expert Consultation. (2003). Recommendations for preventing osteoporosis. In *Population nutrient intake goals for preventing diet-related chronic diseases.* WHO Technical Report Series, no. 916 (pp. 129-33). Geneva: World Health Organization. Retrieved from http://whqlibdoc.who.int/trs/WHO_TRS_916.pdf

13 Joint WHO/FAO Expert Consultation. (2003). Recommendations for preventing osteoporosis. In *Population nutrient intake goals for preventing diet-related chronic diseases.* WHO Technical Report Series, no. 916 (pp. 129-33). Geneva: World Health Organization. Retrieved from http://whqlibdoc.who.int/trs/WHO_TRS_916.pdf

14 Joint WHO/FAO Expert Consultation. (2003). Recommendations for preventing osteoporosis. In *Population nutrient intake goals for preventing diet-related chronic diseases.* WHO Technical Report Series, no. 916 (pp. 129-33). Geneva: World Health Organization. Retrieved from http://whqlibdoc.who.int/trs/WHO_TRS_916.pdf

15 Joint WHO/FAO Expert Consultation. (2003). Recommendations for preventing osteoporosis. In *Population nutrient intake goals for preventing diet-related chronic diseases.* WHO Technical Report Series, no. 916 (pp. 129-33). Geneva: World Health Organization. Retrieved from http://whqlibdoc.who.int/trs/WHO_TRS_916.pdf

16 Joint WHO/FAO Expert Consultation. (2003). Recommendations for preventing osteoporosis. In *Population nutrient intake goals for preventing diet-related chronic diseases.* WHO Technical Report Series, no. 916 (pp. 129-33). Geneva: World Health Organization. Retrieved from http://whqlibdoc.who.int/trs/WHO_TRS_916.pdf

17 Joint WHO/FAO Expert Consultation. (2003). Recommendations for preventing osteoporosis. In *Population nutrient intake goals for preventing diet-related chronic diseases.* WHO Technical Report Series, no. 916 (pp. 129-33). Geneva: World Health Organization. Retrieved from http://whqlibdoc.who.int/trs/WHO_TRS_916.pdf

18 U.S. Department of Health and Human Services, Office of the Surgeon General. (2004, October 14). *Bone health and osteoporosis: A report of the Surgeon General.* Rockville, MD: U.S. Department of Health and Human Services, Office of the Surgeon General. Retrieved from http://www.surgeongeneral .gov/library/reports/bonehealth/full_report.pdf

19 Barrett-Connor, E., Siris, E. S., Wehren, L. E., Miller, P. D., Abbott, T. A., Berger, M. L., . . . Sherwood, L. M. (2005). Osteoporosis and fracture risk in women of different ethnic groups. *Journal of Bone and Mineral Research, 20*(2), 185-94.

20 Hightower, L. (2000). Osteoporosis: Pediatric disease with geriatric consequences [Review]. *Orthopaedic Nursing, 19*(5), 59-62.

21 Landin, L. A. (1983). Fracture patterns in children. *Acta Orthopaedica Scandinavica, 54* (Suppl. 202), 1-109.

22 Khosla, S., Melton, L. J., III, Dekutoski, M. B., Achenbach, S. J., Oberg, A. L., & Riggs, B. L. (2003). Incidence of childhood distal forearm fractures over 30 years: A population-based study. *Journal of the Amercan Medical Association, 290,* 1479-85.

23 Kimmel, D. B., & Recker, R. R. (1994). Clinical assessment of bone strength. In R. Marcus (Ed.), *Osteoporosis* (pp. 49-68). Boston: Blackwell Scientific Publications.

24 Faulkner, K., Cummings, S., Black, D., Palermo, L., Bluer, C., & Genant, H. (1993). Simple measurement of femoral geometry predicts hip fracture: The study of osteoporotic fractures. *Journal of Bone and Mineral Research, 8,* 1211-17.

25 U.S. Department of Health and Human Services, Office of the Surgeon General. (2004, October 14). *Bone health and osteoporosis: A report of the Surgeon General.* Rockville, MD: U.S. Department of Health and Human Services, Office of the Surgeon General. Retrieved from http://www.sur geongeneral.gov/library/reports/bonehealth/full_report .pdf

26 Johnston, C. C., Jr., & Slemenda, C. W. (1994). PBM, bone loss and risk of fracture [Review]. *Osteoporosis International,* (4 Suppl. 1), 43-45.

27 Horsman, A., & Birchall, M. N. (1990). Assessment and modification of hip fracture risk predictions of a stochastic model. In H. F. Deluca & R. Mazess (Eds.), *Osteoporosis: Physiologic basis, assessment and treatment* (pp. 45-54). New York: American Selvier.

28 Bachrach, L. K. (2001). Acquisition of optimal bone mass in childhood and adolescence [Review]. *Trends in Endocrinology and Metabolism, 12*(1), 22-28.

29 Bonjour, J. P., Theintz, G., Buchs, B., Slosman, D., & Rizzoli, R. (1991). Critical years and stages of puberty for spinal and femoral bone mass accumulation during adolescence. *Journal of Clinical Endocrinology & Metabolism, 73,* 555-63.

30 Gilsanz, V., Gibbens, D. T., Roe, T. F., Carlson, M., Senac, M. O., Boechat, M. I., . . . Cann, C. C. (1988). Vertebral bone density in children: Effect of puberty. *Radiology, 166,* 847-50.

31 Recker, R. R., Davies, M., Hinders, S. M., Heaney, R. P., Stegman, M. R., Kimmel, D. B. (1992). Bone gain in young adult women. *Journal of the American Medical Association, 268,* 2403-8.

32 Teegarden, D., Proulx, W. R., Martin, B. R., Zhao, J., McCabe, G. P., Lyle, R. M., . . . Weaver, C. M. (1995). PBM in young women. *Journal of Bone and Mineral Research, 10,* 711-15.

33 Theintz, G., Buchs, B., Rizzoli, R., Slosman, D., Clavien, H., Sizonenko, P. C., & Bonjour, J. P. H. (1992). Longitudinal monitoring of bone mass accumulation in healthy adolescents: Evidence for a marked reduction after 16 years of age at the levels of lumbar spine and femoral neck in female subjects. *Journal of Clinical Endocrinology & Metabolism, 75,* 1060-65.

34 Young, D., Hopper, J. L., Nowson, C. A., Green, R. M., Sherwin, A. J., Kaymakci, B., . . . Wark, J. D. (1995). Determinants of bone mass in 10- to 26-year-old females: A twin study. *Journal of Bone and Mineral Research, 10,* 558-67.

35 Kroger, H., Kotaniemi, A., Kroger, L., & Alhava, E. (1993). Development of bone mass and bone density of the spine and femoral neck: A prospective study of 65 children and adolescents. *Journal of Bone and Mineral Research, 23,* 171-82.

36 Theintz, G., Buchs, B., Rizzoli, R., Slosman, D., Clavien, H., Sizonenko, P. C., & Bonjour, J. P. H. (1992). Longitudinal monitoring of bone mass accumulation in healthy adolescents: Evidence for a marked reduction after 16 years of age at the levels of lumbar spine and femoral neck in female subjects. *Journal of Clinical Endocrinology & Metabolism, 75,* 1060-65.

37 Bailey, D. A., Martin, A. D., McKay, H. A., Whiting, S., & Mirwald, R. (2000). Calcium accretion in girls and boys during puberty: A longitudinal analysis. *Journal of Bone and Mineral Research, 15*(11), 2245-50.

38 Katzman, D. K., Bachrach, L. K., Carter, D. R., & Marcus, R. (1991). Clinical and anthropometric correlates of bone mineral acquisition in healthy adolescent girls. *Journal of Clinical Endocrinology & Metabolism, 73,* 1332-39.

39 Gilsanz, V., Gibbens, D. T., Roe, T. F., Carlson, M., Senac, M. O., Boechat, M. I., . . . Cann, C. C. (1988). Vertebral bone density in children: Effect of puberty. *Radiology, 166,* 847-50.

40 Gilsanz, V., Gibbens, D. T., Carlson, M., Boechat, M. I., Cann, C. C., & Schulz, E. E. (1988). Peak trabecular vertebral density: A comparison of adolescent and adult females. *Calcified Tissue International, 43,* 260-62.

41 Bonjour, J. P., Theintz, G., Buchs, B., Slosman, D., & Rizzoli, R. (1991). Critical years and stages of puberty for spinal and femoral bone mass accumulation during adolescence. *Journal of Clinical Endocrinology & Metabolism, 73,* 555-63.

42 Sabatier, J. P., Guaydier-Souquieres, G., Laroche, D., Benmalek, A., Fournier, L., Guillon-Metz, . . . Denis, A. Y. (1996). Bone mineral acquisition during adolescence and early adulthood: a study in 574 healthy females 10-24 years of age. *Osteoporosis International, 6,* 141-48.

43 Ruiz, J. C., Mandel, C., & Garabedian, M. (1995). Influence of spontaneous calcium intake and physical exercise on the vertebral and femoral bone mineral density of children and adolescents. *Journal of Bone and Mineral Research, 10,* 675-82.

44 Garn, S. M. (1970). *The earlier gain and the later loss of cortical bone.* Springfield, IL: CC Thomas.

45 Matkovic, V., Jelic, T., Wardlaw, G. M., Ilich, J. Z., Andon, M. B., Smith, K. T., & Heaney, R. P. (1993). Timing of PBM in Caucasian females and its implication for the prevention of osteoporosis: inference from a cross-sectional model. *Journal of Clinical Investigation,* 799-808.

46 Recker, R. R., Davies, M., Hinders, S. M., Heaney, R. P., Stegman, M. R., & Kimmel, D. B. (1992). Bone gain in young adult women. *Journal of the American Medical Association, 268,* 2403-8.

47 Rodin, A., Murby, B., Smith, M. A., Caleffi, M., Fentiman, I., Chapman, M. G., & Fogelman, I. (1990). Premenopausal bone loss in the lumbar spine and neck of femur: A study of 225 Caucasian women. *Bone, 11,* 1-5.

48 Teegarden, D., Proulz, W. R., Martin, B. R., Zhao, J., McCabe, G. P., Lyle, R. M., . . . Weaver, C. M. (1995). PBM in young women. *Journal of Bone and Mineral Research, 10,* 711-15.

49 Krall, E. A., & Dawson-Hughes, B. (1993). Heritable and lifestyle determinants of bone mineral density. *Journal of Bone and Mineral Research, 8,* 1-9.

50 Pollitzer, W. S., & Anderson, J. J. B. (1989). Ethnic and genetic differences in bone mass: A review with a hereditary vs environmental perspective. *American Journal of Clinical Nutrition, 50,* 1244-59.

51 Ruiz, J. C., Mandel, C., & Garabedian, M. (1995). Influence of spontaneous calcium intake and physical exercise on the vertebral and femoral bone mineral density of children and adolescents. *Journal of Bone and Mineral Research, 10,* 675-82.

52 Slemenda, C. W., Reister, T. K., Hui, S. L., Miller, J. Z., Christian, J. C., & Johnston, C. C., Jr. (1994). Influences on skeletal mineralization in children and adolescents: evidence for varying effects of sexual maturation and physical activity. *Journal of Pediatrics, 125,* 201-7.

53 Bachrach, L. K. (2001). Acquisition of optimal bone mass in childhood and adolescence [Review]. *Trends in Endocrinology and Metabolism, 12*(1), 22-28.

54 Katzman, D. K., Bachrach, L. K., Carter, D. R., & Marcus, R. (1991). Clinical and anthropometric correlates of bone mineral acquisition in healthy adolescent girls. *Journal of Clinical Endocrinology & Metabolism, 73,* 1332-39.

55 Lu, P. W., Cowell, C. T., Lloyd-Jone, S. A., Briody, J. N., & Howman-Giles, R. (1996). Volumetric bone mineral density in normal subjects, aged 5-27 years. *Journal of Clinical Endocrinology & Metabolism, 81,* 1585-90.

56 McCormick, D. P., Poner, S. W., Fawcett, H. D., & Palmer, J. L. (1991). Spinal bone mineral density in 335 normal and obese children and adolescents: Evidence for ethnic and sex differences. *Journal of Bone and Mineral Research, 6,* 507-13.

57 Teegarden, D., Proulz, W. R., Martin, B. R., Zhao, J., McCabe, G. P., Lyle, R. M., . . . Weaver, C.M. (1995). PBM in young women. *Journal of Bone and Mineral Research, 10,* 711-15.

58 Institute of Medicine. (2011.) *Dietary Reference Intakes for calcium and vitamin D.* Washington, DC: The National Academies Press.

59 Heaney, R. P., Abrams, S., Dawson-Hughes, B., Looker, A., Marcus, R., Matkovic, V., & Weaver, C. (2000). PBM. *Osteoporosis International, 11,* 985-1009.

60 Weaver, C. M., Proulx, W. R., & Heaney, R. (1999). Choices for achieving adequate dietary calcium with a vegetarian diet. *American Journal of Clinical Nutrition, 70*(Suppl.), 543S-548S.

61 Itoh, R., Nishiyama, N., & Suyama, Y. (1998). Dietary protein intake and urinary excretion of calcium: A cross-sectional study in a healthy Japanese population. *American Journal of Clinical Nutrition, 67*(3), 438-44.

62 Institute of Medicine. (2011). *Dietary Reference Intakes for calcium and vitamin D.* Washington, DC: The National Academies Press.

63 Bischoff-Ferrari, H., & Willett, W. (2009). Comment on the IOM vitamin D and calcium recommendations. *The Nutrition Source.* Retrieved from Harvard School of Public Health website, https://www.hsph.harvard.edu/nutritionsource/what-should -you-eat/vitamin-d-fracture-prevention/index.html.

64 Institute of Medicine. (2011). *Dietary Reference Intakes for calcium and vitamin D.* Washington, DC: The National Academies Press.

65 Institute of Medicine. (2011). *Dietary Reference Intakes for calcium and vitamin D.* Washington, DC: The National Academies Press.

66 Institute of Medicine. (2011). *Dietary Reference Intakes for calcium and vitamin D.* Washington, DC: The National Academies Press.

67 Soedamah-Muthu, S. S., Ding, E. L., Al-Delaimy, W. K., Hu, F. B., Engberink, M. F., Willett, W. C., & Geleijnse, J. M. (2010). Milk and dairy consumption and incidence of cardiovascular diseases and all-cause mortality: Dose-response meta-analysis of prospective cohort studies. *American Journal of Clinical Nutrition, 93,* 158-71.

68 Chagas, C. E. A., Rogero, M. M., & Martini, L. A. (2012). Evaluating the links between intake of milk/dairy products and cancer. *Nutrition Reviews, 70,* 294-300.

69 Aune, D., Lau, R., Chan, D. S. M., Vieira, R., Greenwood, D. C., Kampman, E., & Norat, T. (2012). Dairy products and colorectal cancer risk: A systematic review and meta-analysis of cohort studies. *Annals of Oncology, 23,* 37-45.

70 Aune, D., Lau, R., Chan, D. S. M., Vieira, R., Greenwood, D. C., Kampman E., & Norat, T. (2012). Dairy products and colorectal cancer risk: A systematic review and meta-analysis of cohort studies. *Annals of Oncology, 23,* 37-45.

71 Kratz, M., Baars, T., & Guyenet, S. (2012). The relationship between high-fat dairy consumption and obesity, cardiovascular, and metabolic disease. *European Journal of Nutrition, 52*(1), 1-24.

72 McGrane, M. M., Essery, E., Obbagy, J., MacNeil, P., Spahn, J., & Van Horn, L. (2011). Dairy consumption, blood pressure, and risk of hypertension: An evidence-based review of recent literature. *Current Cardiovascular Risk Reports, 5*(4), 287-98.

73 Kratz, M., Baars, T., & Guyenet, S. (2012). The relationship between high-fat dairy consumption and obesity, cardiovascular, and metabolic disease. *European Journal of Nutrition, 52*(1), 1-24.

74 Kratz, M., Baars, T., & Guyenet, S. (2012). The relationship between high-fat dairy consumption and obesity, cardiovascular, and metabolic disease. *European Journal of Nutrition, 52*(1), 1-24.

75 Weaver, C. M. (2008). The role of nutrition on optimizing PBM. *Asia Pacific Journal of Clinical Nutrition, 17*(Suppl. 1), 135-37.

76 Cumming, R. G. (1990). Calcium intake and bone mass: A quantitative review of the evidence. *Calcified Tissue International, 47*, 194-201.

77 Recker, R. R., Davies, M., Hinders, S. M., Heaney, R. P., Stegman, M. R., & Kimmel, D. B. (1992). Bone gain in young adult women. *Journal of the American Medical Association, 268*, 2403-8.

78 Chan, G. M., Hoffman, K., McMurry, M. (1995). Effects of dairy products on bone and body composition in pubertal girls. *Journal of Pediatrics, 126*, 551-56.

79 Johnston, C. C., Miller, J. Z., Slemenda, C. W., Reister, R. K., Hui, S., Christian, J. C., & Peacock, M. (1992). Calcium supplementation and increases in bone mineral density in children. *New England Journal of Medicine, 327*(2), 82-87.

80 Lloyd, T., Andon, M. B., Rollings, N., Martel, J. K., Landis, J. R., Demers, L. M., . . . Kulin, H. E. (1993). Calcium supplementation and bone mineral density in adolescent girls. *Journal of the American Medical Association, 270*, 841-44.

81 Wang, M. C., Crawford, P. B., Hudes, M., Van Loan, M., Siemering, K., & Bachrach, L. K. (2003). Diet in midpuberty and sedentary activity in prepuberty predict PBM. *American Journal of Clinical Nutrition, 77*, 495-503.

82 Johnston, C. C., Miller, J. Z., Slemenda, C. W., Reister, R. K., Hui, S., Christian, J. C., & Peacock, M. (1992). Calcium supplementation and increases in bone mineral density in children. *New England Journal of Medicine, 327*(2), 82-87.

83 Jackman, L. A., Millane, S. S., Martin, B. R., Wood, O. B., McCabe, G. P., Peacock, M., & Weaver, C. M. (1997). Calcium retention in relation to calcium intake and postmenarchal age in adolescent females. *American Journal of Clinical Nutrition, 66*, 327-33.

84 Slemenda, C. W., Reister, T. K., Peacock, M., & Johnston, C. C. (1993). Bone growth in children following the cessation of calcium supplementation. *Journal of Bone and Mineral Research, 8*(Suppl.), S154.

85 Bonjour, J. P., Carrie, A. L., Ferrari, S., Slosman, D., & Rizzoli, R. (1996). Calcium-fortified foods increased bone modeling in prepubertal girls in a double-blind, placebo-controlled, randomized trial. *Osteoporosis International, 6*(Suppl. 1), 88.

86 Bonjour, J. P., Carrie, A. L., Ferrari, S., Slosman, D., & Rizzoli, R. (1996). Calcium-fortified foods increased bone modeling in prepubertal girls in a double-blind, placebo-controlled, randomized trial. *Osteoporosis International, 6*(Suppl. 1), 88.

87 Gafni, R. I., & Baron, J. (2007). Childhood bone mass acquisition and PBM may not be important determinants of bone mass in late adulthood. *Pediatrics, 119*(Suppl. 2), S131-36.

88 Weaver, C. M.(2008). The role of nutrition on optimizing PBM. *Asia Pacific Journal of Clinical Nutrition, 17*(Suppl. 1), 135-37.

89 Vijakainen, H. T., Natri, A. M., Kärkkäinen, M., Huttenen, M. M., Palssa, A., Jakobsen, J., . . . Lamberg Allardt, C. (2006). A positive dose-response effect of vitamin D supplementation on site-specific bone mineral augmentation in adolescent girls: A double-blinded randomized placebo-controlled 1-year intervention. *Journal of Bone and Mineral Research, 21*, 836-44.

90 El-Hajj Fuleihan, G., Nabulsi, M., Tamim, H., Maalouf, J., Salamoun, M., Khalife, H., . . . Veith, R. (2006). Effect of vitamin D replacement on musculoskeletal parameters in school children: A randomized controlled trial. *Journal of Clinical Endocrinology & Metabolism, 91*, 405-12.

91 Heaney, R. P., Dowell, S., Hale, C. A., & Bendict, A. (2003). Calcium absorption varies within the reference range for serum 25-hydroxyvitamin D. *Journal of the American College of Nutrition, 22*, 142-46.

92 Institute of Medicine. (2011). *Dietary Reference Intakes for calcium and vitamin D*. Washington, DC: The National Academies Press.

93 Scrimshaw, N. S., & Murray, E. B. (1988). Prevalence of lactose maldigestion. *American Journal of Clinical Nutrition, 48*(Suppl.), 1086-98.

94 Sahi, T. (1994). Genetics and epidemiology of adult-type hypolactasia. *Scandinavian Journal of Gastroenterology, 29*(Suppl. 202), 7-20.

95 Suarez, F. L., Adshead, J., Furne, J. K., & Levitt, M. D. (1998). Lactose maldigestion is not an impediment to the intake of 1500 mg calcium daily as dairy products. *American Journal of Clinical Nutrition, 68*(5), 118-22.

96 Vesa, T. H., Marteau, P., & Korpela, R. (2000). Lactose intolerance. *American Journal of Clinical Nutrition, 19*, 165S-175S.

97 Weaver, C. M., Proulx, W. R., & Heaney, R. (1999). Choices for achieving adequate dietary calcium with a vegetarian diet. *American Journal of Clinical Nutrition, 70*(Suppl.), 543S-548S.

98 U.S. Department of Health and Human Services, Office of the Surgeon General. (2004, October 14). *Bone health and osteoporosis: A report of the Surgeon General*. Rockville, MD: U.S. Department of Health and Human Services, Office of the Surgeon General.

99 Heaney, R. P., Abrams, S., Dawson-Hughes, B., Looker, A., Marcus, R., Matkovic, V., & Weaver, C. (2000). PBM. *Osteoporosis International, 11*, 985-1009.

100 Recker, R. R., Davies, M., Hinders, S. M., Heaney, R. P., Stegman, M. R., & Kimmel, D. B. (1992). Bone gain in young adult women. *Journal of the American Medical Association, 268*, 2403-8.

101 Snow-Harter, C., Bouxsein, M. L., Lewis, B. T., Carter, D. R., & Marcus, R. (1992). Effects of resistance and endurance exercise on bone mineral status of young women: A randomized exercise intervention trial. *Journal of Bone and Mineral Research, 7*, 761-69.

102 Warren, M. P. (1999). Health issues for women athletes: Exercise-induced amenorrhea [Commentary]. *Journal of Clinical Endocrinology and Metabolism, 84*(6), 1892-96.

103 Heaney, R. P., Abrams, S., Dawson-Hughes, B., Looker, A., Marcus, R., Matkovic, V., & Weaver, C. (2000). PBM. *Osteoporosis International, 11,* 985-1009.

104 Heaney, R. P., Abrams, S., Dawson-Hughes, B., Looker, A., Marcus, R., Matkovic, V., & Weaver, C. (2000). PBM. *Osteoporosis International, 11,* 985-1009.

105 Kannus, P., Haapasalo, H., Sankelo, M., Sievanen, H., Pasanen, M., Heinonen, A., . . . Vuori, I. (1995). Effect of starting age of physical activity on bone mass in the dominant arm of tennis and squash players. *Annals of Internal Medicine, 123*(1), 27-31.

106 Slemenda, C. W., Reister, T. K., Hui, S. L., Miller, J. Z., Christian, J. C., & Johnston, C.C., Jr. (1994). Influences on skeletal mineralization in children and adolescents: Evidence for varying effects of sexual maturation and physical activity. *Journal of Pediatrics, 125,* 201-7.

107 U.S. Department of Health and Human Services, Office of the Surgeon General. (2004, October 14). *Bone health and osteoporosis: A report of the Surgeon General.* Rockville, MD: U.S. Department of Health and Human Services, Office of the Surgeon General.

108 Kannus, P., Haapasalo, H., Sankelo, M., Sievanen, H., Pasanen, M., Heinonen, A., . . . Vuori, I. (1995). Effect of starting age of physical activity on bone mass in the dominant arm of tennis and squash players. *Annals of Internal Medicine, 123*(1), 27-31.

109 Slemenda, C. W., Reister, T. K., Hui, S. L., Miller, J. Z., Christian, J. C., & Johnston, C. C., Jr. (1994). Influences on skeletal mineralization in children and adolescents: Evidence for varying effects of sexual maturation and physical activity. *Journal of Pediatrics, 125,* 201-7.

110 Wang, M. C., Crawford, P. B., Hudes, M., Van Loan, M., Siemering, K., & Bachrach, L. K. (2003). Diet in midpuberty and sedentary activity in prepuberty predict PBM. *American Journal of Clinical Nutrition, 77,* 495-503.

111 Specker, B. L. (1996). Evidence for an interaction between calcium intake and physical activity on changes in bone mineral density. *Journal of Bone and Mineral Research, 11*(10), 1539-44.

112 Heaney, R. P., Abrams, S., Dawson-Hughes, B., Looker, A., Marcus, R., Matkovic, V., & Weaver, C. (2000). PBM. *Osteoporosis International, 11,* 985-1009.

113 Specker, B. L. (1996). Evidence for an interaction between calcium intake and physical activity on changes in bone mineral density. *Journal of Bone and Mineral Research, 11*(10), 1539-44.

114 Lloyd, T., Lin, H. M., Eggli, D. F., Dodson, W. C., Demers, L. M., & Legro, R. S. (2002). Adolescent Caucasian mothers have reduced adult hip bone density. *Fertility and Sterility, 77*(1), 136-40.

115 Sowers, M., Scholl, T., Harris, L., & Jannausch, M, (2000). Bone loss in adolescent and adult pregnant women. *Obstetrics and Gynecology, 96,* 189-93.

116 Lloyd, T., Lin, H. M., Eggli, D. F., Dodson, W. C., Demers, L. M., & Legro, R. S. (2002). Adolescent Caucasian mothers have reduced adult hip bone density. *Fertility and Sterility, 77*(1), 136-40.

117 Lindsay, R., Tohme, J., & Kanders, B. (1986). The effect of oral contraceptive use on vertebral bone mass in pre- and post-menopausal women. *Contraception, 34,* 333-40.

118 Hartard, M., Bottermann, P., Bartenstein, P., Jeschke, D., & Schwaiger, M. (1997). Effects on bone mineral density of low-dosed oral contraceptives compared to and combined with physical activity. *Contraception, 55*(2), 87-90.

119 Albala, C., Yáñez, M., Devoto, E., Sostin, C., Zeballos, L., & Santos, J. L. (1996). Obesity as a protective factor for post-menopausal osteoporosis. *International Journal of Obesity and Related Metabolic Disorders, 20*(11), 1027-32.

120 Ravn, P., Cizza, G., Bjarnason, N. H., Thompson, D., Daley, M., Wasnich, R. D., . . . Christiansen, C. (1999). Low body mass index is an important risk factor for low bone mass and increased bone loss in early postmenopausal women. Early Postmenopausal Intervention Cohort (EPIC) study group. *Journal of Bone and Mineral Research, 14*(9), 1622-27.

121 Khosla, S., Atkinson, E. J., Riggs, B. L., & Melton, L. J., 3rd. (1996). Relationship between body composition and bone mass in women. *Journal of Bone and Mineral Research,* (6), 857-63.

122 Ravn, P., Cizza, G., Bjarnason, N. H., Thompson, D., Daley, M., Wasnich, R. D., . . . Christiansen, C. (1999). Low body mass index is an important risk factor for low bone mass and increased bone loss in early postmenopausal women. Early Postmenopausal Intervention Cohort (EPIC) study group. *Journal of Bone and Mineral Research, 14*(9), 1622-27.

123 Young, D., Hopper, J. L., Macinnis, R. J., Nowson, C. A., Hoang, N. H., & Wark, J. D. (2001). Changes in body composition as determinants of longitudinal changes in bone mineral meeasures in 8 to 26-year-old female twins. *Osteoporosis International, 12,* 506-15.

124 Wang, M. C., Bachrach, L. K., Van Loan, M., Hudes, M., Flegal, K. M., & Crawford, P. B. (2005). The relative contributions of lean tissue mass and fat mass to bone density in young women. *Bone, 37,* 474-81.

Chapter 17

Meeting Adult Nutritional Needs Through Public Health Nutrition Programs

Suzanna A. Young, RD, MPH

"Because of the increasing rates of obesity, unhealthy eating habits, and physical inactivity, we may see the first generation that will have a shorter life expectancy than their parents."–U.S. Surgeon General Richard Carmona, March 2004

Learning Objectives

- Describe how long-term dietary intake affects an individual's risk for developing one or more chronic health conditions.

- Describe the role of dietary guidelines in promoting healthy diets and be able to provide specific examples.

- Understand the increased health risks caused by obesity and be able to describe overall prevalence of adult obesity in the United States.

- Identify at least four social or economic factors that have contributed to the obesity epidemic among adults in the United States.

- Understand the historical, social, and economic factors affecting food consumption patterns and how public policy affects the amount and types of food available to consumers in the United States.

- Explain the benefits of a multilevel strategy and policy/environmental change approach in developing public health nutrition programs to improve dietary intake.

- Give examples of national-, state-, or community-level public policies or programs that might help increase the number of adults making healthy food choices and/or exercising more.

Case Study: Worksite Program to Reduce Employee Risk for Chronic Diseases in North Carolina

Challenges to implementing public health nutrition programs include reaching and actively engaging target populations. Just as schools are ideal settings for nutrition programs for children, workplaces are suitable sites for adult-targeted programs. Worksite wellness programs can reduce costs of employee health care, disability claims, absenteeism, and turnover and generate for employers average savings of $4 for each dollar invested.[1,2] A worksite wellness program in North Carolina is an example of a successful worksite wellness program for government employees.[3]

> Healthy People 2020 Objective ECBP-8: (Developmental) Increase the Proportion of Worksites That Offer an Employee Health Promotion Program to Their Employees

In 2004, North Carolina's self-insured health plan for state employees reported a sharp rise in the proportion of employees with at least one chronic disease, and that of the 132,894 employees, 62% were obese or overweight. Chronic diseases, or noncommunicable diseases (NCDs), accounted for 70% of employee healthcare costs, and the spiraling healthcare costs threatened the state with severe budget shortfalls. To address the diet, physical activity, and tobacco health risk factors linked with chronic disease, the health plan partnered with the largest state agency, the North Carolina Department of Health and Human Services (DHHS), to pilot a worksite wellness program that could serve as a model for all state agencies. The 18,000 employees of the DHHS worked in administrative offices and residential mental health and drug treatment facilities in North Carolina. The Division of Public Health (DPH) led the worksite program.

The program's goal was to create a department-wide, sustainable wellness infrastructure that promoted employee health and wellness and reduced NCD risk factors. Strategies included changing organizational policies and work environments to support employees in making healthier lifestyle choices. Interventions focused on promoting healthy eating habits, exercising, avoiding tobacco, and managing stress.

A public health nutritionist provided program leadership, guided program planning, and helped evaluate the program. Annual employee and agency surveys were used to assess needs, identify concerns, and measure program satisfaction. A wellness leader at each worksite served on a department wellness council that advised management on necessary wellness policy changes. Leaders at each worksite formed wellness committees, developed objectives, and ensured implementation of goal-based programs and activities.

Almost all worksite locations implemented policies and activities to help employees choose healthier diets, exercise more, and avoid tobacco. More than 90% of the worksites offered nutrition education on healthy eating, and over half provided 15-week weight management classes. Additional programs included 30-day challenges to increase consumption of fruits and vegetables, weekly workplace sales of local produce, and healthier vending and cafeteria selections. Indoor fitness areas were created, and fitness classes were offered during employee lunch breaks. Management policies supported flexible work schedules to allow employees to participate in wellness activities, required vending contractors to offer healthy options, and authorized work time for wellness committee work.

Positive outcomes were evident by the program's third year. Over half of employees reported making healthier food choices, with 54% reporting an increased intake of fruits and vegetables. Half reported increased physical activity levels. Eighty percent of employees in weight management classes lost weight, with a mean loss of 8.2 pounds, and 81% of employees maintained or lost additional weight six months later. One-third of participants in weight management classes moved to a lower blood pressure category.

With the pilot program's success, similar worksite programs were implemented throughout the state government. In 2011, the program was one of four successful worksite wellness programs nationwide selected by the federal government as a best practices model to guide public and private employers.

Discussion Questions

- Why is the workplace a potentially effective setting for health interventions among adults? How can employers and employees benefit?

- What are the most salient nutrition-related concerns among adults in industrialized nations? Which does the worksite wellness program address, and how?

- Based on the results of the program evaluations that were conducted, which elements of the program were successful? Which should be modified?

- How would you design a more rigorous program evaluation, and what would you measure?
- How can the North Carolina state worksite wellness program be modified to be applicable to other worksites in the public and private sectors?

Introduction

Two diet-related **chronic diseases**, **cardiovascular disease (CVD)** and **stroke**, are the leading causes of **mortality** worldwide.[4] Their dramatic increase has led global, national, regional, and community public health agencies to focus on developing public health nutrition programs to reduce risk factors for developing these largely preventable diseases.

Obesity is a risk factor for most NCDs, including **diabetes** and CVD.[5] No longer limited to high-income counties, obesity is now a global public health problem prevalent even in low- and middle-income developing counties. Two-thirds of the world's population now lives in countries where obesity causes more deaths than underweight.[6] The **World Health Organization (WHO)** projects that, by 2015, approximately 2.3 billion adults will be **overweight** and more than 700 million will be obese.[7] In the United States, one-third of adults are obese, and almost two-thirds are obese or overweight.[8]

Rising obesity and NCD rates are linked to changes in dietary consumption patterns since World War II. In the United States, federal food policies and rapid industrialization of the food industry created an abundant and inexpensive supply of calorie-dense processed foods, often high in added sugars, salt, and fats. Increasing globalization of the food market has spread Western dietary consumption patterns worldwide. Economic and demographic transitions have also influenced types and quantities of foods and where they are prepared and consumed.[9] Focusing on the United States, this chapter addresses public health nutrition infrastructure and programs designed to meet adult nutrition needs and promote overall health.

Defining the Adult Population

Age of adulthood varies depending on the definition used. An individual is biologically an adult after reaching **puberty** and gaining the ability to reproduce. In industrialized countries, girls typically reach puberty at 10 or 11 years of age, and boys reach it at 12 to 13 years.[10] Poor nutritional status can delay the onset of puberty.[11] Malnutrition can result from lack of access to adequate energy or nutrients, especially in underprivileged populations, but unhealthy dieting practices and exercise causing abnormally low body fat can also delay puberty. More relevant in public health nutrition is the age of complete physical maturation, when calories and nutrients are no longer needed for growth. Girls reach physical maturity about two years after **menarche**,[12] while boys' heights can increase through their early 20s.[13,14]

Social adulthood can be described as the age when young adults establish households that are independent from their parents, and they are responsible for their own food. Nationality, culture, and **socioeconomic status (SES)** are just a few of the factors that can cause the age of social independence to vary widely. In some cultures, men and women live with their parents until they marry. Adults can also be defined legally by age; in many countries, adulthood, which includes the ability to vote and marry, begins at age 18.[15]

World Population Demographic Changes

The proportion of older adults throughout the world is increasing due to declining birthrates and longer life expectancies.[16] The **United Nations (UN)** identifies world population aging as "unprecedented," "pervasive," "enduring," and impactful.[17] The trend increases demands on public health systems and medical and social services. NCDs affect older adults disproportionally and raise healthcare costs.[18] By 2050, the global population over 60 will surpass the number of those under 15.[19] Global strategies must address the health of the aging population.

The "baby boomers" are the 76 million Americans born between 1946 and 1964. Members of this **cohort** reached age 65 years in 2011 and transitioned to government programs, such as **Medicare** health coverage and **Social Security** retirement benefits. Two-thirds of these seniors have at least one NCD, and 20% have five or more.[20] The large size of this cohort raises concern over projected high costs of providing public healthcare coverage under Medicare and **Medicaid**, and of affording individual private coverage.[21] As "boomers" begin to leave the workforce, their poor health status is predicted to overburden the Medicare and Medicaid programs and erode the boomer generation's personal resources.[22]

A cohort study tracked 20,000 U.S. baby boomers over the age of 50 as they approached retirement age. Despite economic affluence and a burgeoning fitness and health industry, participants self-reported poorer health than previous generations, except for having lower smoking rates. Baby boomers were more likely to report trouble with routine activities, pain, excessive drinking, psychiatric problems, stress, and NCDs such as high blood pressure, high cholesterol, and diabetes.[23] The country may encounter an increasing proportion of elderly needing assistance in daily activities, and life expectancy may decline.[24]

Poorer self-reports of health among the boomer generation may have resulted from higher expectations of vitality in older age. However, the cohort rarely achieves recommendations for physical activity or dietary intake. In addition, baby boomers are the first generation exposed from birth to the post–World War II changes in the food supply.

> *Public Health Core Competency 1: Analytical and Assessment Skills 3: Uses variables that measure public health conditions*
>
> *Public Health Core Competency 1: Analytical and Assessment Skills 12: Describes how data are used to address scientific, political, ethical, and social public health issues*
>
> Reproduced from Council on Linkages Between Academia and Public Health Practice. 2010 May. Core Competencies for Public Health Professionals. Washington, DC: Public Health Foundation. http://www.phf.org/resourcestools/Documents/Core_Competencies_for_Public_Health_Professionals_2010May.pdf. Accessed August 13, 2013. This source is used for all Public Health Core Competencies in this chapter.

Global and U.S. Nutrient Standards for Adults

Adults need energy and nutrients to maintain and repair body tissue, support activities, and maintain a healthy weight.[25] Primary nutrition goals for adults are to prevent nutrient deficiencies, maintain a healthy weight, promote a strong immune system, and prevent or slow NCD development.[26]

International Recommendations for Nutrients

WHO's Department of Nutrition for Health and Development and the UN's **Food and Agriculture Organization (FAO)** provide intake recommendations for all life stages for energy, protein, carbohydrates, fats/lipids, vitamins, minerals, and trace elements. Recommendations are updated every 10 to 15 years to reflect new research findings. Many countries use the WHO/FAO nutrient requirement standards to develop food-based dietary guidelines for their populations.[27]

U.S. Nutrient Standards

During World War II, concerns on the part of the U.S. government about ensuring adequate nutrition for the armed forces and the general population led to development of the **Recommended Dietary Allowance (RDA)** standards by the U.S. Academy of Sciences. In 1997, the RDA became one component of the U.S. dietary guidelines called the **Dietary Reference Intakes (DRI)**, developed by the Institute of Medicine (IOM) and Health Canada. The DRIs describe nutrient needs based on age categories, sex, and state of pregnancy or lactation.[28] The **Estimated Average Requirement** is the DRI value of a nutrient that will meet the requirements of half of healthy individuals in a group. These population-based estimated nutrient requirements are useful for calculating the nutrient needs of groups of healthy individuals and provide limited information helpful in assessing the nutrient needs of healthy individuals.

> *Public Health Core Competency 1: Analytical/Assessment Skills 4: Uses methods and instruments for collecting valid and reliable quantitative and qualitative data*

Determining Energy Needs for Adults

Estimated Energy Requirement (EER) is calculated based on an individual's energy intake, energy expenditure, age, sex, weight, height, and physical activity level.[29] Adult energy requirements usually decrease around the mid-40s due to a decrease in lean muscle mass and a drop in **basal metabolic rate (BMR)**.[30] Therefore, caloric intake also needs to decrease to prevent weight gain.[31] Increased physical activity levels and resistance training to build lean muscle mass can also help maintain EER and prevent unwanted weight gain.[32]

Major Health Risk Factors for Adult Populations

WHO identifies 17 top health risk factors for adult populations, listed here in order of significance. Those directly related to nutrition and food safety are in italics.[33]

1. *Hypertension*
2. Tobacco use
3. *High blood glucose*
4. Physical inactivity

5. *Overweight and obesity*

6. *High cholesterol*

7. Unsafe sex

8. *Alcohol use*

9. *Unsafe water, sanitation, hygiene*

10. Low fruit and vegetable intake

11. *Suboptimal breastfeeding (increases maternal risk for breast cancer)*

12. Urban indoor air pollution

13. Occupational risks

14. *Vitamin A deficiency*

15. *Zinc deficiency*

16. Unsafe healthcare injections

17. *Iron deficiency*[34]

Health Problems Related to Nutrition Deficiencies

Obtaining sufficient food and nutrients was the prevailing nutrition concern worldwide until recent decades, and it remains a priority in some developing nations and certain populations, such as refugees and residents of areas experiencing political turmoil or famine.[35] **Protein–energy malnutrition (PEM)** has decreased worldwide, but FAO estimates that 870 million people, or 12% of the world's population, were undernourished between 2010 and 2012. In 2008–2009, nations in sub-Saharan Africa and Southeast Asia had average per capita protein supplies of 58 and 55 grams per day, respectively; in comparison, the value in developed nations was 104 grams.[36]

The United States and other industrialized countries have an abundant supply of affordable food with adequate amounts of protein, calories, and micronutrients. However, **food insecurity** is present in 14.5% of U.S. households.[37] Data on hunger prevalence in the United States often come from indirect sources, such as income data, unemployment percentages, use of emergency food banks, applications for food assistance programs, and surveys with questions on recent food insecurity. These sources do not provide clinical data on health status, and cannot be used as indicators of actual malnutrition. Undernutrition, obesity, and diet-related chronic diseases are superficially distinct nutrition problems, but they can have similar underlying causes, such as poverty, and coexist within countries, communities, and households.[38]

Micronutrient Deficiencies

Many previously common nutrient deficiency diseases, such as **beriberi**, **scurvy**, **pellagra**, and **night blindness**, are now rare in industrialized countries, where they typically occur only in severely malnourished, elderly, and chronically sick populations and individuals with extreme dietary patterns (**Table 17-1**). Mandatory micronutrient fortification has helped virtually eliminate some deficiencies. Fortification can deliver essential nutrients to large segments of the population without changes in food consumption patterns.[39] Enrichment of a wide variety of foods increases nutrient intake among individuals with overall poor dietary habits.[40] Another factor contributing to elimination of these deficiency diseases in affluent countries is a more varied diet due to foods, especially fruits and vegetables, being available year-round.

Deficiencies of iron, folic acid, and iodine remain prevalent, particularly in developing nations. An estimated 3.5 to 5 billion individuals are iron deficient (ID), 2.2 billion have **iodine deficiency disorders (IDD)**, and 140 to 250 million are vitamin A deficient (VAD).[41] As clinical nutrient deficiencies have declined, more attention has been paid to subclinical deficiencies. Vitamin D, for example, was traditionally considered essential only for normal bone mineralization. Now, vitamin D deficiency has been associated with muscle weakness, type 1 diabetes, multiple sclerosis, rheumatoid arthritis, hypertension, cardiovascular heart disease, and certain cancers.[42]

Major Nutrition-Related Health Concerns in the 21st Century

In 2008, NCDs accounted for 63% of all deaths worldwide, making them a focus for local, state, federal, and global public health agencies. In all but the poorest countries, NCDs cause more deaths than communicable diseases and nutrient deficiencies.[43] One-fourth of NCD mortality is among individuals under the age of 60, with 90% of these premature deaths occurring in low- and middle-income countries.[44]

In the United States, NCDs account for 70% of deaths. Over half of all adults have one or more chronic condition, and one in three adults are obese. One-fourth of

Table 17-1 Adult micronutrient deficiency conditions and their global prevalence

Micronutrient	Deficiency Prevalence	Major Deficiency Disorders	Common Sources
Iron	2 billion	Iron deficiency, anemia, reduced learning and work capacity	Red meat, liver, fortified cereals, beans, lentils, eggs
Iodine	2 billion at risk	Goiter, hypothyroidism	Iodized salt, some seafood, naturally occurring in foods grown in some areas of the world
Vitamin D	Widespread in all age groups	Rickets, osteomalacia, osteoporosis, colorectal cancer	Fortified dairy products, fish liver oils, fatty fish, fortified cereals, exposure to ultraviolet rays
Vitamin A	Adult data insufficient	Night blindness, xerophthalmia,	Fortified dairy products
Zinc	Estimated high in developing countries	Decreased resistance to infectious diseases; poor pregnancy outcomes, impaired growth	Red meats, some seafood, fortified cereals
Folate (vitamin B6)	Insufficient data	Megaloblastic anemia, neural tube and other birth defects, heart disease, stroke, impaired cognitive function, depression	Dark, leafy green vegetables; enriched and whole-grain breads; fortified cereals
Cobolamine (vitamin B12)	Insufficient data	Megaloblastic anemia (associated with *Helicobacter pylori*–induced gastric atrophy)	Fish, poultry, meat, fortified cereals
Fluoride	Widespread	Dental decay, poor bone health	Fluoridated water
Thiamine (vitamin B1)	Insufficient data; estimated as common in developing countries and in famines, displaced persons	Beriberi (cardiac and neurologic), Wernicke and Korsakov syndromes (alcoholic confusion and paralysis)	Enriched and whole-grain products, bread, cereals
Riboflavin (vitamin B2)	Insufficient data; estimated to be common in developing countries	Nonspecific: fatigue, eye changes, dermatitis, brain dysfunction, impaired iron absorption	Milk, bread, fortified cereals
Niacin (vitamin B3)	Insufficient data; estimated as common in developing countries and where food shortages exist	Pellagra (dermatitis, diarrhea, dementia, death)	Meat, fish, poultry, enriched and whole-grain breads, fortified cereals
Vitamin B6	Insufficient data; estimated common in developing countries and where food shortages exist.	Dermatitis, neurological disorders, convulsions, anemia, elevated plasma homocysteine	Fortified cereals, fortified soy products, organ meats
Vitamin C	Common in famines, displaced persons	Scurvy (fatigue, hemorrhages, low resistance to infection, anemia)	Citrus, strawberries, potatoes, tomatoes, bell peppers, broccoli
Calcium	Insufficient data; estimated to be widespread	Decreased bone mineralization, rickets, osteoporosis	Dairy products, fortified cereals, spinach
Selenium	Insufficient data; common in Asia, Scandinavia, Siberia	Cardiomyopathy, increased cancer and cardiovascular risk	Organ meats, seafood, some plants if grown in selenium-rich soil

Data from: Tulchinsky, T. (2011). Micronutrient deficiency conditions: global health issues. *Public Health Reviews*, *32*(1), 243–55. Accessed August 26, 2013, from http://www.publichealthreviews.eu/upload/pdf_files/7/13_Micronutrient.pdf.

Americans with chronic diseases have limitations on their daily activities. Arthritis is the most common cause of disability, and diabetes continues to be the leading cause of kidney failure, nontraumatic lower-extremity amputations, and blindness among U.S. adults aged 20 to 74.[45]

Below is a list of the most common diet-related chronic diseases in the United States:

Heart disease: In the United States, 81.1 million people have CVD. Risk factors include **dyslipidemia**, type 2 diabetes, **hypertension**, **metabolic syndrome**, obesity, physical inactivity, and tobacco use. In addition, 74.5 million Americans, or 34% of U.S. adults, have hypertension, which is also a risk factor for stroke and kidney disease, and 36% of American adults have prehypertension.

Diabetes: Nearly 24 million people, or 11% of adults, have diabetes, with the vast majority of cases being type 2 diabetes, which is often related to diet and physical activity. About three times as many adults have prediabetes, or impaired glucose tolerance, which is a risk factor for diabetes.

Cancer: About 41% of Americans will be diagnosed with cancer during their lifetimes. Dietary factors are associated with risk of some types of cancer, including breast, endometrial, colon, kidney, mouth, pharynx, larynx, and esophageal cancer.

Osteoporosis: Half of women and one-quarter of men 50 years and older will have an osteoporotic fracture in their lifetimes. Adequate nutrition and regular participation in physical activity are important factors in achieving and maintaining optimal bone mass.[46]

Chronic Disease and Public Health Nutrition

The rise in chronic diseases is the first major global health crisis not caused by infectious diseases or lack of food or medical care. Policy makers must address the economic and health burdens of NCDs. The Centers for Disease Control and Prevention (CDC) categorizes most chronic diseases as largely preventable and related to behavioral risk factors, including poor diet, physical inactivity, tobacco use, and excessive alcohol consumption.[47] Older age is another risk factor for NCD, and NCD mortality and morbidity will increase as the world's population ages.

Public Health Core Competency 1: Analytical/ Assessment Skills 2: Describes the characteristics of a population-based health problem

Chronic diseases are among the most prevalent, costly, and preventable of all health problems.[48] They are costly because treatment usually requires long-term, multifaceted medical services. For NCDs, the goal is more often to "manage" than to "cure" the condition. The rising cost of providing health care for chronic diseases is contributing to federal and state budget shortfalls in the United States. Furthermore, chronic diseases are increasing the cost burden of private insurance on citizens. Although the United States currently spends more on health care than any other country, its citizens have the lowest life expectancy among the major industrialized countries.[49] The United States must find better solutions; improved access to medical care alone is not sufficient to prevent a continued rise in chronic disease morbidity and mortality. Prevention is likely to be the most effective strategy. Public health programs focusing on prevention from childhood through adulthood should impact multiple levels of the social and built environments, and target lifestyle behaviors related to eating habits, physical activity, and tobacco use.

Diet and the Rise in Chronic Diseases

As mentioned above, the current epidemic of chronic diseases is the first major catastrophic national and worldwide health crisis not caused by a communicable disease, or by a lack of food or medical care. A poor diet, physical inactivity, and tobacco and alcohol use are among the top modifiable causes of chronic diseases.[50] Characteristics of the general diet pattern linked to NCDs include excess calories; low intake of fruits, vegetables, and whole grains; and high consumption of refined carbohydrates, such as sugar, white flour, and white rice; saturated and trans fats; and sodium. Physical inactivity and sedentary lifestyle also contribute to NCDs and obesity.[51]

Public health nutritionists, the medical community, and food policy leadership must address factors that lead to most adults having nutrition-related chronic conditions despite an abundant, affordable, and safe food supply. Changes in types and quantities of foods consumed since World War II contribute to poor diets. As consumers choose more and more processed foods and fast foods, intakes of sugar, sodium, and fat increase dramatically, and consumption of fiber, fruits, and vegetables declines. This is seen in industrialized nations and, increasingly, in less developed countries via globalization and the adoption of Westernized diets.

Screening for Chronic Diseases as Part of Secondary Prevention in Public Health

Routine screening facilitates early detection of many chronic diseases and their risk factors. Treatment is more likely to be effective when it is started sooner. Blood glucose tests can be an example of this form of **secondary prevention**. High blood glucose levels can indicate prediabetes and lead to adoption of an appropriate diet that helps prevent the development of diabetes. Health planners assess the cost-effectiveness of providing screening. Screening is more justified when treatment for a disease is very costly, such as for cancers, and when management can prevent costly complications, as in the case of diabetes. Age categories associated with an elevated risk for the illness are designated for a number of screening tests and procedures such as colonoscopies and mammograms. Even when a test is considered cost-effective, however, many people may not have access to the test because of cost.

Obesity Is a Global Epidemic

As discussed earlier in the chapter, obesity is a global epidemic. It is prevalent in low-, middle-, and high-income counties, and its global burden is expected to continue to increase. Prevalence of overweight varies widely between and within regions (**Figure 17-1**). Central American and Micronesian women have the highest prevalence of overweight worldwide. North American, Australian, and New Zealander males have the highest prevalence of overweight. More females are overweight than males in each WHO subregion except for North America and Europe.[52]

In 2009 to 2010, 35.7% of U.S. adults were obese, and 33.3% were overweight.[53] Obesity prevalence varies by region and state (**Figure** 17-2). Adults aged 60 and over are more likely to be obese.[54] Non-Hispanic blacks, Mexican Americans, and all other Hispanics have higher age-adjusted rates of obesity than non-Hispanic whites.[55] Similar to many other health disparities, obesity is linked to lower income and less education, although the prevalence of obesity has been increasing in adults at all income and education levels. (**Figure 17-3**)

Obesity is a risk factor for multiple NCDs and their risk factors. Overweight and obesity can lead to abnormal blood lipid levels and interfere with normal carbohydrate metabolism. Excess weight stresses the cardiovascular system and joints. By middle age, cumulative effects of a poor diet often lead to onset of clinical symptoms of one or more chronic health conditions.[56,57] Obesity is associated with increased mortality. In the U.S. annually, obesity is associated with 112,000 additional deaths due to CVD, 15,000 additional deaths due to cancer, and 35,000 additional deaths due to other causes.[58]

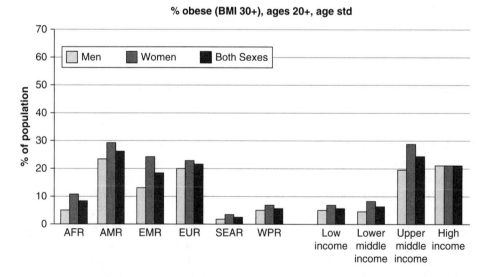

% obese (BMI 30+), ages 20+, age std

Figure 17-1 Global prevalence of obesity and overweight

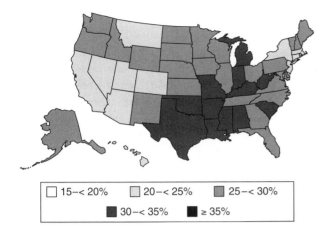

Figure 17-2 Prevalence of self-reported obesity among U.S. adults

Reproduced from Centers for Disease Control and Prevention. (2013). Adult obesity facts. Available at http://www.cdc.gov/obesity/data/adult.html. Accessed September 5, 2013.

Overweight and obesity significantly raises the risk of developing the following health problems:

- Metabolic syndrome and type 2 diabetes
- Coronary heart disease
- Stroke
- Hypertension
- Nonalcoholic fatty liver disease
- Gallbladder disease
- Osteoarthritis (degeneration of cartilage and bone of joints)
- Sleep apnea and other breathing problems
- Many cancers (breast, colorectal, endometrial, and kidney)
- Complications of pregnancy, including gestational diabetes
- Hormonal and menstrual irregularities[59]

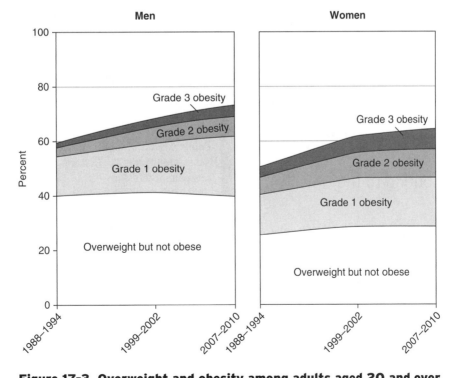

Figure 17-3 Overweight and obesity among adults aged 20 and over, by sex: United States, 1988-1994, 1999-2002, and 2007-2010

Modified from CDC/NCHS, Health, United States, 2012, Table 68.

The Economic Burden of Obesity

Medical costs associated with obesity in the United States were estimated at $147 billion in 2008. In the United States, obesity-related healthcare costs account for 5.5–7.0% of national healthcare expenditures, while in other countries, obesity-related costs account for just 2.0–3.5% of healthcare expenditures.[60] Annual health costs for obese individuals are 42% higher than the costs for people at a healthy weight. On average, an obese individual will pay $1,429 more per year for health care than a normal-weight individual.[61]

Measuring Obesity

Body mass index (BMI) is an inexpensive and easy screening tool to assess body fat.[62] On a population level, this anthropometric measurement is relatively accurate, less expensive, and quicker than more direct measures of body fat such as **skinfold thickness measurement** and use of a **bioelectrical impedance analyzer (BIA)**. However, BMI is not a reliable measure for all individuals.[63] It can overestimate fat levels in individuals such as athletes with high muscle development, and underestimate fat levels in older individuals with less muscle mass or sick individuals with excess body fluid. It does not measure distribution of body fat.

Waist circumference is another anthropometric indicator of obesity-related health risks. Central or abdominal adiposity is more harmful than peripheral adiposity. A waist circumference over 35 inches (88 cm) for women and 40 inches (102 cm) for men is associated with an increased risk for CVD and type 2 diabetes.[64]

Factors Contributing to the Obesity Epidemic

Globalization, industrialization, and urbanization have improved access to food and health care, but have also had some negative effects on dietary patterns,[65,66] with increased consumption of energy-dense processed foods, high in sugar, sodium, and fats, and decreased consumption of locally produced fruits, vegetables, meat, fish, and dairy products. As more countries adopt westernized diets, nations whose primary public health nutrition concerns had been malnutrition due to nutrient deficiency diseases now simultaneously face overnutrition and NCDs.[67,68]

Per capita energy availability in the United States is several hundred more calories per day than in the mid-20th century, and energy expenditure has decreased due to more sedentary work and leisure activities. These factors contribute to positive **energy balance** and weight gain. Fewer than half of U.S. adults participate in recommended levels of physical activity.[69] Foods manufactured with refined carbohydrates and/or added sugars and fats are more palatable and often less expensive per calorie, making them more accessible to low-income populations than fruits, vegetables, lean meats, and fish.[70]

Physiological Factors Contributing to Obesity

The body's capacity to store fat was a survival advantage for most of human history, allowing humans to survive famine and seasonal variations in food availability. For women, fat storage helped meet additional energy requirements in pregnancy and lactation. Fat storage is not an advantage in modern populations with consistent access to nutritious foods.[71]

Physiological factors can affect energy balance. For example, stress and sleep deficits may cause hormonal imbalances and increase weight gain. Multiple genes may increase susceptibility for obesity in individuals and in populations, but an external factor, such as overconsumption of calories, is necessary to result in obesity.[72] Some medical conditions, such as hypothyroid, and some pharmaceuticals, such as prednisone, can also contribute to weight gain. However, these factors are small compared with the environmental factors contributing to obesity.[73]

> *Public Health Core Competency 1: Analytical/ Assessment Skills 10: Collects quantitative and qualitative community data*

Behavioral Factors Contributing to Adult Obesity

Multiple direct and indirect social, psychological, biological, economic, cultural, and environmental variables affect dietary habits and obesity worldwide.

Serving sizes in restaurants and many retail snack foods have continued to rise since the 1970s. In the United States, soft drink servings have increased from 7 to 42 ounces, and hamburgers have tripled in size (**Figure 17-4**).[74] The size of dinner plates in most restaurants has increased to accommodate larger serving sizes, and larger orders are heavily

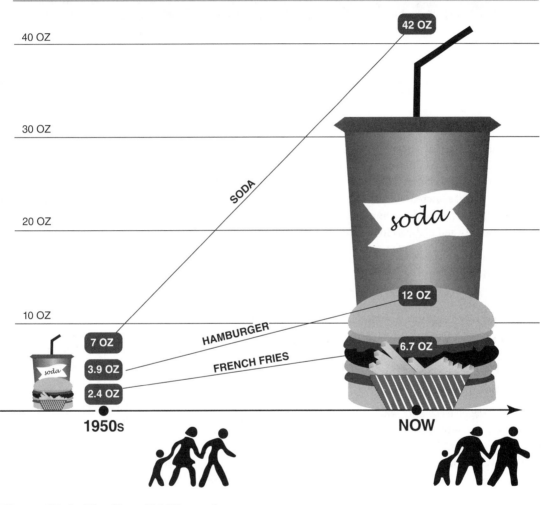

THE NEW (AB)NORMAL

Portion sizes have been growing. So have we. The average restaurant meal today is more than four times larger than in the 1950s. And adults are, on average, 26 pounds heavier. If we want to eat healthy, there are things we can do for ourselves and our community: Order the smaller meals on the menu, split a meal with a friend, or, eat half and take the rest home. We can also ask the managers at our favorite restaurants to offer smaller meals.

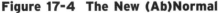

Figure 17-4 The New (Ab)Normal

Reproduced from the Centers for Disease Control and Prevention. (2012). Infographics at CDC. http://www.cdc.gov/socialmedia/tools/infographics. html. Accessed August 12, 2013.

marketed.[75,76] Except for sliced white bread, all of the commonly available food portions exceeded U.S. Department of Agriculture (USDA) and Food and Drug Administration (FDA) standard portion sizes. Virtually all of these products exceed the portion size of the same item prior to 1970. Larger servings contribute to obesity because people tend to eat more when served more.[77]

At all-you-can-eat buffets, individuals with higher BMIs may be more likely to choose larger plates, begin serving themselves before reviewing all options, and sit closer to the buffet.[78]

Carbohydrates and Health

For many years, Americans were told by government nutrition experts to choose **carbohydrates** over fat for health and weight control.[79] However, people increasingly chose refined starches and sugars over highly nutritious **whole grains (Box 17-1).**

Box 17-1 The differences between whole grain, multigrain, and whole wheat

These different terms used to describe grain-based products are confusing to many consumers. Whole grain means that all parts of the grain are used in preparing the bread or other whole-grain product. "Whole" wheat (not flour), oat, or another grain should be listed first in the ingredients when consumers are attempting to purchase whole-grain products. Whole wheat in an ingredients list means whole-wheat flour is used. The term multigrain, by itself, merely means that the food contains more than one type of grain; the term does not imply that the grains used are whole grains.

Data from United States Department of Agriculture. (n.d.). Grains. Retrieved from http://www.choosemyplate.gov/food-groups/grains.html. Accessed August 12, 2013.

Since 1970, grain and cereal consumption increased by almost 60 pounds a year per person, and consumption of caloric sweeteners increased by 30 pounds. Sugar consumption in soft drinks increased 135% between 1977 and 2001. These changes in food consumption paralleled a meteoric rise in obesity and diabetes in the United States.[80]

Refined grain sources, such as white rice, white bread, pasta, and processed breakfast cereals, are generally low-fiber and high-glycemic. They cause a rapid increase in blood glucose (sugar) levels, and stimulate a strong insulin response to remove the excess glucose from the blood.[81] Over time, repeated spikes in insulin levels can make cells insulin resistant, leading to impaired carbohydrate metabolism and high blood sugar levels. This can eventually lead to **metabolic syndrome** and type 2 diabetes.[82]

Choosing fruits, vegetables, and whole grains, such as whole wheat, oats, and brown rice, may help in weight control and NCD prevention.[83] They provide dietary fiber, thus lowering their glycemic index and allowing a slower release of glucose into the bloodstream. Their slow digestion and greater bulk delay the return of hunger.[84] Fruits and vegetables also have higher water contents that help fill the stomach without adding calories. As people increase their intake of these high-fiber foods, they are likely to cut back on less nutritious, high-calorie foods.[85]

Research using biochemical and brain imaging techniques has found that obese individuals appear to have higher desire for high-fat and high-sugar foods. In theory, like addictions to tobacco, narcotics, and alcohol, eating these foods can change brain chemistry and create cravings. Some animal studies confirm this biochemical mechanism and have also showed that even prenatal exposure can pass the unhealthy food cravings on to offspring.[86] However, the food "addiction" theory is not yet proven.

Individual Weight Management Strategies

Healthcare providers can monitor patient BMI and follow-up when necessary, and provide or refer patients for weight management counseling. Earlier detection and treatment of weight problems makes weight control far easier. In addition, delaying treatment can allow deleterious health effects of obesity to manifest.[87] Simply suggesting that the patient "lose some weight" and providing a sample diet sheet is effective in helping people to lose weight.[88] However, many physicians, especially if overweight themselves, hesitate to discuss weight loss with their patients.[89] Specialized exercise programs can be necessary, since excess body weight and related NCDs can make most movement painful or uncomfortable.

Public Health Core Competency 3: Communication Skills 1: Identifies the health literacy of populations serve

Weight loss is a $40 billion annual industry in the United States, although the prevalence of obesity in the United States continues to rise. Americans want products that cause rapid weight loss but do not require behavior change; however, this kind of weight loss is unsustainable in the long term.[90] Weight loss diets are often unsuccessful; on average, half of lost weight is regained after a year.[91]

Achieving and maintaining a healthy weight must include lifelong changes in the types and amounts of foods consumed and increased levels of physical activity. Individuals are more likely to be successful in changing their behaviors when their home, work, community, and social environments encourage and support both healthy eating and daily exercise. Governmental and organizational policies that support those changes can motivate individuals to make and sustain positive changes to health habits.[92]

Box 17-2 Weight management case study

Clinical History

Linda is a 42-year-old-woman whose doctor referred her to a dietitian following diagnoses of metabolic syndrome, hypertension, and overweight. Her blood pressure was 145/92, her triglycerides were 240 mg/dL, HDL cholesterol was 43 mg/dL, and blood glucose was 124 mg/dL. Linda had gained 23 pounds in the past five years. The physician prescribed hydrochlorothiazide for hypertension, and advised dietary changes to address her weight, dyslipidemia, and onset of metabolic syndrome to prevent diabetes and cardiovascular disease. Her family medical history is not remarkable. Linda has recent complaints of excessive fatigue, but no other complaints or medical findings.

Nutrition History

Linda is married with two teenage children and works full-time day shifts as a hospital nurse. She was normal weight through school. She gained weight through two pregnancies, and continued her weight gain over the past 18 years. She lost 15 pounds eight years ago, while on Weight Watchers, but she said she quit because she did not have time to follow the meal plans or go to weekly meetings. She started to gain back weight in the months after her mother passed away four years ago.

Anthropometric Findings

HT 5' 7", 184 lbs. (BMI of 28.8). Waist circumference 38" (high risk).

Dietary Assessment Summary

Notes from her 24-hour dietary recall and food frequency included:

- irregular meal patterns
- often skips breakfast or picks up fast-food breakfast en route to work
- lunches typically in hospital cafeteria—hamburger or sandwich, occasional salad
- dinner as a family meal three times per week due to children's and parents' activities
- feels she does not have time to cook "real" food
- eats meals out or uses take out at least three times a week
- daily meat/protein servings appear more than adequate
- consumes adequate servings of dairy (three servings most days)
- has only three servings of fruits and vegetables daily
- daily servings of bread, cereal, and starchy food servings were high, and none were whole grain
- infrequent desserts with meals, but keeps ice cream for evening snack two to three times per week
- uses sugar substitute in coffee
- takes multivitamin with added calcium

Assessment

Linda is at upper range of overweight category and is at high risk of becoming obese and developing diabetes if present caloric intake and dietary patterns continue without increased physical activity. Dietary intake and low activity also contribute to hyperlipidemia and increased risk for heart disease as well as failure to control hypertension. Caloric intake estimated at 2,200 kcalories, accounting for gradual continued weight gain as physical activity levels are fairly low. Sodium intake is likely high due to use of processed foods and frequent restaurant meals. Through her training as a nurse and time at Weight Watchers, Linda understands the basics of good nutrition and its impact on her health status and knows she could be making better food choices. Work and family time stressors contribute to her feeling she does not have the time to prepare healthier meals.

(continues)

Box 17-2 Weight management case study (*continued*)

Dietary Intervention Plan

Discuss contributing factors to weight gain and that at present caloric intake and activity levels she will continue to gain weight and move into the obese weight category. Discuss the quality of her food choices and the need to increase servings of fruits, vegetables, and whole grains and decrease intake of refined carbohydrates and high-fat and fried foods. Reinforce importance of adequate intake of good sources of potassium to offset losses from hypertension medication. Discuss the importance of eating a healthier breakfast and having more meals prepared at home. Emphasize social and health benefits to entire family of eating home-prepared meals together. Plan a week of quick-to-prepare meals that reflect healthy dietary guidelines for meals and snacks. Discuss heart-healthy food preparation methods and use of monounsaturated fats. Encourage increased time on treadmill of at least 30 minutes, four times a week, and walking outdoors for 30 minutes one or two times a week. Request that patient keep food journal noting types and amount of foods eaten. Provide a MyPlate placemat as reminder of proportions of food groups to include at meals.

Follow-Up

Linda returned in one month to assess weight status, review food diary, and develop strategies to overcome any problems encountered in making dietary changes. Linda was pleased by four-pound weight loss. She had an increased number of meals prepared at home and was eating breakfast five times a week. She reported increased fruit and vegetable servings to six a day and had fewer servings of simple carbohydrate foods. Linda had increased her time on the treadmill to four times a week, but was still not walking outdoors. She was surprised to find she could prepare suggested healthy meals in about 20 minutes, which was less time than it took to go out to eat. Lab values will be retested in another month at follow-up visit with physician to assess effect of dietary improvements and weight loss on blood pressure, blood sugar, and triglycerides. Nutrition counseling will continue monthly to help Linda continue to lose weight and make healthier food choices.

Weight Loss (Bariatric) Surgery for Morbid Obesity

Weight loss or bariatric surgery is an option for morbidly obese individuals who have been unable to lose weight with dietary changes. Multiple types of bariatric surgery can effectively reduce stomach size and limit the volume of food that can be eaten, leading to lower calorie consumption and rapid weight loss. Some types of bariatric surgery induce nutrient malabsorption as well. Side effects of bariatric surgery may include acute or chronic vomiting, nausea, nutrient deficiencies, and more serious complications leading to additional surgeries or mortality. Diabetes is often resolved after gastric bypass surgery. In general, to be eligible for weight loss surgery, individuals must have made multiple previous efforts to lose weight with diet and exercise that were unsuccessful, have a BMI over 40 (morbid obesity), or a BMI over 35 accompanied by a serious weight-related morbidity, such as type 2 diabetes, high blood pressure, or severe sleep apnea.

The long-term success of any type of gastric bypass surgery depends on the patient's ability to make permanent dietary changes. Patients can negate the benefits of the surgery by sipping large quantities of high-calorie liquids or by chronically overeating to stretch the reduced stomach size.[93]

Dietary Guidelines for Adult Populations

Dietary guidelines are science-based guidance on diets to promote health and reduce the risk of NCDs. In contrast to DRIs, which are nutrient values, dietary guidelines are food-based, with information on the types and amounts of foods to eat in order to maintain good health.[94] National and global dietary guidelines are developed through collaboration of governmental agencies, health organizations, and the medical and scientific community. They are used to guide public health nutrition programs and to help shape public health nutrition education and program policies.

Global Dietary Recommendations

WHO's nutrition-related concerns historically emphasized problems with undernutrition and communicable diseases in developing nations, but more recent focus is on reducing risk factors for obesity and diet-related NCDs. In 2004, WHO adopted a global strategy on diet, physical activity, and health with the goal of reducing diet-related morbidity and mortality. The main objectives include:

- *Reduce risk factors for chronic diseases* that stem from unhealthy diets and physical inactivity through public health actions.

- *Increase awareness and understanding* of the influences of diet and physical activity on health and the positive impact of preventive interventions.

- *Develop, strengthen, and implement global, regional, and national policies and action plans* to improve diets and increase physical activity that are sustainable, comprehensive, and actively engage all sectors.

- *Monitor science and promote research* on diet and physical activity.[95]

WHO's scientific reports on nutrition needs in populations worldwide also examine relationships between diet and physical activity patterns and the major nutrition-related chronic diseases. WHO recommendations are intended to assist in the development of regional strategies and national guidelines to reduce the burden of nutrition-related diseases.[96]

> *Public Health Core Competency 6: Basic Public Health Science Skills 1: Describes the scientific foundation of the field of public health*

International Dietary Guidelines

FAO maintains a database of **Food-Based Dietary Guidelines** from various countries. National dietary guidelines have similar messages based on nutrition science, but vary in level of detail and also address the specific nutrition needs and priorities of individual countries.[97] For example, population-wide recommendations in Namibia's dietary guidelines include:

- Eat a variety of foods.
- Eat vegetables and fruit every day.
- Eat more fish.

- Eat beans or meat regularly.
- Use whole-grain products.
- Use only iodized salt, but use less salt.
- Eat at least three meals a day.
- Avoid drinking alcohol.
- Consume clean and safe water and food.
- Achieve and maintain a healthy body weight.

In comparison, guidelines from China and Nigeria include more detailed age-specific recommendations. Dietary guidelines from Japan include similar global messages about energy balance and moderating sodium intake, but place greater emphasis on dietary diversity and making eating a pleasurable social activity in the home, with recommendations to "appreciate home cooking" and "use the mealtime as an occasion for family communication."

U.S. Dietary Guidelines

Since 1980, the Department of Health and Human Services (DHHS) and the USDA have jointly published *Dietary Guidelines for Americans*. Public law requires the *Guidelines* to be reviewed, updated, and published every five years.[98,99] These science-based guidelines focus on promoting health and reducing the risk of developing NCDs in Americans over age 2. Dietary guidelines are intended for populations, and are not always appropriate for a specific individual.[100] The *Dietary Guidelines* influence federal food and nutrition education and assistance programs, and are among the government's strategies to achieve the *Healthy People 2020* objectives related to nutrition and weight management.[101]

The 2010 *Dietary Guidelines for Americans* offer three major dietary goals and recommend eating more of and less of specific types of foods. The main goals are:

- Balance calories with physical activity to manage weight.

- Consume more of certain foods and nutrients, such as fruits, vegetables, whole grains, fat-free and low-fat dairy products, and seafood.

- Consume fewer foods with sodium (salt), saturated fats, trans fats, cholesterol, added sugars, and refined grains.

New recommendations in 2010 advise increased intake of seafood; eating breakfast; choosing healthier snacks; limiting fast-food meals; limiting foods high in sodium, fat, and added sugars; and increasing foods high in certain nutrients, such as calcium, vitamin D, potassium, and fiber. The

Dietary Guidelines include recommendations for physical activity, and call for system-level changes and coordinated efforts to support healthier lifestyles.

MyPlate to Guide Consumers

In 2011, the USDA introduced MyPlate, a nutrition education tool to assist the public in following the *Dietary Guidelines*.[102] The graphic shows the recommended proportions of food on a dinner plate; half the meal is from fruits and vegetables, and one-fourth each is from grains, and meat, fish, poultry, or meat substitute. A glass represents one serving from the dairy group (**Figure 17-5**).

The MyPlate educational campaign includes seven dietary recommendations.

Balancing Calories

- Enjoy your food, but eat less.
- Avoid oversized portions.

Foods to Increase

- Make half your plate fruits and vegetables.
- Make at least half your grains whole grains.
- Switch to fat-free or low-fat (1%) milk.

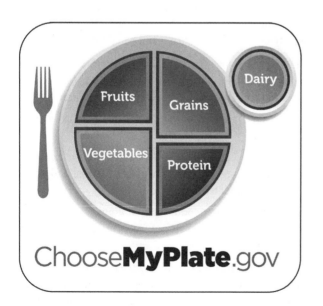

Figure 17-5 MyPlate

Courtesy of USDA.

Foods to Reduce

- Compare sodium in foods like soup, bread, and frozen meals, and choose the foods with lower numbers.
- Drink water instead of sugary drinks.[103]

The Impact of Dietary Guidelines

National and world nutrition guidelines have substantial impacts on policies for federal, state, and county food and nutrition programs. They also affect meal planning in residential facilities, adult day care facilities, and schools. Most nutrition program professionals and clinical staff base educational programs and counseling on the guidelines.[104]

> **Public Health Core Competency 2: Policy Development/Program Planning Skills 2: Describes how policy options can influence public health programs**

The public can become confused and skeptical with changing and conflicting messages due to advances in nutrition knowledge.[105] The public receives most nutrition messages not from government programs promoting healthy eating guidelines, but from commercial media advertising promoting specific products. The U.S. food industry spends billions of dollars annually on advertising, with the majority on processed foods and minimal amounts on fresh meat, fish, fruits, and vegetables.[106] Moderate sums are spent on advertising promoting consumption of general foods; for example, the "Pork, the other white meat" and "Got milk?" campaigns promoted non-branded foods. These media campaigns are usually cooperative efforts of the food producers and food councils. They may include governmental partners, as federal and state governments can authorize generic food promotion programs funded by food producers. Two dairy-promoting programs, authorized by Congress in 1983 and 1990, were generic advertising campaigns that stemmed from the decline in milk consumption.[107]

Mixed Media Messages on Balanced Diets and Dietary Fat

USDA guidance on the optimal balance of protein, fats, and carbohydrates for good health and weight management has changed over recent decades,[108] and commercial advertising of food and diet products, along with popular nutrition books and magazines, present to consumers conflicting information. This is especially true regarding dietary fat. Some popular weight loss diets were high-fat and low-carbohydrate, while others were low-fat and high-carbohydrate. Current dietary guidelines suggest that fats should provide one-third of daily calories, but more specific consideration of types of dietary fats is evident in recommendations that fewer than 10% of calories should come from saturated fats.[109] Further knowledge in the scientific community adds to consumer confusion.[110] Not all polyunsaturated fats are "heart healthy"; rather, the ratio of consumption of **omega-6** to **omega-3** fatty acids appears to be more important for cardiovascular health than total polyunsaturated fat intake. Most Americans consume a higher-than-recommended ratio of omega-6 to omega-3 fatty acids, which are commonly found in fish, walnuts, and flaxseed.[111] Monounsaturated fats, such as those in olive and peanut oils, are likely to be the healthiest choices for added fats, such as cooking oils. Consumption of monounsaturated fats is associated with lower risks of heart disease and other chronic disease risk factors, as seen in Mediterranean regions where intake is high. To further complicate matters, the fat profile of meat and dairy products can vary depending on the animal's diet. Pasture-fed beef cattle have a healthier fat composition, with less saturated fat, than confined cattle fattened on corn.[112]

Factors Influencing Personal Food Choices

Governmental guidelines promoting healthy eating appear to have only a limited direct effect on the dietary choices people make every day. Fewer than half of Americans are aware of the *Dietary Guidelines,* and though the vast majority of adults report that nutrition is important when buying food and say that they know how to choose healthy foods, 2004 surveys suggest that these intentions are not usually reflected in their eating habits.[113]

Although higher education is associated with healthier eating habits, nutrition education by itself has not been significantly correlated with better eating habits. Adults eat for a variety of biological, social, cultural, and psychological reasons other than hunger, and what foods they may choose to eat is affected by even more factors. Cost, income, the type of food available, access to a kitchen and food preparation skills, time to shop and prepare food, and personal health all influence an individual's food choices.[114,115] In addition, preference for sweet-tasting foods is innate.[116] Adding sugars, fats, and salt to processed packaged foods and fast foods increases consumer acceptance.[117]

Childhood eating patterns are strong predictors of adult eating habits. As adults, family and friends' food preferences can also exert a strong influence on food choices. Lack of support of family and friends, higher cost, and time constraints are barriers to purchasing and preparing healthy foods, such as fresh produce.[118] Changes in family structure, with greater proportions of families with both parents working and more single-parent households, have contributed to fewer meals being prepared at home and more food purchased ready to eat.[119]

What is considered edible varies among cultures and religions. These dietary habits may change with assimilation,[120] although cultural factors continue to influence dietary choices. For example, individuals may be nonobservant in practicing the Jewish faith of their parents, but they may still avoid eating some foods, such as pork, prohibited by the **kosher** dietary laws. In addition, food is part of celebrations and social events worldwide, and activities such as watching television or going to sports events trigger food consumption beyond biological hunger.

Adult consumer choices can be positively influenced by information on healthier food choices at the site where they purchase food.[121] The 2010 *Dietary Guidelines for Americans* recognized the role of food environment in consumer dietary choices, and recommended placing **point-of-purchase** cues in supermarkets to remind consumers to select healthier food items.[122] Placing these educational messages throughout supermarkets is a cost-effective way to reach the consumer, though whether these messages significantly change food choices made by American consumers is yet to be determined. Menu labeling and identifying "heart-healthy" and lower-calorie selections on menus also is yet to be confirmed as an effective way to help consumers make better food choices.[123] Cost is a major factor influencing food choice, and subsidizing healthier menu selections so they cost the same or less than less-healthy options can be effective in worksite and other settings;[124] this may not be feasible in many food service venues without aid.

Background on Changes in the U.S. Food Supply and Their Effect on Global Food Consumption Patterns

While each region has its own specific variations, overall, diets worldwide are increasingly energy-dense as processed foods replace whole grains, fruits, and vegetables as staples.[125,126] The United States was among the first nations to experience these changes, which result from multiple factors, such as cheaper food, more disposable income, and more food assistance. American dietary habits have been affected by convenience foods, globalization, food marketing, nutrient fortification, and demographic trends, such as an aging population, more two-income and single-parent households, and greater ethnic diversity.[127]

Circumstances surrounding World War II precipitated many of these trends. In 1941, the U.S. government assessed nutrients in the nation's food supply to evaluate the country's food resources affecting the population's health and readiness for war.[128] Continued nutrient estimates assess the capacity of the U.S. food supply to meet the nation's nutritional needs and analyze dietary trends.[129]

Changes in Food Production Methods Following World War II

Advances in food industry technology, the availability of cheap fossil fuel for the refrigeration and transport of foods, more food safety regulations, and federal food policies subsidizing key food crops widely increased the supply of a wide variety of safe, low-cost foods. The number of different food products offered in U.S. supermarkets increased from 7,800 in 1970 to 38,718 by 2010.[130] Processed products contributing to the increase include sauces, canned soups, packaged mixes, breakfast cereals, frozen meals, and beverages.

The low cost of these products is partly due to government **subsidies** of corn, wheat, soy, and dairy farm products. Subsidies reduce the cost of raw products for the food industry, which passes the savings to consumers. Similarly, the purchase of surplus corn and soy commodities by beef, dairy, and poultry producers lowers production costs and costs to the consumer. Concern has been raised about whether food subsidies encourage less healthy diets.[131]

Increased Use of Infant Formula

Infant formula, or breast milk substitute, is another convenience product that was aggressively marketed. Lay and medical communities believed that formula was at least as good as human milk. Science later provided overwhelming evidence to the contrary, and most public health breastfeeding promotion campaigns were discontinued by the late 20th century.[132] Only one-fourth of newborns in the

United States were breastfed at the time of hospital discharge in the late 1940s.[133]

The decline in breastfeeding may have contributed to the relatively poor health of the baby boomer generation. Breastfed infants have higher cholesterol levels than formula-fed infants, but people who were breastfed as infants have been found to maintain lower cholesterol levels throughout adulthood.[134,135]

> *Public Health Core Competency 6: Basic Public Health Science Skills 2: Identifies prominent events in the history of the public health profession*

U.S. Farm Policies Indirectly Subsidize High-Calorie Foods

U.S. food policy supports the low cost of calories, highlighting a conflict between government dietary guidelines and farm policy. Despite recommendations to increase consumption of vegetables and fruits, federal farm crop subsidies do not support fruits and vegetables, but commodities such as corn, soybeans, and wheat[136] that are primarily incorporated into calorie-dense food products. However, consumers often cite cost as a reason for not buying fresh produce.[137]

The lower cost per calorie of many processed foods is misleading. After adding the costs of subsidizing those foods ($261.9 billion between 1995 and 2010) and those related to the effects of large agribusiness on the environment and the use of cheap farm labor often subsidized by public welfare programs, the price of those foods is considerably higher.[138] If healthcare costs from chronic diseases attributed to consuming too much salt, sugar, and fat were added to the cost of highly processed food products, the price would be staggering.

Added Sugar in the Food Supply: Extra Calories Without Essential Nutrients

Some foods, such as fruits, beets, sugarcane, dates, and agave, are naturally somewhat sweet. However, naturally highly concentrated sugars are rare, such as in honey and maple syrup. For several hundred years, cane or beet sugar was primarily added at home to selected food, such as desserts and as a preservative for fruits and some meats. This limited use of refined sugar changed dramatically with industrialization and a drop in the price of sugar. Federal support of research increased corn crop yields, and farm subsidies for corn production further reduced the price of corn sweeteners. Foreign trade restrictions on cane sugar also made sweeteners manufactured from corn less expensive than imported and domestic cane or beet sugar.

The use of sugar became liberal, adding flavor but also **empty calories** not only to sweets, but also to processed foods such as soup and catsup.[139] Increased consumption of sugars is associated with tooth decay, metabolic syndrome, type 2 diabetes, obesity, and CVD.[140] Worldwide, the consumption of added sugars has increased threefold in the past 50 years, and the average daily intake of added sugars in the United States is 32 teaspoons. Most of the added sugar consumed per year in the United States is in processed foods and beverages.[141] Added sugars listed on food labels may include sugar, corn syrup, high-fructose corn syrup, corn sweetener, fructose, sucrose (sugar), molasses, honey, and maple syrup.

High-Fructose Corn Syrup Controversy

High-fructose corn syrup (HFCS) began to replace sugar in a continually expanding number of food products. In 2008, HFCS accounted for 39% of the 136.3 pounds per person of sweeteners available for consumption.[142] Like sucrose, or table sugar, HFCS is an added sugar without nutrients, and it has the same adverse health risks. Some individuals suspect that HFCS is less healthy than "regular" sugar. Current research is inconclusive about whether the higher ratio of HFCS is more likely to contribute to obesity or metabolic disorders than equal amounts of sucrose, or table sugar.

Public Health Core Competency 6: Basic Public Health Science Skills 7: Discusses the limitations of research findings

Changes in the Quantity and Types of Fat in Food Products

As researchers linked saturated fats and cholesterol to risk for CVD, the food industry responded by substituting vegetable-based oils rich in polyunsaturated fats for animal-based fats high in saturated fat and cholesterol. To preserve the desirable appearance and cooking properties of solid fats such as butter and lard, food manufacturers processed oils to make them partially hydrogenated, leading to the production of trans fatty acids. These became common

Nutrition Facts

Serving Size 1 cup (228g)
Servings Per Container about 2

Amount Per Serving

Calories 250   Calories from Fat 110

% Daily Value*

Total Fat 12g	**18%**
Saturated Fat 3g	**15%**
Trans Fat 3g	
Cholesterol 30mg	**10%**
Sodium 470mg	**20%**
Total Carbohydrate 31g	**10%**
Dietary Fiber 0g	**0%**
Sugars 5g	
Proteins 5g	

Vitamin A	4%
Vitamin C	2%
Calcium	20%
Iron	4%

* Percent Daily Values are based on a 2,000 calorie diet. Your Daily Values may be higher or lower depending on your calorie needs:

	Calories:	2,000	2,500
Total Fat	Less than	65g	80g
Saturated Fat	Less than	20g	25g
Cholesterol	Less than	300mg	300mg
Sodium	Less than	2,400mg	2,400mg
Total Carbohydrate		300g	375g
Dietary Fiber		25g	30g

For educational purposes only. This label does not meet the labeling requirements described in 21 CFR 101.9.

Figure 17-6 Sample nutrition label that conforms to the Nutrition Labeling and Education Act of 1994

Reproduced from the U.S. Food and Drug Administration. Food: Nutrition Facts Label. http://www.fda.gov/Food/IngredientsPackagingLabeling/LabelingNutrition/ucm114155.htm. Accessed September 6, 2013.

in snack foods and fast food. The industry began efforts to remove trans fats from products in 2007 with increasing evidence that trans fats are likely the most harmful fats for the heart.[143]

Social and Economic Changes After World War II

The last half of the 20th century saw an increased consumer demand for convenience foods[144] and a significant increase in the proportion of foods consumed outside the home. These changes are partly due to social and economic changes following World War II.

During World War II, women increasingly entered the workforce. The average number of hours worked per week also increased. Increased consumer expectations fueled the perceived need for two incomes. Larger homes, more appliances, air conditioning, and owning two cars added to the pressure of maintaining two full-time incomes, leaving less time for shopping and home food preparation.

Foods Away from Home and Fast Food

The amount and frequency of food eaten away from home is increasing. Currently, over half of all Americans eat out on a given day, although individuals over 60 eat out less often.[145] Food consumed away from home claimed half of the average food budget and provided almost one-third of total calories consumed from 1994 to 1996, an 18% increase over 20 years. Longer work hours and commutes have decreased frequency of eating breakfast and lunch at home.[146] Meals at restaurants and fast-food venues are usually larger and higher in fat, salt, and added sugars.

McDonald's now has restaurants in 179 countries, and its golden arches are the most recognized symbol in the world.[147] Nearly all small towns offer one or more fast-food options.[148] By now, fast-food franchises have expanded into many schools, universities, public attractions, airports, and even hospitals. Fast-food meals are routine for many people, and drive-throughs even allow diners to eat without exiting the car. Foods typically offered at fast-food restaurants are generally high in calories, fat, and sugar, and low in nutrients. Young adults who eat frequently at fast-food restaurants gain more weight and have increased insulin resistance by early middle age.[149,150]

Concerns About Toxins in Foods Create Organic Movement

World War II was also pivotal for U.S. agriculture. Chemicals developed for war use were used in insecticides, with the invention of DDT in 1939. These toxins reduce crop loss due to insects and plant diseases. By the 1960s, however, U.S. consumer concerns about the increasing use of food additives and pesticide residues, along with a desire to improve the overall quality and taste of foods, created a demand for organically produced foods and fueled the green movement with its focus on environmental issues.[151] The **organic** movement had begun in Europe early in the 20th century as a countermovement to the increasing industrialization of agriculture.

Until the 1990s, organically produced food products were sold primarily in small health food stores or directly from farms. By the end of the 20th century, a variety of fresh, frozen, and canned organic foods were available in chain supermarkets, albeit usually at a higher shelf cost than similar nonorganic food products. Sales of organic food and beverages in the United States increased from $1 billion in 1990 to $26.7 billion in 2010 but still account for only approximately 4% of the sale of food and beverages.[152]

Food Availability in the 21st Century

Food Scarcity in the Midst of Adequate Food Stores Worldwide

Access to sufficient, affordable food remains a global concern. In 2010, hunger affected nearly one in seven of the world's population, with nearly all of these people living in underdeveloped counties. Chronic hunger is almost always tied to poverty, and acute shortages can result from war, civil disruption, and natural disasters.[153,154] Lack of support for local agriculture in poor areas, volatility in food costs,[155] and political turmoil can worsen food shortages and prevent distribution of emergency food supplies to the most needy.

Global food production is sufficient to feed everyone in the world, but distribution is inadequate. In 2011, FAO reported that an estimated one-third of food produced worldwide for human consumption (1.3 billion tons) is lost during production, transport, and manufacturing levels or is wasted at the retail or consumer levels. Consumers in wealthier countries account for the preponderance of waste and annually throw away almost as much food as the entire net food production of sub-Saharan Africa.[156,157,158]

Differences in the Proportion of Income Needed to Purchase Food

The proportion of income needed to purchase sufficient food varies considerably worldwide. As a nation's or individual's wealth decreases, the percentage of disposable income that must be spent on food increases, making higher food commodity prices in poorer counties devastating. Not only do Americans have a higher average income than people in most other countries, but they also spend the smallest percentage of their income on food (**Figure 17-7**). Americans on average spend 6% of income on food. The French spend 14%, and poorer populations, such as those in India and Kenya, spend one-third to almost one-half of their incomes on food.[159] These percentages vary within countries, and low-income households spend a higher percentage than the average. Low-income U.S. households spend 30% of income on food.

Contributing to the ability of Americans to spend less money on food is the low cost of food in the United States compared with many other nations. Unfortunately, unhealthier food items are most likely to be low cost. From 1985 to 2000, the prices of fresh fruits and vegetables rose 40%, while prices of fats and soft drinks decreased by 15% and 25%, respectively. On a per-calorie basis, energy-dense foods are 10% of the price of more nutritious foods, such as fruits and vegetables.[160] Besides cost, accessibility affects food choices. Many low-income individuals are residents of **food deserts**.[161] These areas are without full-service supermarkets, and residents rely on small convenience stores with little or no produce, and poorer selections of

other items, such as dairy products, at higher costs than supermarkets.

Current Data and Trends on Nutrition Status

Monitoring the Dietary Intake and Nutritional Status of Populations

"Nutritional surveillance" means "to watch over nutrition." Nutrition surveillance systems typically monitor the prevalence of malnutrition and provide dietary intake and clinical data to assist in long-term program planning and program evaluation. Data collected can also uncover concerning trends, such as food shortages or poor nutritional status. Nutrition surveillance information may include nutritional outcome indicators, such as the prevalence of iron-deficiency anemia in a particular population. It may also collect data from other sources indirectly related to nutrition status, such as crop and water supplies.[162] WHO compiles national, regional, and local information on the prevalence of anemia and deficiencies of iron, vitamin A, and iodine. Differences in methodologies can lead to some inconsistency in the data and interpretation of the data by individual countries and nongovernmental organizations (NGOs).[163]

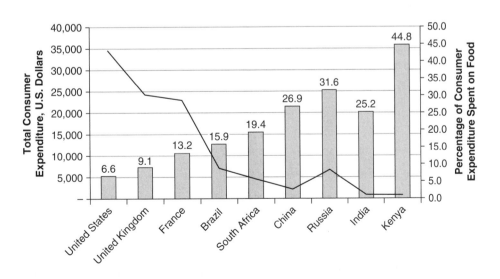

Figure 17-7　The poor spend a high percentage of their income on food

Data from USDA. (2013). Percent of household food consumption spent on food, alcoholic beverages, and tobacco that were consumed at home, by selected countries, 2012. http://www.ers.usda.gov/data-products/food-expenditures.aspx#26654. Accessed September 5, 2013.

Nutrition Surveillance in the United States

The largest nutrition surveillance survey in the United States is the **National Health and Nutrition Examination Survey (NHANES)**, which includes a detailed phone survey on the health and dietary habits of individuals from all states. The survey uses two-year data collection cycles to provide sufficient sample sizes for analysis.[164] The USDA uses **food availability** data to estimate the nation's food consumption. Overall, Americans consume more than adequate amounts of grain and meat products, but less than recommended levels of vegetables, dairy, and fruit products (**Figure 17-8**).[165]

The average American today eats 47 more pounds of poultry, seven more pounds of red meat, and four more pounds of fish per year than in the 1950s. Total grain consumption is high, but only 7% of the population reported meeting recommendations for whole-grain products. Less than one-fourth of adults eat five servings of fruits and vegetables daily.[166]

Based on NHANES data, Americans have adequate intakes of carbohydrates, selenium, niacin, and riboflavin. Nutrients of concern for men and women are vitamins A, C, and K, as well as magnesium, potassium, calcium, and dietary fiber. Intakes of iron and folate may be low in

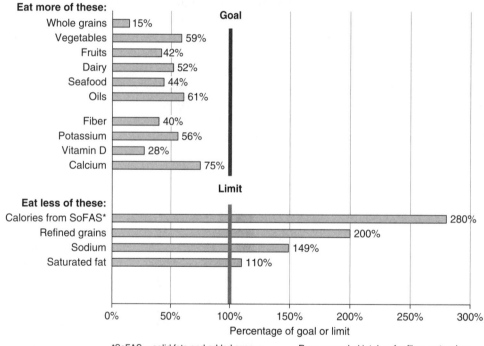

Usual Intake as a Percentage of Goal or Limit

*SoFAS = solid fats and added sugars.
Note: Bars show average intakes for all individuals (ages 1 or 2 years or older, depending on the data source) as a percent of the recommended intake level or limit. Recommended intakes for food groups and limits for refined grains and solid fats and added sugars are based on amounts in the USDA 2000-calorie food pattern.

Recommended intakes for fiber, potassium, vitamin D, and calcium are based on the highest AI or RDA for ages 14 to 70 years. Limits for sodium are based on the UL and for saturated fat on 10% of calories. The protein foods group is not shown here because, on average, intake is close to recommended levels.

Figure 17-8 How do typical american diets compare to recommended intake levels or limits?

Reproduced from Department of Health and Human Services and Department of Agriculture. *Dietary Guidelines for Americans, 2010.* 7th Edition, Washington, DC: US Government Printing Office, 2010. http://www.health.gov/dietaryguidelines/dga2010/DietaryGuide lines2010.pdf. Accessed August 28, 2013.

women. Dietary intake data from NHANES do not include intake of multivitamins, which could considerably affect the proportion of groups at risk.[167,168]

Alcohol Use

Each year, the average American consumes 9.44 liters of alcohol, or half of the per capita consumption in countries with the highest rates. Half of U.S. adults are categorized as regular alcohol users, based on the CDC's criterion of having at least 12 drinks in the past year.[169] This is a modest amount, and not useful in assessing excess consumption. Of more concern is that that 17% of U.S. adults report binge drinking, with an average of eight drinks per binge. Excessive alcohol consumption is associated with accidents and health conditions, including cancers of the mouth, throat, esophagus, liver, colon, and breast; liver diseases; and certain cardiovascular, neurological, psychiatric, and gastrointestinal health problems.[170] Since moderate consumption of alcoholic beverages, particularly red wine, may confer cardiovascular health benefits, the *Dietary Guidelines for Americans* advise "if you drink alcoholic beverages, do so in moderation," which is defined as no more than one drink per day for women and no more than two drinks per day for men. Alcoholic drinks provide significant calories without offering any essential nutrients to the diet.[171] For some people these added calories contribute to unwanted weight gain. A 12-ounce beer has 150–200 calories, 5 ounces of wine has 120 calories, and a mixed drink such as a 7-ounce gin and tonic has 200 calories. Added sugars and juices in mixed drinks further increase calorie content.[172]

Use of Dietary Supplements

Dietary supplements are increasingly common in the United States and other developed countries. Over half of American adults take supplements, and the supplement industry is a $61 billion industry,[173] previously dominated by multivitamin/mineral supplements for children and pregnant women. Multivitamin/mineral products remain most common, but many adults also take a variety of supplements. Supplemental calcium use has increased in older women, folic acid supplementation has increased in younger women, and vitamin D supplement use has increased in most age groups. Individuals should inform healthcare providers about all of their dietary supplements.[174]

The FDA regulates dietary supplement products not as foods or drugs, but under less stringent regulations resulting from the Dietary Supplement Health Education Act (DSHEA). Under DSHEA, supplement manufacturers are responsible for ensuring the safety and efficacy of supplements. To prevent supplements from being classified and regulated as drugs, manufacturers may not market supplements as treatments or cures for diseases.[175] However, the FDA permits certain health claims, such as for the cardiovascular benefits of omega-3 fatty acids.[176] Proper use of certain supplements can potentially lead to substantial cost savings from disease prevention.[177]

Drug Nutrient Interactions

Over-the-counter and prescription medications can interfere with nutrient digestion and absorption, appetite, and energy metabolism. Almost half of Americans, including 90% of older adults, take at least one prescribed drug; 31% of Americans take two or more; and 10% take at least five medications.[178] The most commonly prescribed drugs in the United States are analgesics, statins for lowering blood cholesterol, and antidepressants.[179,180,181,182]

Special Nutritional Needs of Older Adults

Proper nutrition is critical for maintaining health and independence in old age. Eighty-five percent of elderly individuals living outside an institution are estimated to have one or more chronic health problems that could be improved by a better diet.[183] Aging is associated with decreased lean body mass and reduced metabolic rate. A reduction in caloric intake and/or increase in physical activity is necessary to prevent unwanted weight gain.[184] Preventing malnutrition is also a priority for maintaining functionality among older adults in or out of institutions.[185] Low income and lack of transportation often make access to nutritious foods difficult for elderly individuals.[186] Social isolation, depression, and disabilities can also affect an older individual's interest in preparing and eating a balanced diet.[187] Furthermore, health conditions may interfere with nutrient absorption and contribute to deficiencies.

Global Nutrition Strategies

WHO's Department of Nutrition for Health and Development is charged with preventing, reducing, and eliminating malnutrition worldwide (especially protein–energy malnutrition and nutrient deficiencies for vitamin A, iodine, and iron), obesity, and diet-related diseases. These strategies to address global nutrition are more focused on undernutrition and specific nutrient deficiencies than the U.S. *Healthy People 2020* objectives.[188]

Objectives of the WHO Department of Nutrition

The WHO Department of Nutrition is organized into four areas of work with the following objectives:

1. Nutrition policy and scientific advice

- Help regions and countries address nutrition challenges through evidence-based policies and actions
- Develop user-friendly databases and decision-making tools
- Provide scientific advice on diet and health

2. Growth assessment and surveillance

- Set child growth standards and develop measurement tools
- Collect and share information on nutritional status

3. Micronutrients

- Monitor the vitamin and mineral status of populations globally
- Help Member States and their partners design and implement effective strategies to achieve vitamin and mineral balance in diets
- Advocate for the importance of vitamins and minerals in health and nutrition

4. Nutrition in the life course

- Improve maternal, infant, and young child nutrition
- Help countries prevent and treat malnutrition using evidence-based guidance
- Support nutrition action in emergencies
- Promote adequate nutrition for people affected by infections such as HIV/AIDS or tuberculosis[189]

Development of Global Policies and Strategies to Address Obesity

The International Obesity Task Force (IOTF) is a policy and advocacy "think tank," composed of scientists and health experts, within the International Association for the Study of Obesity (IASO). It was created in 1996 to report on the global obesity epidemic for WHO.[190] A follow-up report offered broad policy and environmental strategies at all levels of society to prevent obesity and improve nutritional health.

The objectives of the IOTF are related to:

1. policy and leadership development needed for obesity prevention,
2. facilitating knowledge exchange systems between individuals and organizations working in obesity prevention,
3. supporting research, training, and projects to advance obesity prevention, and
4. advocating for evidence-based obesity prevention policies at national, regional, and global levels.

To help identify best practices in obesity prevention and facilitate information exchange on effective strategies, the IOTF identified England as the world's leader on obesity prevention because of its obesity surveillance systems, control of marketing of unhealthy food to children, movement to reformulate processed foods to make them healthier, nutrition labeling methods, and targeted social marketing campaigns to increase public awareness and action to prevent obesity.[191]

U.S. Federal and State Strategies to Promote Good Nutrition and Weight Management

In 1980, the U.S. government began developing 10-year objectives, known as Healthy People, for improving the health of Americans. Healthy People collaborators include the CDC, the National Institutes of Health (NIH), and other agencies. Public comments and feedback from private and public stakeholders are solicited before objectives are finalized.[192]

> *Public Health Core Competency 5: Community Dimension of Practice Skills 9: Gathers input from the community to inform the development of public health policy and programs*

Objectives are based on scientific data and surveillance studies. Each includes benchmarks to assess progress toward meeting goals, and identifies data sources to be used in monitoring progress. The objectives are intended to encourage collaborations across communities and public and private sectors, empower individuals to make informed health decisions, and measure the impact of prevention activities.[193] Healthy People objectives offer federal agencies, states, and communities tools and resources for planning successful public health interventions to meet the objectives. A section of the Healthy People website provides specific guidance on the basics of planning and implementing public health programs using **evidence-based interventions**.[194]

> *Public Health Core Competency 5: Community Dimension of Practice Skills 7: Describes the role of governmental and nongovernmental organizations in the delivery of community health services*

In 2005, the Association of State and Territorial Public Health Nutrition Directors (ASTPHND) published a Blueprint for Nutrition and Physical Activity to provide additional state and local-level strategies for achieving the 2010 Healthy People objectives related to nutrition and weight management. The Blueprint strategies and actions are based on the Healthy People objectives and the *Dietary Guidelines for Americans*.[195]

Healthy People 2020 Nutrition and Weight Management Objectives

The following *Healthy People 2020* nutrition and weight management objectives are intended for the general population over the age of 2. The nutrition-related objectives for 2020 are categorized into five areas:

1. Healthier Food Access
2. Food Insecurity
3. Healthcare and Worksite Settings
4. Weight Status
5. Food and Nutrient Consumption

Overall, the nutrition objectives focus on the following changes:

- Increasing consumption of fruits, vegetables, whole grains, and foods high in calcium.
- Decreasing consumption of added sugar, fats, and sodium.
- Decreasing the prevalence of obesity and increasing efforts to prevent obesity.
- Increasing the number of healthcare providers measuring BMI, and counseling obese patients on healthy eating and exercise.

- Increasing the number of worksites that offer nutrition or weight management education or counseling.
- Improving consumer access to healthy foods at the retail level and reducing the number of people without resources to purchase sufficient food.[196]

Progress Toward Achieving *Healthy People 2020* Objectives

In 2011, the DHHS reported that 23% of the 733 *Healthy People 2010* objectives had been met. Little progress was made toward meeting nutrition and weight targets. The proportion of obese adults actually increased from 23% at baseline to 34%.[197]

The Healthy People objectives outline a national health improvement strategy and influence policy makers and programs. Federal, state, and local agencies can use the Healthy People objectives to guide their agency strategic plans and align their budgets to address the objectives, but the objectives do not come with a guarantee that funds will be made available to support programs designed to meet objectives.[198]

Factors and components needed as part of a strategy to achieve the desired goals (outcomes) include health determinants, interventions, assessment, monitoring, and program evaluation actions needed to achieve behavior changes and reduce health risks (**Figure 17-9**).

Public Health Nutrition Infrastructure

Global Public Health Organizations

Public health infrastructure, from the community level through the global level, has the primary leadership role in preventing and managing public health concerns through surveillance and the promotion of healthy behaviors and communities and environments that support healthy behaviors. WHO is the agency within the UN that coordinates global public health initiatives. WHO's Department of Nutrition for Health and Development focuses on global nutrition concerns.[199]

Public Health Organizations Within Nations

National public health systems vary in their structures of governmental agencies responsible for domestic health and

Determinants of Health

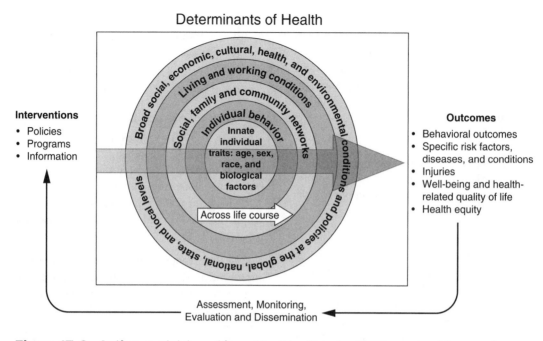

Figure 17-9   Action model to achieve *Healthy People 2020* overarching goals

Reproduced from: Department of Health and Human Services. (2008, October 28). The secretary's advisory committee on national health promotion and disease prevention objectives for 2020: Phase 1 report: recommendations for the framework and format of Healthy People 2020. http://healthypeople.gov/2020/about/advisory/Phase1.pdf. Accessed August 28, 2013.

nutrition programs. Public health infrastructure and range of programs and services remain vastly different between industrialized and developing countries. The poorest countries lack resources to provide even basic public health prevention programs.

The U.S. Department of Health and Human Services is the main federal body responsible for protecting the health of Americans. The DHHS funds many services through grants to state, county, and private-sector agencies. The DHHS consists of 11 divisions, including the U.S. Public Health Service under the U.S. Surgeon General, the CDC, and the NIH.[200] State and local health departments conduct surveillance and implement public health programs, although administration of public health programs varies widely between states. Only 30% of U.S. states have centralized structures in which state staff oversee local programs and services, and the state retains control over budget decisions. Many states have decentralized structures with nearly complete localized autonomy, except in limited areas where the state has statutory authority. In all states, federal allocations are the largest source of state public health revenue for most programs.[201]

> *Public Health Core Competency 7: Financial Planning and Management Skills 1: Describes the local, state, and federal public health and health care systems*

Designing Public Health Programs and Services to Meet Nutrition Objectives

Overview of Public Health Nutrition Programs

Public health nutrition efforts focus on high-risk populations and on major concerns, such as malnutrition and obesity.[202] Most early nutrition programs were part of maternal and child programs to ensure adequate nutrition for high-risk pregnant women and young children. Efforts in the 19th century built a foundation for public health nutrition services to address infant and childhood morbidity and mortality. By 1980, public health programs expanded to focus on health promotion and disease prevention throughout the life cycle. Separate adult or community health programs began to emerge in state public health agencies. New programs were also developed to focus on nutrition, physical activity, and tobacco, and to assist the chronically ill and disabled, older adults, and recent immigrant populations. Graduate-level nutrition training programs and professional practice standards and guidelines were established. Public health nutrition leadership focused on nutrition policy, program planning, and evaluation of public health nutrition programs.[203]

Public health nutrition policy makers and program administrators must consider various factors when developing strategies to effectively address nutrition objectives. Some considerations include:

1. What public and private policies and intervention programs would most effectively encourage individuals to choose more healthful foods and fewer unhealthful foods?

2. What types of public and private policies and programs would be cost-effective strategies to help change the community and work environments to encourage and support people making healthier food choices every day?

3. What are the diverse cultural factors that might affect the impact of any public health nutrition program?

4. What public and private policies and programs would be most effective in ensuring that the poor have access to sufficient amounts of healthy food?

> *Public Health Core Competency 4: Financial Planning and Management Skills 13: Describes how cost-effectiveness, cost-benefit, and cost-utility analyses affect programmatic prioritization and decision making*

Developing Effective Public Health Nutrition Programs

Public health professionals often use models that can guide development of programs that can lead to desired positive behavior changes among large numbers of individuals. The socioecological model, for example, can be used to describe how food choices are influenced by a complex interaction of factors at various levels, including personal (taste, physiology, knowledge, and skills), social (friends and family), cultural (norms and beliefs), and environmental (organizational, community, and public policy). The socioecological approach applies a broader focus than just considering population risk factors and individual behavior change.[204]

> *Public Health Core Competency 4: Cultural Competency Skills 2: Recognizes the role of cultural, social, and behavioral factors in the accessibility, availability, acceptability, and delivery of public health services*

The multilevel approach, derived from the socioecological model, describes a strategy of program interventions at multiple vertical layers.[205] For example, in addition to a statewide media campaign with individual nutrition messages on the benefits of increasing fruit and vegetable intake, a multilevel program could also include interventions to increase access to fresh produce through state policy changes to allow roadside produce stands in urban and suburban locations and efforts to promote private organizational changes that would allow worksites to offer weekly onsite produce sales to their employees.

Multilevel interventions are most effective when they include changes to policy, such as formal and informal changes to laws, ordinance, regulations, or rules, and to the environment, such as material changes to the built, social, or economic environment.[206] This dual approach can reach the greatest number of adults at the least cost and be more effective than strategies aimed primarily at the individual level.

Evidence-Based Practice

Evidence-based practice is the gold standard for clinical and public health policy, protocols, and programs. It uses scientific research as the basis for developing public health programs that also use resources optimally.[207] Programs should be effective in the long term and should not cause significant harm. With further research and/or evaluation, interventions originally deemed effective may later be modified.

In evidence-based public health practice, decisions are made using the best available peer-reviewed quantitative and qualitative research. Data and information systems are used systematically, and program-planning frameworks, often with a foundation in behavioral science, are applied. The community is engaged in assessment and decision making, and evaluations are conducted regularly, with results disseminated to key stakeholders and decision makers.[208]

> **Public Health Core Competency 3: Communication Skills 3: Solicits community-based input from individuals and organizations**

A survey of 107 U.S. public health practitioners found that only 58% of practices in their public health agency programs were considered evidence-based. However, estimating the use of evidence-based approaches is difficult.[209]

Many evidence-based programs for improving the dietary habits of Americans include policies to promote good dietary habits and access to healthy foods, such as *Healthy People 2020*, and environmental changes to encourage healthy eating habits. For example, the work environment can be altered to encourage employees to eat healthier if the worksite cafeteria offers attractive, well-prepared healthier food options at a cost comparable to fast-food options.

The Role of Nutrition Education in Improving Dietary Habits

Assessing the impact of government-sponsored nutrition education programs remains difficult, but government accountability rules and public scrutiny are leading to a closer evaluation of the effectiveness of educational programs.[210] It appears that nutrition education on its own is less effective in changing dietary habits than if, in addition to imparting information or teaching skills, it is accompanied by strategies that (1) address beliefs and attitudes to increase motivation to change individual dietary behaviors, (2) set goals for actions to improve dietary intake, and (3) work with local policy makers, such as at the worksite or in the community, to effect environmental changes that support positive dietary changes.[211] The latter might involve getting worksites to offer healthier snack or meal options, or working with city officials to ensure that water fountains and bottled water are available at community events where soft drinks are sold. Nutrition education programs and media messages must consider a variety of factors,[212] including the provision of culturally appropriate information.[213]

Web- and computer-based nutrition education programs are emerging channels for nutrition education. They are less effective than one-on-one counseling, but can be more effective than providing printed materials, largely because computer-based programs can be interactive and can provide tailored messages to specifically address the needs and interests of the patient or consumer. Another advantage of web-based programs over printed materials is their ability to reach more individuals at a lower cost.[214]

> **Public Health Core Competency 3: Communication Skills 4: Conveys public health information using a variety of approaches**

Evaluating Public Health Nutrition Programs

Program evaluation uses a systematic process to assess the impact of programs and use that information to improve programs and services.[215] External evaluation of interventions and outcomes can assess public health programs. Such evaluations may involve **quantitative** or **qualitative evaluation**, or both. Many state and local programs lack the resources needed to fund a rigorous external evaluation process, and instead evaluate programs through internal efforts to collect and analyze program data. An advantage of evidence-based programs is that they require less rigorous evaluation.

Data may be collected to assess the effectiveness of an entire program or a specific intervention within the program. For example, in the North Carolina worksite wellness case study described earlier, changes in employees' fruit and vegetable consumption were correlated with program participation, but not to any specific component of the overall program. A separate analysis examined one intervention, a series of 15-week weight management classes. Detailed data, pre- and post-intervention, were collected to assess whether the classes promoted weight loss.

Public health nutrition program evaluation can occur at multiple levels. Process evaluation is the lowest level. The North Carolina worksite program collected and analyzed program implementation indicators, such as the number of wellness committees created, how often the committee met, and the types and numbers of activities offered. A higher level of evaluation in the study involved collecting data on changed health behaviors, such as employees reporting improved dietary habits. A more rigorous level of evaluation of the entire program would have attempted to correlate clinical evidence of improved health status (health outcomes) with employee participation in the program. This more intensive level of program evaluation is more costly and slower.

Some evaluation efforts include qualitative evidence, such as **anecdotal evidence** volunteered by program participants. The North Carolina worksite program collected employee feedback though anonymous surveys that provided testimonials of positive health outcomes. Some employee participants reported lower blood pressure or that they no longer needed their diabetes medications. Program evaluation can guide decisions on the program's future existence and any necessary modifications.

Findings from regular program evaluation can inform management and focus agency efforts on the most effective and economical ways to achieve the overall objectives of the program and agency. The CDC recommends the following steps in program evaluation:

1. *Engage all stakeholders*—those involved in program operations, those served or affected by the program, and primary users of the evaluation.

2. *Describe the program,* including the need, expected effects, activities, resources, stage, context, and logic model.

3. *Focus the evaluation design* to assess the issues of greatest concern to stakeholders while using time and resources as efficiently as possible. Consider the purpose, users, uses, questions, methods, and agreements.

4. *Gather credible evidence* (data) to strengthen evaluation judgments and the recommendations that follow. These aspects of evidence gathering typically affect perceptions of credibility: indicators, sources, quality, quantity, and logistics.

5. *Justify conclusions* by linking them to the evidence gathered and by judging them against agreed-upon values or standards set by the stakeholders. Justify conclusions on the basis of evidence using these five elements: standards, analysis/synthesis, interpretation, judgment, and recommendations.

6. *Ensure use of evaluation and share lessons learned* though design, preparation, feedback, follow-up, and dissemination.[216]

Evaluation of public health food assistance programs can include broader outcomes that indirectly impact health status. For example, in 2009 the USDA released a nine-year evaluation of its **Supplementary Nutrition Assistance Program (SNAP)**. The report concluded that SNAP reduced the poverty rate by nearly 8% in 2009 and on average lifted an individual's income by 6%.[217]

As planners design their own programs, they can review successful programs that serve as models of "best practices." Best practices are usually experience-based programs that have been evaluated and found effective. Report summaries of best practice model programs provide additional program details and anecdotal information not included in descriptions of evidence-based interventions. For example, weight management programs at worksites are considered an evidence-based strategy. Reviewing examples of programs identified as best practice models of worksite weight management programs can provide the public health program planner with practical information on how to implement effective weight-loss programs. The weight management classes offered as part of the North Carolina model worksite were identified as a best practices model by the DHHS and reported to assist other worksites in implementing similar programs.

Social Marketing Used to Promote Good Nutrition to Consumers

Public health nutrition programs can apply social marketing, which is the use of the principles and methods of commercial product and services marketing to persuade individuals to change behavior to benefit their own health, that of their family, or that of society in general. Social marketing has progressed from simple radio and television announcements and billboards to more high-tech approaches. Social marketing uses consumer research for program development and implementation. Conducting small focus groups to elicit information from health consumers is often the first step in developing media campaigns or nutrition intervention programs.[218,219]

Overview of Nutrition Assistance and Education Programs for Adults

Global Nutrition Programs to Prevent Malnutrition

Global nutrition programs increasingly must address the **double burden of nutrition** that includes undernutrition and obesity. Major micronutrient concerns include deficiencies of iron, folic acid, vitamin A, and iodine.[220] International and national governmental and nongovernmental agency programs may include nutrition assistance programs to improve the chronic situation, and emergency food relief in areas distressed by political turmoil, natural disasters, or economic situations.

Malnutrition and micronutrient deficiencies are a priority of the Global Alliance for Improved Nutrition (GAIN), established in 2002 by the UN. The foundation collaborates with governments and other agencies in 30 countries to provide 610 million people with nutritionally enriched food products.[221]

WHO's Department of Nutrition for Health and Development provides advice to regions and nations to address nutrition challenges through evidence-based policies and interventions. The department compiles global data on nutritional status, and provides guidance on maintaining adequate nutrition throughout the life cycle and in the presence of special situations such as famine and HIV or tuberculosis.

The World Food Programme (WFP) is the UN's food aid agency and is governed by a board representing 36 member states. Using donated funds, the program includes food assistance programs responding to emergency situations and community-based programs that use food assistance to help education, support economic and social development, and build capacity for self-sufficiency in poor countries.[222,223]

Nongovernmental Programs Providing Hunger Relief

Faith-based and other nonprofit international relief organizations help alleviate world hunger. These groups sponsor programs ranging from direct food aid in crisis situations to projects that promote and support sustainable agriculture in underdeveloped countries. Examples of these organizations include World Hunger Relief, Inc.,[224] Action Against Hunger,[225] Heifer International,[226] ELCA World Hunger,[227] and CARE.[228]

International Food Assistance Programs Supported by the U.S. Government

The United States has administered various international food assistance programs since World War II, and it currently funds over half of international food aid. Some

NGOs, think-tanks, UN organizations, and academics have suggested that providing funds rather than shipping food may be more cost effective; the issue can affect agricultural policy in the United States.[229]

U.S. Food Assistance Programs

The USDA Food for Progress and the McGovern–Dole International Food for Education and Child Nutrition programs provided international food assistance to more than 9.7 million people in 2012. The USDA purchases U.S. farm surplus commodities and, in Food for Progress, donates these commodities to government and nongovernmental agencies in developing countries. Revenue from the sale of the food in those countries is intended to support the introduction of expansion of free markets in the countries' farm sectors. The McGovern–Dole program uses funds raised from the sale of donated U.S. food commodities to support food security and education. Involved commodities include corn and soy products, dried potatoes and beans, rice, wheat, and vegetable oils.[230]

The **U.S. Agency for International Development (USAID)** is a governmental agency offering international support to over 100 countries to promote long-term, equitable economic development, and to advance U.S foreign policy objectives related to global health, maternal and child health, and nutrition. Programs address the root causes of hunger and poverty by supporting development of agricultural growth and providing nutrition interventions.[231]

The CDC's International Micronutrient Malnutrition Prevention and Control Program is a global effort to eliminate micronutrient malnutrition by assisting the establishment of micronutrient interventions, and building surveillance systems to monitor projects.

Federal Food Assistance Programs Within the United States

Supplemental Nutrition Assistance Program

The largest federal food assistance program is the Supplemental Nutrition Assistance Program (SNAP), formerly the Food Stamp Program. In 2012, the program provided food assistance to 46 million individuals monthly.[232]

SNAP is a federal assistance means-tested program, with an income limit of 130% of the poverty level. It is available to most low-income households of U.S. citizens and refugees. Without categorical eligibility, participants need not fall into a category, such as children, pregnant women, the elderly, or the disabled. Most college students, workers out on strike, immigrants without documentation, and certain legal immigrants regardless of income are not eligible. Individual states may modify the income eligibility criteria. To receive benefits, unemployed nondisabled and nonelderly adults must register for work and accept a job if offered. Eligibility screening occurs at the local level, and states issue an electronic benefits transfer (EBT) card that can be used for food purchases.[233]

The amount of the SNAP food assistance benefit depends on family size and income. A family of four in 2012 could receive up to $668 per month.[234] SNAP benefits can be used only to purchase food items. Originally, prepared foods were not eligible, but concern about the homeless and others not able to prepare foods expanded program approval to prepared food items. Although it provides nutrition information to participants, SNAP does not limit the types or cost of foods that may be purchased. Participants can therefore use the SNAP assistance to purchase expensive low-nutrient, high-calorie foods such as chips, candy, and soft drinks.[235] SNAP is often referenced as a barometer reflecting changes in the economy. As unemployment increases, more families apply for program assistance. As employment figures rise, fewer households participate in the program.

The Emergency Food Assistance Program (TEFAP) provides states with **commodity foods** to allocate to local agencies—usually food banks—that distribute the food to emergency food pantries providing assistance to eligible low-income households and "soup kitchens" that serve low-income individuals.[236]

The USDA **Food Security Action Resources** assist organizations working to alleviate food insecurity. The program offers guidance to help public and private program providers overcome barriers to making the nutrition assistance programs available to all of those eligible in their local communities.[237]

Food Assistance Program for Low-Income Elderly Populations

The **Elderly Nutrition Program** helps fund food and nutrition programs such as congregate meals and home-delivered meals for older Americans. The Meals On Wheels Association of America has 5,000 community-based Senior Nutrition Programs in all 50 U.S. states, as well as the U.S. Territories. These community-organized programs daily provide over one million low-cost or free hot meals per day to seniors at home and at community centers. The association has approximately two million volunteers.[238]

The **Senior Farmers' Market Nutrition Program (SFMNP)** is a categorical, means-tested program of the Food and Nutrition Services of the USDA. The program awards grants to state, territories, and tribal governments to provide coupons to low-income older Americans to purchase certain foods at farmers' markets and stands and community agriculture programs.[239]

The **Commodity Supplemental Food Program (CSFP)** is a federal program providing supplemental foods to low-income adults age 60 and over, mothers, and children. States receive commodity food and funds from the federal government and distribute them to eligible households.[240]

The **Nutrition Services Incentive Program (NSIP)** offers incentives to states and tribal nations to assist them in the delivery of nutritious meals to older adults.[241]

The **Children and Adult Care Food Program (CACFP)** provides nutrition assistance for 3.3 million children in day care and emergency shelters, and to 120,000 older adults in day care.[242]

Community Nutrition Program Partners at the local level are thousands of community organizations and agencies that partner with state and federal food and nutrition programs. For example, local Council on Aging Congregate Meal programs can apply for CACFP food assistance. Some local organizations provide food assistance to the needy independently of any state or county program. Local resources include faith-based programs, many of whom run food pantries, local Councils on Aging, and neighborhood assistance centers. Local organizations can also assist low-income people who are applying for county and state food assistance programs.

Government Nutrition Education Programs

The USDA's **Expanded Food and Nutrition Education Program (EFNEP)** assists limited-resource populations in acquiring the knowledge, skills, attitudes, and changed behavior necessary for nutritionally sound diets. The program is offered as a series of 10 to 12 hands-on learning sessions led by paraprofessional peer educators and volunteers from the community. Participants learn how to make food choices that can improve the nutritional quality of the meals they purchase and prepare for their families. County extension nutrition professionals train and supervise the program instructors. Local EFNEP programs are provided under the umbrella of one of the country's Land Grant colleges and universities. These traditionally agricultural-oriented institutions of higher learning have a special mission of reaching out to serve public needs though informal programs. These programs are typically administered through local county and regional extension offices.[243]

Public Health Nutrition and Healthy Weight Programs

The CDC develops and promotes nutrition education and obesity prevention programs and campaigns.

- The **State-Based Nutrition and Physical Activity Program** provides grants to states to support programs aimed at preventing obesity and chronic diseases.[244]
- **Fruits and Veggies—More Matters** is an initiative to assist states and communities in promoting increased consumption of fruits and vegetables.[245]
- The **Healthier Worksite Initiative** website has resources for worksite program planners at federal, state, and local levels.[246]
- The **Lean Works** website, for employees and employers, identifies science-based interventions effective in preventing and controlling obesity. For example, it identifies as "promising practices" weight loss competitions and incentives to reward employees for weight loss. Rewards can be in-kind, financial, or the honor of winning. Incentives can be used to promote screening, enrollment, compliance, and maintenance of the changes after program completion.[247]

The Michigan 4 × 4 Plan to Reduce Obesity

The state of Michigan developed the 4 × 4 Plan to reduce obesity and encourage its citizens to adopt four key health behaviors: (1) maintain a healthy diet, (2) engage in regular physical activity, (3) have an annual health exam, and (4) avoid exposure to tobacco. The statewide initiative attempts to make policy, social, and infrastructure changes.

The 4 × 4 Plan uses a multilevel approach involving:

- a multimedia public awareness campaign to reduce obesity and promote a social movement encouraging every Michigan resident to adopt the four key health behaviors.
- community coalitions throughout the state to support implementation of the plan.
- partnerships (employers, trade and professional organizations, educational system, state government agencies) to help coalitions implement the 4 × 4 Plan.
- infrastructure within the Department of Community Health to support the plan.
- efforts to identify funding to finance the plan for a projected first-year cost of $18.25 million.

Michigan's Nutrition, Physical Activity, and Obesity (NPAO) program is one component of the 4 × 4 Plan. This CDC state-based program works to prevent and control obesity and other chronic diseases through strategic public health efforts aimed at increasing the number of policies in place to support physical activity and healthful eating, increasing access to and use of environments to support healthful eating and physical activity, and increasing the number of social and behavioral approaches that complement policy and environmental strategies to promote healthful eating and physical activity.

Michigan's program encourages implementation of local and statewide interventions based on the sociolecological model, a framework that takes a more holistic approach to the obesity problem, looking at all levels of influence (societal, community, organizational, interpersonal, and individual) that can be addressed to support long-term, healthful eating and physical activity choices. This "systems approach" to overweight and obesity helps communities to develop interventions that include a wide range of individual and institutional stakeholders.

Goals of NPAO:

- Increase the consumption of fruits and vegetables
- Decrease the consumption of sugar-sweetened beverages
- Reduce the consumption of high-energy-dense foods
- Increase breastfeeding initiation, duration, and exclusivity
- Increase physical activity
- Decrease television viewing

Examples of interventions include:

Local food policy councils: Local food system stakeholders, citizens, and government officials provide ideas for public policy change to improve local food systems.

Farmers' markets: Markets are placed in neighborhoods where fruits and vegetables cannot be easily purchased. Counties enable farmers' markets to accept SNAP EBT and provide coupons for fruits and vegetables at farmers' markets.

Community gardens: Community gardens may be managed by neighborhood residents, community-based organizations, government agencies, or coalitions and are often located on vacant lots re-zoned for gardens, on school or community center property, or in parks. Some programs also teach participants about preparing food from the garden.

Emergency food sites: These provide hunger relief through food banks, food rescue programs, emergency food organizations, emergency kitchens, food pantries, and homeless shelters.

Nutrition education: The Building Healthy Communities Program provides funding to local health departments to incorporate nutrition education and physical activity promotion into their policy and environmental change interventions.

Public Health Core Competency 8: Leadership and Systems Thinking Skills 3: Participates with stakeholders in identifying key values and a shared vision as guiding principles for community action

Worksites Offer Ideal Settings for Adult Nutrition Programs

Worksites can deliver nutrition and wellness programs to a large proportion of adults. Policies to promote health can be simple and cost-free; for example, employees can be encouraged to take walks during lunch or break times. Basic programs might consist of subsidizing gym memberships for employees; other programs can include education, worksite policies, and services, such as early screening programs.

In 2013 employer-sponsored healthcare premiums were rising two to three times as fast as wages and inflation.[248] For employers, workplace wellness programs are important,

cost-effective methods to address the rising cost of providing healthcare coverage for employees increasingly impacted by NCD. The return on investment (ROI) of wellness programs can be more than two dollars for every one invested in the program.[249,250,251] Employees can see reduced out-of-pocket healthcare expenses and improved health. Another benefit of comprehensive wellness programs is that they can improve employee and recruitment retention.

Logic Models

Graphic logic models are increasingly used as part of the process of developing and evaluating public health programs. The following logic model developed for the North Carolina worksite wellness case study described earlier shows the overall design of the program and the flow of expected outcomes (**Box 17-3**). Logic models are primarily for internal use by program administrators and for academic evaluation and presentation purposes. Logic models are not generally useful in explaining the program to participants or community partners.

Public-Private Partnerships to Promote Healthy Eating

The chair of the UN Standing Committee on Nutrition (UNSCN) wrote in the 2011 UN Report on Nutrition and Business, "We are entering a new era of cooperation with new stakeholders working closely with national governments to support better nutrition in effective and innovative ways."[252] Successful food and nutrition initiatives must involve new business models and collaborative approaches that promote public- and private-sector stakeholder partnerships and engage target populations.[253]

The private sector is an important partner in nutrition programs. Businesses provide funds and bring marketing expertise and venues often lacking in public agencies. The private sector benefits from increased public exposure and markets for their products.

Some nutrition stakeholders fear conflict of interest between private and public partners. A risk for the government entity is that the public sector may perceive a certain company as better because of its involvement with the government, even though it may also promote unhealthy products. A risk to private industry is potential governmental pressure to make additional costly commitments beyond the scope of the original collaboration.

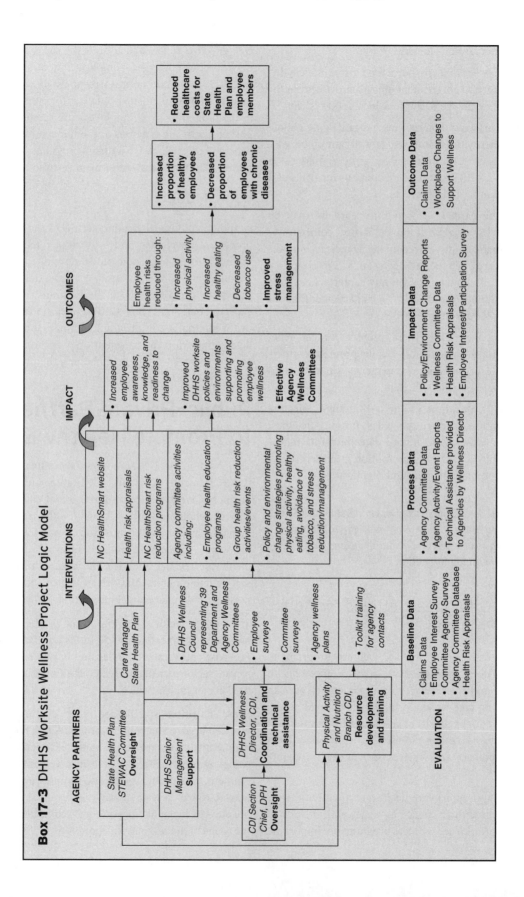

Box 17-3 DHHS Worksite Wellness Project Logic Model

Public collaborations with private industries and corporations may be established on global, national, state, and community levels. An international nutrition partnership is the European Technology Platform Food for Life sponsorship by food industry companies to promote the development of new and reformulated food products.[254] Canada's national Work Group on Sodium included representatives from private industry.[255] At the other end of the spectrum, local community wellness fairs in the United States typically include private companies and healthcare corporations that participate as vendors or as sponsors for the events.

Public–private collaboration can involve formal contractual agreements or more informal collaborations, such as industry representation on government advisory committees. The UNSCN report identifies the following strategies for public–private healthy eating initiatives:

1. Conduct health promotion and communication campaigns (e.g., distributing information leaflets and posters)

2. Provide diet and nutrition education in formal and informal learning venues (e.g., teaching cooking skills)

3. Communicating information on food products (e.g., through nutrition labeling and "healthy food" logos)

4. Controlling advertising and marketing of food products (e.g., through advertising codes on marketing)

5. Increasing or decreasing access to food products (e.g., fruits, vegetables, vending machines)

6. Conducting or supporting research (e.g., on development of novel foods)

7. Developing or reformulating food products (e.g., reducing salt in processed foods)

8. Developing recommendations, guidelines, advice, and strategies for governments and industry (e.g., convening a government forum that includes the food industry)

9. Encouraging private-sector action in general, such as providing a forum for commitments

10. Providing funding for the above activities connected to healthy eating[256]

National Models to Guide Nutrition Policies and Programs: The French Paradox and Collaborative Efforts in France

When applied in settings different from the original one, model programs must be adapted to meet any cultural, economic, organizational, and environmental differences. This is also true when nations look to a nation with better health status to generate ideas for improving the health and nutrition status of their own populations. Not all factors are likely to be reproducible, but many insights are likely to be gained by looking at the dietary patterns of other populations.

For years, the U.S. *Dietary Guidelines* have emphasized restricting consumption of fatty meats, butter, cream, and full-fat cheeses because of their high contents of saturated fat and cholesterol, which are associated with increased risk of CVD.[257,258] The "French paradox" is that a traditional French diet includes these foods, but the French have lower rates of CVD and obesity, and longer average life expectancies, than Americans.

Some ascribe lower CVD rates to the greater consumption of wine in France,[259] but additional factors likely are also influential.[260] Better health outcomes among the French may result partly from their focus on enjoying food.[261] Compared with Americans, the French spend over twice the percentage of their disposable income on food, and are more willing to spend more of their income on smaller quantities of high-quality food.[262] Other characteristics of the French diet are a wide variety of fresh seasonal produce and other freshly prepared foods, and three meals a day with small portions of meats and starches and larger servings of fruits and vegetables. Sweets are occasional. The pattern includes drinking water or wine rather than sweetened beverages. Restaurant portion sizes in France are almost all smaller than American and British restaurant meals.

While the obesity rate in France is increasing, the rate is slower than that in the United States, and is associated with increasing imports of U.S. food products and fast-food franchises in many areas of France. Some nutrition researchers believe that the higher smoking rates in France may account for lower adult obesity rates, although this theory would not explain France's lower childhood obesity rates.[263]

A possibly important difference in dietary habits between the French and Americans is that the French more often enjoy their meals in relaxed social settings, with formal meal times and less snacking than Americans, who spend more than half their food budget on prepared foods. In France and in many other European countries, people eating at work, in public areas, or in transit are less common than in the United States.

Multi-course meals are more common in France. Breaking meals into several small courses offering a variety of foods slows down the eating process and satisfies the appetite with less food. A typical meal might include small portions of soup, followed by a main course, then salad with fresh fruit and/or cheese for dessert.

The French eat more "mindfully" than Americans, with fewer distractions such as television or smartphones during meals, and greater concentration on chewing food slowly and enjoying each bite. Mindful eating has become a weight management technique in the United States. Slowing down the eating process in a social setting and being aware of how much is being eaten have been shown to help control a tendency to overeat. Pleasure is also important. In a multinational study, participants "from the U.S. associated food most with health and least with pleasure, while the French group were the most food–pleasure orientated and the least food–health orientated."[264]

The French government has played a role in combating obesity. French policies on healthy eating date back 80 years when maternal nutrition education stressed adopting healthy food patterns for children. These eating patterns continue to be a norm today in French culture.[265] In 2001, the Programme National Nutrition Santé (PNNS) was created to promote healthy eating nationwide.[266] Stakeholders from ministries, research and educational institutions, the food industry, the healthcare industry, and consumer groups helped develop nine objectives focused on diet, nutritional status, and physical activity. Because childhood weight is often predictive of adult weight, additional actions were taken specifically to target French youth.[267] Strategies to achieve PNNS objectives were based on nutritional sciences and maintenance of traditional gastronomy and enjoyment of food.

- Increase fruit and vegetable consumption
- Reduce prevalence of overweight and obesity
- Increase daily activity levels
- Increase consumption of calcium
- Reduce vitamin D deficiency by 25%
- Reduce consumption of saturated fats
- Increase consumption of carbohydrates
- Decrease consumption of simple sugars, and increase fiber and complex carbohydrates
- Reduce alcohol intake to no more than two drinks per day
- Reduce blood cholesterol and blood pressure

The program's core approach is centered on six strategies:

1. Educate and inform consumers about healthy food choices and create an environment that encourages good choices.
2. Prevent, screen for, and limit nutritional illnesses in the healthcare system.
3. Involve multiple stakeholders, including the food industry and consumer organizations.
4. Implement dietary and nutritional surveillance systems.
5. Develop research on the clinical, behavioral, and epidemiological aspects of nutrition.
6. Target specific population groups through other related public health initiatives.

The PNNS works closely with the food industry and requires that advertising of any food product include a health message such as "exercise every day." Food manufacturers and retailers are encouraged to formalize intended changes in producing, selling, and marketing foods to reach the national PNNS goals. In exchange, they can use the PNNS logo in marketing their food products.[268] The French nutritional guidelines appear to help prevent metabolic syndrome.[269]

Over 75% of the planned PNNS actions were accomplished or in progress by the end of 2005, with many of the advances seen in areas of nutrition communication, education, research, and nutritional surveillance. Success of this type of public health program required "synergistic and complementary actions, measures, regulations, and laws."[270]

A major part of promoting healthier dietary patterns in the United States includes increasing the amount of nutritional information provided on food label (**Figure 17-6**), but most European nations have less government influence on food nutrition labels. The European Union (EU) does not require such labeling unless the food product makes nutritional claims. If a food does make a health or nutrition claim, then it must contain minimum levels of relevant nutrients.

Conclusion

While malnutrition and nutrient deficiencies remain critical issues in developing nations, overnutrition, leading to obesity and NCD risk, is an increasing threat in low-, middle-, and high-income nations alike. Industrialization and globalization have led to changes in dietary patterns characterized by higher intakes of processed foods, solid fats, added sugars and sodium, and lower consumption of

unprocessed foods, such as fruits, vegetables, and whole grains. Proper nutrition during adulthood supports a healthy weight and helps reduce NCD risk. Public health nutrition programs can promote good dietary choices through education, policy change, nutrition assistance, and food fortification. For adults, the worksite is an important potential location for delivery of nutrition programs.

Changing the types and amounts of foods consumed, how and where the foods are prepared, the amount of income spent on food, the setting where most meals are consumed, and the amount of time and attention devoted to meals require radical lifestyle changes. Positive changes include having more home-prepared food, eating smaller portions of better quality and more nutritious foods, and enjoying more formal meal times in a relaxed social setting.[271,272]

References

1 Goetzel, R. Z., Juday, T. R., & Ozminkowski, R. J. (1999). What's the ROI? A systematic review of return-on-investment studies of corporate health and productivity management initiatives. *AWHP's Worksite Health, 6*(3), 12-21.

2 Aldana, S. G. (2001). Financial impact of health promotion programs: A comprehensive review of the literature. *American Journal of Health Promotion, 15*(5), 296-320.

3 Young, S., Halladay, J., Plescia, M., Herget, C., & Dunn, C. (2011). Establishing worksite wellness programs for North Carolina government employees, 2008. *Preventing Chronic Disease, 8*(2), A48. Retrieved from http://www.cdc.gov/pcd/issues/2011/mar/10_0069.htm

4 World Health Organization. (2011, June). *The 10 leading causes of death by broad income group, 2008.* Retrieved from http://www.who.int/mediacentre/factsheets/fs310/en/index.html

5 World Health Organization Consultation on Obesity. (1999). *Obesity: Preventing and managing the global epidemic.* WHO Technical Report Series, no. 894. Geneva, Switzerland: World Health Organization. Retrieved from http://apps.who.int/iris/bitstream/10665/42330/1/WHO_TRS_894.pdf

6 World Health Organization. (2013, March). *Obesity and overweight.* Media Centre Fact sheet 311. Retrieved from http://www.who.int/mediacentre/factsheets/fs311/en

7 Coutsoukis, P. (n.d.). *Obesity and overweight.* Retrieved from http://www.allcountries.org/health/obesity_and_overweight.html

8 Centers for Disease Control and Prevention. (2012, August 13). *Overweight and obesity: Adult obesity facts.* Retrieved from http://www.cdc.gov/obesity/data/adult.html

9 Swinburn, B. A., Sacks, G., Hall, K. D., McPherson, K., Finegood, D. T., Moodie, M. L., & Gortmaker, S. L. (2011). The global obesity pandemic: Shaped by global drivers and local environments. *Lancet, 378*(9793), 804-14. doi:10.1016/S0140-6736(11)60813-1

10 Palo Alto Medical Foundation Sutter Health. (2001). *Teenage growth and development, Years 11 to 14.* Retrieved from http://www.pamf.org/teen/parents/health/growth-11-14.html

11 Altchek, A., & Deligdisch, L. (2009). *Pediatric, adolescent and young adult gynecology.* Hoboken, NJ: Wiley-Blackwell.

12 Stang, J. (2000). Adolescent physical growth and development: Implications for pregnancy. In M. Story & J. Stang (Eds.). *Nutrition and the pregnant adolescent: A practical reference guide* (pp. 31-36). Minneapolis, MN: Center for Leadership, Education, and Training in Maternal and Child Nutrition, University of Minnesota. Retrieved from http://www.epi.umn.edu/let/pubs/img/NMPA_31-36.pdf

13 Steinberg, L. (2011). The fundamental changes of adolescence. In *Adolescence* (9th ed.) (pp. 21-57). Columbus, OH: McGraw-Hill. Retrieved from http://highered.mcgraw-hill.com/sites/dl/free/0072414561/16698/ch01.pdf

14 Centers for Disease Control and Prevention. (2009, August 4). *Clinical growth charts.* http://www.cdc.gov/growthcharts/clinical_charts.htm

15 ChartsBin. (2011). *Age of majority.* Retrieved from http://chartsbin.com/view/545

16 Kinsella, K., & Phillips, D. R. (2005). Global aging: The challenge of success. *Population Bulletin, 60*(1). Retrieved from http://www.prb.org/Publications/PopulationBulletins/2005/GlobalAgingTheChallengeofSuccessPDF575KB.aspx

17 United Nations, Department of Economic and Social Affairs, Population Division. (n.d.). *World population ageing: 1950-2050.* Prepared by the Population Division as a contribution to the 2002 World Assembly on Ageing and its follow-up. Retrieved from http://www.un.org/esa/population/publications/worldageing19502050

18 Centers for Disease Control and Prevention. (2003). Public health and aging: Trends in aging—United States and worldwide. *Morbidity*

and Mortality Weekly Report, 52(6), 101-6. Retrieved from http://www.cdc.gov/mmwr/preview/mmwrhtml/mm5206a2.htm

19 United Nations, Department of Economic and Social Affairs, Population Division. (n.d.). *World population ageing: 1950-2050.* Prepared by the Population Division as a contribution to the 2002 World Assembly on Ageing and its follow-up. Retrieved from http://www.un.org/esa/population/publications/worldageing19502050

20 Hoven, A. D. (2010). *Coping with baby boomers, and staggering statistics.* Retrieved from American Medical Association, American Medical News, website, http://www.ama-assn.org/amednews/2010/09/20/edca0920.htm

21 Ganim, L. J. (2004). Baby boomers and Medicare. *Health Affairs, 23*(2), 282-83. doi:10.1377/hlthaff.23.2.282-a

22 Robison, J., Shugrue, N., Fortinsky, R. H., Gruman, C. (2013). Long-term supports and services planning for the future: implications from a statewide survey of baby boomers and older adults. *The Gerontologist.*

23 Soldo, B. J., Mitchell, O. S., Tfaily, R., & McCabe, J. F. (2006). *Cross-cohort differences in health on the verge of retirement.* National Bureau of Economic Research working paper 12762. Cambridge, MA: National Bureau of Economic Research. Retrieved from www.nber.org/papers/w12762

24 Stein, R. (2007, April 20). Baby boomers appear to be less healthy than parents. *Washington Post.* Retrieved from http://www.washingtonpost.com/wp-dyn/content/article/2007/04/19/AR2007041902458.html

25 Food and Agriculture Organization of the United Nations. (2011, May 5). *Nutritional requirements: Dietary energy.* Retrieved from http://www.fao.org/ag/humannutrition/nutrition/63139/en

26 Nutrition Academic Award Program Curriculum Committee. (n.d.). *Nutrition curriculum guide for training physicians. Lifespan: Young adulthood/middle age.* Retrieved from http://www.nhlbi.nih.gov/funding/training/naa/curr_gde/c2_youngadult.htm

27 World Health Organization. (2013). *Dietary recommendations /Nutritional requirements.* Retrieved from http://www.who.int/nutrition/topics/nutrecomm/en/index.html

28 Food and Nutrition Board, Institute of Medicine, National Academies. (n.d.). *Dietary reference intakes (DRIs): Estimated average requirements.* Retrieved from http://www.iom.edu/Activities/Nutrition/SummaryDRIs/~/media/Files/Activity%20Files/Nutrition/DRIs/5_Summary%20Table%20Tables%201-4.pdf

29 Food and Nutrition Board, Institute of Medicine, National Academies. (n.d.). *Dietary reference intakes (DRIs): Estimated average requirements.* Retrieved from http://www.iom.edu/Activities/Nutrition/SummaryDRIs/~/media/Files/Activity%20Files/Nutrition/DRIs/5_Summary%20Table%20Tables%201-4.pdf

30 Poelman, E. T., Goran, M. I., Gardner, A. W., Ades, P. A., Arciero, P. J., Katzman-Rooks, S., & Sutherland, P. T. (1993). Determinants of decline in resting metabolic rate in aging females. *American Journal of Physiology, Endocrinology, and Metabolism, 264*(3), E450-E455.

31 Evans, W. J., & Campbell, W. W. (1993). Sarcopenia and age-related changes in body composition and functional capacity. *Journal of Nutrition, 123*(2 Suppl.), 465-68.

32 Roberts, S. B., & Rosenberg, I. (2006). Nutrition and aging: Changes in the regulation of energy metabolism with aging. *Physiological Reviews, 86*(2), 651-67. doi: 10.1152/physrev.00019.2005. Retrieved from http://physrev.physiology.org/content/86/2/651.full

33 World Health Organization. (2009). *World global health risks: Mortality and burden of disease attributable to selected major risks.* Retrieved from http://www.who.int/healthinfo/global_burden_disease/GlobalHealthRisks_report_full.pdf

34 World Health Organization. (2009). *World global health risks: Mortality and burden of disease attributable to selected major risks.* Retrieved from http://www.who.int/healthinfo/global_burden_disease/GlobalHealthRisks_report_full.pdf

35 Food and Agriculture Organization of the United Nations. (2012). *The state of food insecurity in the world.* Retrieved from http://www.fao.org/docrep/016/i2845e/i2845e00.pdf

36 Food and Agricultural Organization. (2013). *Food security indicators.* Retrieved from http://www.fao.org/economic/ess/ess-fs/ess-fadata/en

37 Coleman-Jensen, A., Nord, M., Andrews, M., & Carlson, S. (2011). *Household food security in the United States in 2010.* Economic research report ERR-125. Washington, DC: United States Department of Agriculture, Economic Research Service. Retrieved from http://www.ers.usda.gov/Publications/err125

38 United Nations System, Standing Committee on Nutrition. (2011). Nutrition and business: How to engage? *SCN News, 39.* Retrieved from http://www.unscn.org/files/Publications/SCN_News/SCNNEWS39_10.01_low_def.pdf

39 Allen, L., de Benoist, B., Dary, O., & Hurrell, R. (Eds.). (2006). *Guidelines on food fortification with micronutrients.* Geneva: World Health Organization; Rome: Food and Agricultural Organization of the United Nations. Retrieved from http://www.who.int/nutrition/publications/micronutrients/9241594012/en/index.html

40 Backstrand, J. R. (2002). The history and future of food fortification in the United States: A public health perspective. *Nutrition Reviews, 60*(1), 15-26.

41 World Health Organization. (1990). *Diet, nutrition and the prevention of chronic diseases.* Technical Report Series 797. Retrieved from http://www.iaso.org/site_media/uploads/WHO_TRS_797_part1.pdf

42 World Health Organization. (1990). *Diet, nutrition and the prevention of chronic diseases.* Technical Report Series 797. Retrieved from http://www.iaso.org/site_media/uploads/WHO_TRS_797_part1.pdf

43 Centers for Disease Control and Prevention, Office of the Associate Director for Program. (2011). *Chronic disease prevention.* Retrieved from http://www.cdc.gov/program/performance/fy2000plan/2000vii.htm

44 Centers for Disease Control and Prevention, Office of the Associate Director for Program. (2011). *Chronic disease prevention*. Retrieved from http://www.cdc.gov/program/performance/fy2000plan/2000vii.htm

45 Centers for Disease Control and Prevention. (2012). *Chronic diseases and health prevention*. Retrieved from http://www.cdc.gov/chronicdisease/overview/index.htm#ref1#ref1

46 United States Department of Agriculture & United States Department of Health and Human Services. (2010). *Dietary guidelines for Americans, 2010* (7th ed., pp. 1-7). Washington, DC: U.S. Government Printing Office. Retrieved from http://www.cnpp.usda.gov/Publications/DietaryGuidelines/2010/PolicyDoc/Chapter1.pdf

47 Centers for Disease Control and Prevention. National Center for Chronic Disease Prevention and Health Promotion (NCCDPHP). (2009). Chronic disease: The public health challenge of the 21st century. Atlanta, GA: Centers for Disease Control and Prevention.

48 Centers for Disease Control and Prevention. (2012). *Chronic diseases and health promotion*. Retrieved from http://www.cdc.gov/chronicdisease/overview/index.htm

49 World Health Organization. (2007). *Spending on health: A global overview*. Fact sheet no. 319. Retrieved from http://www.who.int/mediacentre/factsheets/fs319/en/index.html

50 Popkin, B. M. (2006). Global nutrition dynamics: The world is shifting rapidly toward a diet linked with noncommunicable diseases. *American Journal of Clinical Nutrition, 84*(2), 289-98. Retrieved from http://students.med.mcgill.ca/sites/default/files/content/clubs/mighc/2008/readings/popkin.pdf

51 Remington, P. L., & Brownson, R. C. (2011). Fifty years of progress in chronic disease epidemiology and control. Centers for Disease Control and Prevention. *Morbidity and Mortality Weekly Report (MMWR), Suppl. 60*(4), 70-77.

52 World Health Organization. (2010). *A review of nutrition policies*. Draft report. Retrieved from http://www.who.int/nutrition/EB128_18_Backgroundpaper1_A_review_of_nutrition policies.pdf

53 Centers for Disease Control and Prevention. (2012). *FastStats: Obesity and overweight*. Retrieved from http://www.cdc.gov/nchs/fastats/overwt.htm

54 Ogden, C. L., Carroll, M. D., Kit, B. K., & Flegal, K. M. (2012). *Prevalence of obesity in the United States, 2009-2010*. NCHS Data Brief No. 82. Hyattsville, MD: Centers for Disease Control and Prevention, National Center for Health Statistics. Retrieved from http://www.cdc.gov/nchs/data/databriefs/db82.pdf

55 Flegal, K. M., Carroll, M. D., Kit, B. K., & Ogden, C. L. (2012). Prevalence of obesity and trends in the distribution of body mass index among U.S. adults, 1999-2010. *Journal of the American Medical Association, 307*(5), 491-97. doi:10.1001/jama.2012.39]

56 Mokdad, A. H., Ford, E. S., Bowman, B. A., Dietz, W. H., Vinicor, F., Bales, V. S., & Marks, J. S. (2003). Prevalence of obesity, diabetes, and obesity-related health risk factors, 2001. *Journal of the American Medical Association. 289*(1), 76-79.

57 World Health Organization. (2000). *Obesity: Preventing and managing the global epidemic*. Retrieved from http://libdoc.who.int/trs/WHO_TRS_894.pdf

58 Flegal, K. M., Graubard, B. I., Williamson, D. F., & Gail, M. H. (2007). Cause-specific excess deaths associated with underweight, overweight, and obesity. *Journal of the American Medical Association, 298*(17), 2028-37.

59 Centers for Disease Control and Prevention. (2012). *Overweight and obesity: Causes and consequences*. Retrieved from http://www.cdc.gov/obesity/adult/causes/index.html

60 Thompson, D., & Wolf, A. M. (2001). The medical-care cost burden of obesity. *Obesity Reviews, 2*(3), 189-97. Retrieved from http://onlinelibrary.wiley.com/doi/10.1046/j.1467-789x.2001.00037.x/abstract

61 Finkelstein, E. A., Trogdon, J. G., Cohen, J. W., & Dietz, W. (2009). Annual medical spending attributable to obesity: Payer- and service-specific estimates. *Health Affairs, 28*(5), w822-w831.

62 Centers for Disease Control and Prevention. (2012). *Overweight and obesity: Defining overweight and obesity*. Retrieved from http://www.cdc.gov/obesity/adult/defining.html

63 Prentice, A. M., & Jebb, S. A. (2001). Beyond body mass index. *Obesity Reviews, 2*(3), 141-147. doi:10.1046/j.1467-789x.2001.00031.x

64 National Institute of Health & National Heart Lung and Blood Institute. (n.d.). *Assessing your weight and health risk*. Retrieved from http://www.nhlbi.nih.gov/health/public/heart/obesity/lose_wt/risk.htm

65 Southgate, D. D., Jr., Graham, D. H., & Tweeten, L. G. (2011). *The world food economy* (2nd ed.). Hoboken, NJ: Wiley.

66 Popkin, B. M. (2001). The nutrition transition and obesity in the developing world. *Journal of Nutrition, 131*(3), 871S-873S.

67 Swinburn, B. A., Sacks, G., Hall, K. D., McPherson, K., Finegood, D. T., Moodie, M. L., & Gortmaker, S. (2011). The global obesity pandemic: Shaped by global drivers and local environments. *Lancet, 378*(9793), 804-14. Retrieved from http://www.thelancet.com/journals/lancet/article/PIIS0140-6736(11)60813-1

68 United States Department of Agriculture, Office of Communications. (2003). Profiling food consumption in America. In *Agriculture fact book, 2001-2002* (pp. 13-21). Washington, DC: U.S. Government Printing Office. Retrieved from http://www.usda.gov/factbook/chapter2.pdf

69 Centers for Disease Control and Prevention. (2005). Adult participation in recommended levels of physical activity: United States, 2001 and 2003. *Morbidity and Mortality Weekly Report, 54*(47), 1208-12.

70 Drewnowski, A., & Spector, S. E. (2004). Poverty and obesity: The role of energy density and energy costs. *American Journal of Clinical Nutrition, 79*(1), 6-16.

71 Wells, J. C. K. (2006). The evolution of human fatness and susceptibility to obesity: An ethological approach. *Biological Reviews, 81*(2), 183-205.

72 Centers for Disease Control and Prevention. (2011). *Healthy weight: It's not a diet, it's a lifestyle!* Retrieved from http://www.cdc.gov/healthyweight/calories/other_factors.html

73 National Institutes of Health & National Heart, Lung, and Blood Institute. (2012). *What causes overweight and obesity?*

Retrieved from http://www.nhlbi.nih.gov/health/health-topics/topics/obe/causes.html

74 Young, L. R., & Nestle, M. (2002). The contribution of expanding portion sizes to the U.S. obesity epidemic. *American Journal of Public Health, 92*(2), 246-49.

75 Wansink, B., & Van Ittersum, K. (2007). Portion size me: Downsizing our consumption norms. *Journal of the American Dietetic Association, 107*(7), 1103-6. Retrieved from http://mindlesseating.org/lastsupper/pdf/portion_size_me_JADA_2007.pdf

76 Young, L. R., & Nestle, M. (2002). The contribution of expanding portion sizes to the U.S. obesity epidemic. *American Journal of Public Health, 92*(2), 246-49. http://www.ncbi.nlm.nih.gov/pmc/articles/PMC1447051

77 Young, L. R., & Nestle, M. (2002). The contribution of expanding portion sizes to the U.S. obesity epidemic. *American Journal of Public Health, 92*(2), 246-49.

78 Wansink, B,. & Payne, C. R. (2012). Eating behavior and obesity at Chinese buffets. Obesity, 16(8), 1957-60.

79 Taubes, G. (2012, November 19). *What would happen if . . . ? Thoughts (and thought experiments) on the calorie issue.* Retrieved from http://garytaubes.com

80 Taubes, G. (2001). The soft science of dietary fat. *Science, 291*(5513), 2536-45. doi:10.1126/science.291.5513.2536

81 Centers for Disease Control and Prevention. (2012). *Nutrition for everyone: Carbohydrates.* Retrieved from http://www.cdc.gov/nutrition/everyone/basics/carbs.html

82 National Center for Biotechnology Information, United States National Library of Medicine. (2012). *Metabolic syndrome: Insulin resistance syndrome; Syndrome X.* Retrieved from http://www.ncbi.nlm.nih.gov/pubmedhealth/PMH0004546

83 Liu, S., & Manson, J. E. (2001). Dietary carbohydrates, physical inactivity, obesity, and the "metabolic syndrome" as predictors of coronary heart disease. *Current Opinion in Lipidology, 12*(4), 395-404.

84 Burton-Freeman, B., Davis, P. A., & Schneeman, B. O. (2002). Plasma cholecystokinin is associated with subjective measures of satiety in women. *American Journal of Clinical Nutrition, 76*(3), 659-67.

85 Mozaffarian, D., Hao, T., Rimm, E. B., Willett, W. C., & Hu, F. B. (2011). Changes in diet and lifestyle and long-term weight gain in women and men. *New England Journal of Medicine, 364*, 2392-2404. doi:10.1056/NEJMoa1014296

86 Chang, G. Q., Gaysinskaya, V., Karatayev, O., & Leibowitz, S. F. (2008). Maternal high-fat diet and fetal programming: Increased proliferation of hypothalamic peptide-producing neurons that increase risk for overeating and obesity. *Journal of Neuroscience, 28*(46), 12107-19. doi:10.1523/JNEUROSCI.2642-08.2008

87 Harvard School of Public Health. (2013). *Writing a prescription for obesity prevention.* Retrieved from http://www.hsph.harvard.edu/obesity-prevention-source/obesity-prevention/healthcare

88 Simkin-Silverman, L. R., & Wing, R. R. (1997). Management of obesity in primary care. *Obesity Research, 5*(6), 603-12.

89 Hash, R., Munna, R. K., Vogel, R. L. & Bason, J. J. (2003). Does physician weight affect perception of health advice? *Preventive Medicine, 36*(1), 41-44.

90 The diet industry: A big fat lie. (2008). *Bloomberg Businessweek.* Retrieved from http://www.businessweek.com/debateroom/archives/2008/01/the_diet_indust.html

91 Curioni, C. C., & Lourenço, P. M. (2005). Long-term weight loss after diet and exercise: A systematic review. *International Journal of Obesity, 29*, 1168-74. doi:10.1038/sj.ijo.0803015

92 Swinburn, B., & Egger, G. (2002). Preventive strategies against weight gain and obesity. *Obesity Reviews, 3*(4), 289-301.

93 MedlinePlus. (n.d.). *Weight loss surgery.* Retrieved from http://www.nlm.nih.gov/medlineplus/weightlosssurgery.html

94 Food and Agriculture Organization of the United Nations. (2009). *Food-based dietary guidelines.* Retrieved from http://www.fao.org/ag/humannutrition/nutritioneducation/fbdg/en

95 World Health Organization Global Strategy. (n.d.). *Global strategy on diet, physical activity and health.* Retrieved from http://www.who.int/dietphysicalactivity/strategy/en

96 World Health Organization. (2003). *Diet, nutrition and the prevention of chronic diseases.* Technical report series, No. 916 (TRS 916). Retrieved from http://www.who.int/dietphysicalactivity/publications/trs916/en

97 Food and Agriculture Organization of the United Nations. (2009). *Food-based dietary guidelines.* Retrieved from http://www.fao.org/ag/humannutrition/nutritioneducation/fbdg/en

98 Public Law 101-445, Title III, 7 U.S.C. 5301 et seq.

99 United States Department of Agriculture & United States Department of Health and Human Services. (2010). *Dietary guidelines for Americans: An overview* (7th ed.). Retrieved from http://www.nationaldairycouncil.org/Research/DairyCouncilDigestArchives/Pages/dcd82-3Page2.aspx

100 United States Department of Agriculture & United States Department of Health and Human Services. (2010). *Dietary guidelines for Americans 2010* (7th ed.). Washington, DC: U.S. Government Printing Office. Retrieved from http://www.health.gov/dietaryguidelines

101 U.S. Department of Health and Human Services. (n.d.). *History of dietary guidelines of America.* Retrieved from http://www.health.gov/dietaryguidelines/history.htm

102 United States Department of Agriculture, Center for Nutrition Policy and Promotion. (2013). *MyPlate.* Retrieved from http://www.cnpp.usda.gov/MyPlate.htm

103 United States Department of Agriculture. (n.d.). *Selected messages for consumers.* Retrieved from http://www.choosemyplate.gov/print-materials-ordering/selected-messages.html

104 United States Food and Drug Administration. (2008). *Health and diet survey: Dietary guidelines supplement—Report of findings (2004 & 2005).* Retrieved from http://www.fda.gov

/Food/ScienceResearch/ResearchAreas/ConsumerResearch/ucm080331.htm#overall

105 Should a low-fat, high-carbohydrate diet be recommended for everyone? Clinical debate. (1997). *New England Journal of Medicine, 337*(8), 562-67.

106 Gallo, A. E. (1999). Food advertising in the United States. In E. Frazao, *America's eating habits: Changes and consequences* (pp. 173-80). Agriculture Information Bulletin (AIB-750). Washington, DC: United States Department of Agriculture. Economic Research Service. Retrieved from http://www.ers.usda.gov/media/91050/aib750i_1_.pdf

107 Blisard, N. (1999). Advertising and what we eat: The case of dairy products. In E. Frazao, *America's eating habits: Changes and consequences* (pp. 181-88). Agriculture Information Bulletin (AIB-750). Washington, DC: United States Department of Agriculture, Economic Research Service. Retrieved from http://www.ers.usda.gov/media/91054/aib750j_1_.pdf

108 Gifford, K. D. (2002). Dietary fats, eating guides, and public policy: History, critique, and recommendations. *American Journal of Medicine, 113*(9 Suppl. 2), 89-106.

109 Centers for Disease Control and Prevention. (2012). *Dietary fat.* Retrieved from http://www.cdc.gov/nutrition/everyone/basics/fat/index.html

110 McNamara, D. J. (2000). Dietary cholesterol and atherosclerosis. *Biochimica et Biophysica Acta (BBA)—Molecular and Cell Biology of Lipids, 1529*(1-3), 310-20.

111 Simopoulos, A. P. (2002). The importance of the ratio of omega-6/omega-3 essential fatty acids. *Biomedicine & Pharmacotherapy, 56*(8), 365-79.

112 Daley, C. A., Abbott, A., Doyle, P. S., Nader, G. A., & Larson, S. (2010). A review of fatty acid profiles and antioxidant content in grass-fed and grain-fed beef. *Nutrition Journal, 9*, 10. doi:10.1186/1475-2891-9-10

113 U.S. Food and Drug Administration. (2008). *Health and diet survey: Dietary guidelines supplement—Report of findings (2004 & 2005).* Retrieved from http://www.fda.gov/Food/ScienceResearch/ResearchAreas/ConsumerResearch/ucm080331.htm#overall

114 European Food Information Council. (2005). *The determinants of food choice.* Retrieved from http://www.eufic.org/article/en/expid/review-food-choice

115 European Food Information Council. (2005). The determinants of food choice. Retrieved from http://www.eufic.org/article/en/expid/review-food-choice

116 European Food Information Council. (2005). *The determinants of food choice.* Retrieved from http://www.eufic.org/article/en/expid/review-food-choice

117 Nestle, M. (2007). *Food politics: How the food industry influences nutrition, and health* (Revised and expanded ed.). Berkeley, CA: University of California Press.

118 Anderson, A. S., Cox, D. N., McKellar, S., Reynolds, J., Lean, M. E., & Mela, D. J. (1998). Take Five, a nutrition education intervention to increase fruit and vegetable intakes: Impact on attitudes towards dietary change. *British Journal of Nutrition, 80*(2), 133-40.

119 Tillotson, J. E. (2002). Business and nutrition: Our ready-prepared ready-to-eat nation. Nutrition Today, 37(1), 36-38.

120 Kittler, P. G., Sucher, K. P., & Nelms, M. (2011). *Food and culture.* Pacific Grove, CA: Brooks/Cole.

121 Ernst, N. D., Wu, M., Frommer, P., Katz, E., Matthews, O., Moskowitz, J., . . . Zifferblatt. (1986). Nutrition education at the point of purchase: The foods for health project evaluated. *Preventative Medicine, 15*(1), 60-73. Retrieved from http://www.ncbi.nlm.nih.gov/pubmed/3714660

122 United States Department of Agriculture, Center for Nutrition Policy and Promotion. (2010). *Dietary guidelines for Americans 2010.* Retrieved from http://www.cnpp.usda.gov/dietaryguidelines.htm

123 Healthy Eating Research. (n.d.). *Menu labeling.* Retrieved from http://www.healthyeatingresearch.org/research-results-mainmenu-35/menu-labeling

124 Ruopeng, A. (2013). Effectiveness of subsidies in promoting healthy food purchases and consumption: a review of field experiments. *Public Health Nutrition, 16*(7), 1215-28

125 Popkin, B. M. (2006). Global nutrition dynamics: The world is shifting rapidly toward a diet linked with noncommunicable diseases. *American Journal of Clinical Nutrition, 84*(2), 289-98. Retrieved from http://students.med.mcgill.ca/sites/default/files/content/clubs/mighc/2008/readings/popkin.pdf

126 Antar, M. A., Ohlson, M. A., & Hodges, R. E. (1964). Changes in retail market food supplies in the United States in the last seventy years in relation to the incidence of coronary heart disease, with special reference to dietary carbohydrates and essential fatty acids. *American Journal of Clinical Nutrition, 14*(3), 169-78. Retrieved from http://ajcn.nutrition.org/content/14/3/169.short

127 United States Department of Agriculture, Office of Communications. (2003). Profiling food consumption in America. In *Agriculture fact book, 2001-2002* (pp. 13-21). Washington, DC: U.S. Government Printing Office.

128 Gerrior, S., Bente, L., & Hiza, H., (2004). *Nutrient content of the U.S. food supply, 1909-2000.* Home economics research report 56. Washington, DC: United States Department of Agriculture, Center for Nutrition Policy and Promotion. Retrieved from http://www.cnpp.usda.gov/publications/foodsupply/foodsupply1909-2000.pdf

129 Gerrior, S., Bente, L., & Hiza, H., (2004). *Nutrient content of the U.S. food supply, 1909-2000.* Home economics research report 56. Washington, DC: United States Department of Agriculture, Center for Nutrition Policy and Promotion. Retrieved from http://www.cnpp.usda.gov/publications/foodsupply/foodsupply1909-2000.pdf

130 Food Marketing Institute. (n.d.). *Supermarket facts: Industry overview 2011.* http://www.fmi.org/research-resources/supermarket-facts

131 Alston, J. M., Sumner, D. A., & Vosti, S. A. (2006). Are agricultural policies making us fat? Likely links between agricultural

policies and human nutrition and obesity, and their policy implications. *Applied Economic Perspectives and Policy, 28*(3), 313-22. doi:10.1111/j.1467-9353.2006.00292.x

132 Stevens, E. E., Patrick, T. E., & Pickler, R. (2009). A history of infant feeding. *Journal of Perinatal Education, 18*(2), 32-39.

133 Hirschman, C., & Butler, M. (1981). Trends and differentials in breastfeeding: An update. *Demography, 18*(1), 39-54.

134 Owen, C. G., Whincup, P. H., Odoki, K., Gilg, J. A., & Cook, D. G. (2002). Infant feeding and blood cholesterol: A study in adolescents and a systematic review. *Pediatrics, 110*(3), 597-608. doi:10.1542/peds.110.3.597

135 Owen, C. G., Whincup, P. H., Kaye, S. J., Martin, R. M., Smith, G. D., Cook, D. G., . . . Williams, S. M. (2008). Does initial breastfeeding lead to lower blood cholesterol in adult life? A quantitative review of the evidence. *American Journal of Clinical Nutrition, 88*, 305-14. Retrieved from http://www.allattamentoalseno.it/lavori/Does%20initial%20breastfeeding%20lead%20to%20lower%20blood%20cholesterol%20in%20adult.pdf

136 Environmental Working Group. (n.d.). *Farm subsidy primer.* Retrieved from http://farm.ewg.org/subsidyprimer.php

137 Ard, J. D., Fitzpatrick, S., Desmond, R. A., Sutton, B. S., Pisu, M., Allison, D. B., . . . Baskin, M. L. (2007). The impact of cost on the availability of fruits and vegetables in the homes of schoolchildren in Birmingham, Alabama. *American Journal of Public Health, 97*(2), 367-72.

138 Nestle, M. (2007). *Food politics: How the food industry influences nutrition, and health* (Revised and expanded ed.). Berkeley, CA: University of California Press.

139 Popkin, B. M. & Nielsen, S. J. (2003). The sweetening of the world's diet. *Obesity Research, 11*, 1325-32.

140 Mardis, A. L. (2001). Current knowledge of the health effects of sugar intake. *Family Economics & Nutrition Review, 13*(1), 87-91.

141 United States Department of Agriculture, Office of Communications. (2003). Profiling food Consumption in America. In *Agriculture fact book, 2001-2002* (pp. 13-21). Washington, DC: U.S. Government Printing Office.

142 Morrison, R. M., Buzby, J. C., & Wells, H. F. (2010). Guess who's turning 100? Tracking a century of American eating. *Amber Waves, United States Department of Agriculture Economic Research Service, 8*(1), 12-19. Retrieved from http://ageconsearch.umn.edu/bitstream/122141/2/01TrackingACentury.pdf

143 Harvard School of Public Health. (n.d.). *Shining the spotlight on trans fats.* Retrieved from http://www.hsph.harvard.edu/nutritionsource/transfats

144 United States Department of Agriculture, Office of Communications. (2003). Profiling food consumption in America. In *Agriculture fact book, 2001-2002* (pp. 13-21). Washington, DC: U.S. Government Printing Office.

145 McBride, J. (1996). *USDA finds more and more Americans eat out, offers tips for making healthier food choices.* Retrieved from the United States Department of Agriculture, Agricultural Research Service website, http://www.ars.usda.gov/is/pr/1996/eatout1196.htm

146 United States Department of Agriculture, Office of Communications. (2003). Profiling food consumption in America. In *Agriculture fact book, 2001-2002* (pp. 13-21). Washington, DC: U.S. Government Printing Office.

147 Lubin, G., & Badkar, M. (2010). *15 facts about McDonald's that will blow your mind.* Retrieved from http://www.businessinsider.com/amazing-facts-mcdonalds-2010-12?op=1#ixzz26ZUGVHvi

148 Schlosser, E. (2001). *Fast food nation: The dark side of the all-American meal.* Boston, MA: Houghton Mifflin.

149 Pereira, M. A., Kartashov, A. I., Ebbeling, C. B., Van Horn, L., Slattery, M. L., Jacobs, D. R., & Ludwig, D. S. (2005). Fast-food habits, weight gain, and insulin resistance (the CARDIA study): 15-year prospective analysis. *Lancet, 365*(9453), 36-42. doi:10.1016/S0140-6736(04)17663-0

150 United States Department of Agriculture, Economic Research Service. (2010). *Tracking the American diet for 100 years.* Retrieved from www.worldebooklibrary.org/eBooks/WPLBN0002111636-Amber_Waves___Tracking_the_American_Diet_for_100_Years__Issue_March_2010-by_Usda__Economic_Research_Service.aspx

151 Callaghan, P. (2011). *What is organic food? A brief history of organic food.* Retrieved from http://world.edu/organic-food-history-organic-food

152 Organic Trade Association. (2011). *2011 organic industry survey.* Brattleboro, VT: Organic Trade Association. Highlights retrieved from http://www.ota.com/pics/documents/2011OrganicIndustrySurvey.pdf

153 World Hunger Education Service. (n.d.). *2012 world hunger and poverty facts and statistics.* Retrieved from http://www.worldhunger.org/articles/Learn/world%20hunger%20facts%202002.htm

154 Food and Agriculture Organization. (2011). *The state of food and agriculture: Women in agriculture: Closing the gender gap for development.* Rome, Italy: Food and Agriculture Organization.

155 United Nations Food and Agriculture Organization 2010 Report

156 Food and Agriculture Organization. (2011). *Cutting food waste to feed the world.* Retrieved from http://www.fao.org/news/story/en/item/74192/icode

157 Gustavsson, J., Cederberg, C., Sonesson, U., van Otterdijk, R., & Meybeck, A. (2011). *Global food losses and food waste.* Rome, Italy: Food and Agriculture Organization of the United Nations.

158 World Hunger Education Service. (n.d.). *2012 world hunger and poverty facts and statistics.* Retrieved from http://www.worldhunger.org/articles/Learn/world%20hunger%20facts%202002.htmx

159 Washington State University. (2011). *Annual income spent on food.* Retrieved from http://wsm.wsu.edu/researcher/WSMaug11_billions.pdf

160 Traub, A. (2011). *Farmers markets as a healthy food access strategy: Assessing Baltimore's farmers markets and proposing recommendations to increase access* (MPH Capstone thesis, Johns Hopkins Bloomberg School of Public Health). Retrieved

from http://ocw.jhsph.edu/courses/capstone2011/PDFs/Traub_Arielle_2011.pdf

161 United States Department of Agriculture, Economic Research Service. (2013). *Food desert locator*. Retrieved from http://www.ers.usda.gov/data-products/food-desert-locator/go-to-the-locator.aspx

162 Mason, J. B., & Mitchell, J. T. (1983). Nutritional surveillance. *Bulletin of the World Health Organization, 61*(5), 745–55.

163 World Health Organization. (n.d.). *Programmes and projects: Nutrition*. Retrieved from http://www.who.int/nutrition/about_us/en

164 Centers for Disease Control and Prevention. (n.d.). *National health and nutrition examination survey*. Retrieved from http://www.cdc.gov/nchs/nhanes.htm

165 United States Department of Agriculture. Office of Communications. (2003). Profiling food consumption in America. In *Agriculture fact book, 2001–2002* (pp. 13–21). Washington, DC: U.S. Government Printing Office.

166 Centers for Disease Control and Prevention. (n.d.). *National health and nutrition examination survey*. Retrieved from http://www.cdc.gov/nchs/nhanes.htm

167 Centers for Disease Control and Prevention. (n.d.). *National health and nutrition examination survey*. Retrieved from http://www.cdc.gov/nchs/nhanes.htm

168 Moshfegh, A. J., Goldman, J. D., Ahuja, J. K., Rhodes, D. G., & Lacomb, R. P. (2009). *What we eat in America, NHANES 2005–2006: Usual nutrient intakes from food and water compared to 1997 Dietary Reference Intakes for vitamin D, calcium, phosphorus, and magnesium*. Beltsville, MD: United States Department of Agriculture, Agricultural Research Service. Retrieved from http://www.ars.usda.gov/SP2UserFiles/Place/12355000/pdf/0506/usual_nutrient_intake_vitD_ca_phos_mg_2005-06.pdf

169 Centers for Disease Control and Prevention. (2013). *Alcohol and public health*. Retrieved from http://www.cdc.gov/alcohol

170 Centers for Disease Control and Prevention. (2012). *Chronic diseases and health promotion*. Retrieved from http://www.cdc.gov/chronicdisease/overview/index.htm

171 Centers for Disease Control and Prevention. (2012). *Alcohol-related public health objectives and guidelines*. Retrieved from http://www.cdc.gov/alcohol/ph_objectives.htm

172 U.S. Department of Agriculture. (2012). *National nutrient database for standard reference, release 25*. Retrieved from http://www.ars.usda.gov/ba/bhnrc/ndl

173 Natural Products Foundation. (2010). *Dietary supplement industry contributes more than $60 billion to national economy*. Retrieved from http://www.naturalproductsfoundation.org/index.php?src=news&srctype=detail&category=News&refno=20

174 Gahche, J., Bailey, R., Burt, V., Hughes, J., Yetley, E., Dwyer, J., . . . Sempos, C. (2011). *Dietary supplement use among U.S. adults has increased since NHANES III (1988–1994)*. NCHS Data Brief

61. Retrieved from http://www.cdc.gov/nchs/data/databriefs/db61.pdf

175 U.S. Food and Drug Administration. (2013). *Dietary supplements*. Retrieved from http://www.fda.gov/Food/DietarySupplements/default.htm

176 United States Food and Drug Administration. (2004). *FDA announces qualified health claims for omega-3 fatty acids*. Retrieved from http://www.fda.gov/NewsEvents/Newsroom/PressAnnouncements/2004/ucm108351.htm

177 Isaacson, M. (2009). *The missing link in healthcare reform: Why healthy living and prevention aren't part of the plan . . . but need to be*. Managed Healthcare Executive Whitepapers. Retrieved from http://managedhealthcareexecutive.modernmedicine.com/managed-healthcare-executive/category/managed-healthcare-executive/whitepapers

178 Goulding, M. R. (2005). Trends in prescribed medicine use and spending by older Americans, 1992–2001. *Aging Trends, 5*. Hyattsville, MD: National Center for Health Statistics. Retrieved from http://www.cdc.gov/nchs/data/ahcd/agingtrends/05medicine.pdf

179 Centers for Disease Control and Prevention. (2012). *Therapeutic drug use*. Retrieved from http://www.cdc.gov/nchs/fastats/drugs.htm

180 Gu, Q., Dillon, C. F., & Burt, V. L. (2010). *Prescription drug use continues to increase: U.S. prescription drug data for 2007–2008*. NCHS Data Brief no. 42. Retrieved from http://www.cdc.gov/nchs/data/databriefs/db42.pdf

181 United States Department of Health and Human Services, Centers for Disease Control and Prevention, National Center for Health Statistics. (2012). Table 99. Prescription drug use in the past 30 days, by sex, age, race and Hispanic origin: United States, selected years 1988–1994 through 2005–2008. In *Health, United States, 2011: With special feature on socioeconomic status and health* (pp. 321–22). Hyattsville, MD: U.S. Government Printing Office. Retrieved from http://www.cdc.gov/nchs/data/hus/hus11.pdf

182 Gu, Q., Dillon, C. F., & Burt, V. L. (2010, September). *Prescription drug use continues to increase: U.S. prescription drug data for 2007–2008*. NCHS Data Brief no. 42. Retrieved from http://www.cdc.gov/nchs/data/databriefs/db42.pdf

183 Posner, B. M., Jette, A. M., Smith, K. W., & Miller, D. R. (1993). Nutrition and health risks in the elderly: The nutrition screening initiative. *American Journal of Public Health, 83*(7), 972–78. Retrieved from http://www.ncbi.nlm.nih.gov/pmc/articles/PMC1694757/pdf/amjph00531-0046.pdf

184 Rivlin, R. S. (2007). Keeping the young-elderly healthy: Is it too late to improve our health through nutrition? *American Journal of Clinical Nutrition, 86*(5), 1572S–1576S.

185 Mobarhan, S., & Trumbore, L. S. (1991). Nutritional problems of the elderly. *Clinics in Geriatric Medicine, 7*(2), 191–214. Retrieved from http://www.ncbi.nlm.nih.gov/pubmed/1906772

186 Lee, J. S., & Frongillo, E. A., Jr. (2001). Nutritional and health consequences are associated with food insecurity among U.S. elderly persons. *Journal of Nutrition, 131*(5), 1503–9.

187 Culross, B. (2008). Nutrition: Meeting the needs of the elderly. *ARN Update, 7.* Retrieved from http://www.rehabnurse.org/pdf/GeriatricsNutrition.pdf

188 World Health Organization. (n.d.). *Programmes and projects: Nutrition.* Retrieved from http://www.who.int/nutrition/about_us/en

189 World Health Organization. (n.d.). *Programmes and projects: Nutrition.* Retrieved from http://www.who.int/nutrition/about_us/en

190 World Health Organization Consultation on Obesity. (2000). *Obesity: Preventing and managing the global epidemic.* World Health Organization Technical Report Series 894. Geneva, Switzerland: World Health Organization. Retrieved from http://www.bvsde.paho.org/bvsacd/cd66/obeprev/indice.pdf

191 International Obesity Taskforce. (n.d.). *Welcome to IOTF.* Retrieved from http://www.iaso.org/iotf

192 Centers for Disease Control and Prevention. (1989). Health objectives for the nation. *Morbidity and Mortality Weekly Report, 38*(37), 629-33. Retrieved from http://www.cdc.gov/mmwR/preview/mmwrhtml/00001462.htm

193 *History and development of healthy people.* (2011). Retrieved from HealthyPeople.gov website, http://www.healthypeople.gov/2020/about/history.aspx

194 United States Preventive Services Task Force (USPSTF). (2011). *Guide to clinical preventive services, 2012: Recommendations of the U.S. Preventive Services Task Force.* Rockville, MD: Agency for Healthcare Research and Quality. Retrieved from http://www.ahrq.gov/professionals/clinicians-providers/guidelines-recommendations/guide/index.html

195 Association of State & Territorial Public Health Nutrition Directors (ASTPHND). (n.d.). Blueprint for nutrition and physical activity: Cornerstones of a healthy lifestyle. Retrieved from http://www.astphnd.org/resource_files/42/42_resource_file1.pdf

196 U.S. Department of Health and Human Services. (2012). *Nutrition and weight status.* Retrieved from http://www.healthypeople.gov/2020/topicsobjectives2020/objectiveslist.aspx?topicId=29

197 Moyer, C. S. (2011). *Healthy People 2010 misses targets on obesity and health disparities.* Retrieved from http://www.amednews.com/article/20111024/health/310249947/4

198 U.S. Department of Health and Human Services, The Secretary's Advisory Committee on National Health Promotion and Disease Prevention Objectives for 2020. (2008). *Phase 1 report: Recommendations for the framework and format of Healthy People 2020.* Retrieved from http://healthypeople.gov/2020/about/advisory/Phase1.pdf

199 World Health Organization, Department of Nutrition for Health and Development (NHD). (n.d.). *Nutrition.* Retrieved from http://www.who.int/nutrition/about_us/en

200 U.S. Department of Health and Human Services. (n.d.). *About HHS.* Retrieved from http://www.hhs.gov/about

201 Association of State and Territorial Health Officials. (2011). *ASTHO profile of state public health* (Vol. 2). Arlington, VA: ASTHO. Retrieved from http://www.astho.org/profiles

202 Egan, M. C. (1994). Public health nutrition: A historical perspective. *Journal of the American Dietetic Association, 94*(3), 298-304.

203 Egan, M. C. (1994). Public health nutrition: A historical perspective. *Journal of the American Dietetic Association, 94*(3), 298-304.

204 Robinson, T. (2008). Applying the socio-ecological model to improving fruit and vegetable intake among low-income African Americans. *Journal of Community Health, 33*(6), 395-406. doi: 10.1007/s10900-008-9109-5. Retrieved from http://unix.cc.wmich.edu/~lewisj/pdf/health.pdf

205 Huang, T. T., Drewnowski, A., Kumanyika, S. K., & Glass, T. A. (2009). A systems-oriented multilevel framework for addressing obesity in the 21st century. *Preventing Chronic Disease, 6*(3), A82. Retrieved from http://www.cdc.gov/pcd/issues/2009/jul/09_0013.htm.

206 Ahlquist, B. (n.d.). *Understanding policy, systems, and environmental change to improve health.* Presentation at the Minnesota Department of Health. Retrieved from http://www.health.state.mn.us/ommh/committees/ommhadvcomm/policypres0110.pdf

207 *Overview: From evidence-based medicine to evidence-based public health.* (2013). Retrieved from Public Health Information & Data Tutorial website, http://phpartners.org/tutorial/04-ebph/2-keyConcepts/4.2.1.html

208 Brownson, R. C., Fielding, J. E., & Maylahn, C.M. (2009). Evidence-based public health: A fundamental concept for public health practice. *Annual Review of Public Health, 30,* 175-201. doi:10.1146/annurev.publhealth.031308.100134

209 Dreisinger, M., Leet, T. L., Baker, E. A., Gillespie, K. N., Haas, B., & Brownson, R. C.(2008). Improving the public health workforce: Evaluation of a training course to enhance evidence-based decision making. *Journal of Public Health Management and Practice, 14*(2), 138-43. doi:10.1097/01.PHH.0000311891.73078.50

210 Jones, W. A., Nobles, C. J., & Larke, A., Jr. (2006). The effectiveness of a public nutrition education and wellness system program. *Journal of Extension, 44*(3). Retrieved from http://www.joe.org/joe/2006june/rb5.php

211 Contento, I. R. (2008). Nutrition education: Linking research, theory, and practice [review article]. *Asia Pacific Journal of Clinical Nutrition, 17*(1), 176-79.

212 Anderson, J. E. L. (1994). What should be next for nutrition education? *Journal of Nutrition, 124*(9s), 1828s-1832s.

213 Blank, R. M. (1997). *It takes a nation: A new agenda for fighting poverty.* Princeton, NJ: Princeton University Press.

214 Aldridge, D. K. (2006). Interactive computer-tailored nutrition education. In B. F. Realine (Ed.), *Nutrition education and change* (pp. 51-69). Hauppauge, NY: Nova Science Publishers. Retrieved from http://www.fns.usda.gov/ora/MENU/Published/NutritionEducation/Files/LitReview_Tailoring.pdf

215 Milstein, R. L., Wetterhall, S. F., & CDC Evaluation Working Group. (1999, September 17). Framework for program evaluation in public health. *Morbidity and Mortality Weekly Report, Recommendations and Reports, 48*(RR11), 1–40. Retrieved from http://www.cdc.gov/mmwr/preview/mmwrhtml/rr4811a1.htm

216 Centers for Disease Control and Prevention. (2011). *Evaluation steps.* Retrieved from http://www.cdc.gov/eval/steps/index.htm

217 U.S. Department of Agriculture, Office of Inspector General. (2009). *Supplemental Nutrition Assistance Program benefits and the Thrifty Food Plan.* Audit Report 27703-1-KC. Retrieved from http://www.usda.gov/oig/webdocs/27703-1-KC.pdf

218 Grier, S., & Bryant, C.A. (2005). Social marketing in public health. *Annual Review of Public Health, 26,* 319–39. doi:10.1146/annurev.publhealth.26.021304.144610

219 Grier, S., & Bryant, C.A. (2005). Social marketing in public health. *Annual Review of Public Health, 26,* 319–39. doi: 10.1146/annurev.publhealth.26.021304.144610

220 World Health Organization. (2012). *2012 in review: Key health issues.* Retrieved from http://www.who.int/features/2012/year_review/en/index.html

221 Global Alliance for Improved Nutrition (GAIN). (2012). *About GAIN: Investing in partnerships to end malnutrition.* Retrieved from http://www.gainhealth.org/about-gain

222 World Food Programme. (n.d.). *Mission statement.* Retrieved from https://www.wfp.org/about/mission-statement

223 World Food Programme. (n.d.) *Our work.* Retrieved from http://www.wfp.org/our-work

224 World Hunger Relief, Inc. (n.d.) *Mission statement.* Retrieved from http://worldhungerrelief.org/who-we-are/mission-statement

225 Action Against Hunger. (n.d.). *About.* Retrieved from http://www.actionagainsthunger.org/about

226 Heifer International. (n.d.). *Our mission.* Retrieved from http://www.heifer.org/ourwork/mission

227 Evangelical Lutheran Church in America. (n.d.). *ELCA world hunger.* Retrieved from http://www.elca.org/Our-Faith-In-Action/Responding-to-the-World/ELCA-World-Hunger.aspx

228 Care. (n.d.). *About Care.* Retrieved from http://www.care.org/about/index.asp

229 Barrett, C. B. (2007). U.S. international food assistance programs: Issues and Options for the 2007 Farm Bill. In B. L. Gardner & D.A. Summer (Eds.), *The 2007 Farm Bill and beyond* (pp. 97–102). Washington, DC: American Enterprise Institute for Public Policy Research. Retrieved from http://aic.ucdavis.edu/research/farmbill07/aeibriefs/20070516_Summary.pdf

230 U.S. Department of Agriculture, Foreign Agricultural Service. (n.d.). *Food aid.* Retrieved from http://www.fas.usda.gov/food-aid.asp

231 U.S. Agency for International Development. (2012). *Who we are.* Retrieved from http://www.usaid.gov/who-we-are

232 U.S. Department of Agriculture, Food and Nutrition Service. (2013). *Supplemental Nutrition Assistance program: Number of persons participating.* Retrieved from http://www.fns.usda.gov/pd/29snapcurrpp.htm

233 U.S. Department of Agriculture, Food and Nutrition Service. (2013). *Supplemental Nutrition Assistance program: Eligibility.* Retrieved from http://www.fns.usda.gov/snap/applicant_recipients/eligibility.htm#employment

234 U.S. Department of Agriculture, Food and Nutrition Service. (2013). *Supplemental Nutrition Assistance program: Eligibility.* Retrieved from http://www.fns.usda.gov/snap/applicant_recipients/eligibility.htm#employment

235 U.S. Department of Agriculture, National Agriculture Library, Food and Nutrition Information Center. (2013). *Reports and studies.* Retrieved from http://fnic.nal.usda.gov/nutrition-assistance-programs/us-nutrition-assistance-programs/reports-and-studies

236 U.S. Department of Agriculture, Food and Nutrition Service. (2013). *The Emergency Food Assistance Program.* Retrieved from http://www.fns.usda.gov/fdd/programs/tefap

237 U.S. Department of Agriculture, Food and Nutrition Service. (n.d.). *Food security action resources.* Retrieved from http://www.fns.usda.gov/fsec/Resources.htm

238 The Meals on Wheels Association of America. (2013). *About us.* Retrieved from http://www.mowaa.org/about

239 U.S. Department of Agriculture, Food and Nutrition Service. (n.d.). *Senior Farmers' Market Nutrition Program (SFMNP).* Retrieved from http://www.fns.usda.gov/sfmnp

240 U.S. Department of Agriculture, Food and Nutrition Service. (2013). *Commodity Supplemental Food Program.* Retrieved from http://www.fns.usda.gov/fdd/programs/csfp

241 U.S. Department of Agriculture, Food and Nutrition Service. (2013). *Nutrition Services Incentive Program.* Retrieved from http://www.fns.usda.gov/fdd/programs/nsip/default.htm

242 U.S. Department of Agriculture, Food and Nutrition Service. (2013). *Child & Adult Care Food Program.* Retrieved from http://www.fns.usda.gov/cnd/care

243 U.S. Department of Agriculture, National Institute of Food and Agriculture. (2011). *About us: Extension.* Retrieved from http://www.nifa.usda.gov/qlinks/extension.html

244 Centers for Disease Control and Prevention. (2012). *Overweight and obesity: State and community programs.* Retrieved from http://www.cdc.gov/obesity/stateprograms/index.html

245 Centers for Disease Control and Prevention. (n.d.). *Fruits and veggies: More matters.* Retrieved from http://www.fruitsandveggiesmorematters.org/cdc-resources

246 Centers for Disease Control and Prevention. (2010). *Healthier worksite initiative: Introduction.* Retrieved from http://www.cdc.gov/nccdphp/dnpao/hwi/index.htm

247 Centers for Disease Control and Prevention. (2011). *CDC's LEAN Works! A workplace obesity prevention program.* Retrieved from http://www.cdc.gov/leanworks/resources/communityguide.html

248 The Henry J. Kaiser Family Foundation and Health Research and Educational Trust. (2013). *2013 employer health benefits survey.* Retrieved from http://kaiserfamilyfoundation.files .wordpress.com/2013/08/8465-employer-health-benefits -20131.pdf

249 Goetzel, R. Z., & Ozminkowski, R. J. (2008). The health and cost benefits of work site health-promotion programs. *Annual Review of Public Health, 29,* 303-23.

250 Centers for Disease Control and Prevention. (2010). *Healthier worksite initiative: About us.* Retrieved from http://www.cdc .gov/nccdphp/dnpao/hwi/aboutus/index.htm

251 Berry, L. L., Mirabito, A. M., & Baun, W. B. (2010). What's the hard return on employee wellness programs? *Harvard Business Review.* Retrieved from http://hbr.org/2010/12 /whats-the-hard-return-on-employee-wellness-programs/ar/1

252 Lopes da Silva, R. (2011). Chair's round-up. *SCN News, 39,* 3. Retrieved from http://www.unscn.org/files/Publications/SCN _News/SCNNEWS39_10.01_low_def.pdf

253 McLachlan, M., & Garrett, J. (2008). Nutrition change strategies: The new frontier. *Public Health Nutrition, 11*(10), 1063-75. Traitler, H., Watzke, H. J., & Saguy, I. S. (2011). Reinventing R&D in an open innovation ecosystem. *Journal of Food Science, 76*(2), R62-68. doi:10.1111/j.1750-3841.2010.01998.x

254 FoodDrinkEurope. (2012). *ETP Food for Life places innovation at heart of research.* Retrieved from http:// www.fooddrinkeurope.eu/publication/etp-food-for-life -places-innovation-at-heart-of-research

255 Health Canada. (2010). *Sodium reduction strategy for Canada.* Retrieved from http://www.hc-sc.gc.ca/fn-an/nutrition/sodium /related-info-connexe/strateg/index-eng.php

256 Hawkes, C., & Buse, K. (2011). Public-private engagement for diet and health: Addressing the governance gap [commentary]. *SCN News, 39,* 6-10. Retrieved from http://www.unscn .org/files/Publications/SCN_News/SCNNEWS39_10.01_low _def.pdf.

257 U.S. Department of Health and Human Services. (2011). *Dietary guidelines for Americans, 2010: Choose sensibly.* Retrieved from http://www.health.gov/dietaryguidelines/dga2000/document /choose.htm

258 Lichtenstein, A. H., Appel, L. J., Brands, M., Carnethon, M., Daniels, S., . . . Wylie-Rosett, J. (2006). Diet and lifestyle recommendations revision 2006: A scientific statement from the American Heart Association Nutrition Committee. *Circulation, 114*(1), 82-96.

259 Renaud, S., & de Lorgeril, M. (1992). Wine, alcohol, platelets, and the French paradox for coronary heart disease. *Lancet, 339*(8808), 1523-26.

260 Ferrières, J. (2004). The French paradox: Lessons for other countries. *Heart, 90*(1), 107-11. Retrieved from http://www.ncbi .nlm.nih.gov/pmc/articles/PMC1768013

261 Guiliano, M. (2005). *French women don't get fat.* New York, NY: Knopf.

262 Perry, M. (2010). *As share of income, Americans have the cheapest food in history and cheapest food on the planet.* Retrieved from http://www.dailymarkets.com/economy/2010/07/03/as-share -of-income-americans-have-the-cheapest-food-in-history-and- cheapest-food-on-the-planet

263 WebMD. (2010). *French women don't get fat diet review.* Retrieved from http://www.webmd.com/diet/features/french -women-dont-get-fat-diet?page=3

264 Rozin, P., Fischler, C., Imada, S., Sarubin, A., & Wrzesniewski, A. (1999). Attitudes to food and the role of food in life in the U.S.A., Japan, Flemish Belgium and France: Possible implications for the diet-health debate. *Appetite, 33*(2), 163-80.

265 Critser, G. (2003). *Fat land: How Americans became the fattest people in the world.* Boston, MA: Houghton Mifflin.

266 Hercberg, S., Chat-Yung, S., & Chauliac, M. (2008). The French National Nutrition and Health Program: 2001-2006-2010. *International Journal of Public Health, 53,* 68-77.

267 Global Knowledge Exchange Network. (n.d). *French National Nutrition and Health Program (France-Public-Private).* Retrieved from http://www.gken.org/Synopses/CI_10008.pdf

268 Manger Bouger. (n.d.). *Programme National Nutrition Santé.* Retrieved from http://www.mangerbouger.fr/pnns

269 Kesse-Guyot, E., Fezeu, L., Galan, P., Hercberg, S., Czernichow, S., & Castetbon, K. (2011). Adherence to French Nutritional Guidelines is associated with lower risk of metabolic syndrome. *Journal of Nutrition, 141*(6), 1134-39.

270 Hercberg, S., Chat-Yung, S., & Chauliac, M. (2008). The French National Nutrition and Health Program: 2001-2006-2010. *International Journal of Public Health, 53,* 68-77.

271 *Eat well Monday.* (2011). Retrieved from Johns Hopkins Bloomberg School of Public Health website, http://www.jhsph .edu/news/stories/2011/healthy-monday-2011/03282011_home- cooked.html.

272 *Top 12 ways to eat green.* (n.d.). Retrieved from A Well-Fed World website, http://awellfedworld.org/eatinggreen/top12.

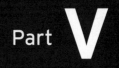

Obesity and Chronic Diseases: Global and Community Public Health Approaches

Chapter 18

Obesity: An Ecologic Perspective on Challenges and Solutions

Rebecca E. Lee, PhD
Heather J. Leach, PhD
Erica G. Soltero, BA
Kirstin R. Vollrath, RD, LD
Allen M. Hallett, BS
Nathan H. Parker, MPH
Matthew B. Cross, MA
Scherezade K. Mama, DrPH
Tracey A. Ledoux, PhD, RD

Overweight and obesity are the fifth leading risk for global deaths. At least 2.8 million adults die each year as a result of being overweight or obese. In addition, 44% of the diabetes burden, 23% of the ischaemic heart disease burden and between 7% and 41% of certain cancer burdens are attributable to overweight and obesity.

Reproduced from: WHO. Fact sheet Number 311. http://www.who.int/mediacentre/factsheets/fs311/en/index.html

Learning Objectives

- Recognize the behavioral, political, and environmental determinants and consequences of obesity.
- Understand how energy balance may be maintained to promote healthy weight.
- Describe the environmental levels of influence within an ecologic model of obesity.
- Identify individual, environmental, and policy-oriented solutions to reverse the obesity epidemic.

Case Study: David from Kansas City, Kansas

David's mother, Juanita, had always been concerned about her son's weight status. She and David's father were not overweight. Before David was born, Juanita had lived in an older home with David's father; his father's parents from Monterrey, Mexico; and their daughter. The home was large, but was in an older part of town near oil refineries and a plastics factory. Aging paint was peeling off the walls. Juanita worried that these conditions were not very good for a new baby, so after David was born, she moved to a small but newer apartment in a better part of town. In a year, David's father left her, and she had to assume financial responsibility for the household.

To make ends meet, Juanita worked as a receptionist by day and in a fast-food restaurant in the evenings. She received free meals from work. She often took these meals home to make sure David had enough to eat, since no supermarkets were nearby and she had little time to prepare meals. In those early years, her mother, David's grandmother, or *abuela,* took care of him. Abuela encouraged him to eat whatever he liked, often giving him soda and sweets to keep him smiling. She lived in a crime-ridden area of town and did not feel safe taking David outside. Instead, they watched television. David was a very sweet but nonathletic boy. His mother could not pay for sports teams or extra-curricular activities. Abuela did not feel safe taking David to the nearby park, and David's mother was so tired from working and cleaning the house that she did not take him, either.

As a schoolchild, David liked to get to school early so he could walk to the nearby convenience store for sodas and snack cakes with his friends. He enjoyed the before-school socializing, soda, and snack, although he ate breakfast at home. He usually prepared himself sugar-sweetened cereal and a fruit-flavored drink while his mother got his little sisters ready for preschool and kindergarten. His sisters were the daughters of his mother's boyfriend, who often stayed over at the apartment. Neither girl was as overweight as David was, likely a result of her boyfriend's cooking skills and assistance in caregiving.

David was a good student who told his friends that his secret was staying quiet and working on his homework during class so that he didn't have to do it after school. This strategy kept him out of trouble. Another habit was to come in early from recess to finish his homework. This was partly because several kids outdoors would call him *gordo* (fat), and also because he didn't want to miss his favorite after-school television programs. His mother had recently bought a new computer, which he used to play online games. He was home alone after school on most days because his mother worked, his sisters had an after-school or day care program, and his mother's boyfriend usually worked afternoons and evenings at a restaurant.

David became obese and developed related health problems. When David's mother finally married her boyfriend, an important benefit to the legal marriage was the health insurance David received to cover his frequent trips to the pediatrician. Although David did well in school, he was not as popular as his two normal-weight sisters. David's mother worried about his health and well-being and wondered how one child had turned out so differently from the other two.

Discussion Questions

- How did factors beyond David's control contribute to David's obesity?
- How did David's micro-environments (home, neighborhood, school) contribute to his obesity?
- What are the individual and public health physical, psychosocial, and other consequences of obesity?
- What types of public health interventions could have prevented David's obesity? Which interventions could still be effective in reducing the effects?
- How do David's daily habits contribute to an imbalance in his overall energy balance? How can public health programs help David and his family become healthier?

Introduction

Obesity Trends

Obesity may be the most serious and challenging public health issue in the world today. In the United States, obesity has become alarmingly more prevalent among all age groups over the past several decades. The prevalence of obesity in children has tripled since 1980, and approximately 17% of children and adolescents aged 2–19 are obese.[1] Obesity prevalence exceeds 12% among American preschoolers aged 2–5, 18% among children aged 6–11, and 18% among adolescents aged 12–19. These figures represent respective increases of 7%, 12%, and 13% since the 1970s.[2,3] The prevalence of obesity among U.S. adults exceeded 35% in 2010.[4] With an additional 33.3% of American adults overweight, fewer than one-third of Americans are classified as "normal weight."[5]

> *Healthy People 2020: NWS-10: Reduce the proportion of children and adolescents who are considered obese*
>
> *Healthy People 2020: NWS-11: (Developmental) Prevent inappropriate weight gain in youth and adults*
>
> Reproduced from the U.S. Department of Health and Human Services. Healthypeople.gov. Retrieved from http://www.healthypeople.gov/2020/default.aspx. Last updated July 30, 2013. Accessed August 13, 2013. All HP 2020 in this chapter are from this source.

Efforts to curb obesity in the United States have fallen short of goals. Not a single U.S. state met the Healthy People 2010 goal to lower rates of adult obesity to 15%; in fact, 12 states currently have rates of adult obesity greater than 30%.[6] Age-adjusted obesity rates, demonstrating nationwide ethnic and socioeconomic disparities, are highest among non-Hispanic blacks (49.5%), followed by Mexican Americans (40.4%), all Hispanics (39.1%), and non-Hispanic whites (34.3%).[7] Low-income women are more likely to be obese than their higher-income peers, and the same relationship exists among non-Hispanic black and Hispanic men.[8] Women who have lower levels of education are also more likely to be obese.

These distressing statistics are paralleled on a global level; the worldwide obesity prevalence has more than doubled since 1980. Once considered a problem of high-income countries, obesity is quickly becoming a serious threat in many low- and middle-income countries, particularly in urban areas. Only eight million of the world's 43 million overweight and obese children live in high-income countries. The risk of dying due to overweight- or obesity-related conditions exceeds the risk of dying due to underweight-related conditions for 65% of the world's population.[9] Lifestyle changes, such as increased calorie consumption and sedentary behavior, are widely accepted as causes of these increases in obesity. Obesity has clearly reached pandemic status, and it has debilitating repercussions.

> *Public Health Core Competency 1: Analytical/ Assessment Skills 2: Describes the characteristics of a population-based health problem*
>
> *Public Health Core Competency 1: Analytical/ Assessment Skills 3: Uses variables that measure public health conditions*
>
> Reproduced from Council on Linkages Between Academia and Public Health Practice. 2010 May. Core Competencies for Public Health Professionals. Washington, DC: Public Health Foundation. http://www.phf.org/resourcestools/Documents/Core_Competencies_for_Public_Health_Professionals_2010May.pdf. Accessed August 13, 2013. This source is used for all Public Health Core Competencies in this chapter.

Consequences of Obesity

The obesity epidemic has dire consequences for the physical health and economic well-being of populations across the globe. Obesity is a risk factor for many noncommunicable diseases. **Cardiovascular diseases (CVD)**, such as heart disease and stroke, are the world's leading causes of death and are commonly linked to obesity. Obesity also increases risk for **type 2 diabetes**, musculoskeletal disorders such as osteoarthritis, and certain cancers, including those of the colon, breast, and endometrium. Children who are overweight or obese are more likely to be obese in adulthood, to die prematurely, and to experience disability than their normal-weight peers. Rising rates of breathing difficulties, **hypertension**, and early diabetes among children and adolescents reflect increases in childhood and adolescent obesity.[10]

In the United States, obesity-related costs account for more than 20% of total healthcare expenditures, with overweight and obese people costing, on average, $2,700 more per year than those who are normal weight.[11] America's poor—those who most often face **food insecurity**—confront obesity due to limited availability of nutritious foods. In many developing countries, overweight and obesity coexist with **undernutrition** and **malnutrition**, adding a significant obstacle to economic progress.[12] Obesity is a complex global health phenomenon with multifaceted causes and impacts, and myriad stakeholders.

> *Public Health Core Competency 1: Analytical/ Assessment Skills 2: Describes the characteristics of a population-based health problem*
>
> *Public Health Core Competency 5: Community Dimension of Practice Skills 1: Recognizes community linkages and relationships among multiple factors (or determinants) affecting health*

Obesity also has economic consequences. In addition to being less likely to secure employment, obese individuals who do work tend to receive lower wages than nonobese people. These disparities may result from discrimination or **comorbidities**. Obesity-related changes in posture, muscle strength, work capacity, and physical mobility reduce employee productivity. Obesity is associated with more work-related injuries, such as carpal tunnel syndrome and back pain.[13] Desks, chairs, and other amenities can be too small for obese individuals. Larger seats, as on airplanes and public transportation, are expensive. Furthermore, clothing sizes have expanded with the increase in obesity. Obesity-related needs such as wheelchairs, larger blood pressure cuffs, and longer needles to penetrate excess fat increase healthcare delivery costs.[14] Obesity has also required changes in ambulances and gurneys to accommodate larger people in medical transport.[15]

> *Public Health Core Competency 4: Cultural Competency Skills 2: Recognizes the role of cultural, social, and behavioral factors in the accessibility, availability, acceptability, and delivery of public health services*

Obesity has even been implicated in climate change. Using a hypothetical population with a 40% obesity rate, Edwards and Roberts (2009) projected a 19% increase in the food energy needs, contributing to an annual increase in greenhouse gas emissions.[16] Similarly, increases in population weight may further contribute to climate change by demanding greater amounts of fuel to haul heavier people.

What Is Obesity?

Overweight and **obesity** are conditions characterized by excessive accumulation of fat in adipose tissue. **Body mass index (BMI)** is the ratio of a person's weight in kilograms to height in meters squared. It is a common measure of nutritional status used to assess body composition and the associated risk for morbidity and mortality. Adults with a BMI between 25 and 29.9 kg/m^2 are considered overweight, whereas adults with a BMI greater than or equal to 30 kg/m^2 are classified as obese. For children and adolescents, BMI is adjusted for age and sex and reported as a percentile. Normative values from a nationally representative sample, taken from the **National Health and Nutrition Examination Survey (NHANES)**, categorize overweight children and adolescents as having a BMI between the 85th and 94.9 percentiles.[17,18] Children and adolescents identified as obese have a BMI greater than or equal to the 95th percentile. BMI scores classified as overweight or obese are associated with higher incidence of chronic diseases, such as cardiovascular disease and type 2 diabetes, and increased risk of death.[19]

Public Health Core Competency 1: Analytical/Assessment Skills 3: Uses variables that measure public health conditions

Public Health Core Competency 1: Analytical/Assessment Skills 9: Describes the public health applications of quantitative and qualitative data

Public Health Core Competency 3: Communication Skills 6: Applies communication and group dynamic strategies in interactions with individuals and groups

Public Health Core Competency 6: Basic Public Health Science Skills 5: Describes the scientific evidence related to a public health issue, concern, or intervention

The location of body fat, or **regional adiposity distribution**, affects the risk of developing obesity and related comorbidities. Regional adiposity distribution is determined in part by genetic predisposition and in part by unhealthy lifestyle habits. Eating foods higher in saturated fats and cholesterol has been closely associated with gains in visceral fat and upper-body subcutaneous fat, particularly in the abdominal area, resulting in an "apple shape." The "apple" shape is associated with greater risk for a number of obesity-related health-compromising conditions. A "pear" shape, characterized by more fat stored in the lower body, chiefly in the hips and thighs, is associated with decreased risk for chronic disease.[20] Regardless of genetic predisposition, regular moderate to vigorous aerobic physical activity (MVPA) is associated with reduced likelihood of being overweight or obese and having related health conditions.[21]

Public Health Core Competency 3: Communication Skills 4: Participates in the development of demographic, statistical, programmatic, and scientific presentations

Public Health Core Competency 4: Cultural Competency Skills 2: Recognizes the role of cultural, social, and behavioral factors in the accessibility, availability, acceptability, and delivery of public health services

Public Health Core Competency 6: Basic Public Health Science Skills 1: Describes the scientific foundation of the field of public health

Energy Balance

Consuming and metabolizing food provides the human body with the energy necessary to function. Energy in food is measured in **kilocalories**, commonly referred to as **calories**. During digestion, food is broken down into macro- and micronutrients. **Macronutrients** include carbohydrate, protein, and fat. Carbohydrates and protein provide 4 calories per gram, while fat supplies 9 calories per gram. Alcohol supplies 7 calories per gram.[22] **Micronutrients**, or vitamins and minerals, do not supply the body with energy.

Energy balance is the concept that body weight will remain the same if the number of calories consumed equals the number of calories expended. Obesity can result from positive energy imbalance, or when the amount of energy consumed exceeds the amount expended. Many nations enjoy a food supply with more than sufficient calories. Furthermore, modern technological conveniences have reduced the amount of necessary daily physical activity and therefore calorie expenditure.[23]

An accumulation of approximately 3,500 extra calories is stored by the body as 1 pound of fat. Expenditure of approximately 3,500 calories more than consumed will lead to the reduction of body fat by 1 pound. This conversion of calories to body tissue explains why gaining and losing body weight are often slow and gradual. On a daily basis, perfect energy balance is unlikely, but the average intake versus expenditure over time equates to energy balance, or a stable weight.

With abundant opportunities to eat and reduced need for physical activity, energy balance can easily become unbalanced over time. Because of environmental influences on energy balance, the most effective strategies for helping to stabilize energy balance, thereby reducing weight gain and preventing obesity, may be policy and environmental strategies. These changes can improve available food choices to feature lower-calorie nutrient-dense options and increase opportunities for physical activity, making sedentary choices more difficult.[24]

> *Public Health Core Competency 2: Policy Development/ Program Planning Skills 2: Describes how policy options can influence public health programs*

Energy Needed for Optimal Health

Many methods are available to predict total daily energy needs in adults. The most commonly used calculation predicts **resting energy expenditure**[25] **(REE)** based on age, gender, height, and weight, and individual physical activity levels. REE considers **basal metabolic rate (BMR)**, or the energy needed to sustain bodily functions, such as the heart beating, as well as the **thermic effect of food (TEF)**, or the energy required for metabolizing food.

The following gender-specific equations are used to calculate REE in adults.[26]

Males: REE $= 10 \times$ weight (kg) $+ 6.25 \times$ height (cm) $- 5 \times$ age $(y) + 5$

Females: REE $= 10 \times$ weight (kg) $+ 6.25 \times$ height (cm) $- 5 \times$ age $(y) - 161$

To calculate total energy expenditure, this REE calculation is then multiplied by an **activity factor (AF)** that considers gender and the amount of occupational activity regularly performed, as shown in **Table 18-1**. The TEE is calculated using this equation:

TEE $=$ REE $\times$ AF

Table 18-1 Activity factor (AF) based on intensity of occupational work

	Light	Moderate	Heavy
Men	1.55	1.78	2.10
Women	1.56	1.64	1.82

Adapted from World Health Organization. (1991). Energy and protein requirements. Report of a joint FAO/WHO/UNU Expert Consultation. Geneva. Accessed August 27, 2013, from http://www.fao.org/docrep/003 /AA040E/AA040E00.htm.

Physical Activity Recommendations

All adults should do some form of physical activity on most days of the week in addition to the light-intensity activities of daily living, such as sweeping and climbing a flight of stairs. Low or light amounts of physical activity include moderate exercise fewer than 150 minutes per week. Medium or moderate amounts of activity include moderate exercise 150–300 minutes per week or 75 minutes per week of vigorous exercise, and high or heavy amounts of activity include greater than 300 minutes of moderate activity per week or 150 minutes of vigorous exercise per week. Examples of moderate exercise are bicycling (less than 10 miles per hour), dancing, and walking 3.5 miles per hour. Examples of vigorous exercise are aerobic dancing, jogging at 6 miles per hour, and heavy yard work.[27] Individuals trying to lose weight or maintain a weight loss should get 60 to 90 minutes of physical activity every day.[28]

The concept of energy balance is the same for children as for adults, although children need additional energy for growth. The 2010 *Dietary Guidelines for Americans* estimate that a moderately active 2-year-old child requires 1,000 kcal/day,[29] with this number increasing by about 100 calories per year until age 8. Beginning at age 9, girls require an additional 50 calories per year of age until age 18, while boys require an additional 110 calories per year of age until 18. More active children require a greater number of calories, while less active children require fewer.

Physical activity is as important a factor in determining children's energy needs as it is for those of adults. The *Physical Activity Guidelines for Americans 2008* strongly recommend that children engage in moderate to vigorous physical activity for 60 minutes per day. This includes any rhythmic activity, such as swimming, running, bicycling, and dancing, which uses major muscle groups. An additional three days per week of muscle and bone-strengthening exercises is recommended as well.[30] Examples include climbing trees, playing hopscotch, playing tennis, or playing on playground equipment. Compared with physically inactive children, children who participate in physical activity have stronger muscles, higher levels of cardiovascular fitness, less body fat, and stronger bones. Physical activity in children is linked to lower levels of depression and anxiety and a lower risk for developing chronic diseases such as hypertension, type 2 diabetes, and cardiovascular disease.

Determinants of Obesity

Obesity has complex **determinants**, or factors, elements, or circumstances that influence an outcome. Identifying and understanding the most significant and modifiable determinants of obesity helps public health nutritionists develop effective interventions. Conceptual or theoretical **models** can help with this understanding of the complex determinants of obesity.

Public Health Core Competency 8: Leadership and Systems Thinking Skills 2: Describes how public health operates within a larger system

Ecologic models conceptualize individual and environmental determinants and can serve as useful frameworks for understanding the multiple factors that contribute to obesity.[31,32,33,34] Intra-individual factors (that is, biological, behavioral, or cognitive) are relatively small influences on human health in the context of the ecological model.[35] Outcomes suggested in these models can include individual-level health behaviors, such as physical activity and dietary habits, and disease states, such as obesity.[36,37,38,39,40] A limitation of ecologic models is that they artificially categorize factors.

The Ecologic Model of Physical Activity (EMPA) includes individual biologic and behavioral determinants of physical activity and categorizes environmental factors into four levels of influence (micro, meso, exo, and macro).[41] This chapter describes an adaptation of the EMPA for studying human obesity and offers determinants and solutions for the obesity epidemic framed within the EMPA. **Figure 18-1** presents an EMPA adapted for conceptualizing determinants of human obesity.

Public Health Core Competency 2: Policy Development/ Program Planning Skills 4: Gathers information that will inform policy decisions

Micro-environmental factors are actual places, such as the home, school, or workplace. Meso- and exo-environmental factors serve as dynamic physical and social connections between micro-environments and behavioral outcomes. **Meso-environmental** factors describe a link that directly connects one micro-environment with another

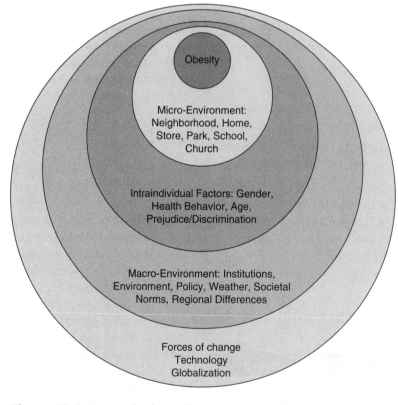

Figure 18-1 An ecologic systems framework for studying human obesity

Data from Lee, R. E., & Cubbin, C. (2009). Striding toward social justice: The ecologic milieu of physical activity. *Exercise and Sport Sciences Reviews, 37*(1), 10-17.

micro-environment and a behavioral outcome, while **exo-environmental** factors are indirect links between two micro-environments and a behavioral outcome. **Macro-environmental** factors have broad implications for most of the population. **Forces of change** are cross-level phenomena, such as globalization and technology, which can potentially impact all other levels directly and indirectly in measurable and nonmeasurable ways.

Individual Determinants

Personal determinants of obesity include age, gender, ethnicity, and psychological factors such as personality, attitude constructs, self-efficacy, and motivation.[42] These personal factors are directly related to the behaviors, such as physical inactivity and overeating, that affect obesity. Cognitive control and self-regulatory behaviors may also have a role in obesity in adults and children.[43] Recent research suggests that sedentary adolescents have less self-regulation and motivation than active and healthy adolescents.[44]

Many factors contribute to individual food preferences and consumption. One study looked at taste, cost, convenience, nutrition, and weight control as factors in food preference. Taste and cost were found to be the greatest contributing factor to food preference among American adults overall, while cost was the most important factor for younger age groups, women, and people with lower incomes.[45] Processed, energy-dense, nutrient-poor foods are often lowest in cost. Another study found that after controlling for moderate to vigorous physical activity overall energy intake, refined grains, vegetables, total fat, total protein, and total carbohydrate were all associated with adiposity in children. Vegetables were likely included in this group due to butter, cheese, and other high-fat, energy-dense condiments.[46]

> *Public Health Core Competency 5: Community Dimension of Practice Skills 8: Identifies community assets and resources*

Micro-Environment

An individual's immediate surroundings define the micro-environment. The eating environments and opportunities for physical activity that are available in these daily settings directly contribute to dietary behaviors and levels of physical activity.

One's neighborhood is an example of a micro-environment that affects obesity. Having healthful, economically priced food located in close proximity to one's residence can increase the probability of having healthful food available in the home,[47] which may lead to increased consumption of healthier, lower-calorie food. For example, living in a neighborhood with nearby supermarkets that offer affordable fruits and vegetables may lead to increased consumption of these low-calorie options, while residents in **food deserts**, or neighborhoods without much access to healthy foods, may have poorer diets and higher risk of obesity.[48,49,50,51,52]

The Micro-Environment and Food Choices

Worksites and schools are additional micro-environments that affect weight. Most Americans spend at least eight hours per working day at work,[53] and food and beverage consumption is more common at work than anywhere except the home.[54] Therefore, calories consumed at work are significant factors in weight status. Low-status jobs, poor occupational conditions, and high workloads and demands are associated with less healthful employee diets compared with high-status jobs and low job demands.[55,56] Employees may be less likely to consume low-calorie, nutrient-rich food if the workplace lacks accessible, healthy options. Consider these two hypothetical workplaces:

Company A allows 30 minutes for lunch. On-site vending machines primarily dispense snack items, such as chips, candy, and soda. The only accessible alternative is a hamburger stand across the street. Employees can go to the stand, eat, and return to work on time.

Company B also allows its employees 30 minutes for lunch. A cafeteria on the main floor offers a daily lunch special consisting of a lean protein source, such as chicken or fish, a whole grain, and seasonal vegetables. Other available items include salads, sandwiches, low-fat yogurt, and fresh fruit.

Compared with Company A, the food environment at Company B promotes healthier employee diet choices. School environments and children's dietary behaviors are analogous to this example; school lunch programs that provide nutritionally dense and calorically appropriate meals improve children's access to healthy food and create an environment that encourages healthy eating. Students who participate in the **National School Lunch Program (NSLP)**, whose regulations include certain nutritional standards, are more likely than nonparticipants to consume milk, fruit, and vegetables, and less likely to consume desserts, snack items, and beverages other than milk or 100% juice.[57] Another study found that the **School Breakfast Program (SBP)** may reduce childhood obesity, but found opposite effects of the NSLP.[58] Furthermore, a different study comparing NSLP participants with nonparticipants found no difference in BMI, but faster weight gain for girls on NSLP, with no difference among boys.[59]

> *Healthy People 2020: NWS-2: Increase the proportion of schools that offer nutritious foods and beverages outside of school meals*

The home environment is another micro-environment and determinant of obesity. Food available in the home affects dietary intake.[60,61,62] For example, children whose homes contain prepared fresh fruits and vegetables at eye level in the refrigerator can eat more healthfully than children whose options are potato chips or cookies.[63]

The Micro-Environment and Physical Activity

The micro-environment also influences obesity through physical activity. Safer, more pleasant neighborhoods promote physical activity. For example, residents of neighborhoods with lower speed limits do more physical activity.[64] Research among adults has consistently found that living in attractive areas, with a high population density, greater street connectivity, greater access to goods and services, and greater access to high-quality physical-activity resources, is associated with more physical activity and lower BMIs.[65,66,67] Children who live in neighborhoods that have more parks or parkland and are safer are more likely to engage in physical activity and less likely to be overweight or obese.[68,69,70,71]

Living in lower **socioeconomic status**, or SES, areas is associated with negative effects on health and promotes obesity. These neighborhoods often pose safety concerns and other physical characteristics that reduce quality of life. Even when high-quality physical activity resources are available, residents are discouraged from using these resources if they perceive their neighborhoods as unsafe or unappealing. Engaging in physical activity or actively transporting to work, church, or quality supermarkets and grocery stores becomes hindered, negatively impacting physical activity and dietary habits.[72,73]

Sedentary Time and Obesity

In the home environment, the television is strongly related to childhood obesity. Increased "screen" time may have a stronger association with overweight and obesity in children than even physical activity.[74] One study found that each extra hour per day of watching television was associated with an extra 1 kg of body fat in preschool children.[75]

Access to, and nighttime use of, electronic entertainment and communication devices such as video games, computers, and smartphones may be associated with poorer diet quality and shortened sleep duration, which is linked to childhood overweight.[76,77,78] Weight gain can also result when children consume high-calorie snacks while watching television or playing video games.[79]

Meso-Environment

The interaction between two or more settings can influence behaviors that affect obesity. The dynamic linkages and interactive processes that occur between individual environments are referred to as the meso-environment.[80]

Distance to Supermarkets

The relationship between the places where food is purchased and consumed is an important meso-environment linkage. Low access to a supermarket due to distance, traffic, or lack of transportation makes keeping fresh foods available at home more difficult, thereby decreasing fruit and vegetable consumption and facilitating unhealthy food decisions such as consuming processed foods or dining out.[81,82] In addition, long commutes to the supermarket require sedentary time en route, not only decreasing physical activity, but also reducing available time to prepare nutritious food. Further, this commuting linkage can reduce social connectivity by limiting the amount of time spent engaging with others socially—for example, reducing shared family meal time, and further contributing to obesity.[83]

The route of the daily commute may provide exposure to marketing materials for food and opportunities to buy food. Lower SES neighborhoods tend to have more convenience, liquor, or small grocery stores with lower-quality fruits and vegetables, which often have higher-priced foods than higher-SES neighborhoods.[84] Individuals in these low-SES areas have more opportunities to make poor nutritional choices, including considering fast food while in transit.[85]

Social Meso-Environmental Links

Meso-environmental links can be social. Shared interactions between people can link separate settings, causing events in one setting to influence events in another setting. Children may receive similar messages about the importance of eating fruits and vegetables in the school environment and the home environment. Receiving these messages in two different settings may encourage fruit and vegetable consumption in either setting.

Exo-Environment

Indirect links between a micro-environment and a person's behavior can contribute to obesity.[86] Like meso-environmental factors, the exo-environment describes the dynamic factors that link occurrences in one micro-environment to occurrences in another micro-environment. In contrast to the meso-environment, the exo-environment describes a link from one micro-environment to another. The person from the first micro-environment does not usually interact directly with the second micro-environment.

Consider a workplace wellness program aimed at increasing fruit and vegetable consumption. The program could lead employees to provide more of these foods in their children's lunches, leading to increased fruit and vegetable consumption by the child. In this case, the linkage between events at the parent's workplace and the food eaten by the child at school demonstrate an exo-environmental link between the parent and the child by connecting the workplace, a micro-environment in which the child does not interact, with the school, a micro-environment where the parent does not typically interact.[87]

These interactive environmental processes are frequent and influential, but rarely consciously recognized. Employees working at separate companies may share workout plans and recipes via email. Their communication via email serves as a social exo-environmental link between their separate micro-environments, allowing their correspondence to influence their dietary and physical activity behavior. Another example of a social exo-environmental linkage might be while traveling in a vehicle between micro-environmental settings. For example, while on a public bus, a passenger may discuss current events involving nutrition. This social exo-environmental linkage then can influence choices that another passenger who overhears the conversation may make for meals later that day or the next. Similarly, friends can influence each others' eating habits through exo-environmental links.

Media and Exo-Environmental Links

The media provide additional exo-environmental links. Children are exposed to a high volume of television commercials advertising food products for children. These advertisements encourage children to ask their parents to purchase these foods, which are often high-calorie. Most children tend to request that their parents purchase these products, and parents often indulge children in their requests, succumbing to their pestering and nagging.[88,89] If parents purchase the food without the child being present at the store, then the advertisement stimulated an exo-environmental linkage between the child in the home environment with the parent in the grocery store environment.

Macro-Environment

The macro-environment includes determinants that impact a large segment of the population. Examples include policies, social norms, technological innovations, and weather patterns.

Policies at the municipal, state, and federal levels have the potential to affect health for many people, and even one effective policy can improve many people's health without individual effort. Previous examples include school meal programs improving access to healthful foods,[90,91] neighborhood coalitions promoting physical activity–friendly programs[92] and campaigns increasing awareness of healthy eating.[93] Some policies, such as agricultural subsidies, indirectly affect obesity by affecting cost and availability of certain crops.[94]

> *Healthy People 2020: NWS-1: Increase the number of states with nutrition standards for foods and beverages provided to preschool-aged children in child care*
>
> *Healthy People 2020: NWS-3: Increase the number of states that have state-level policies that incentivize food retail outlets to provide foods that are encouraged by the* Dietary Guidelines for Americans

Transportation Policies

Transportation policies can promote physical activity to target obesity. An initiative known as the "Complete Streets Policy" alters the design of streets to accommodate not only automobile traffic, but also public transit, bicycles, and pedestrians. These streets are designed to improve safety for *all* users by allowing pedestrians to safely cross busy streets, reducing left-turning motorist crashes and creating designated bike lanes.[95] These streets create more walkable neighborhoods, which are associated with more physical activity and lower likelihood of being overweight or obese. Less driving saves fuel, reduces carbon emissions, and improves air quality, which in turn makes outdoor exercise more enjoyable.

> *Millennium Development Goal 7: Ensure Environmental Sustainability. Target 7.A: Integrate the principles of sustainable development into the country policies and programs and reverse the loss of environmental resources*
>
> Reproduced from the United Nations. (n.d.). 2015 Millennium Development Goals. Retrieved from http://www.un.org/millenniumgoals/. Accessed August 13, 2013. This source is used for all Millennium Development Goals in this chapter.

Discrimination

Discrimination is another macro-environmental factor that can affect obesity. The effects of **institutional discrimination**, often manifested in disparities in political and civic representation, education, and occupational opportunities, are substantial but hard to measure. In one example, gender discrimination leads to lower wages for women compared with men doing the same work.[96,97] This can contribute to obesity and poor diet quality among women who limit more nutritious but expensive food options.[98,99,100,101]

> *Millennium Development Goal 3: Promote Gender Equality and Empower Women. Target 3.A: Eliminate gender disparity in primary and secondary education, preferably by 2005, and in all levels of education by 2015*

Additional disparities in health behaviors and outcomes may reflect the lack of health promoting urban planning in deprived areas compared with higher-income areas. As discussed earlier, differences in type, quantity, quality, and cost of healthful food by neighborhood income and ethnic composition are evident. Many low-SES, high-ethnic minority neighborhoods have primarily convenience, liquor, or small grocery stores; lower produce quality; and higher prices of some foods.[102] Fewer accessible supermarkets implies less opportunity to select low-calorie foods, contributing to poor dietary choices and obesity.

Toxic Exposure and Obesity

Superficially unrelated toxin exposure can also influence obesity. For example, low levels of maternal lead exposure have been associated with obesity in offspring in mice.[103] This phenomenon of early metabolic programming that occurs in utero has also been documented with maternal exposure to numerous environmental toxins that are by-products of many modern-day production processes.[104] Commonly occurring toxins such as cigarette smoke, diesel exhaust, pharmaceuticals, and pesticides have been implicated as possible obesogens that may be widely present in the macro-environment.

Forces of Change and Other Determinants

Forces of change that can affect obesity include weather, technology, and globalization. Poor weather conditions can be a barrier to participation in physical activity.[105] Weather patterns can also affect accessibility of foods. Fruit and vegetable availability varies naturally by season, and extreme weather can influence the cost, types, and selection available to consumers, especially disadvantaged ones.[106] Droughts and extreme weather patterns can also increase costs of grains and animal products.

Technological innovations have led to methodologies that allow reduced physical activity. Examples include agricultural machines and personal vehicles.

Globalization

Despite some health benefits,[107] **globalization** has largely facilitated obesity's spread from being exclusively a Western problem to becoming a global problem. An estimated 1.5 billion adults worldwide are overweight or obese.[108] Global trade liberalization policies have led to cheaper, more readily available high-calorie processed food, which is often chosen instead of traditional, healthier foods. This increases risk of overweight or obesity.[109] Much of the rise in obesity worldwide has been attributed to the Westernization of diets, with fast food replacing traditional meals.[110,111,112]

Current Solution Strategies

Obesity is a grave public health issue with high relapse rates and modest effects even in the most successful treatment and prevention programs.[113,114,115] However, repeated weight loss efforts and small weight losses can have health benefits.[116] Data from NHANES and the National Weight Control Registry, which is a database of people who have sustained weight loss of at least 30 pounds for at least one year, suggest significant long-term weight loss is achievable.[117] Sustained weight loss is relatively uncommon. Continuation of obesogenic behavior choices likely results from causes discussed so far in this chapter. Public health strategies should be based on time-tested interventions to change behavior.[118]

Individual Solutions (Behavioral Interventions)

Weight loss diet and exercise plans are well developed and widely researched. These individual antiobesity strategies use one-on-one or group approaches to change an individual's obesity-related behaviors. Often the initial results are quite promising, but maintaining weight loss is challenging. Relapse rates are high. Some recently developed programs simultaneously target micro-, meso-, exo-, or macro-environmental factors along with individual factors.

Behavioral interventions involve counseling and education to improve dietary habits and physical activity, using techniques such as reducing barriers to change, self-monitoring, goal setting, nutrition education, stress management, stimulus control, problem solving, contingency management, cognitive restructuring, and social support.[119,120] Multicomponent interventions use multiple behavioral techniques tailored to individual needs and preferences to achieve behavior change and prevent relapse.[121] Intensive interventions consist of 12 to 26 group or individual sessions in the first year.[122] The Academy of Nutrition and Dietetics recommends comprehensive weight management programs with regular patient contact for six or more months or until goals are reached.[123] Research shows that high-quality multicomponent intensive behavioral interventions produce a 4–6% decrease in body weight in one year at a rate of 1–2 pounds per week.[124,125] Other positive outcomes from multicomponent behavioral interventions are improved **glucose tolerance** and cardiovascular health.[126]

Micro-Environment Solutions

Like individually focused solutions, community-level interventions target obesity by aiming to change obesity-related behaviors such as eating, physical activity, sleep, and screen time. Community-level interventions are sometimes called public health interventions, because of their focus on populations, rather than individuals, and on prevention, rather than treatment. They focus on preventing obesity in normal-weight individuals. In overweight and obese individuals, the focus may be on weight loss to prevent or mitigate obesity-related health problems. The hope of these strategies is to shift the population average, so that their impact is broader than individually focused strategies. Community interventions to treat or prevent obesity may be delivered through micro-environments such as worksites, healthcare systems, and schools.

Worksite Solutions

Employed U.S. adults spend the majority of their waking hours at the worksite,[127] and multilevel worksite programs can effectively promote weight loss and maintenance.[128,129] Individual workplace strategies can include dissemination of health information via seminars and educational software, and behavioral techniques, such as individual counseling, skills building, reward reinforcement, and social support of coworkers. Strategies affecting the micro-environment include offering healthier choices in cafeterias and vending machines.[130,131,132] Worksite programs have demonstrated cost savings from $1.44 to $4.16 saved per pound of loss in body weight.[133]

> *Healthy People 2020: NWS-7: (Developmental) Increase the proportion of worksites that offer nutrition or weight management classes or counseling*
>
> *Healthy People 2020: PA-12: (Developmental) Increase the proportion of employed adults who have access to and participate in employer-based exercise facilities and exercise programs*

Worksite wellness programs in the United States typically depend on individually focused strategies peppered with social and physical environmental supports. Providence College introduced free health screenings in the worksite micro-environment, measured body composition and related health indicators during health fairs, and provided information on weight control through nationally recognized programs such as Weight Watchers. The program's 12-week fitness challenge capitalized on social connections in the meso-level environment. Farmers' markets hosted in March and October improved healthy food access in the micro-environment.[134] This multicomponent strategy showed that careful monitoring of health and information at the individual level, partnered with meso- and micro-environmental change, could be more sustainable and even reach people beyond the worksite.

Finnair, whose employees work in nontraditional settings, implemented its program upon finding that 30% of its employees were at risk for developing diabetes. The voluntary program features health screenings and follow-up information and counseling. Program participants had modestly improved health and lower risk for obesity and type 2 diabetes compared with nonparticipants.[135] Many multinational companies are beginning to take worksite wellness very seriously because of the impact that obesity has on the workforce,[136] particularly because of absenteeism and reduced productivity. Most current programs emphasize individual approaches, but the use of public health approaches targeting environmental change is increasing. Altering the environment can be less costly and more effective than changing individual behaviors.

Healthcare Setting Interventions

Healthcare settings are another micro-environment where obesity prevention and treatment strategies can combine strategies. The U.S. Preventive Task Force (USPTF) recommends that healthcare providers refer overweight or obese children for intensive behavioral interventions. Research shows that effective weight management programs for children include parent involvement,[137] as a meso- or exo-environment pathway, and individual behavioral counseling,[138,139] to address physical activity and diet, and at least 25 hours of provider contact in six months.[140] Behavioral counseling should include techniques such as self-monitoring, stimulus control, eating management, contingency management, and cognitive behavioral techniques.[141] Success is greater when more behavior change techniques are used in child obesity prevention interventions.[142] The USPTF Expert Committee recommends clinicians provide counseling to children and families to promote evidence-based obesity prevention behaviors among all children annually. The Expert Panel also recommends a staged approach in which treatment intensity increases as treatment resistance is demonstrated. Counseling should be delivered using patient-centered communication, with the goal of promoting the following evidence-based behaviors among all children and their families starting at birth:

1. Limit consumption of sugar-sweetened beverages.
2. Encourage consumption of diets with recommended quantities of fruits and vegetables.
3. Limit television and other screen time to no more than 2 hours per day.
4. Eat breakfast daily.
5. Limit eating out at restaurants, particularly fast-food restaurants.
6. Encourage family meals.
7. Limit portion sizes to those recommended by the U.S. Department of Agriculture.
8. Eat a diet rich in calcium.
9. Eat a high-fiber diet.
10. Eat a diet with balanced macronutrients (i.e., fat, protein, and carbohydrate).
11. Encourage exclusive breastfeeding until children are 6 months of age.
12. Promote moderate to vigorous physical activity for at least 60 minutes per day.
13. Limit consumption of **energy-dense** foods.[143]

The USPTF also recommends that healthcare providers screen all adults for obesity and that those with a BMI of at least 30 kg/m^2 receive intensive multicomponent behavioral intervention.[144] However, most physicians are not trained in counseling techniques, and medical school curricula are typically lacking in education on nutrition and physical activity. For most providers, discussing healthy dietary habits and physical activity during the office visit is not routine.[145]

> *Healthy People 2020: NWS-5: Increase the proportion of primary care physicians who regularly measure the body mass index of their patients*
>
> *Healthy People 2020: NWS-6: Increase the proportion of physician office visits that include counseling or education related to nutrition or weight*

Strategies for Childhood Obesity

As gatekeepers of the home, parents should be involved in programs to reduce child obesity. In addition, children spend significant time in schools, where modifications can be made in available foods, such as in the cafeteria, classrooms, and foods brought from home; classroom, homework, and web-based nutrition education; activities, such as taste testing, school gardens, and cooking classes; and role models, such as teachers and peers. The community also contains multiple influences on children's eating behaviors. The physical built neighborhood includes food stores, farmer's markets, and vending machines.

Reducing screen time, which includes television viewing, video games, movies, computers, and Internet, is among the most effective strategies for combating childhood obesity.[146] Programs should include behavioral techniques such as skills building, advice, goal setting, reinforcement, family support, and stimulus control, such as removing screen time prompts in the immediate environment. Some interventions have reduced daily screen time by 26 to 55 minutes, with associated reductions in adiposity.[147]

Healthy People 2020: PA-8: Increase the proportion of children and adolescents who do not exceed recommended limits for screen time

Intervention Strategies Based on the Traffic Light Diet

The Traffic Light Diet is among the most successful and widely adopted strategies developed for children.[148,149,150] Based on the familiar red, yellow, and green colors of traffic lights to help children and families make better health choices, the diet is part of a package with family and behaviorally based, therapeutic interventions.

Foods are divided into five food groups and color coded in terms of nutrient density. Low-nutrient and high-fat or high-sugar foods, such as sweets, sodas, French fries, and chips, are coded red. Yellow-coded foods include grains, meats, and other nutritious foods. Low in fat and added sweeteners, most green foods have fewer than 20 calories per serving and include many vegetables and fruits. Children and families are advised to consume red foods no more than four times per week, consume some yellow foods, and choose more green foods to achieve a particular calorie range. The individual behavior change strategy is teamed with an environmental strategy to reduce the availability of red foods in the home and increase the availability of green foods to foster healthy choices. Another advantage is that it is easy to understand, and is useful among diverse ages and income levels. The Academy of Nutrition and Dietetics and other groups have adopted the program.[151]

Healthy People 2020: NWS-17: Reduce consumption of calories from solid fats and added sugars in the population aged 2 years and older

Several countries have adopted the traffic light strategy for food labeling systems to help guide consumer food choices. A traffic signal is printed on the front of the packaging of the product with a red, yellow, or green light to indicate the healthfulness of the particular product at a glance. The United Kingdom Food Standards Agency recommended such a policy in 2006. An early evaluation of this macro-environmental policy strategy aimed at improving the supermarket micro-environment found little impact of traffic light labels on consumer sales of ready-to-eat meals and sandwiches.[152] A more recent analysis suggested that traffic light labeling could be cost effective in improving consumer awareness and ultimately food choices and dietary habits.[153] Similarly contradictory findings have also been reported in Australia, which adopted a different color-coded front-of-package labeling strategy.[154] All three of these evaluations were conducted by the same research group, who suggested that these findings are inconclusive owing to the short duration of the programs and research studies. The effectiveness that a modest micro-environment intervention such as food labeling can have on its own is also unclear. A comprehensive, ecologic approach that includes multiple levels of environment coupled with improvements in individual knowledge and skills that includes improved food labeling is likely best.

Solutions Based on the Meso- and Exo-Environments

The dynamic linkages between micro-environments that drive behavior are complex, difficult to quantify, and not extensively described in the research literature. However, work on ecologic momentary assessment and transportation studies shows some promise at measuring social and physical interactions.

In **ecologic momentary assessment (EMA)**, participants carry handheld communication devices, such as phones.[155] Researchers periodically send participants messages asking what they are doing, where and with whom they are, and what feelings they are experiencing. Access to conversations or experiences throughout the day allows researchers to understand how experiences in one micro-environment can influence behaviors in another micro-environment. One recent study using EMA found that compared with people who rarely overeat, regular overeaters are more likely be influenced by the presence of appealing foods.[156] Studies in clinical pharmacology have demonstrated improvements in compliance and tracking,[157] and EMA has the potential to prompt physical activities and improved dietary habits, but more research on applications for obesity is necessary.

Combining EMA data with GPS tracking and accelerometer-measured physical activity monitoring devices provides detailed objective information on daily activities that can contribute to exposures to obesity-affecting environmental cues. For example, GPS and accelerometry together can detect whether people are riding bikes, walking, or driving between locations.[158] Many mobile smartphones contain GPS tracking, and retailers take advantage of this information via mobile apps. When consumers enter stores, retailers can send messages to the consumers offering information about products available and promotions at the point of purchase. This information could also be used by health promoters to help consumers avoid poor nutritional choices or to help motivate people to try new physical activities when in an appropriate environment.

Macro-environment strategies can be combined to help influence meso- and exo-environmental change. Changing norms to facilitate healthy choices via community campaigns, public service announcements, and changes in the workplace or school culture can help increase communication about healthy choices. Word of mouth and lay information gathering can contribute significantly to decisions about healthy eating and physical activity. Most Americans and millions of other users participate in Internet social networks. For example, over 54% of Americans are registered on Facebook, which has been broadly adopted throughout most of the Americas, Europe, and Australia, with additional users worldwide. This platform increases popular access to lay health information.

Transportation networks in municipalities affect micro-environment (street-scale) and macro-environment factors. Reducing sprawl, improving roads and complete streets, and multiple transportation options can make transit better, lower rates of obesity, and increase physical activity. Strategies include reducing the number of cars per household, increasing active transportation and improving air quality.[159,160] Improving roads and making more complete streets increases capacity to support all potential users, including drivers, transit users, cyclists, and walkers. The city of Moses Lake, Washington, has adopted a comprehensive community plan that includes rezoning of streets to make them complete streets. This is in response to mounting data that suggest that people who can walk or bicycle in their neighborhoods do, increasing physical activity and reducing obesity.[161] Simultaneous reductions in automobile emissions can improve air quality that may yield further health boons.

Strategies at the Macro-Environment

Policy is an important component of public health approaches to prevent obesity and improve dietary habits. Policies developed to encourage healthy choices include state bans on trans fats in restaurants,[162,163] and outlawing the sale of soft drinks larger than 16 ounces.[164] To be effective, policies must be implemented, enforced, evaluated, and revised to accommodate unexpected consequences, technological

innovation, and secular trends. Policies aimed at improving dietary habits and decreasing obesity prevalence are recent developments, and their impacts remain to be seen.

CATCH Intervention for Children

The Coordinated Approach to Child Health (CATCH), which aims to increase physical activity and healthy dietary habits while reducing tobacco use, has improved children's health habits.[165,166,167] CATCH combines individual educational and behavioral strategies and attempts to impact the micro-, meso-, and exo-environments. The program emphasizes changing the school environment to foster physical activity and nutritious choices and includes a family component to help to increase communication and norms around health behaviors that can help to reinforce and buffer individual choices. CATCH has been effective at producing population-level measurable effects in obesity prevention and control where it was implemented county-wide.[168]

Healthy People 2020

Healthy People is a federal initiative to provide evidence-based health benchmarks for all Americans to achieve in 10-year increments. Current nutrition and obesity-related objectives of Healthy People are to reduce the proportion of adults and children who are obese by 10% by 2020. Healthy People recommends communities work toward achieving this benchmark through community-setting interventions.[169]

Nationally Coordinated Programs

Federally funded nutrition programs promote outreach and education for low-income families. The Special Supplemental Nutrition Program for Women, Infants, and Children (WIC) and Supplemental Nutrition Assistance Program (SNAP) aim to reduce and prevent food insecurity and hunger in underserved communities. WIC provides coupons for healthy foods, such as whole grains, fruits, vegetables, and dairy products. SNAP participants use an electronic benefit card (EBT) to purchase foods in eligible stores.[170] These programs influence better dietary choices on a limited budget by creating a culturally supportive climate for eligible participants in a comprehensive linkage of the micro-, meso-, and exo-environments.

Federal programs in a community enhance obesity prevention messages by mobilizing grassroots organizations to collaborate with local and state governments. The 2012 Institute of Medicine (IOM) report, "Accelerating

Progress in Obesity Prevention: Solving the Weight of the Nation," affirms that federal assistance policies should be aligned closely with the *Dietary Guidelines for Americans* to encourage healthy eating choices and reduce consumption of certain types of food among socioeconomically disadvantaged populations.[171] Multinational collaboration can potentially impact obesity. However, few global examples exist of integrated clinical care teams dedicated to nutrition support and education.[172]

> *Healthy People 2020: NWS-14: Increase the contribution of fruits to the diets of the population aged 2 years and older*
>
> *Healthy People 2020: NWS-15: Increase the variety and contribution of vegetables to the diets of the population aged 2 years and older*
>
> *Healthy People 2020: NWS-16: Increase the contribution of whole grains to the diets of the population aged 2 years and older*
>
> *Healthy People 2020: NWS-20: Increase consumption of calcium in the population aged 2 years and older*

Ecologic models posit interactive relationships among individual, social, and each level of environmental factors.[173,174,175,176,177,178] For example, individual and social factors may contribute to efforts aimed at policy changes that afford construction of a community garden to provide residents with fresh fruits and vegetables. In this example, individual residents of a neighborhood may unite socially to petition the local government to allocate funds to build the garden, provide maintenance, and promote educational activities about gardening. If local pressure is strong enough, it may succeed in changing policies that consequently improve the lives of individual residents. Policies aimed at improving quality of life in one domain may have additional consequences in other domains. A congestion road tax was implemented in Stockholm, Sweden, in the hope of reducing automobile traffic and increasing the use of public transportation. The outcomes of the road tax included increased physical activity, reduced traffic congestion, and improved air quality.[179] Thus, pressure at one level of an ecologic system can influence change at another level of the ecologic system, which may, in turn, influence still another level of the ecologic system. Although environments may change as a result of individual and social factors, this change may take a long time, years or even

decades. On the upside, slow growth is often more sustainable than rapid change, benefiting more people for a longer period of time.

Solutions Based on Forces of Change

Forces of change that influence obesity are vast and varied. Innovations in technology and discovery of new biomedical health factors seem to be daily events. This discussion will consider solutions related to technology, keeping in mind that many other forces of change exist that could influence obesity. The Community Preventive Services Task Force found sufficient evidence for the effectiveness of technology-supported interventions to reduce weight. Technology-supported interventions include computers, video conferencing, personal digital assistants, and mobile phones; and nontechnology components such as face-to-face counseling or classes or printed materials. The research on interventions relying solely on technology components is inconclusive to date,[180] but text messaging interventions have promise.[181,182]

Social Networking to Reduce Obesity

Other work looks at interventions to improve health using social networking and virtual environments.[183,184,185] Virtual interventions do not require face-to-face communication, but may still establish communication networks that help people to make healthy choices, discuss personal struggles, share resources, and overcome daily barriers to good health. Virtual interventions may potentially be easily deployed for people across a wide geographic area and may be easily scalable and modularized to facilitate customizable public health interventions.

Health Information and Obesity

Another technological innovation that has the potential to change obesity prevention and treatment is the ready telemetry of health information between devices. It is easy for consumers to track their physical activity and eating behaviors online, or via virtual monitors. For example, some running shoe manufacturers have integrated telemetry into their shoes that tracks distance and speed and transmits this information to a nearby smartphone. This information can also be easily transmitted to healthcare providers or promoters to help monitor progress and provide feedback. To take this a step further, feedback can be automated and designed to respond to a variety of preset goals and responses. Another application of this kind of technology is the use of "smart appliances" that sense when food supplies are low. These could also link to healthy recipes in a database to tell consumers what ingredients are needed to complete the menu. This strategy might also work in reverse, where the smart appliance can search through existing ingredients and suggest recipes that follow a particular menu plan.

Integrating Physical Activity into Sedentary Lifestyles

Another intriguing technological innovation is the advent of the stand-up desk and the treadmill desk ("Walking Workstation"). This is not unlike the concept of the television that is activated by an exercise station. Simply by standing or walking slowly during routine tasks (e.g., answering email), consumers can increase caloric expenditure, and improve their health. Small amounts of physical activity throughout the day may reduce the risk of obesity. Some research has found that short, intermittent sessions of moderate-intensity physical activity (the equivalent of fast walking) that equal the same duration of one long session of physical activity may have similar effects on weight loss and may be more sustainable for some people.[186,187]

Recommendations for Policy, Research, and Practice

Obesity is exceedingly difficult to treat, is becoming increasingly prevalent among youth, tracks into adulthood, and poses serious threats to health. Health behaviors that influence obesity are developed early in life and are largely shaped by environmental factors beyond the control of the individual. Therefore, obesity prevention programs for youth have become the focus of most public health obesity reduction efforts.[188] Most major national health advisory panels and health organizations recommend all children be screened for excess adiposity starting at birth.[189] The conclusion from multiple comprehensive reviews of child obesity prevention and intervention studies is that there is no single effective program available for widespread use; however, there are components of programs that seem to be consistently effective.[190] An Expert Committee of representatives from 15 national healthcare organizations convened by the U.S. Department of Health and Human Services first published evidence-based recommendations for addressing child obesity in health care in 1998. The most recent update was published in 2007.

Specific behaviors for weight loss among adults include the following:

1. Reducing calories in the diet. While some evidence suggests low-carbohydrate (CHO) diets (less than 35% total kcal from CHO) promote more weight and fat loss in the first six months than low-fat diets, these differences are not evident after one year. There is no evidence that low-glycemic-index diets are effective for weight loss or maintenance.[191] Fruit and vegetable consumption has a weak but positive effect on obesity prevention among adults.[192]

2. Spreading daily food consumption over four to five eating episodes per day.

3. Controlling food portions, with the aid of meal replacements if necessary.

4. Consuming sufficient calcium and eating breakfast.[193]

5. Engaging in physical activity, an important part of a comprehensive weight-management program. For health benefits, a minimum of 150 minutes of moderate physical activity per week is recommended, and additional benefits occur with more physical activity.[194]

> *Healthy People 2020: NWS-20: Increase consumption of calcium in the population aged 2 years and older*

The lack of consistently effective programs or clear guidance on "best practices" for promoting behavior change among children suggests we need to better understand where the breakdowns are likely occurring. A challenge to multifaceted school-based interventions is in maintaining fidelity of intervention delivery to their original design or intent; the more components, staff, and school personnel support needed, the less ability researchers have to tightly control implementation. Low participation and high attrition are problematic in obesity interventions.[195] Lack of interest, boredom, inconvenience, low perceived value, and low personal relevance can lead to low participation and high attrition, but enlisting feedback from members of the target audience during intervention planning and development should increase the likelihood of creating appealing, applicable, relevant, convenient, and engaging interventions.

Targeting Group Settings

Behavioral and environmental interventions should begin by focusing on groups of people who are already in an accessible setting. It may be easier to implement changes among groups of people in worksites or at schools rather than in community settings. Recent data have suggested that one strategy to increasing sustainability of interventions on an individual level is the introduction of preintervention skills and executive function training.[196] This technique involves helping people to learn the skills necessary to change and maintain a new behavior, before they attempt the behavior change. Similar is the ability to plan for high-risk situations, in order to improve brain executive function and reduce impulsivity. This method involves helping people to remember why they decided to change their behavior in the first place, and to avoid making poor dietary or physical inactivity choices.

Coordination and Collaboration

Coordination among agencies that deliver health promotion interventions is needed. Many people may expect that their healthcare providers will provide information about dietary habits and physical activity, when in fact, few physicians provide this information. Those who do, often provide it after it is too late—when people are already overweight or obese.[197] Medical education does not typically include sufficient information about counseling patients about daily health habits that are critical to maintaining good health. Many healthcare providers may not realize the important role they can play in preventing obesity as part of a larger ecologic system. Additional collaboration might come from health insurance companies, who could offer lower rates for individuals who maintain a healthy weight, include diet counseling services, or reduce rates for employers that have worksite wellness programs. Worksites could offer wellness programs with healthy foods available on site, ample time for physical activity at lunch, and incentives for participation in educational sessions.

Implementing Obesity-Specific Policies

There is a clear need for policies that are specifically developed to improve health outcomes, rather than to promote economic gains. This approach will not only be more effective in reducing obesity and improving health outcomes, but will ultimately support economic gains. Obesity is a tremendous economic burden. Long-term benefits of obesity prevention include reduced costs. Many current policies save money in the short term, but will be expensive in the long term because they promote obesity and lead to higher

costs in the longer term. For example, agricultural policies in the United States focus on food security rather than nutritional adequacy, resulting in an oversupply of wheat, corn, soy, and other grains. This abundance contributes to very low cost, nutritionally limited foods such as commercial baked goods, and salty and sweet snacks and sugar-sweetened beverages. This availability of inexpensive and filling foods makes it easy to consume many more calories than are needed while still not meeting basic nutritional standards.[198]

Another obvious policy arena with room for improvement is transportation. There has long been a focus on the automobile, with little regard for cyclists, public transit, and pedestrians. Existing policies could be relatively easily enhanced to improve streets for multiple forms of transit, thereby increasing physical activity, reducing environmental toxins, reducing commuter stress, and creating greater attention to the many forms of transportation available for consumers. These results from improved policy could contribute to obesity prevention and control efforts.[199]

> *Healthy People 2020: PA-15: (Developmental) Increase legislative policies for the built environment that enhance access to and availability of physical activity opportunities*

As there are many levels of influence on human health, multiple levels of environments that are ripe for intervention exist. A strategy that coordinates among levels and intervenes strategically at multiple levels will have the greatest impact and sustainability. It makes sense that a coordinated strategy to increase individual knowledge and behavioral skills, improve communication around healthy living, improve community infrastructure, and improve policies that contribute to human health will have the best results in the long term.

> *Public Health Core Competency 7: Financial Planning and Management Skills 5: Operates programs within current and forecasted budget constraints*
>
> *Public Health Core Competency 7: Financial Planning and Management Skills 6: Identifies strategies for determining budget priorities based on federal, state, and local financial contributions*

Conclusion

Obesity may be the most significant health challenge facing the world today. Obesity is not solely a health issue; it has become an economic and societal issue, impacting the world at multiple levels. Ultimately the result of energy imbalance, the challenge of obesity goes beyond focusing on an individual's calories consumed and expended. Genetic tendencies and individual behavioral and attitudinal lifestyle choices are important starting points and well researched. However, obesity represents a true complex system challenge, because of failures at every level of the ecologic system. Micro-, meso-, exo-, and macro-environments all

tend to foster obesity, and forces of change have shaped each of these levels into obesogenic influences.

Policy and environmental intervention strategies may offer the greatest sustainability for reversing the obesity epidemic; however, limited research has investigated these strategies. Therefore, research is needed to provide evidence about which policy and environmental strategies are most effective not only for reducing the burden of obesity, but also for reducing its economic and societal impacts. Once strategies have been identified as conclusively helpful, multisector coordination is needed to implement and sustain them to enhance health and well-being for future generations.

References

1 Ogden, C. L., Carroll, M. D., Kit, B. K., & Flegal, K. M. (2012). Prevalence of obesity and trends in body mass index among U.S. children and adolescents, 1999-2010. *JAMA, 307*(5), 483-90.

2 Ogden, C. L., Carroll, M. D., Kit, B. K., & Flegal, K. M. (2012). Prevalence of obesity and trends in body mass index among U.S. children and adolescents, 1999-2010. *JAMA, 307*(5), 483-90.

3 Ogden, C. L., Carroll, M. D., Curtin, L. R., Lamb, M. M., & Flegal, K. M. (2010). Prevalence of high body mass index in U.S. children and adolescents, 2007-2008. *JAMA, 303*(3), 242-49.

4 Flegal, K. M., Carroll, M. D., Kit, B. K., & Ogden, C. L. (2012). Prevalence of obesity and trends in the distribution of body mass index among U.S. adults, 1999-2010. *JAMA, 307*(5), 491-97.

5 Centers for Disease Control and Prevention. (2010). *FastStats obesity and overweight.* Retrieved from http://www.cdc.gov/nchs/fastats/overwt.htm

6 Centers for Disease Control and Prevention. (2012). *Adult obesity facts.* Retrieved from http://www.cdc.gov/obesity/data/adult.html

7 Flegal, K. M., Carroll, M. D., Kit, B. K., & Ogden, C. L. (2012). Prevalence of obesity and trends in the distribution of body mass index among U.S. adults, 1999-2010. *JAMA, 307*(5), 491-97.

8 Flegal, K. M., Carroll, M. D., Kit, B. K., & Ogden, C. L. (2012). Prevalence of obesity and trends in the distribution of body mass index among U.S. adults, 1999-2010. *JAMA, 307*(5), 491-97.

9 World Health Organization. (2012). *Obesity and overweight.* Retrieved from http://www.who.int/mediacentre/factsheets/fs311/en

10 World Health Organization. (2012). *Obesity and overweight.* Retrieved from http://www.who.int/mediacentre/factsheets/fs311/en

11 Cawley, J., & Meyerhoefer, C. (2012). The medical care costs of obesity: An instrumental variables approach. *Journal of Health Economics, 31*(1), 219-30.

12 Lee, R. E., McAlexander, K. M., & Banda, J. A. (2011). *Reversing the obesogenic environment.* Champagne, IL: Human Kinetics.

13 Capodaglio, P., Castelnuovo, G., Brunani, A., Vismara, L., Villa, V., & Capodaglio, E. M. (2010). Functional limitations and occupational issues in obesity: A review. *International Journal of Occupational Safety and Ergonomics, 16*(4), 507-23.

14 Lee, R. E., McAlexander, K. M., & Banda, J. A. (2011). *Reversing the obesogenic environment.* Champagne, IL: Human Kinetics.

15 Zezima, K. (2008, April 8). Increasing obesity requires new ambulance equipment. *New York Times,* F5.

16 Edwards, P., & Roberts, I. (2009). Population adiposity and climate change. *International Journal of Epidemiology, 38*(4), 1137-40.

17 Centers for Disease Control and Prevention. (n.d.). *Healthy weight—it's not a diet, it's a lifestyle!* Retrieved from http://www.cdc.gov/healthyweight/assessing/bmi/childrens_bmi/about_childrens_bmi.html

18 Ogden, C. L., & Flegal, K. M. (2010). Changes in terminology for childhood overweight and obesity. *National Health Statistics Report,* (25), 1-5.

19 Lee, R. E., McAlexander, K. M., & Banda, J. A. (2011). *Reversing the obesogenic environment.* Champagne, IL: Human Kinetics.

20 Lebovitz, H. E. (2003). The relationship of obesity to the metabolic syndrome. *International Journal of Clinical Practice,* (134), 18-27.

21 Garber, C. E., Blissmer, B., Deschenes, M. R., Franklin, B. A., Lamonte, M. J., Lee, I. M., . . . Swain, D. P.; American College of Sports Medicine. (2011). American College of Sports Medicine position stand. Quantity and quality of exercise for developing and maintaining cardiorespiratory, musculoskeletal, and neuromotor fitness in apparently healthy adults: Guidance for prescribing exercise. *Medicine and Science in Sports and Exercise, 43*(7), 1334-59.

22 Merrill, A. L., & Watt, B. K. (1955). *Energy value of foods, basis and derivation* (Vol. 74). Washington, DC: U.S. Government Printing Office.

23 Lee, R. E., McAlexander, K. M., & Banda, J. A. (2011). *Reversing the obesogenic environment*. Champagne, IL: Human Kinetics.

24 Lee, R. E., McAlexander, K. M., & Banda, J. A. (2011). *Reversing the obesogenic environment*. Champagne, IL: Human Kinetics.

25 Ogden, C. L., Carroll, M. D., Kit, B. K., & Flegal, K. M. (2012). Prevalence of obesity and trends in body mass index among U.S. children and adolescents, 1999-2010. *JAMA, 307*(5), 483-90.

26 Mifflin, M. D., St. Jeor, S. T., Hill, L. A., Scott, B. J., Daugherty, S. A., & Koh, Y. O. (1990). A new predictive equation for resting energy expenditure in healthy individuals. *American Journal of Clinical Nutrition, 51*(2), 241-47.

27 U.S. Department of Health and Human Services. (2008). *Physical activity guidelines for Americans*. Retrieved from http://www.health.gov/paguidelines/guidelines/default .aspx

28 Institute of Medicine. (2012). *Accelerating progress in obesity prevention: Solving the weight of the nation*. Retrieved from http://www.iom.edu/Reports/2012/Accelerating-Progress-in-Obesity-Prevention.aspx

29 U.S. Department of Agriculture & U.S. Department of Health and Human Services. (2010). *Dietary guidelines for Americans*. Washington, DC: Government Printing Office.

30 U.S. Department of Health and Human Services. (2008). *Physical activity guidelines for Americans*. Retrieved from http://www.health.gov/paguidelines/guidelines/default.aspx

31 Egger, G., Swinburn, B., & Rossner, S. (2003). Dusting off the epidemiological triad: Could it work with obesity? *Obesity Reviews, 4*(2), 115-19.

32 Lee, R. E., & Cubbin, C. (2009). Striding toward social justice: The ecologic milieu of physical activity. *Exercise and Sport Science Reviews, 37*(1), 10-17.

33 Sallis, J. F., & Owen, N. (1997). *Ecological models* (2nd ed.). San Francisco, CA: Jossey-Bass.

34 Spence, J. C., & Lee, RE. (2003). Toward a comprehensive model of physical activity. *Psychology of Sport and Exercise, 4*, 7-24.

35 Spence, J. C., & Lee, RE. (2003). Toward a comprehensive model of physical activity. *Psychology of Sport and Exercise, 4*, 7-24.

36 Lee, R. E., & Cubbin, C. (2009). Striding toward social justice: The ecologic milieu of physical activity. *Exercise and Sport Science Reviews, 37*(1), 10-17.

37 Spence, J. C., & Lee, RE. (2003). Toward a comprehensive model of physical activity. *Psychology of Sport and Exercise, 4*, 7-24.

38 Bronfenbrenner, U. (1977). Toward an experimental ecology of human development. *American Psychologist, 32*, 513-31.

39 Bronfenbrenner, U. (1979). *The ecology of human development: Experiments by nature and design*. Cambridge, MA: Harvard University Press.

40 McLeroy, K. R., Bibeau, D., Steckler, A., & Glanz K. (1988). An ecological perspective on health promotion programs. *Health Education Quarterly, 15*(4), 351-77.

41 Spence, J. C., & Lee, RE. (2003). Toward a comprehensive model of physical activity. *Psychology of Sport and Exercise, 4*, 7-24.

42 Sallis, J. F., & Owen N. (1999). *Physical activity and behavioral medicine* (Vol. 3). Thousand Oaks, CA: Sage Publications.

43 Skoranski, A. M., Most, S. B., Lutz-Stehl, M., Hoffman, J. E., Hassink, S. G., & Simons, R. F. (2012). Response monitoring and cognitive control in childhood obesity. *Biological Psychology, 92*(2), 199-204.

44 Veloso, S. M., Matos, M. G., Carvalho, M., & Diniz, J. A. (2012). Psychosocial factors of different health behaviour patterns in adolescents: Association with overweight and weight control behaviours. *Journal of Obesity, 2012*, 852672.

45 Glanz, K., Basil, M., Maibach, E., Goldberg, J., & Snyder, D. (1998). Why Americans eat what they do: Taste, nutrition, cost, convenience, and weight control concerns as influences on food consumption. *Journal of the American Dietetic Association, 98*(10), 1118-26.

46 Ledoux, T. A., Watson, K., Barnett, A., Nguyen, N. T., Baranowski, J. C., & Baranowski, T. (2011). Components of the diet associated with child adiposity: A cross-sectional study. *Journal of the American College of Nutrition, 30*(6), 536-46.

47 Lee, R. E., Heinrich, K. M., Medina, A. V., Regan, G. R., Reese-Smith, J. Y., Jokura, Y., & Maddock, J. E. (2010). A picture of the healthful food environment in two diverse urban cities. *Environmental Health Insights, 4*, 49-60.

48 Buscher, L. A., Martin, K. A., & Crocker, S. (2001). Point-of-purchase messages framed in terms of cost, convenience, taste, and energy improve healthful snack selection in a college food-service setting. *Journal of the American Dietetic Association, 101*(8), 909-13.

49 Horgen, K. B., & Brownell, K. D. (2002). Comparison of price change and health message interventions in promoting healthy food choices. *Health Psychology, 21*(5), 505-12.

50 Hunt, M. K., Lefebvre, R. C., Hixson, M. L., Banspach, S. W., Assaf, A. R., & Carleton, R. A. (1990). Pawtucket Heart Health Program point-of-purchase nutrition education program in supermarkets. *American Journal of Public Health, 80*(6), 730-32.

51 Morland, K., Wing, S., & Diez Roux A. (2002). The contextual effect of the local food environment on residents' diets: The atherosclerosis risk in communities study. *American Journal of Public Health, 92*(11), 1761-67.

52 Morland, K., Wing, S., Diez Roux, A., & Poole, C. (2002). Neighborhood characteristics associated with the location of food stores and food service places. *American Journal of Preventive Medicine, 22*(1), 23-29.

53 Bureau of Labor Statistics. (2011). *American time use survey*. Retrieved from http://www.bls.gov/tus/charts/chart1.pdf

54 Hamrick, K. S., Andrews, A., Guthrie, J., Hopkins, D., & McClelland K. (2011). *How much time do Americans spend on food?* Economic Information Bulletin No. EIB-86. Retrieved

from U.S. Department of Agriculture website, http://www.ers.usda.gov/publications/eib-economic-information-bulletin/eib86.aspx#.UoUEmxUo4y8

55 Cohen, N. L., Stoddard, A. M., Sarouhkhanians, S., & Sorensen, G. (1998). Barriers toward fruit and vegetable consumption in a multiethnic worksite population. *Journal of Nutrition Education, 30*(6), 381-86.

56 Ng, D. M., & Jeffery, R. W. (2003). Relationships between perceived stress and health behaviors in a sample of working adults. *Health Psychology, 22*(6), 638-42.

57 Condon, E. M., Crepinsek, M. K., & Fox, M. K. (2009). School meals: Types of foods offered to and consumed by children at lunch and breakfast. *Journal of the American Dietetic Association, 109*(2 Suppl.), S67-78.

58 Millimet, D. L., Tchernis, R., & Husain, M. (2009). School nutrition programs and the incidence of childhood obesity. *Journal of Human Resources, 45*(3), 640-54.

59 Hernandez, D. C., Francis, L. A., & Doyle, E. A. (2001). National School Lunch Program participation and sex differences in body mass index trajectories of children from low-income families. *Archives of Pediatric and Adolescent Medicine, 165*(4), 346-53.

60 Jago, R., Baranowski, T., & Baranowski, J. C. (2007). Fruit and vegetable availability: A micro environmental mediating variable? *Public Health Nutrition, 10*(7), 681-89.

61 Ledoux, T. A., Mama, S. K., O'Connor, D. P., Adamus, H., Fraser, M. L., & Lee, R. E. (2012). Home availability and the impact of weekly stressful events are associated with fruit and vegetable intake among African American and Hispanic/Latina women. *Journal of Obesity, 2012,* 737891.

62 Van Ansem, W. J., Schrijvers, C. T., Rodenburg, G., & van de Mheen, D. (2012). Is there an association between the home food environment, the local food shopping environment and children's fruit and vegetable intake? Results from the Dutch INPACT study. *Public Health Nutrition, 2012,* 1-9.

63 Cullen, K. W., Baranowski, T., Owens, E., Marsh, T., Rittenberry, L., & de Moor, C. (2003). Availability, accessibility, and preferences for fruit, 100% fruit juice, and vegetables influence children's dietary behavior. *Health Education and Behavior, 30*(5), 615-26.

64 Lee, R. E., Mama, S. K., McAlexander, K. P., Adamus, H., & Medina, A. V. (2011). Neighborhood and PA: Neighborhood factors and physical activity in African American public housing residents. *Journal of Physical Activity and Health, 8*(Suppl. 1), S83-90.

65 Heinrich, K. M., Lee, R. E., Regan, G. R., Reese-Smith, J. Y., Howard, H. H., Haddock, C. K., . . . Ahluwalia, J. S. (2008). How does the built environment relate to body mass index and obesity prevalence among public housing residents? *American Journal of Health Promotion, 22*(3), 187-94.

66 Lee, R. E., Mama, S. K., Medina, A. V., Ho, A., & Adamus, H. J. (2012). Neighborhood factors influence physical activity among African American and Hispanic or Latina women. *Health Place, 18*(1), 63-70.

67 Sallis, J. F., Saelens, B. E., Frank, L. D., Conway, T. L, Slymen, D. J., Cain, K. L., . . . Kerr, J. (2009). Neighborhood built environment and income: Examining multiple health outcomes. *Social Science and Medicine, 68*(7), 1285-93.

68 Epstein, L. H., Raja, S., Daniel, T. O., Paluch, R. A., Wilfley, D. E., Saelens, B. E., & Roemmich, J. N. (2012). The built environment moderates effects of family-based childhood obesity treatment over 2 years. *Annals of Behavioral Medicine, 44*(2), 248-58.

69 Lovasi, G. S., Jacobson, J. S., Quinn, J. W., Neckerman, K. M., Ashby-Thompson, M. N., & Rundle, A. (2011). Is the environment near home and school associated with physical activity and adiposity of urban preschool children? *Journal of Urban Health, 88*(6), 1143-57.

70 Miranda, M. L., Edwards, S. E., Anthopolos, R., Dolinsky, D. H., & Kemper, A. R. (2012). The built environment and childhood obesity in Durham, North Carolina. *Clinical Pediatrics, 51*(8), 750-58.

71 Sandy, R., Tchernis, R., Wilson, J., Liu, G., & Zhou, X. (2013). Effects of the built environment on childhood obesity: The case of urban recreational trails and crime. *Economics and Human Biology, 11*(1), 18-29.

72 Adamus-Leach, H. J., Mama, S. K., O'Connor, D. P., & Lee, R. E. (2012). Income differences in perceived neighborhood environment characteristics among African American women. *Environmental Health Insights, 6,* 33-40.

73 Lee, R., & Ho, A. (2011). Physical activity and socioeconomic status. In F. Mooren & J. Skinner (Eds.), *Encyclopedia of exercise medicine in health and disease.* Berlin: Springer-Verlag.

74 Maher, C., Olds, T. S., Eisenmann, J. C., & Dollman, J. (2012). Screen time is more strongly associated than physical activity with overweight and obesity in 9- to 16-year-old Australians. *Acta Paediatrica, 101*(11), 1170-74.

75 Jackson, D. M., Djafarian, K., Stewart, J., & Speakman, J. R. (2009). Increased television viewing is associated with elevated body fatness but not with lower total energy expenditure in children. *American Journal of Clinical Nutrition, 89*(4), 1031-36.

76 Chahal, H., Fung, C., Kuhle, S., & Veugelers, P. J. (2013). Availability and night-time use of electronic entertainment and communication devices are associated with short sleep duration and obesity among Canadian children. *Pediatric Obesity, 8*(1), 42-51.

77 De Jong, E., Stocks, T., Visscher, T. L., Hirasing, R. A., Seidell, J. C., & Renders, C. M. (2012). Association between sleep duration and overweight: The importance of parenting. *International Journal of Obesity, 36*(10), 1278-84.

78 Chaput, J. P., Brunet, M., & Tremblay, A. (2006). Relationship between short sleeping hours and childhood overweight/obesity: Results from the "Quebec en Forme" Project. *International Journal of Obesity, 30*(7), 1080-85.

79 Jackson, D. M., Djafarian, K., Stewart, J., & Speakman, J. R. (2009). Increased television viewing is associated with elevated body fatness but not with lower total energy expenditure in children. *American Journal of Clinical Nutrition, 89*(4), 1031-36.

80 Spence, J. C., & Lee, R. E. (2003). Toward a comprehensive model of physical activity. *Psychology of Sport and Exercise, 4,* 7-24.

81 Morland, K., Wing, S., & Diez Roux, A. (2002). The contextual effect of the local food environment on residents' diets: The atherosclerosis risk in communities study. *American Journal of Public Health, 92*(11), 1761–67.

82 Ledoux, T. A., Mama, S. K., O'Connor, D. P., Adamus, H., Fraser, M. L., & Lee, R. E. (2012). Home availability and the impact of weekly stressful events are associated with fruit and vegetable intake among African American and Hispanic/Latina women. *Journal of Obesity, 2012,* 737891.

83 Lee, R. E., McAlexander, K. M., & Banda, J. A. (2011). *Reversing the obesogenic environment.* Champagne, IL: Human Kinetics.

84 Lee, R. E., Heinrich, K. M., Medina, A. V., Regan, G. R., Reese-Smith, J. Y., Jokura, Y., & Maddock, J. E. (2010). A picture of the healthful food environment in two diverse urban cities. *Environmental Health Insights, 4,* 49–60.

85 Heinrich, K. M., Li, D., Regan, G. R., Howard, H. H., Ahluwalia, J. S., Lee, R. E. (2012). Store and restaurant advertising and health of public housing residents. *American Journal of Health Behavior, 36*(1), 66–74.

86 Spence, J. C., & Lee, R. E. (2003). Toward a comprehensive model of physical activity. *Psychology of Sport and Exercise, 4,* 7–24.

87 Spence, J. C., & Lee, R. E. (2003). Toward a comprehensive model of physical activity. *Psychology of Sport and Exercise, 4,* 7–24.

88 Aktas Arnas, Y. (2006). The effects of television food advertisement on children's food purchasing requests. *Pediatrics International, 48*(2), 138–45.

89 Mehta, K., Coveney, J., Ward, P., Magarey, A., Spurrier, N., & Udell, T. (2010). Australian children's views about food advertising on television. *Appetite, 55*(1), 49–55.

90 U.S. Department of Agriculture Food and Nutrition Service. (2009). *National School Lunch Program.* Retrieved from www.fns.usda.gov/cnd/Lunch/default.htm

91 U.S. Department of Agriculture Food and Nutrition Service. (2009). *National School Breakfast Program.*

92 National Complete Street Coalition website, http://www.smartgrowthamerica.org/complete-streets

93 NHS Choices. (n.d.). *5 A Day.* Retrieved from NHS website, http://www.nhs.uk/LiveWell/5ADAY/Pages/5ADAYhome.aspx

94 Rickard, B. J., Okrent, A. M., & Alston, J. M. (2013). How have agricultural policies influenced caloric consumption in the United States? *Health Economics, 22*(3), 316–39.

95 National Complete Street Coalition website, http://www.smartgrowthamerica.org/complete-streets

96 U.S. Bureau of Labor Statistics. (2011). *Women in the labor force: A databook.* Report 1034. Retrieved from http://www.bls.gov/cps/wlf-databook-2011.pdf

97 U.S. Bureau of Labor Statistics. (2010). *Highlights of women's earnings in 2009.* Report 1025. Retrieved from http://www.bls.gov/cps/cpswom2009.pdf

98 Coleman-Jensen, A., Nord, M., Andrews, M., & Carlson, S. (2011). *Household food security in the United States in 2010.* Retrieved from U.S. Department of Agriculture website, http://www.ers.usda.gov/publications/err-economic-research-report/err125.aspx#.UoUNhxUo4y8

99 Drewnowski, A. (2004). Obesity and the food environment: Dietary energy density and diet costs. *American Journal of Preventive Medicine, 27*(3 Suppl):154-162.

100 Eisenmann, J. C., Gundersen, C., Lohman, B. J., Garasky, S., & Stewart, S. D. (2011). Is food insecurity related to overweight and obesity in children and adolescents? A summary of studies, 1995-2009. *Obesity Review, 12*(5), e73-83.

101 Larson, N. I., & Story, M, T. (2011). Food insecurity and weight status among U.S. children and families: A review of the literature. *American Journal of Preventive Medicine, 40*(2), 166-73.

102 Lee, R. E., Heinrich, K. M., Medina, A. V., Regan, G. R., Reese-Smith, J. Y., Jokura, Y., & Maddock, J. E. (2010). A picture of the healthful food environment in two diverse urban cities. *Environmental Health Insights, 4,* 49-60.

103 Leasure, J. L., Giddabasappa, A., Chaney, S., Johnson, J. E., Jr., Pothakos, K., Lau, Y. S., & Fox, D. A. (2008). Low-level human equivalent gestational lead exposure produces sex-specific motor and coordination abnormalities and late-onset obesity in year-old mice. *Environmental Health Perspectives, 116*(3), 355-61.

104 La Merrill, M., & Birnbaum, L. S. (2011). Childhood obesity and environmental chemicals. *Mount Sinai Journal of Medicine, 78*(1), 22-48.

105 Tucker, P., & Gilliland, J. (2007). The effect of season and weather on physical activity: A systematic review. *Public Health, 121*(12), 909-22.

106 Locke, E., Coronado, G. D., Thompson, B., & Kuniyuki, A. (2009). Seasonal variation in fruit and vegetable consumption in a rural agricultural community. *Journal of the American Dietetic Association, 109*(1), 45-51.

107 Institute of Medicine. (2010). *Promoting cardiovascular health in the developing world: A critical challenge to achieve global health.* Washington, DC: National Academies Press.

108 Finucane, M. M., Stevens, G. A., Cowan, M. J., Danaei, G., Lin, J. K., Paciorek, C. J., . . . Ezzati, M.; Global Burden of Metabolic Risk Factors Collaborating Group. (2011). National, regional, and global trends in body-mass index since 1980: Systematic analysis of health examination surveys and epidemiological studies with 960 country-years and 9.1 million participants. *Lancet, 377*(9765), 557-67.

109 Duffey, K. J., Gordon-Larsen, P., Shikany, J. M., Guilkey, D., Jacobs, D. R., Jr., & Popkin, B. M. (2010). Food price and diet and health outcomes: 20 years of the CARDIA Study. *Archives of Internal Medicine, 170*(5), 420-26.

110 Monteiro, C. A., & Cannon, G. (2012). The impact of transnational "big food" companies on the South: A view from Brazil. *PLoS Medicine, 9*(7), e1001252.

111 Odegaard, A. O., Koh, W. P., Yuan, J. M,, Gross, M. D., & Pereira, M. A. (2012). Western-style fast food intake and cardiometabolic risk in an Eastern country. *Circulation, 126*(2), 182-88.

112 Popkin, B. M., Adair, L. S., & Ng, S. W. (2012). Global nutrition transition and the pandemic of obesity in developing countries. *Nutrition Review, 70*(1), 3-21.

113 Gill, T., King, L., & Caterson, I. (2005). Obesity prevention: necessary and possible: A structured approach for effective planning. *Proceedings of the Nutrition Society, 64*(2), 255-61.

114 Glenny, A. M., O'Meara, S., Melville, A., Sheldon, T. A., & Wilson, C. (1997). The treatment and prevention of obesity: A systematic review of the literature. *International Journal of Obesity and Related Metabolic Disorders, 21*(9), 715-37.

115 Lemmens, V. E., Oenema, A., Klepp, K. I., Henriksen, H. B., & Brug, J. (2008). A systematic review of the evidence regarding efficacy of obesity prevention interventions among adults. *Obesity Review, 9*(5), 446-55.

116 Stevens, M., Paans, N., Wagenmakers, R., van Beveren, J., van Raay, J. J., van der Meer, K., . . . van den Akker-Scheek, I. (2012). The influence of overweight/obesity on patient-perceived physical functioning and health-related quality of life after primary total hip arthroplasty. *Obesity Surgery, 22*(4), 523-29.

117 Nicklas, J. M., Huskey, K. W., Davis, R. B., & Wee, C. C. (2012). Successful weight loss among obese U.S. adults. *American Journal of Preventive Medicine, 42*(5), 481-85.

118 Lee, R. E., McAlexander, K. M., & Banda, J. A. (2011). *Reversing the obesogenic environment.* Champagne, IL: Human Kinetics.

119 Academy of Nutrition and Dietetics. (n.d.). *How effective is MNT provided by Registered Dietitians in the management of type 1 and type 2 diabetes?* Retrieved from http://andevidencelibrary.com/evidence.cfm?evidence_summary_id=250466

120 Moyer, V. A. (2012). Screening for and management of obesity in adults: U.S. Preventive Services Task Force recommendation statement. *Annals of Internal Medicine, 157*(5), 373-78.

121 Academy of Nutrition and Dietetics. (n.d.). *How effective is MNT provided by Registered Dietitians in the management of type 1 and type 2 diabetes?* Retrieved from http://andevidencelibrary.com/evidence.cfm?evidence_summary_id=250466

122 Moyer, V. A. (2012). Screening for and management of obesity in adults: U.S. Preventive Services Task Force recommendation statement. *Annals of Internal Medicine, 157*(5), 373-78.

123 Academy of Nutrition and Dietetics. (n.d.). *How effective is MNT provided by Registered Dietitians in the management of type 1 and type 2 diabetes?* Retrieved from http://andevidencelibrary.com/evidence.cfm?evidence_summary_id=250466

124 Academy of Nutrition and Dietetics. (n.d.). *How effective is MNT provided by Registered Dietitians in the management of type 1 and type 2 diabetes?* Retrieved from http://andevidencelibrary.com/evidence.cfm?evidence_summary_id=250466

125 Moyer, V. A. (2012). Screening for and management of obesity in adults: U.S. Preventive Services Task Force recommendation statement. *Annals of Internal Medicine, 157*(5), 373-78.

126 Moyer, V. A. (2012). Screening for and management of obesity in adults: U.S. Preventive Services Task Force recommendation statement. *Annals of Internal Medicine, 157*(5), 373-78.

127 Anderson, L. M., Quinn, T. A., Glanz, K., Ramirez, G., Kahwati, L. C., Johnson, D. B., . . . Katz, D. L.; Task Force on Community Preventive Services. (2009). The effectiveness of worksite nutrition and physical activity interventions for controlling employee overweight and obesity: A systematic review. *American Journal of Preventive Medicine, 37*(4), 340-57.

128 Anderson, L. M., Quinn, T. A., Glanz, K., Ramirez, G., Kahwati, L. C., Johnson, D. B., . . . Katz, D. L.; Task Force on Community Preventive Services. (2009). The effectiveness of worksite nutrition and physical activity interventions for controlling employee overweight and obesity: A systematic review. *American Journal of Preventive Medicine, 37*(4), 340-57.

129 Task Force on Community Preventive Services. (2009). A recommendation to improve employee weight status through worksite health promotion programs targeting nutrition, physical activity, or both. *American Journal of Preventive Medicine, 37*(4), 358-59.

130 Anderson, L. M., Quinn, T. A., Glanz, K., Ramirez, G., Kahwati, L. C., Johnson, D. B., . . . Katz, D. L.; Task Force on Community Preventive Services. (2009). The effectiveness of worksite nutrition and physical activity interventions for controlling employee overweight and obesity: A systematic review. *American Journal of Preventive Medicine, 37*(4), 340-57.

131 Hennrikus, D. J., & Jeffery, R. W. (1996). Worksite intervention for weight control: A review of the literature. *American Journal of Health Promotion, 10*(6), 471-98.

132 Hersey, J., Williams-Piehota, P., Sparling, P. B., Alexander, J., Hill, M. D., Isenberg, K. B., . . . Dunet, D. O. (2008). Promising practices in promotion of healthy weight at small and medium-sized U.S. worksites. *Preventing Chronic Disease, 5*(4), A122.

133 Guide to Community Preventive Services. (2007). *Obesity prevention and control: Worksite programs.* Retrieved from www.thecommunityguide.org/obesity/workprograms.html

134 *Providence College wins "exemplary" worksite health award.* (2012). Retrieved from Providence College website, http://www.providence.edu/news/headlines/Pages/Healthy-Workplace-Award.aspx

135 Finnair. (2011). *Corporate responsibility report.* Retrieved from http://www.finnairgroup.com/linked/Finnair_Corporate-ResponsibilityReport_2011.pdf

136 Togami, T. (2008). Interventions in local communities and work sites through Physical Activity and Nutrition Programme. *Obesity Review, 9*(Suppl. 1), 127-29.

137 Golley, R., Baines, E., Bassett, P., Wood, L., Pearce, J., & Nelson, M. (2010). School lunch and learning behaviour in primary schools: An intervention study. *European Journal of Clinical Nutrition, 64*(11), 1280-88.

138 Golley, R., Baines, E., Bassett, P., Wood, L., Pearce, J., & Nelson, M. (2010). School lunch and learning behaviour in primary schools: An intervention study. *European Journal of Clinical Nutrition, 64*(11), 1280-88.

139 Summerbell, C. D., Douthwaite, W., Whittaker, V., Ells, L. J., Hillier, F., Smith, S., . . . Macdonald, I. (2009). The association between diet and physical activity and subsequent excess weight gain and obesity assessed at 5 years of age or older: A systematic review of the epidemiological evidence. *International Journal of Obesity, 33*(Suppl. 3), S1-92.

140 U.S. Preventive Services Task Force. (2010). Screening for obesity in children and adolescents: U.S. Preventive Services Task Force recommendation statement. *Pediatrics, 125*(2), 361-67.

141 U.S. Preventive Services Task Force. (2010). Screening for obesity in children and adolescents: U.S. Preventive Services Task Force recommendation statement. *Pediatrics, 125*(2), 361-67.

142 Hendrie, G. A., Brindal, E., Corsini, N., Gardner, C., Baird, D., & Golley, R. K. (2012). Combined home and school obesity prevention interventions for children: What behavior change strategies and intervention characteristics are associated with effectiveness? *Health Education and Behavior, 39*(2), 159-71.

143 Ledoux, T. A., Hingle, M. D., & Baranowski, T. (2011). Relationship of fruit and vegetable intake with adiposity: A systematic review. *Obesity Review, 12*(5), e143-50.

144 Moyer, V. A. (2012). Screening for and management of obesity in adults: U.S. Preventive Services Task Force recommendation statement. *Annals of Internal Medicine, 157*(5), 373-78.

145 Anis, N. A., Lee, R. E., Ellerbeck, E. F., Nazir, N., Greiner, K. A., & Ahluwalia, J. S. (2004). Direct observation of physician counseling on dietary habits and exercise: Patient, physician, and office correlates. *Preventive Medicine, 38*(2), 198-202.

146 Guide to Community Preventive Services. (2008). *Obesity prevention and control: Behavioral interventions to reduce screen time.* Retrieved from www.thecommunityguide.org/obesity/behavorial.html

147 Guide to Community Preventive Services. (n.d.). *Obesity prevention and control: Behavioral interventions to reduce screen time.* Retrieved from www.thecommunityguide.org/obesity/behavorial.html

148 Epstein, L. H. (1996). Family based behavioural intervention for obese children. *International Journal of Obesity, 20,* S14-S21.

149 Epstein, L. H., Valoski, A., Wing, R. R., & Mccurley, J. (1990). 10-year follow-up of behavioral, family-based treatment for obese children. *JAMA, 264*(19), 2519-23.

150 Johnston, C. A., Steele, R. G. Treatment of pediatric overweight: An examination of feasibility and effectiveness in an applied clinical setting. *Journal of Pediatric Psychology, 32*(1), 106-10.

151 Academy of Nutrition and Dietetics. (2012). *The Traffic Light Diet and treating childhood obesity.* Retrieved from http://andevidencelibrary.com/evidence.cfm?evidence_summary_id=250033&auth=1

152 Sacks, G., Rayner, M., & Swinburn, B. (2009). Impact of front-of-pack "traffic-light" nutrition labelling on consumer food purchases in the UK. *Health Promotion International, 24*(4), 344-52.

153 Sacks, G., Veerman, J. L., Moodie, M., & Swinburn, B. (2011). "Traffic-light" nutrition labelling and "junk-food" tax: A modelled comparison of cost-effectiveness for obesity prevention. *International Journal of Obesity, 35*(7), 1001-9.

154 Sacks, G., Tikellis, K., Millar, L., & Swinburn, B. (2011). Impact of "traffic-light" nutrition information on online food purchases in Australia. *Australian and New Zealand Journal of Public Health, 35*(2), 122-26.

155 Rofey, D. L., Hull, E. E., Phillips, J., Vogt, K., Silk, J. S., Dahl, R. E. (2010). Utilizing Ecological momentary assessment in pediatric obesity to quantify behavior, emotion, and sleep. *Obesity, 18*(6), 1270-72.

156 Thomas, J. G., Doshi, S., Crosby, R. D., & Lowe, M. R. (2011). Ecological momentary assessment of obesogenic eating behavior: Combining person-specific and environmental predictors. *Obesity, 19*(8), 1574-79.

157 Moskowitz, D. S., & Young, S. N. (2006). Ecological momentary assessment: What it is and why it is a method of the future in clinical psychopharmacology. *Journal of Psychiatry and Neuroscience, 31*(1), 13-20.

158 Kerr, J., Norman, G., Godbole, S., Raab, F., Demchak, B., & Patrick, K. (2012). Validating GPS data with the PALMS system to detect different active transportation modes. *Medicine and Science in Sports and Exercise, 44*(5 Suppl.), S2529.

159 Smart Growth America. (2003). *Measuring sprawl and its impact.* Retrieved from http://www.smartgrowthamerica.org/research/measuring-sprawl-and-its-impact

160 Vandegrift, D., & Yoked, T. (2004). Obesity rates, income, and suburban sprawl: An analysis of U.S. states. *Health Place, 10*(3), 221-29.

161 Smart Growth America. (2010). *National Complete Streets Coalition.*

162 Manion-Fischer, K. (2009). *States consider trans fat bans, menu labeling.* Retrieved from http://www.stateline.org/live/details/story?contentId=383615

163 *New York restaurants nearly all trans-fat free.* (2009). Retrieved from Reuters Health website, http://www.reuters.com/article/2009/07/20/us-new-york-restaurants-trans-fat-free-idUSTRE56J5HQ20090720

164 Grynbaum, M. M. (2012, September 14). Health panel approves restriction on sale of large sugary drinks. *New York Times,* A24.

165 Hamrick, K. S., Andrews, A., Guthrie, J., Hopkins, D., & McClelland K. (2011). *How much time do Americans spend on food?* Economic Information Bulletin No. EIB-86. Retrieved from U.S. Department of Agriculture website, http://www.ers.usda.gov/publications/eib-economic-information-bulletin/eib86.aspx#.UoUEmxUo4y8

166 Centers for Disease Control and Prevention. (2007, June 15). *CATCH—A coordinated approach to child health* [national satellite broadcast and webcast]. Retrieved from http://www.cdc.gov/news/2007/06/Catch.html

167 Perry, C. L., Stone, E. J., Parcel, G. S., Ellison, R. C., Nader, P. R., Webber, L. S., & Luepker, R. V. (1990). School-based cardiovascular health promotion: The child and adolescent trial for cardiovascular health (CATCH). *Journal of School Health, 60*(8), 406-13.

168 Hoelscher, D. M., Kelder, S. H., Perez, A., Day, R. S., Benoit, J. S., Frankowski, R. F., . . . Lee, E. S. (2010). Changes in the regional prevalence of child obesity in 4th, 8th, and 11th grade students in Texas from 2000-2002 to 2004-2005. *Obesity, 18*(7), 1360-68.

169 Healthy People 2020. (2010). *Summary of objectives: Nutrition and weight status.* http://www.healthypeople.gov/2020/topicsobjectives2020/pdfs/NutritionandWeight.pdf

170 Lee, R. E., McAlexander, K. M., & Banda, J. A. (2011). *Reversing the obesogenic environment.* Champagne, IL: Human Kinetics.

171 Institute of Medicine. (2012). *Accelerating progress in obesity prevention: Solving the weight of the nation.* Retrieved from http://www.iom.edu/Reports/2012/Accelerating-Progress-in-Obesity-Prevention.aspx

172 Shang, E., Hasenberg, T., Schlegel, B., Sterchi, A. B., Schindler, K., Druml, W., . . . Meier, R. (2005). An European survey of structure and organisation of nutrition support teams in Germany, Austria and Switzerland. *Clinical Nutrition, 24*(6), 1005-13.

173 Sallis, J. F., & Owen, N. (1997). *Ecological models* (2nd ed.). San Francisco, CA: Jossey-Bass.

174 Spence, J. C., & Lee, R. E. (2003). Toward a comprehensive model of physical activity. *Psychology of Sport and Exercise, 4,* 7-24.

175 Bronfenbrenner, U. (1977). Toward an experimental ecology of human development. *American Psychologist, 32,* 513-31.

176 Bronfenbrenner, U. (1979). *The ecology of human development: Experiments by nature and design.* Cambridge, MA: Harvard University Press.

177 McLeroy, K. R., Bibeau, D., Steckler, A., & Glanz, K. (1988). An ecological perspective on health promotion programs. *Health Education Quarterly, 15*(4), 351-77.

178 Sallis, J. F., & Owen, N. (1999). *Physical activity and behavioral medicine* (Vol. 3). Thousand Oaks, CA: Sage Publications.

179 Bergman, P., Grjibovski, A. M., Hagstromer, M., Patterson, E., & Sjostrom, M. (2010). Congestion road tax and physical activity. *American Journal of Preventive Medicine, 38*(2), 171-77.

180 Arem, H., & Irwin, M. (2011). A review of web-based weight loss interventions in adults. *Obesity Review, 12*(5), e236-43.

181 Mahmud, N., Rodriguez, J., & Nesbit, J. (2010). A text message-based intervention to bridge the healthcare communication gap in the rural developing world. *Technology and Health Care, 18*(2), 137-44.

182 Schwerdtfeger, A. R., Schmitz, C., & Warken, M. (2012). Using text messages to bridge the intention-behavior gap? A pilot study on the use of text message reminders to increase objectively assessed physical activity in daily life. *Front Psychology, 3,* 270.

183 Coons, M. J., Roehrig, M., & Spring, B. (2011). The potential of virtual reality technologies to improve adherence to weight loss behaviors. *Journal of Diabetes Science and Technology, 5*(2), 340-44.

184 Lee, R. E., Layne, C. S., McFarlin, B. K., O'Connor, D. P., & Siddiqi, S. (2010). Obesity prevention in Second Life: The International Health Challenge. In *Cases on collaboration in virtual learning environments.* Hershey, PA: Information Science Reference.

185 Siddiqi, S., & Lee, R. E. (2010). Building virtual communities for health promotion: Emerging best practices through an analysis of the International Health Challenge and related literature in Second Life. In S. Mohammed & J. Fiaidhi (Eds.), *Ubiquitous health and medical informatics: The ubiquity 2.0 trend and beyond.* Hershey, PA: Information Science Reference.

186 Jakicic, J. M., Wing, R..R., Butler, B. A., & Robertson, R. J. (1995). Prescribing exercise in multiple short bouts versus one continuous bout: Effects on adherence, cardiorespiratory fitness, and weight loss in overweight women. *International Journal of Obesity and Related Metabolic Disorders, 19*(12), 893-901.

187 Schmidt, W. D., Biwer, C. J., & Kalscheuer, L. K. (2001). Effects of long versus short bout exercise on fitness and weight loss in overweight females. *Journal of the American College of Nutrition, 20*(5), 494-501.

188 White House Task Force on Childhood Obesity Report to the President. (2010). *Solving the problem of childhood obesity within a generation.* Retrieved from http://www.letsmove.gov/white-house-task-force-childhood-obesity-report-president

189 U.S. Preventive Services Task Force. (2010). Screening for obesity in children and adolescents: U.S. Preventive Services Task Force recommendation statement. *Pediatrics, 125*(2), 361-67.

190 Summerbell, C. D., Douthwaite, W., Whittaker, V., Ells, L. J., Hillier, F., Smith, S., . . . Macdonald, I. (2009). The association between diet and physical activity and subsequent excess weight gain and obesity assessed at 5 years of age or older: A systematic review of the epidemiological evidence. *International Journal of Obesity, 33*(Suppl. 3), S1-92.

191 Academy of Nutrition and Dietetics. (2012). *The Traffic Light Diet and treating childhood obesity.* Retrieved from http://andevidencelibrary.com/evidence.cfm?evidence_summary_id=250033&auth=1

192 Ledoux, T. A., Hingle, M. D., & Baranowski, T. (2011). Relationship of fruit and vegetable intake with adiposity: A systematic review. *Obesity Review, 12*(5), e143-50.

193 Academy of Nutrition and Dietetics. (2012). *The Traffic Light Diet and treating childhood obesity.* Retrieved from http://andevidencelibrary.com/evidence.cfm?evidence_summary_id=250033&auth=1

194 U.S. Department of Health and Human Services. (2008). *Physical activity guidelines for Americans.* Retrieved from http://www.health.gov/paguidelines/guidelines/default.aspx

195 Moroshko, I., Brennan, L., & O'Brien, P. (2011). Predictors of dropout in weight loss interventions: a systematic review of the literature. *Obesity Review, 12*(11), 912-34.

196 Kiernan, M., Brown, S. D., Schoffman, D. E., Lee, K., King, A. C., Taylor, C. B., . . . Perri, M. G. (2013). Promoting healthy weight with "stability skills first": A randomized trial. *Journal of Consulting and Clinical Psychology, 81*(2), 336-46.

197 Anis, N. A., Lee, R. E., Ellerbeck, E. F., Nazir, N., Greiner, K. A., & Ahluwalia, J. S. (2004). Direct observation of physician counseling on dietary habits and exercise: Patient, physician, and office correlates. *Preventive Medicine, 38*(2), 198-202.

198 Lee, R. E., McAlexander, K. M., & Banda, J. A. (2011). *Reversing the obesogenic environment.* Champagne, IL: Human Kinetics.

199 Lee, R. E., McAlexander, K. M., & Banda, J. A. (2011). *Reversing the obesogenic environment.* Champagne, IL: Human Kinetics.

Chapter 19

Nutrition and Cardiovascular Disease: A Global Public Health Concern

Shweta Khandelwal, PhD, MSc
Mohammed K. Ali, MBchB, MSc, MBA
Karen R. Siegel, MPH

"... Replacement of red meat with alternative protein sources including fish and nuts will reduce risk of CHD [coronary heart disease]. Additional reduction in risk will be achieved by a diet generous in fruits, vegetables and whole grains and low in refined starches, sugar-sweetened beverages, potatoes and salt."–W. C. Willett

Reproduced from Willett, W. C. (2012). Dietary fats and coronary heart disease. *Journal of Internal Medicine, 272*, 13–24.

Learning Objectives

- Understand the role of dietary nutrients and patterns associated with the development of or protection against cardiovascular diseases (CVD).

- Understand the significance of CVD worldwide.

- Describe examples of apparently cardioprotective diets and the evidence demonstrating the beneficial effects.

- Discuss the role of public health nutrition policy in supporting dietary patterns that reduce the impact of CVD.

Case Study: Dietary Guidelines Amidst a Transitioning Global Nutritional Landscape

In every corner of the world, food is central to people's lives. Worldwide, diets are changing to be lower in high-fiber grains and higher in processed goods. In low- and middle-income countries (LMIC), these changes are described by the **nutrition transition** model, which is a framework for explaining these dietary shifts and how they relate to economic, demographic, and epidemiological changes. The nutrition transition is characterized by the shift from traditional diets based on unprocessed foods to "Western" diets that are high in sugars, fat, and animal-source foods (ASF).

Until recently, disease risks were distinct in high-income countries (HIC) versus LMIC. HIC had high noncommunicable chronic disease burdens, while LMIC had high infectious disease and maternal–child disease burdens. Within countries, differences in disease burdens exist across socioeconomic groups, with traditionally distinct patterns between HIC and LMIC. In HIC, poorer individuals generally have less access to fresh foods and physical activity opportunities, and higher chronic disease risks. In LMIC, poorer sections tended be more physically active due to labor-intensive occupations, leading to lower chronic disease risk. High socioeconomic status was traditionally linked to high-fat foods and sedentary lifestyles and higher chronic disease burden. However, this socioeconomic gradient of noncommunicable disease (NCD) burden may be diminishing.[1] The trickle-down theory suggests that low-socioeconomic-status individuals aspire to the lifestyles of wealthier counterparts. Other forces at play include urbanization, better purchasing power, different physical activity patterns in contemporary jobs, access to cheaper cooking oils, and nutrition policies.

NCD burden and deteriorating dietary quality have led nutrition researchers and public health experts to examine diet–disease relationships, often through **nutritional epidemiology**, and to provide dietary guidance for decreasing NCD risk. Accumulations in scientific evidence, however, do not always translate into more effective public health messages. For example, controversies surrounding specific nutrients, such as sodium, calcium, and dietary fats, and their respective roles in CVD cultivate doubt within the public domain.

Discussion Questions

- Which characteristics of Westernized diets lead to their associations with CVD?

- How might public health nutrition programs to reduce CVD be designed differently in developing and industrialized nations?

- Which nutrients and dietary patterns are considered risk factors for CVD, and which are health promoting?

- How can public health programs promote heart-healthy dietary changes among populations?

Introduction

Cardiovascular diseases (coronary heart disease, stroke, peripheral vascular disease) are the leading causes of mortality and disability worldwide. The Global Burden of Disease Study reported that in 2010, CVD accounted for 30% of global mortality, or over 15.6 million deaths,[2] and was the leading cause of **disability-adjusted life years (DALY)** lost.[3] This disease burden is largely caused by modifiable risk factors. Such risk behaviors include dramatic transitions toward poorer diets and lower physical activity levels.[4,5] In recent decades, diets have become higher in preprocessed foods, ASF, added sugars and fats, and alcohol.[6,7] High consumption of these "unhealthy" components, low consumption of protective nutrients, and sedentary lifestyles are associated with increased risks of CVD, some cancers, diabetes, and mortality.

Together, dietary risk factors and physical inactivity accounted for nearly 10% of global mortality due to all causes in 2010.[8]

Dietary risk factors may cause up to 40% of DALY due to coronary heart disease (CHD).[9] Acknowledging that the relationships among diet, nutrition, and diseases are complex, the chapter summarizes the most current evidence regarding the associations between dietary risks and CVD, with the aim of presenting a comprehensive overview for readers. This chapter sequentially describes nutrient groups, foods, and even dietary patterns such that readers are able to disentangle the relationships between diet and disease with greater perspective.

Macronutrients and CVD

Carbohydrates, proteins, and fats constitute the group of **macronutrients**, and they should be consumed in recommended proportions. Over time, high-fat, high-carbohydrate diets with excess calories cause weight gain and **obesity**. Obesity-associated comorbidities include type 2 diabetes mellitus, hypertension, cardiovascular diseases, sleep, and breathing disorders.[10]

Dietary Fats: Lipids and Fatty Acids

Chemically, fatty acids consist of the elements carbon (C), hydrogen (H), and oxygen (O) arranged as a carbon chain skeleton with a carboxyl group (–COOH) at one end. Fatty acids can be classified as saturated fatty acids (SFA), monounsaturated fatty acids (MUFA), and polyunsaturated fatty acids (PUFA) (**Box 19-1**). Most foods contain a combination of these different types of fats. Fats provide a concentrated source of energy, help maintain healthy skin, and are involved in production of reproductive hormones, immune function, as well as the development of the brain and visual systems. Fatty acids serve as carriers for the fat-soluble vitamins A, D, E, and K to allow proper absorption.

However, overconsumption of total, saturated, trans fats, and/or dietary cholesterol can harm the body. Fat deposited around the heart, or epicardial adipose tissue,[11,12] has the function of storing triglycerides to supply free fatty acids for production of myocardial energy. However, it is **metabolically active**, generating inflammatory **adipokines** and exerting paracrine, or locally active signaling, effects on heart function.[13,14,15] It can also interfere with cardiac function mechanically or through generation of bioactive compounds.[16,17,18] Fat deposited around the organs, or visceral adipose tissue, is also metabolically active, secreting adipokines that can cause atherosclerosis of blood vessels in the heart, brain, and peripheral vasculature, leading to CVD.[19]

Excess dietary fat and calories can result in **dyslipidemia** and increased risk for **atherosclerosis** in arteries supplying the heart, brain, limbs, and other organs (**Box 19-2**). Higher

Box 19-1 Saturated, monounsaturated, and polyunsaturated fatty acids

The carbon chains of saturated fatty acids (SFA) are "saturated" because they hold as much hydrogen as chemically possible. Examples of dietary SFA include lauric, myristic, palmitic, and stearic acids. Animal fats have high proportions of SFA.

The carbon chains of monounsaturated fatty acids (MUFA) contain one unsaturated site, where the two surrounding carbons are attached to each other by a double bond. The other carbons are saturated with hydrogen and attached to each other with single bonds, thereby making the fatty acid monounsaturated (one site of unsaturation). Oleic acid is the main dietary MUFA. High-MUFA foods include vegetable oils such as olive, canola, peanut, sunflower, and sesame; avocados; peanut butter; and many nuts and seeds.

Polyunsaturated fatty acids (PUFA) have multiple sites of unsaturation or more than one double bond. Two of the main types of PUFA, omega-3 and omega-6 fatty acids, are found in oily fish, vegetable oils, and nuts and seeds. The omega-3 PUFA alpha-linolenic acid (ALA) and the omega-6 PUFA linoleic acid (LA) are essential fatty acids. Most diets provide more than enough omega-6 PUFA in relationship to their low amounts of omega-3 PUFA. Ideally, these two fats should be consumed in a ratio of 1:1 or less, but Americans often consume 10 or more times the amount of omega-6 PUFA compared to omega-3 PUFA. Ratios smaller than 5:1 omega-6:omega-3 are linked to health benefits and protection from CVD.

The position of the hydrogen atoms around the double bond determines the geometric configuration of the MUFA and hence whether it is the naturally predominant *cis* form, in which both of the hydrogen atoms are on the same side of the chain, or the uncommon-in-nature trans isomer, in which the hydrogen atoms are on opposite sides. Most dietary trans fats are formed from PUFA during food processing or frying. Small amounts of trans fats are naturally present in beef, and are unlikely to have the negative health consequences of artificially produced trans fats.

Data from American Heart Association. (Updated May 1, 2013). Know your fats. Accessed August 27, 2013, from http://www.heart.org/HEARTORG/Conditions/Cholesterol/PreventionTreatmentofHighCholesterol/Know-Your-Fats_UCM_305628_Article.jsp.

Box 19-2 Types and roles of various cholesterol fractions

Cholesterol is a fat-like substance produced endogenously by the liver and also obtained from ASF, including meat, dairy, seafood, and egg yolks. Although the body uses cholesterol to produce hormones and as components of cell membranes, cholesterol is not an essential nutrient from the diet because the liver can produce sufficient quantities of cholesterol endogenously. Excess cholesterol in the body can lead to CVD.

In the blood, cholesterol combines with proteins to form lipoproteins.

- Low-density lipoproteins (LDL) carry cholesterol and other lipids from the liver to other parts of the body. LDL is known as "bad cholesterol" because excess amounts can lead to atherosclerosis. "Optimal" LDL is under 100 mg/dL, according to the American Heart Association.
- High-density lipoprotein (HDL) removes cholesterol and other fats from the tissues to the liver for breakdown. HDL is known as "good cholesterol," and levels over 60 mg/dL are considered cardioprotective. A ratio of total to HDL cholesterol of more than 3.5:1 is considered a risk factor for heart disease.
- Very-low-density lipoproteins (VLDL) include cholesterol, triglycerides, and protein. High blood VLDL levels are a risk factor for stroke and CVD.
- Triglycerides are fats carried by VLDL cholesterol and stored in fat cells. Excess calories consumed from sugars and alcohol are converted into triglycerides. Recommended levels are below 100 mg/dL.

Data from American Heart Association. (Updated September 8, 2013). What your cholesterol levels mean. Accessed August 27, 2013, from http://www.heart.org/HEARTORG/Conditions/Cholesterol/AboutCholesterol/What-Your-Cholesterol-Levels-Mean_UCM_305562_Article.jsp intakes of sources of saturated fat are associated with elevated risk of CHD.[20] Sources of saturated fat include fatty red meat, skin from poultry, butter, other high-fat dairy products, and coconut and palm oil.

Effects of Modifying Dietary Fat Intake and Intake Recommendations

Effects of reducing quantity or modifying the quality of dietary fats consumed on cardiovascular risk factors, such as serum cholesterol, are complex.[21] Experts currently emphasize replacing SFA and trans fats with unsaturated fats, or MUFA and PUFA, and urge that all recommendations be embedded within the overarching message of achieving and maintaining **energy balance**.[22] Furthermore, fat should provide 37% or less of total calorie intake to prevent increased risk of CVD.[23,24] Shifting toward plant-based diets also appears cardioprotective.[25] For example, replacing red meat with some combination of nuts and legumes, and replacing animal fats with vegetable oils, lowers the diet's ratio of SFA to unsaturated fat. No epidemiological or clinical evidence currently supports replacing calories from saturated fats with calories from carbohydrates.[26,27,28,29]

To maintain optimal cardiovascular health, the World Health Organization (WHO) recommends that SFA contribute 10% or less of total energy, or 7% or less for high-risk groups, such as individuals with diabetes or CVD.[30,31,32] For a 2,000-calorie diet, this range is equivalent to 140 to 200 kcalories (kcal) from SFA, or 15 to 22 grams of SFA per day, since fat provides 9 kcal per gram.

Demographic and physiological factors can impact recommendations for an individual's diet. For example, LDL cholesterol is a significant CVD risk factor among younger, leaner individuals who exercise.[33] Recommendations include reducing SFA and increasing fiber intake. For older, overweight, and inactive individuals, insulin resistance, low HDL cholesterol, and high triglyceride levels may be more important risk factors. Programs for this population might emphasize weight control, physical activity, and lower consumption of refined carbohydrates.

Omega-6 and Omega-3 PUFA: Evidence and Recommendations

In general, PUFA are associated with benefits both for early health, such as promoting cognitive development, and for later life diseases, such as mitigating Alzheimer's disease.[34] However, omega-3 and omega-6 PUFA have differential health effects.[35,36,37] Omega-6 (n-6) polyunsaturated fatty acids include linoleic acid (LA), an essential fatty acid, and arachidonic acid (AA). Omega-3 (n-3) PUFA include alpha-linolenic acid (ALA), an essential fatty acid, as well as eicosapentaenoic acid (EPA) and docosahexaenoic acid (DHA). These PUFA are precursors to signaling molecules called **eicosanoids**. In general, eicosanoids derived from n-6 PUFA are proinflammatory, while n-3-derived eicosanoids are anti-inflammatory (**Table 19-1**).[38] Fatty fish is an important source of EPA and DHA.

Omega-3 PUFA confer cardioprotective benefits.[39,40,41,42] Eating fish at least once a week has been associated with a lower risk of fatal CHD.[43] In contrast, EPA and DHA from supplements do not appear to reduce risk of death from CHD. Therefore, dietary recommendations for primary and secondary prevention of CHD are to eat fatty fish once or lean fish twice a week,[44] while no advice is given about supplemental EPA and DHA (**Box 19-3**).[45,46,47,48]

Table 19-1 Classification of unsaturated fatty acids

	Unsaturated Fatty Acids		
	Omega-3	**Omega-6**	**Omega-9**
Examples	Essential fatty acid: α-linolenic acid (ALA) Nonessential fatty acids: Eicosapentanoic acid (EPA) and docosahexaenoic acid (DHA)	Essential fatty acid: Linoleic acid (LA) Nonessential fatty acid: Arachidonic acid (AA)	Nonessential fatty acid: Oleic acid
Sources	Seafood: (tuna, salmon, fish oil) flaxseed oil, walnuts	Safflower, canola, sunflower oil, nuts, peanuts	Olive oil, avocado, olives, peanuts
Functions	Reduces inflammation, plays important roles in brain development and function, helps improve HDL level, reduces triglycerides	Shows beneficial effects in atherosclerosis, asthma, arthritis, vascular diseases	Helps promote healthy inflammatory responses and lower LDL cholesterol

Data from American Heart Association. Know your fats. http://www.heart.org/HEARTORG/Conditions/Cholesterol/PreventionTreatmentofHighCholesterol/Know-Your-Fats_UCM_305628_Article.jsp. Updated May 1, 2013. Accessed August 27, 2013.

Box 19-3 Mercury in seafood

Seafood, or fish and shellfish, provide high-quality protein, DHA and EPA, and essential nutrients. They are also low in saturated fats. However, nearly all seafood contains traces of mercury, an environmental contaminant, in the form of methylmercury, which can accumulate in animal and human tissues. Mercury can adversely affect the nervous systems of fetuses and young children, and it may harm adults' cardiovascular, reproductive, and immune systems.

To reduce mercury exposure, the Food and Drug Administration (FDA) recommends that women who may become pregnant, pregnant and lactating mothers, and young children avoid consuming species of fish and shellfish highest in mercury, and limiting weekly low-mercury seafood consumption to 12 ounces (340 grams).

Larger fish, such as shark, swordfish, and king mackerel, have higher methylmercury contents. Lower-mercury choices include shrimp, canned light tuna, salmon, catfish, and pollock. The European Union (EU) has developed a comprehensive strategy with 20 steps to environmental reduce mercury levels and human exposure to mercury. The recommendation to consume a variety of low-mercury seafood currently remains in place to balance the risks of mercury with the benefits consuming of DHA, EPA, and other nutrients from seafood.

Data from: the U.S. Food and Drug Administration & U.S. Environmental Protection Agency. (2004.) What you need to know about mercury in fish and shellfish: Advice for women who might become pregnant, women who are pregnant, nursing mothers, young children. http://water.epa.gov/scitech /swguidance/fishshellfish/outreach/advice_index.cfm and http://www.fda.gov/downloads/Food/FoodborneIllnessContaminants/UCM182158.pdf

The American Heart Association (AHA) has published an advisory summarizing the evidence on the consumption of omega-6 PUFAs, particularly LA, and CHD risk.[49] Consuming at least 5–10% of energy from omega-6 PUFA appears cardioprotective. In addition, the ratio of n-3 to n-6 PUFA also provides cardioprotective benefits.[50] Clearly, generic recommendations for consumption of "fats" as a broad category should be avoided.[51]

Healthy People 2020: NWS-18: Reduce consumption of saturated fat in the population aged 2 years and older

Reproduced from the U.S. Department of Health and Human Services. Healthypeople.gov. Retrieved from http://www.healthypeople.gov/2020/default.aspx. Last updated July 30, 2013. Accessed August 13, 2013. All HP 2020 in this chapter are from this source.

Carbohydrates

Dietary **carbohydrates** provide energy. They are also found on cell membranes and are essential components of the genetic materials DNA and RNA and, in the form of cellulose, structural materials in plants.[52] The name "carbohydrates" reflects their chemical structures consisting of hydrated carbons, or carbon atoms bound to molecules of water. The chemical formula is $C_n(H_2O)_n$.

Carbohydrates can be classified as simple sugars, which include **monosaccharides** and **disaccharides**, and complex carbohydrates, which include **oligosaccharides** and **polysaccharides**. Monosaccharides, such as glucose and fructose, consist of one molecule of sugar. Disaccharides are short chains of two monosaccharides. They include sucrose, made up of glucose and fructose, and lactose, which consists of glucose and galactose. Oligosaccharides consist of 3 to 10 monosaccharides, and are important for the absorption of certain minerals and the formation of fatty acids. Polysaccharides, with more than 10 sugars, include cellulose, dextrin, glycogen, and starch.[53]

Most dietary carbohydrates supply 4 kcal per gram, and these macronutrients provide the greatest proportion of energy in most diets. During digestion, dietary carbohydrates are broken down into glucose, which is released into the bloodstream to provide energy for body functions.

A food with carbohydrates has a **glycemic index (GI)**, which is a measure of the body's blood glucose response upon eating that food.[54] A higher GI value indicates a higher, more rapid peak blood glucose level after consumption. The **glycemic load (GL)** is the product of dietary GI and total dietary carbohydrate intake. It is a measure of both the quality and quantity of carbohydrate intake.[55] Whole fruits, vegetables, legumes, nuts, and whole grains are low-GI foods. In general, more added sugars and refined grains and less fat, protein, and fiber raise a food's GI content (**Table 19-2**). Low-GI plant-based foods are often high in dietary fiber, a unique carbohydrate that reduces total and LDL cholesterol levels. Fiber also helps improve glycemic

Table 19-2 Glycemic index and glucose contents of commonly consumed food items

Food Item	Glycemic Index (glucose = 100)
High	
Cornflakes	93
Pretzels	83
White rice	89
White potato, boiled	82
White bread	72
Watermelon	72
Raisins	64
Banana, ripe	62
Medium	
White pasta, cooked	58
Oatmeal	55
High-fiber bran cereal	55
Green peas	51
Potato chips	51
Brown rice	50
Whole grain pasta, cooked	42
Low	
Apple, raw	39
Pizza, with cheese and meat	36
Milk, skim	32
Carrots, raw	35
Black beans	30
Kidney beans	29
Lentils	29
Cashews	27
Soybeans	15
Chickpeas (garbanzo beans)	10
Peanuts	7

Data from Harvard Health Publications. Harvard Medical School. (2008). Glycemicindexandglycemicloadfor100+foods.http://www.health.harvard.edu/newsweek/Glycemic_index_and_glycemic_load_for_100_foods.htm. Accessed August 12, 2013.

control in individuals with diabetes by binding to glucose and slowing its release in the body. Frequent consumption of low-GI foods provides these benefits, and ongoing research examines if these benefits are independent of the dietary fiber content.

Also uncertain is whether manufactured low-GI foods confer the same long-term benefits as plant-based low-GI foods. Findings from the Framingham study suggest that dietary GI is associated with fasting triglycerides and fasting insulin, and inversely associated with HDL cholesterol.[56] Total carbohydrate intake is also associated with fasting triglycerides and inversely associated with HDL cholesterol concentrations. This evidence suggests possible benefits of substituting low-GI for high-GI foods to reduce CVD risk.[57] Current information supports choosing whole-grain cereals, fruits, vegetables, and legumes as carbohydrate sources to reduce lipoprotein-mediated risk of CVD, especially in individuals who have one or more CVD risk factors.[58]

> *Healthy People 2020: NWS-16: Increase the contribution of whole grains to the diets of the population aged 2 years and older*

Proteins

Proteins are large molecules consisting of one or more chains of **amino acids**. They provide 4 kcal per gram and have multiple structural and chemical functions in the body. A protein's unique amino acid sequence determines its three-dimensional structure and physiological function. Dietary sources of protein include meat, poultry, seafood, dairy products, eggs, legumes, and nuts.

Some protein sources, such as fatty red meat, are high in SFA, while others, such as skinless chicken, legumes, and fish, are leaner. Although high in total fat, nuts are low in SFA and are considered lean. Data from the Nurses' Health Study of over 80,000 women demonstrated that consumption of lean protein from poultry, fish, and nuts was associated with lower risk of atherosclerotic vascular diseases.[59,60,61,62] Each daily serving of nuts instead of red meat was associated with a 30% lower risk of CHD. Replacing red meat with other protein sources, such as nuts and fish, led to lower SFA, heme iron, and sodium intake.[63] The cardioprotective benefits from reducing red meat are thus likely due to multiple changes in nutrient intake.[64]

Meta-analyses examining red meat and processed meat consumption found a 42% increase in heart disease risk with each 50-gram (1.8-oz.) daily serving of processed meat, or the equivalent of about one to two slices of deli meats or one hot dog. Eating unprocessed red meat was not associated with CVD or diabetes.[65] Further studies have confirmed these results. The high fat and sodium contents in processed meats may be responsible for the negative health effects. Recommendations to limit intake of processed meats seem prudent.[66]

Optimal Combination of Macronutrients to Consume

Much research has focused on the optimal combination of the three principal dietary macronutrients, or fat, protein, and carbohydrate, to prevent CVD. A recent study among Swedish women[67] suggests that after adjusting for variables such as **body mass index (BMI)** and SFA intake, low-carbohydrate, high-protein diets increase CVD risk. In the study, a 20-gram decrease in daily carbohydrate intake and a 5-gram increase in daily protein intake were associated with a 5% increase in CVD risk.[68]

The Optimal Macronutrient Intake Trial to Prevent Heart Disease (OmniHeart)[69,70] was a randomized crossover study investigating effects on blood pressure and LDL-C of consuming three different diets over six-week periods. The first diet included 58% of kcal from carbohydrates; the other two diets included 48% of kcal from carbohydrates, and unsaturated fats or protein provided an additional 10% of kcal. Half of the protein in the third diet was plant-based. Diets were low in SFA and sodium and rich in fruits, vegetables, fiber, and potassium. Participants were 164 prehypertensive adults. Following each diet for six weeks was associated with lower blood pressure, LDL cholesterol, and 10-year risk of CHD. Compared with the carbohydrate diet, the MUFA and protein-rich diets led to greater decreases is CVD risk.

Micronutrients, Antioxidants, and CVD

The **micronutrients** include vitamins and minerals. Many are essential for cardiovascular health, with functions including homeostatic regulation. **Antioxidants**, including vitamins A, C, and E, may have additional cardioprotective benefits.

Fat-Soluble Vitamins

Vitamins are classified as fat-soluble or water-soluble. The fat-soluble vitamins, or vitamins A, D, E, and K, are stored in liver and fat tissues and mobilized as needed. Vitamins A and E have antioxidant properties and are protective against cellular damage due to **free radicals**. Free radicals are highly reactive molecules with an unpaired electron, often formed by interacting with **reactive oxygen species (ROS)**. Free radicals can damage DNA and cell membranes

and cause loss of cellular function and cell death. Results can include heart disease, diabetes, and cancer. Free radicals promote atherosclerosis, often through oxidation of LDL cholesterol by ROS.

Antioxidant vitamins, such as **beta-carotene**, can reduce effects of oxidation and potentially lower CVD risk. Current evidence shows cardiovascular benefits in **observational studies**, but no incremental benefit in **randomized controlled trials (RCT)**. Following is a summary of current evidence on links between heart health and the carotenoids and vitamins D, E, and K.

Dietary Carotenoids

Beta-carotene is a form of provitamin A, and the body converts dietary beta-carotene to the active form of vitamin A. Ecological, cohort, and case-control studies suggest that consumption of carotenoid-rich foods is associated with a reduced risk of heart disease, but clinical trials show that supplemental beta-carotene does not prevent CHD. Other carotenoids, such as lycopene, cryptoxanthin, and lutein, could be beneficial.[71] Fruits and vegetables are sources of carotenoids.

Public Health Core Competency 6: Basic Public Health Science Skills 5: Describes the scientific evidence related to a public health issue, concern, or intervention

Reproduced from Council on Linkages Between Academia and Public Health Practice. 2010 May. Core Competencies for Public Health Professionals. Washington, DC: Public Health Foundation. http://www.phf.org/resourcestools/Documents/Core_Competencies_for_Public_Health_Professionals_2010May.pdf. Accessed August 13, 2013. This source is used for all Public Health Core Competencies in this chapter.

Vitamin D

Vitamin D has effects on a variety of tissues, including cardiomyocytes, vascular smooth muscle cells, and endothelial cells. It inhibits inflammation and alters cell proliferation and differentiation.[72] Vitamin D deficiency may contribute to the development of CVD through its association with CVD risk factors such as diabetes and hypertension. However, this evidence is insufficient for making general recommendations regarding vitamin D supplementation for the prevention and treatment of CVD. RCTs are needed to better understand possible links.[73] Sunlight stimulates endogenous vitamin D production, and food sources of the vitamin include salmon, fortified milk, egg yolks, and certain mushrooms. Older adults or people having less exposure to the sun due to vocational, personal, or medical reasons are prone to developing vitamin D deficiency.

Vitamin E

Vitamin E is a fat-soluble antioxidant vitamin whose most naturally abundant and active form is alpha-tocopherol. Vitamin E has in vitro antioxidant properties, and it prevents atherosclerotic plaque formation in mouse models.[74] Consumption of vitamin E–rich foods is linked to lower CHD risk in middle-aged and older men and women. However, RCTs have not found a benefit of vitamin E in primary or secondary CVD prevention.[75] The AHA does not recommend vitamin E supplements to prevent CVD, but does support consumption of foods abundant in antioxidant vitamins. Nuts, seeds, peanuts, and vegetable oils provide vitamin E.

Vitamin K

Vitamin K–dependent proteins, including matrix Gla-protein, inhibit vascular calcification.[76] Leafy greens and other plant foods provide vitamin K1, or phylloquinone. Menaquinone, or vitamin K2, is in animal organs and aged or fermented products, such as cheeses, sauerkraut, miso, and natto, or fermented soybeans. The population-based Rotterdam Study linked consumption of vitamins K1 and K2 to decreased aortic calcification and CHD.[77] However, in the European Prospective Investigation into Cancer and Nutrition (EPIC) study, there was no relationship between K1 intake and incidence of myocardial infarction over 8.1 years of follow-up. Each 10-microgram increase in daily vitamin K2 consumption, however, was associated with a 9% lower incidence of myocardial infarction.[78]

Water-Soluble Vitamins

Water-soluble vitamins dissolve in water and are cofactors of enzymes involved in metabolism. With the exceptions of vitamins B6 and B12, water-soluble vitamins cannot be stored in the body in large quantities.

Folate, Vitamin B6, and Vitamin B12

Folate, vitamin B6, and vitamin B12 are necessary for preventing the buildup of homocysteine by converting it into the amino acid methionine (**Figure 19-1**). High homocysteine levels may raise CVD risk, while higher dietary folate and vitamin B6 intakes appear to lower risk of CHD.[79,80] However, several large RCTs investigating B vitamin supplementation have failed to find any benefit.[81] A recent meta-analysis suggests that folic acid supplements can reduce the risk of first-time stroke in people, but they do not reduce the risk of second stroke in people who have already had one.[82] Folate is in spinach, asparagus, lettuce,

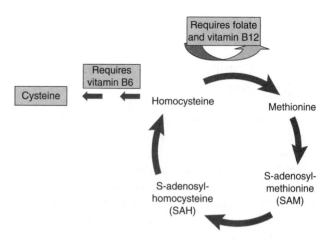

Figure 19-1 Methionine cycle

Data from Miller, A. L. (2003). The methionine-homocysteine cycle and its effects on cognitive diseases. *Alternative Medicine Review, 8*(1), 7-19. Available at http://www.altmedrev.com/publications/8/1/7.pdf. Accessed September 6, 2013.

and avocado, while sources of vitamin B6 include chicken, turkey, beef, pork, bell peppers, broccoli, peanuts, and hazelnuts. Vitamin B12 is in ASF, such as fish, shellfish, meat, chicken, eggs, and milk.

Intakes of folate above 400 micrograms per day and vitamin B6 above 3 milligrams per day appear to be protective against high homocysteine levels.[83] Therefore, the current **recommended daily allowance (RDA)** for folate (400 µg/day for nonlactating adults) and vitamin B6 (1.5 mg/day) can prevent deficiency among nonpregnant women, but may not be high enough to minimize CHD risk. Furthermore, up to 90% of the U.S. population has dietary intakes below 400 micrograms per day. Studies have shown that folic acid supplementation is most protective when taken for at least three years and when there is also supplementation with vitamins B6 and B12.[84,85,86,87,88,89,90] Current evidence does not suggest a benefit of B vitamin supplementation in people who already have heart disease.

Vitamin C

Vitamin C is the most prevalent natural antioxidant vitamin. Food sources include guava, peppers, tomatoes, broccoli, and citrus fruits, such as oranges and grapefruit. Observational studies suggest that vitamin C supplements may lower the risk for coronary events, but several large RCTs have failed to confirm this. Vitamin C supplementation may, however, help lower systolic and diastolic blood pressure in the short term.[91] Before vitamin C supplementation can be recommended for the prevention of hypertension or as adjuvant antihypertensive therapy, additional trials are needed, designed with large sample sizes, and with attention to quality of outcomes assessment.

Polyphenols

Polyphenols (PPHs) are a group of phytochemicals characterized by the presence of more than one phenol unit. The most common and best studied group of PPHs are flavonoids, whose sources include dark chocolate, tea, citrus fruit, berries, and grapes. Naturally occurring dietary PPH have potential therapeutic value as antioxidants and anti-inflammatory agents.[92,93] They reduce LDL oxidation, induce nitric oxide (NO) production to lower blood pressure, and inhibit platelet aggregation, thereby helping to prevent blood clots and reducing the risk of stroke and heart attack.[94] However, experimental evidence regarding PPH and CVD is still lacking.[95]

Sodium

Sodium is an essential electrolyte for maintaining proper blood pressure, but excessive sodium in the bloodstream can lead to fluid imbalance, with increased water within and outside of cells. This causes an increase in blood pressure. **Hypertension** is the leading risk factor for mortality worldwide,[96] raising risk for CHD, stroke, and kidney disease.

Among 2,657 participants (36% men; 21% white, 24% black, and 53% Hispanic) aged over 40 years in the Northern Manhattan Study, those consuming at least 4,000 milligrams (mg) of sodium per day had a 2.6-fold higher risk of stroke compared with those who consumed no more than 1,500 milligrams per day.[97] Furthermore, each 500 milligram per day increase in sodium intake increased the risk of ischemic stroke by 16%. In a study of 421 Inuit adults in Canada, higher consumption of salt, which is 39% sodium by weight, was associated with higher blood pressure.[98] Urinary sodium excretion is a more accurate measure of excess sodium intake than dietary assessments. Studies have consistently found associations between higher sodium excretion and adverse cardiovascular outcomes, such as death, myocardial infarction, and stroke.[99] Interestingly, lower rates of sodium excretion are also associated with increased risk of the composite CVD outcome.[100]

Public Health Recommendations for Sodium Intake

Debate continues regarding appropriate recommendations for sodium intake.[101,102,103,104,105,106] Current WHO recommendations are to consume less than 5 grams of salt, or less than 2,300 milligrams of sodium, per day. The AHA encourages a maximum daily intake of 1,500 milligrams of sodium. Major dietary sources of sodium include salt, added at the table and in cooking, as well as processed and prepared foods, bakery items, and salty seasonings.

Potassium

A diet high in potassium and low in sodium reduces blood pressure,[107,108,109] and potassium intake is inversely related to incidence of stroke.[110] Increasing daily potassium intake by 1,000 milligrams may lower relative risk of stroke by 11%.[111,112] To reduce risk of stroke, public health recommendations should include high dietary intake of potassium-rich foods,[113] such as fruits, vegetables, avocadoes, baked potatoes, lentils, beans, and nuts.

Calcium

Calcium is an essential mineral that acts predominantly as a second messenger, transmitting signals between the plasma membrane and the intracellular machinery. Extracellular calcium is also an essential cofactor in clotting and proper function of adhesion molecules, such as platelets. In bone, calcium provides the structural strength that allows the bone to support the body's weight and anchor the muscles, and more than 99% of the calcium in the human body is in the bones and teeth. Bone calcium also serves as a reservoir that can be tapped to maintain extracellular calcium concentration when dietary calcium intake is insufficient. Other functions that require calcium include muscle contraction, exocytosis, nerve conduction, regulation of enzyme activity, and formation of cell membranes. Recent evidence suggests that calcium has direct effects in the parathyroid gland, the kidney, and the brain.[114] Dietary sources of calcium include milk and milk products, tofu, canned fish, such as sardine and salmon, and leafy green vegetables, such as kale.

Calcium and vitamin D are often considered together because of vitamin D's role in regulating blood calcium levels. When blood calcium levels decrease, calcitriol, the active form of vitamin D, increases calcium absorption and reduces excretion to raise serum calcium levels. Calcium supplementation consumption is increasingly common, as is the prevalence of vitamin D deficiency. Calcium supplements are often recommended for postmenopausal women to prevent or treat **osteoporosis**. However, there is also great interest in the potential role of calcium supplementation in reducing CVD risk. A 2012 review linked calcium supplementation to reductions in systolic and diastolic blood pressure and found high intakes of milk and/or dairy products to be associated with reduction in CVD risk.[115] However, in the Heidelberg cohort, calcium supplementation was associated with increased risk of myocardial infarction.[116] The current tentative inference is that calcium supplementation may slightly increase the risk of myocardial infarction along with other CVD,[117] supporting cardioprotective effects of dietary calcium obtained from low-fat dairy sources, and possible deleterious effects of calcium supplements, especially in the absence of adequate vitamin D.[118,119]

Iron

The mineral iron is involved in enzymatic action, is part of **hemoglobin**, and helps regulate the immune system. **Anemia**[120] is a well-known consequence of iron deficiency. Among heart failure patients, iron-deficiency anemia increases the risk of cardiovascular mortality.[121] Prospective studies have shown a positive relationship between **heme** iron intake and the risk of CVD,[122,123,124] while an increased intake of **non-heme** iron may lower homocysteine levels and also attenuate risk of CHD.[125]

The Japan Collaborative Cohort Study demonstrated that the dietary intake of total iron was positively associated with mortality from total and ischemic stroke and total CVD in men, but found no association in women.[126] However, data from the Atherosclerosis Risk in Communities (ARIC) Study, with a matched case-control design,[127] did not find a relationship between higher iron status and progression of heart disease.[128]

Mineral Balance

Interactions between minerals in the body impact their overall bioavailability, functionality, and effects on CVD risk.[129] One study, for example, investigated the effect of dietary iron reduction on salt-induced cardiovascular pathophysiology using Dahl salt-sensitive rats, which are particularly susceptible to hypertension.[130] Iron reduction reduced oxidative stress and the development of hypertension, left-ventricular hypertrophy, and heart failure.

While this chapter has examined each nutrient individually, it is important to note that mineral nutrients, such as calcium, potassium, and magnesium, collectively act to lower blood pressure. A deficiency of any one of the essential minerals can result in severe metabolic disorders and compromise cardiovascular health. Thus, the interactions, synergies, and biological pathways of action of the micronutrients need to be understood and examined holistically.

Dietary Patterns and Composite Dietary Interventions

This chapter so far has focused on single nutrients. However, people eat mixed diets, not single nutrients, and nutrient interactions influence their bioavailability, absorption, and effects.[131,132] Therefore, investigating dietary patterns is necessary, especially when considering public health implications. The next sections of this chapter focus on cardioprotective dietary patterns, such as the Mediterranean, Dietary Approaches to Stopping Hypertension (DASH), Japanese, and vegetarian diets, and cardiovascular health, including implications for policies and recommendations. These diets have notable differences from Western-style diets, whose high levels of SFA, refined carbohydrates, and animal proteins may increase the risk of heart disease.

> *Public Health Core Competency 2: Policy Development/ Program Planning Skills 4: Gathers information that will inform policy decisions*

Mediterranean Diet

The Mediterranean diet refers not to a specific diet, but to a general dietary pattern. It emphasizes minimally processed, seasonally fresh, locally grown plant-based foods, or fruit, vegetables, breads, cereals, potatoes, beans, nuts, and seeds. Consumption of red meat and sweets with refined sugars or honey is limited. The diet is rich in MUFA because olive oil is the main fat source. Dairy products, mainly cheese and yogurt, are consumed daily. The diet includes fish and poultry at least twice weekly, up to four eggs per week, and low to moderate wine consumption.[133,134] Locations where the Mediterranean diet prevails are known for a reduced premature cardiac death. In addition, countries with high consumption of plant foods and fish, such as Scandinavia, Switzerland, and Austria, also have low CVD mortality.

Cardioprotective Factors in the Mediterranean Diet

A high ratio of MUFA to SFA likely contributes to the Mediterranean diet's health benefits. In addition, the diet is rich in omega-3 PUFA as DHA and EPA from seafood, and as their precursor, alpha-linolenic acid (ALA), from walnuts, flaxseed, and many vegetable oils. Protective mechanisms of omega-3 PUFAs include anti-arrhythmic and anti-inflammatory effects, lowering triglycerides, reducing platelet aggregation, and decreasing heart rate.

Fruits and vegetables in the Mediterranean diet provide heart-healthy compounds, such as fiber, antioxidants, potassium, and phytosterols, which have antioxidative, antithrombotic, and serum **cholesterol**–lowering effects.[135] Folate, present in many fruits and vegetables, can also provide cardiovascular protection through its homocysteine-lowering effects. With abundant vegetables, fruits, unrefined cereals, legumes, nuts, garlic, olive oil, and red wine, this diet is rich in PPH. It is higher in potassium and lower in sodium than Western diets high in processed foods.

Evidence Suggests That the Mediterranean Diet Reduces Morbidity and Mortality

The Seven Countries Study was the first to draw attention to beneficial effects of the Mediterranean diet on lipid metabolism, blood pressure, BMI, inflammation, and coagulation.[136] Prospective population studies in Greece, Denmark, and Australia have subsequently supported the protective effects of the Mediterranean diet on overall mortality.[137] Data from RCTs associate a Mediterranean-style diet with reductions in BMI, blood pressure, fasting plasma glucose, total cholesterol, and high-sensitivity C-reactive protein, or CRP. Each of these may affect CVD incidence.[138,139] In a secondary prevention trial in patients who had suffered a heart attack, an ALA-enriched Mediterranean diet lowered risk of cardiac death and nonfatal myocardial infarction compared with a prudent diet (described below).[140,141] Additionally, a cohort study showed that adherence to the Mediterranean diet and was strongly associated with survival among Greek cardiac patients.[142]

Mediterranean Diet Score and Health Benefits

The Mediterranean Diet Score (MDS) is a novel way of representing the cumulative benefits of the sum of its components. The MDS recognizes that the diet's benefits result from the cumulative impact of multiple components rather than from a single nutrient, and that individuals can follow this diet pattern to varying extents. The MDS assigns scores of 0 or 1 to each of the diet's nutrition components, including consumption of vegetables, fruits, legumes and nuts combined, grains, fish and seafood combined, meat and dairy products, and alcohol, and the ratio of unsaturated to saturated fatty acids. Sex-specific medians are used as cutoff values. Intakes equal to or above the median receive a value of 1, and intakes below that median are assigned a value of 0; thus, possible scores range from 0 to 9. In one meta-analysis, each two-unit increment in MDS was associated with a 10% lower incidence of fatal and nonfatal CVD endpoints.[143,144] Disease-specific associations were strongest for incident myocardial infarction, stroke, and pulmonary embolism.

DASH Diet

The DASH diet is similar to a Mediterranean-style diet in its emphasis on fruits, vegetables, reduced-fat dairy products, whole grains, nuts, fish, and poultry, as well as minimal consumption of total and saturated fats.[145] The standard DASH diet limits daily sodium intake to 2,300 milligrams, and the low-sodium version limits daily intake to 1,500 milligrams. The DASH diet is rich in potassium, calcium, and magnesium, and is widely recommended for reducing hypertension and the risk of heart disease and stroke.

In two RCTs, the DASH diet rapidly reduced blood pressure among people with moderate or prehypertension.[146,147] In the original DASH trial, 459 subjects with hypertension were randomized to a control diet, a diet rich in fruits and vegetables, or the DASH diet. Within two weeks, blood pressure was reduced among individuals on the DASH diet, but only minimally changed among those on the control diet.[148,149] Further investigation of the effects of sodium restriction, albeit measured by self-report, was performed in the DASH-Sodium Trial, which found that restriction of sodium to 1.2 grams per day further reduced diastolic blood pressure. However, such strict sodium consumption is unlikely to be achieved without major changes in food processing and manufacturing.

> *Healthy People 2020: NWS-19: Reduce consumption of sodium in the population aged 2 years and older*

Vegetarian Diet

Vegetarians avoid meat, fish, and poultry. Lacto-ovo vegetarians consume dairy products and eggs, while vegans consume no ASF. Ecological and case-control studies report that vegetarian diets are associated with reduced risks of

CVD in both developed[150,151,152] and developing countries.[153] The protective effect is likely due in part to consuming more fruit, vegetables, nuts, and cereals. Furthermore, the absence of animal-derived foods results in lower SFA intake, resulting in lower total and LDL cholesterol levels and lower CVD risk. The high intake of fiber may also lower cholesterol levels. In the EPIC-Oxford cohort study, vegetarians had a 32% lower risk of ischemic heart disease than nonvegetarians. This finding is likely due to lower HDL cholesterol and systolic blood pressure.[154]

Not all vegetarian diets are healthful, per se. Even while avoiding high-SFA ASF, vegetarians can potentially have high intakes of added sugars and trans fats if they consume high levels of processed foods.[155] Additionally, without nutrient supplementation, vegetarians are at risk for B12 and sulfur deficiency and may have a higher risk of heart disease.

Cooking is another issue surrounding vegetable consumption and heart health. Griddle and microwave cooking generally help maintain the highest levels of antioxidants, while pressure-cooking and boiling lead to the greatest losses.[156] To further complicate matters, although raw, uncooked vegetables are often perceived as healthier, cooking may offer certain benefits. One study found that individuals following a strict raw food diet had normal to high levels of vitamin A and beta-carotene, but low levels of lycopene.[157] In fact, cooking boosts lycopene content of tomatoes.[158] Additionally, cooked carrots, spinach, mushrooms, asparagus, cabbage, peppers, and many other vegetables supply more antioxidants, such as carotenoids and ferulic acid, than raw forms.[159,160] This may be because boiling and steaming without throwing away the water better preserves antioxidants in the vegetables.

Prudent Versus Western Diet Patterns

Defining other scoring systems and dietary patterns has allowed researchers to examine diet–disease relationships. For example, as part of the Health Professionals Follow-up Study, researchers identified two major dietary patterns based on results from food frequency questionnaires (FFQ). The "prudent pattern" included higher intake of vegetables, fruit, legumes, whole grains, fish, and poultry, and the "Western pattern" was characterized by higher intake of red meat, processed meat, refined grains, sweets and dessert, French fries, and high-fat dairy products.[161] The prudent pattern was associated with lower risk of CVD, while increasing Western pattern scores were linked to higher CVD risk.

Japanese Diet

The Japanese have the world's highest life expectancies and low CVD mortality rates, leading to interest in the traditional Japanese diet for its potential health benefits.[162,163,164] The traditional Japanese diet is high in plant-based and seafood components that are naturally low in SFA and sugars. Consumption of cruciferous vegetables, such as cabbage, broccoli, Brussels sprouts, Chinese cabbage, cauliflower, kale, watercress, radishes, parsnips, and turnips, is high. Shitake mushrooms, which symbolize longevity in Japan, lower cholesterol, have antioxidant effects, and are common. Consumption of seaweed, which is rich in iodine and other minerals, approaches one-half pound per day. As described earlier, fish is rich in essential fatty acids (EPA and DHA), which are known for a myriad of health benefits, including reduced heart disease and lowered cholesterol. Tofu and green tea are rich in antioxidants, can lower cholesterol and blood pressure, and improve cardiovascular function.[165]

> *Public Health Core Competency 4: Cultural Competency Skills 4: Describes the dynamic forces that contribute to cultural diversity*

Polymeal

Mimicking the concept of a "Polypill," or single pill combining several therapeutic agents to lower CVD risk, a "polymeal" to reduce CVD risk has also been proposed. The meal consists of a daily regimen of wine, fish, dark chocolate, fruits, vegetables, garlic, and almonds,[166] as a "tastier and safer alternative to the Polypill." It is estimated that the polymeal—just like the Polypill—could reduce heart attacks and strokes in people over age 50 by three-quarters, increasing longevity by about seven years for men and five years for women.[167] The "polymeal" essentially includes many of the protective dietary components present in the dietary patterns described above.

Although each of the diets described in this section originated in diverse regions of the world and varies slightly in its components, many similarities across the Mediterranean, Japanese, vegetarian, DASH, and the proposed "polymeal" diets are apparent. Each is low in animal products, thereby reducing SFA, and high in fruits, vegetables, fiber, MUFA, and PUFA.

Implications for Policy

The previous sections of this chapter have focused on the major dietary risk factors that contribute to the development of CVD. The following section translates these healthy dietary patterns into some policy recommendations (**Table 19-3**).

Evidence-Based Recommendations for Different Dietary Components

Fat: Recognizing the differential effects on health of SFA, trans fats, MUFA, PUFA, and cholesterol, recommendations include limiting SFA and trans fats, restricting dietary cholesterol, and getting adequate PUFA and MUFA.[168,169]

Fruits and vegetables: The recommendation for fruits and vegetables is a minimum of 400 to 500 grams, or five servings, per day.[170] Greater benefits occur at intake of nine servings per day.

Sodium and potassium: Current evidence suggests an intake of 70 mmol, or 1.7 grams, of sodium per day,

can be consumed without adverse effects.[171] Daily potassium levels of 70–80 mmol per day, or 1.7 grams, which will keep the sodium–potassium ratio close to 1, are recommended.

Fiber: Adequate intake of fiber[172] can protect against CHD and help to lower blood pressure. Fruits, vegetables, whole grains, legumes, or beans, peas and lentils, nuts, and peanuts are sources.

Seafood: Regular fish consumption to provide an average of 200 milligrams per day of DHA and EPA protects against CHD and stroke.[173] Approximately two servings of seafood per week achieve this recommendation.

Alcohol: Regular low to moderate alcohol consumption, or one to two drinks per day for men and one drink for women, is protective against CHD. Overconsumption may increase risk of stroke and hypertension. One drink is equivalent to one 12-ounce beer, 4 ounces of wine, 1.5 ounces of 80-proof spirits, or 1 ounce of 100-proof spirits.

Table 19-3 Evidence for diet and risk of CVD

	Increase in Risk	**Decrease in Risk**	**No Relation**
Convincing	Myristic and palmitic acids	LA	Vitamin E supplements
	Trans-fats	Fruits, berries, and vegetables	
	High sodium intake	Fish and fish oils (EPA and DHA)	
	High alcohol intake (for stroke)	Potassium	
		Low to moderate alcohol intake (for CHD)	
Probable	Dietary cholesterol	ALNA	Stearic acid
	Unfiltered boiled coffee	OA	
	Beta-carotene supplements	Nonstarch polysaccharides (fiber)	
		Whole grain cereals	
		Nuts (unsalted)	
		Folate	
		Plant sterols	
Possible	Fats rich in lauric acid	Flavonoids	
	Impaired fetal nutrition	Soy products	
Insufficient evidence: carbohydrates, iron, calcium, magnesium, vitamin C			

Reproduced from Srinath Reddy, K., & Katan, M. B. (2004). Diet, nutrition and the prevention of hypertension and cardiovascular diseases. *Public Health Nutrition*, 7(1a), 167-186.

Individual (High-Risk) Versus Population-Wide Approaches: Building a Case for Government Intervention

Development of effective public health programs to reduce CVD on a population level requires consideration of current knowledge of encouraging cardiovascular health through societal-level interventions that act through policy or by changing environments to make healthier choices easier. Geoffrey Rose famously noted, "The efforts of individuals are only likely to be effective when they are working with societal trends."[174] While consumer education and individualized lifestyle modifications can help to encourage individual behavior change to consume healthier diets, these approaches often have limited effects due to a food environment in which unhealthy foods are readily accessible, affordable, and acceptable. To combat the effects of globalization and the modern food environment, researchers have explored approaches to preventing CVD through population-level nutritional interventions.

Ecological Studies Indicating Population-Wide Effects of Dietary Change

Multiple ecological studies explore the potential impacts of population-wide policies. For example, demonstrating the effect of food availability on heart health, sharp declines in CHD mortality accompanied the changes in type of dietary fat and increased supplies of fresh fruit and vegetables in Poland in 1991.[175] Analogously in Mauritius, a developing island country off the coast of Africa, a government program led to shifts from using high-SFA palm oil to low-SFA soybean oil in 1987. By 1992, cholesterol levels among adults living in Mauritius declined by 19%.[176] In 1972 in Finland, the North Karelia Project was launched in response to the local petition for urgent and effective help to reduce the great burden of locally high mortality from heart disease. Within the program, dairy farmers, who were major contributors to the country's economy, were encouraged to switch to berry production. Over time, berry consumption in Finland increased while dairy consumption decreased, as did population cholesterol levels and CVD mortality.[177]

Sample Policies to Reduce CVD: Examples in Denmark, the United Kingdom, and the United States

Because of the current strength of evidence relating quality of dietary fat and quantity of dietary sodium, the most common policy discussions revolve around regulation of fat and sodium (salt) intake. In 2004, Denmark became the first country to ban nonnatural trans fats. This regulation is attributed with helping to reduce CVD by over 30%. In 2011, the Danish government went a step further by imposing a "fat tax" on saturated fats, or those largely found in animal products such as butter, cream, and meat. The tax, which, like the trans-fat ban, is the first of its kind, raises the price of any food that contains more than 2.3% saturated fat by 16 krone (U.S. $2.85) per kilogram of saturated fat, or per 43 kilograms of food. The tax had been implemented without any plans for formal evaluation of its impacts. However, no evidence linked the tax to reductions in CVD. Danes may have switched to lower-cost fat alternatives, such as lower-fat cheeses and dairy products, or purchased their goods in bordering nations, where fats were cheaper. Within a year, citing fears over job losses, the Danish government announced that it would remove the tax.[178,179]

Salt legislation from 2006 provides evidence that policies based on collaboration and pragmatic implementation can promote health. The United Kingdom's Food Standards Agency spearheaded an effort that involved food manufacturers, retailers, and scientists to agree to lower the sodium content of consumer foods. By 2008, average daily salt consumption in the United Kingdom declined to 8.6 grams from 9.5 grams in 2006; this is expected to prevent 6,000 premature deaths in coming years.[180]

Other targets for public health policy are soda and sugar-sweetened beverages, whose high calorie and sugar content make them nutritional risk factors for CVD through their effects on weight gain and adiposity. One article setting out a public policy case for soda taxation reported that consumption may decrease by up to 7.8% for every 10% increase in price.[181] It has also been estimated that a penny-per-ounce excise tax would raise an estimated $1.2 billion in New York State alone.[182,183] In 2012, New York City passed legislation banning the sale of sodas over 16 ounces in restaurants, movie theaters, and stadiums.[184] However, a state judge blocked the ban in 2013.

Policy formulation to positively impact dietary habits has tended to be top-down. However, policies with greater public buy-in may have a greater chance of success and sustainability, and this process should involve representative voices/views from all sections of society. In particular, consumer demand can influence which foods companies produce. These shifts occur gradually, though, and depend on improved awareness regarding nutrition among consumers. Mandating nutrition labels and advocacy approaches alone are not enough, especially where they may result in the provision of misinformation, such as false claims regarding the nutrient benefits of a food without informing the population about poor bioavailability/absorption.[185]

Though all of these policy initiatives are attractive and offer high population reach, the impacts and externalities associated with each of these measures are, as yet, untested. And while ecological data are promising, more rigorous quasi-experimental designs may offer a more robust approach to evaluating these population-level initiatives.[186,187]

Conclusion

Understanding of the health benefits and risks of food and nutrient consumption is continually evolving. While the associations between dietary risk factors and CVD have been extensively studied, the findings are largely derived from observational studies. Experimental rather than observational studies are gold standards for determining causal relationships.

This chapter contains several important messages. Consideration of quality and quantity of nutrients is critical. Appropriate energy balance is also essential and requires sustained approaches to improving portion size control, engaging in physical activity, and enhancing local environments such that they support these positive lifestyle choices.[188] Another important consideration is that people do not consume nutrients in isolation, but rather entire diets, which include both nutrients and antinutrients. Diet disease relationships likely result from combined effects of foods, including quantities, combinations, and preparation methods, rather than isolated nutrient content.[189]

The core of effective primary prevention of CVD at the population level consists of interventions to reduce four common behavioral risk factors: tobacco use, unhealthy diet, low physical activity, and excess alcohol consumption.[190] This chapter reinforces the scientific evidence to date that indicates it is better to prioritize whole foods and overall dietary patterns rather than focus on individual nutrients when providing nutritional guidance for CVD prevention, and to emphasize the quality of a nutrient in addition to its quantity. Rigorous nutritional epidemiological research and effective communication are required to engage all stakeholders—including policy makers, manufacturers, consumers, and scientists—to collectively work toward combating the huge global CVD burden by making improved and healthier dietary options available and accessible across all socioeconomic groups. Such win-win solutions permit stakeholder groups to work toward their respective individual goals, while contributing to the collective goal of improving human health and well-being.

References

1   Kinra, S., Bowen, L. J., Lyngdoh, T., Prabhakaran, D., Reddy, K. S., Ramakrishnan, L., . . . & Ebrahim, S. (2010). Sociodemographic patterning of non-communicable disease risk factors in rural India: A cross sectional study. *BMJ, 341*, c4974. doi:10.1136/bmj.c4974

2   Lozano, R., Naghavi, M., Foreman, K., Lim, S., Shibuya, K., Aboyans, V., . . . Murray, C. J. L. (2012). Global and regional mortality from 235 causes of death for 20 age groups in 1990 and 2010: A systematic analysis for the Global Burden of Disease Study 2010. *Lancet, 380*(9859), 2095-2128.

3   Murray, C. J., Vos, T., Lozano, R., Naghavi, M., Flaxman, A. D., Michaud, C., . . . Memish, Z. A. (2012). Disability-adjusted life years (DALYs) for 291 diseases and injuries in 21 regions, 1990-2010: A systematic analysis for the Global Burden of Disease Study 2010. *Lancet, 380*(9859), 2197-2223.

4   Lozano, R., Naghavi, M., Foreman, K., Lim, S., Shibuya, K., Aboyans, V., . . . Murray, C. J. L. (2012). Global and regional mortality from 235 causes of death for 20 age groups in 1990 and 2010: A systematic analysis for the Global Burden of Disease Study 2010. *Lancet, 380*(9859), 2095-2128.

5   Popkin, B. M. (2011). Contemporary nutritional transition: Determinants of diet and its impact on body composition. *Proceedings of the Nutrition Society, 70*(1), 82-91. doi:10.1017/S0029665110003903

6   Lozano, R., Naghavi, M., Foreman, K., Lim, S., Shibuya, K., Aboyans, V., . . . Murray, C. J. L. (2012). Global and regional mortality from 235 causes of death for 20 age groups in 1990 and 2010: A systematic analysis for the Global Burden of Disease Study 2010. *Lancet, 380*(9859), 2095-2128.

7   Popkin, B. M. (1998). The nutrition transition and its health implications in lower-income countries. *Public Health Nutrition, 1*(1), 5-21.

8   Lim, S. S., Vos, T., Flaxman, A. D., Danaei, G., Shibuya, K., Adair-Rohani, H., . . . Memish, Z. A. (2012). A comparative risk assessment of burden of disease and injury attributable to 67 risk factors and risk factor clusters in 21 regions, 1990-2010: A systematic analysis for the Global Burden of Disease Study 2010. *Lancet, 380*(9859), 2224-60.

9   Lim, S. S., Vos, T., Flaxman, A. D., Danaei, G., Shibuya, K., Adair-Rohani, H., . . . Memish, Z. A. (2012). A comparative risk

assessment of burden of disease and injury attributable to 67 risk factors and risk factor clusters in 21 regions, 1990-2010: A systematic analysis for the Global Burden of Disease Study 2010. *Lancet, 380*(9859), 2224-60.

10 Noria, S. F., & Grantcharov, T. (2013). Biological effects of bariatric surgery on obesity-related comorbidities. *Canadian Journal of Surgery, 56*(1), 47-57. doi:10.1503/cjs.036111

11 D'Avila, A., Scanavacca, M., Sosa, E., Ruskin, J. N., & Reddy, V. Y. (2003). Pericardial anatomy for the interventional electrophysiologist. *Journal of Cardiovascular Electrophysiology, 14*(4), 422-30.

12 Iacobellis, G., Corradi, D., & Sharma, A. M. (2005). Epicardial adipose tissue: Anatomic, biomolecular and clinical relationships with the heart. *Nature Clinical Practice Cardiovascular Medicine, 2*(10), 536-43. doi:10.1038/ncpcardio0319

13 Iacobellis, G., & Leonetti, F. (2005). Epicardial adipose tissue and insulin resistance in obese subjects. *Journal of Clinical Endocrinology & Metabolism, 90*(11), 6300-6302. doi:10.1210/jc.2005-1087

14 Mazurek, T., Zhang, L., Zalewski, A., Mannion, J. D., Diehl, J. T., Arafat, H., . . . Shi, Y. (2003). Human epicardial adipose tissue is a source of inflammatory mediators. *Circulation, 108*(20), 2460-66.

15 Iacobellis, G., Corradi, D., & Sharma, A.M. (2005). Epicardial adipose tissue: Anatomic, biomolecular and clinical relationships with the heart. *Nature Clinical Practice Cardiovascular Medicine, 2*(10), 536-43. doi:10.1038/ncpcardio0319

16 Rokey, R., Mulvagh, S. L., Cheirif, J., Mattox, K. L., & Johnston, D. L. (1989). Lipomatous encasement and compression of the heart: Antemortem diagnosis by cardiac nuclear magnetic resonance imaging and catheterization. *American Heart Journal, 117*(4), 952-53.

17 De Scheerder, I., Cuvelier, C., Verhaaren, R., De Buyzere, M., De Backer, G., & Clement, D. (1987). Restrictive cardiomyopathy caused by adipositas cordis. *European Heart Journal, 8*(6), 661-63.

18 Willett, W. C. (2012). Dietary fats and coronary heart disease. *Journal of Internal Medicine, 272*, 13-24.

19 Boscaro, M., Giacchetti, G., & Ronconi, V. (2012). Visceral adipose tissue: Emerging role of gluco- and mineralocorticoid hormones in the setting of cardiometabolic alterations. *Annals of the New York Academy of Sciences, 1264*(1), 87-102. doi:10.1111/j.1749-6632.2012.06597.x

20 Oh, K., Hu, F. B., Manson, J. E., Stampfer, M. J., & Willett, W.C. (2005). Dietary fat intake and risk of coronary heart disease in women: 20 years of follow-up of the nurses' health study. *American Journal of Epidemiology, 161*(7), 672-79.

21 Willett, W. C. (2012). Dietary fats and coronary heart disease. *Journal of Internal Medicine, 272*(1), 13-24. doi:10.1111/j.1365-2796.2012.02553.x

22 Mozaffarian, D. (2011). The great fat debate: Taking the focus off of saturated fat. *Journal of the American Dietetic Association, 111*(5), 665-66.

23 Lichtenstein, A. H. (2011). The great fat debate: The importance of message translation. *Journal of the American Dietetic Association, 111*(5), 667-70.

24 Willett, W. C. (2011). The great fat debate: Total fat and health. *Journal of the American Dietetic Association, 111*(5), 660-62.

25 Willett, W. C. (1999). Convergence of philosophy and science: The third international congress on vegetarian nutrition. *American Journal of Clinical Nutrition, 70*(3 Suppl.), 434S-438S.

26 Astrup, A., Dyerberg, J., Elwood, P., Hermansen, K., Hu, F. B., Jakobsen, M. U., . . . Willett, W. C. (2011). The role of reducing intakes of saturated fat in the prevention of cardiovascular disease: Where does the evidence stand in 2010? *American Journal of Clinical Nutrition, 93*(4), 684-88. doi:10.3945/ajcn.110.004622

27 Siri-Tarino, P. W., Sun, Q., Hu, F. B., & Krauss, R. M. (2010). Meta-analysis of prospective cohort studies evaluating the association of saturated fat with cardiovascular disease. *American Journal of Clinical Nutrition, 91*(3), 535-46.

28 Siri-Tarino, P. W., Sun, Q., Hu, F. B., & Krauss, R. M. (2010). Saturated fatty acids and risk of coronary heart disease: Modulation by replacement nutrients. *Current Atherosclerosis Reports, 12*(6), 384-90.

29 Siri-Tarino, P. W., Sun, Q., Hu, F. B., & Krauss, R. M. (2010). Saturated fat, carbohydrate, and cardiovascular disease. *American Journal of Clinical Nutrition, 91*(3), 502-9.

30 Mozaffarian, D. (2011). The great fat debate: Taking the focus off of saturated fat. *Journal of the American Dietetic Association, 111*(5), 665-66.

31 Zelman, K. (2011). The great fat debate: A closer look at the controversy: Questioning the validity of age-old dietary guidance. *Journal of the American Dietetic Association, 111*(5), 655-58.

32 Gifford, K. D. (2002). Dietary fats, eating guides, and public policy: History, critique, and recommendations. *American Journal of Medicine, 113* (Suppl. 9B), 89S-106S.

33 Willett, W. C. (2011). The great fat debate: Total fat and health. *Journal of the American Dietetic Association, 111*(5), 660-62.

34 Freund-Levi, Y., Eriksdotter-Jönhagen, M., Cederholm, T., Basun, H., Faxén-Irving, G., Garlind, A., . . . Palmblad, J. (2006). Omega-3 fatty acid treatment in 174 patients with mild to moderate Alzheimer disease: OmegAD study: A randomized double-blind trial. *Archives of Neurology, 63*(10), 1402-8.

35 Willett, W. C. (2012). Dietary fats and coronary heart disease. *Journal of Internal Medicine, 272*(1), 13-24. doi:10.1111/j.1365-2796.2012.02553.x

36 De Lorgeril, M., & Salen, P. (2012). New insights into the health effects of dietary saturated and omega-6 and omega-3 polyunsaturated fatty acids. *BMC Medicine, 10,* 50.

37 Patterson, E., Wall, R., Fitzgerald, G. F., Ross, R. P., & Stanton, C. (2012). Health implications of high dietary omega-6 polyunsaturated fatty acids. *Journal of Nutrition and Metabolism, 2012,* 539426. doi:10.1155/2012/539426

38 Patterson, E., Wall, R., Fitzgerald, G. F., Ross, R. P., & Stanton, C. (2012). Health implications of high dietary omega-6 polyunsaturated fatty acids. *Journal of Nutrition and Metabolism, 2012*, 539426. doi:10.1155/2012/539426

39 Kromhout, D., Yasuda, S., Geleijnse, J. M., & Shimokawa, H. (2012). Fish oil and omega-3 fatty acids in cardiovascular disease: Do they really work? *European Heart Journal, 33*(4), 436-43.

40 Burillo, E., Martin-Fuentes, P., Mateo-Gallego, R., Baila-Rueda, L., Cenarro, A., Ros, E., & Civeira, F. (2012). Omega-3 fatty acids and HDL: How do they work in the prevention of cardiovascular disease? *Current Vascular Pharmacology, 10*(4), 432-41.

41 Kromhout, D., Geleijnse, J. M., de Goede, J., Oude Griep, L. M., Mulder, B. J. M., de Boer, M.-J., . . . Giltay, E. J. (2011). N-3 fatty acids, ventricular arrhythmia-related events, and fatal myocardial infarction in postmyocardial infarction patients with diabetes. *Diabetes Care, 34*(12), 2515-20.

42 Massaro, M., Scoditti, E., Carluccio, M. A., Campana, M. C., & De Caterina, R. (2010). Omega-3 fatty acids, inflammation and angiogenesis: Basic mechanisms behind the cardioprotective effects of fish and fish oils. *Cellular and Molecular Biology, 56*(1), 59-82.

43 Mozaffarian, D. (2008). Fish and n-3 fatty acids for the prevention of fatal coronary heart disease and sudden cardiac death. *American Journal of Clinical Nutrition, 87*(6), 1991S-1996S.

44 Kromhout, D., Yasuda, S., Geleijnse, J. M., & Shimokawa, H. (2012). Fish oil and omega-3 fatty acids in cardiovascular disease: Do they really work? *European Heart Journal, 33*(4), 436-43.

45 Kromhout, D. (2012). Omega-3 fatty acids and coronary heart disease: The final verdict? *Current Opinion in Lipidology, 23*(6), 554-59.

46 Kromhout, D., Geleijnse, J. M., de Goede, J., Oude Griep, L. M., Mulder, B. J. M., de Boer, M.-J., . . . Giltay, E. J. (2011). n-3 fatty acids, ventricular arrhythmia-related events, and fatal myocardial infarction in postmyocardial infarction patients with diabetes. *Diabetes Care, 34*(12), 2515-20.

47 Kromhout, D., Giltay, E. J., & Geleijnse, J. M. (2010). n-3 fatty acids and cardiovascular events after myocardial infarction. *New England Journal of Medicine, 363*(21), 2015-26.

48 Kromhout, D., Yasuda, S., Geleijnse, J. M., & Shimokawa, H. (2012). Fish oil and omega-3 fatty acids in cardiovascular disease: Do they really work? *European Heart Journal, 33*(4), 436-43.

49 Harris, W. S., Mozaffarian, D., Rimm, E., Kris-Etherton, P., Rudell, L. L., Appel, L. J., . . . Sacks, F. (2009). Omega-6 fatty acids and risk for cardiovascular disease: A science advisory from the American Heart Association Nutrition Subcommittee of the Council on Nutrition, Physical Activity, and Metabolism; Council on Cardiovascular Nursing; and Council on Epidemiology and Prevention. *Circulation, 119*(6), 902-7. doi:10.1161/CIRCULATIONAHA.108.191627

50 Ramsden, C. E., Hibbeln, J. R., Majchrzak, S. F., & Davis, J. M. (2010). n-6 fatty acid-specific and mixed polyunsaturate dietary interventions have different effects on CHD risk: A meta-analysis of randomised controlled trials. *British Journal of Nutrition, 104*(11), 1586-1600. doi:10.1017/S0007114510004010

51 Khandelwal, S., Kelly, L., Malik, R., Prabhakaran, D., & Reddy S. (2013). Impact of omega-6 fatty acids on cardiovascular outcomes: A review. *Journal of Preventive Cardiology, 2*(3), 325-36.

52 Ramesh, H. P., & Tharanathan, R. N. (2003). Carbohydrates: The renewable raw materials of high biotechnological value. *Critical Reviews in Biotechnology, 23*(2), 149-73.

53 Tharanathan, R. N. (2002). Food-derived carbohydrates: Structural complexity and functional diversity. *Critical Reviews in Biotechnology, 22*(1), 65-84.

54 Brand-Miller, J., McMillan-Price, J., Steinbeck, K., & Caterson, I. (2009). Dietary glycemic index: Health implications. *Journal of the American College of Nutrition, 28*(4 Suppl. 1), 446S-449S.

55 Venn, B. J., & Green, T. J. (2007). Glycemic index and glycemic load: Measurement issues and their effect on diet-disease relationships. *European Journal of Clinical Nutrition, 61*(Suppl. 1), S122-31.

56 McKeown, N. M., Meigs, J. B., Liu, S., Rogers, G., Yoshida, M., Saltzman, E., & Jacques, P. F. (2009). Dietary carbohydrates and cardiovascular disease risk factors in the Framingham offspring cohort. *Journal of the American College of Nutrition, 28*(2), 150-58.

57 McKeown, N. M., Meigs, J. B., Liu, S., Rogers, G., Yoshida, M., Saltzman, E., & Jacques, P. F. (2009). Dietary carbohydrates and cardiovascular disease risk factors in the Framingham offspring cohort. *Journal of the American College of Nutrition, 28*(2), 150-58.

58 Brand-Miller, J., McMillan-Price, J., Steinbeck, K., & Caterson, I. (2009). Dietary glycemic index: Health implications. *Journal of the American College of Nutrition, 28*(4 Suppl. 1), 446S-449S.

59 Kromhout, D. (2012). Omega-3 fatty acids and coronary heart disease: The final verdict? *Current Opinion in Lipidology, 23*(6), 554-59.

60 Kromhout, D., Geleijnse, J. M., de Goede, J., Oude Griep, L. M., Mulder, B. J. M., de Boer, M.-J., . . . Giltay, E. J. (2011). n-3 fatty acids, ventricular arrhythmia-related events, and fatal myocardial infarction in postmyocardial infarction patients with diabetes. *Diabetes Care, 34*(12), 2515-20.

61 Hu, F. B., Stampfer, M. J., Manson, J. E., Rimm, E., Colditz, G. A., Rosner, B. A., . . . Willett, W. C. (1997). Dietary fat intake and the risk of coronary heart disease in women. *New England Journal of Medicine, 337*(21), 1491-99.

62 Hu, F. B., Stampfer, M. J., Manson, J. E., Rimm, E. Colditz, G. A., Speizer, F. E., . . . Willett, W. C. (1999). Dietary protein and risk of ischemic heart disease in women. *American Journal of Clinical Nutrition, 70*(2), 221-27.

63 Bernstein, A. M., Sun, Q., Hu, F. B., Stampfer, M. J., Manson, J. E., & Willett, W. C. (2010). Major dietary protein sources and risk of coronary heart disease in women. *Circulation, 122*(9), 876-83.

64 Oh, K., Hu, F. B., Manson, J. E., Stampfer, M. J., & Willett, W. C. (2005). Dietary fat intake and risk of coronary heart disease in women: 20 years of follow-up of the Nurses' Health Study. *American Journal of Epidemiology, 161*(7), 672-79.

65 Micha, R., Wallace, S. K., & Mozaffarian, D. (2010). Red and processed meat consumption and risk of incident coronary heart disease, stroke, and diabetes mellitus: A systematic review and meta-analysis. *Circulation, 121*(21), 2271-83.

66 Micha, R., Michas, G., & Mozaffarian, D. (2012). Unprocessed red and processed meats and risk of coronary artery disease and type 2 diabetes: An updated review of the evidence. *Current Atherosclerosis Reports, 14*(6), 515-24.

67 Lagiou, P., Sandin, S., Lof, M., Trichopoulos, D., Adami, H. O., & Weiderpass, E. (2012). Low carbohydrate-high protein diet and incidence of cardiovascular diseases in Swedish women: Prospective cohort study. *BMJ, 344*, e4026. doi:10.1136/bmj.e4026

68 Lagiou, P., Sandin, S., Lof, M., Trichopoulos, D., Adami, H. O., & Weiderpass, E. (2012). Low carbohydrate-high protein diet and incidence of cardiovascular diseases in Swedish women: Prospective cohort study. *BMJ, 344*, e4026. doi:10.1136/bmj.e4026

69 Swain, J. F., McCarron, P. B., Hamilton, E. F., Sacks, F. M., & Appel, L. J. (2008). Characteristics of the diet patterns tested in the optimal macronutrient intake trial to prevent heart disease (OmniHeart): Options for a heart-healthy diet. *Journal of the American Dietetic Association, 108*(2), 257-65.

70 Carey, V. J., Bishop, L., Charleston, J., Conlin, P., Erlinger, T., Laranjo, N., . . . Appel, L. J. (2005). Rationale and design of the Optimal Macro-Nutrient Intake Heart Trial to Prevent Heart Disease (OMNI-Heart). *Clinical Trials, 2*(6), 529-37.

71 De Waart, F. G., Schouten, E. G., Stalenhoef, A. F., & Kok, F. J. (2001). Serum carotenoids, alpha-tocopherol and mortality risk in a prospective study among Dutch elderly. *International Journal of Epidemiology, 30*(1), 136-43.

72 Samuel, S., & Sitrin, M. D. (2008). Vitamin D's role in cell proliferation and differentiation. *Nutrition Reviews, 66*(10 Suppl. 2), S116-24.

73 Gouni-Berthold, I., Krone, W., & Berthold, H. K. (2009). Vitamin D and cardiovascular disease. *Current Vascular Pharmacology, 7*(3), 414-22.

74 Peluzio Mdo, C., Teixeira, T. F., Oliveira, V. P., Sabarense, C. M., Dias, C. M., Abranches, M. V., & Maldonado, I. R. (2011). Grape extract and α-tocopherol effect in cardiovascular disease model of Apo E -/- mice. *Acta Cirurgica Brasiliera / Sociedade Brasileira para Desenvolvimento Pesquisa em Cirurgia, 26*(4), 253-60.

75 Lee, I. M., Cook, N. R., Gaziano, J. M., Gordon, D., Ridker, P. M., Manson, J. E., . . . Juring, J. E. (2005). Vitamin E in the primary prevention of cardiovascular disease and cancer: The Women's Health Study: A randomized controlled trial. *JAMA, 294*(1), 56-65.

76 Schurgers, L. J., Dissel, P. E., Spronk, H. M., Soute, B. A., Dhore, C. R., Cleutjens, J. P., & Vermeer, C. (2001). Role of vitamin K and vitamin K-dependent proteins in vascular calcification. *Zeitschrift für Kardiologie, 90* (Suppl. 3), 57-63.

77 Geleijnse, J. M., Vermeer, C., Grobbee, D. E., Schurgers, L. J., Knapen, M. H., van der Meer, I. M., . . . Witteman, J. C. (2004). Dietary intake of menaquinone is associated with a reduced risk of coronary heart disease: The Rotterdam Study. *Journal of Nutrition, 134*(11), 3100-3105.

78 Gast, G. C. M., de Roos, N. M., Sluijs, I., Bots, M. L., Beulens, J. W. J., Geleijnse, J. M., . . . van der Schouw, Y. T. (2009). A high menaquinone intake reduces the incidence of coronary heart disease. *Nutrition, Metabolism, and Cardiovascular Diseases, 19*(7), 504-10.

79 Rimm, E. B., Willett, W. C., Hu, F. B., Sampson, L., Colditz, G. A. Manson, J. E., . . . Stampfer, M. J. (1998). Folate and vitamin B6 from diet and supplements in relation to risk of coronary heart disease among women. *JAMA, 279*(5), 359-64.

80 Koutoubi, S., & Huffman, F. G. (2004). Serum total homocysteine levels, folate, and B-vitamins intake and coronary heart disease risk factors among tri-ethnic college students. *Ethnicity & Disease, 14*(1), 64-72.

81 Abraham, J. M., & Cho, L. (2010). The homocysteine hypothesis: Still relevant to the prevention and treatment of cardiovascular disease? *Cleveland Clinic Journal of Medicine, 77*(12), 911-18.

82 Lee, M., Hong K.-S., Chang., S.-C., & Saver, J. L. (2010). Efficacy of homocysteine-lowering therapy with folic acid in stroke prevention: A meta-analysis. *Stroke. 41*(6), 1205-12. doi:10.1161/STROKEAHA.109.573410

83 Riddell, L. J., Chisholm, A., Williams, S., & Mann, J. I. (2000). Dietary strategies for lowering homocysteine concentrations. *American Journal of Clinical Nutrition, 71*(6), 1448-54.

84 VITATOPS Trial Study Group. (2002). The VITATOPS (Vitamins to Prevent Stroke) Trial: Rationale and design of an international, large, simple, randomised trial of homocysteine-lowering multivitamin therapy in patients with recent transient ischaemic attack or stroke. *Cerebrovascular Diseases, 13*(2), 120-26. doi:10.1159/000047761

85 VITATOPS Trial Study Group. (2010). B vitamins in patients with recent transient ischaemic attack or stroke in the VITAmins TO Prevent Stroke (VITATOPS) trial: A randomised, double-blind, parallel, placebo-controlled trial. *Lancet Neurology, 9*(9), 855-65.

86 Cavalieri, M., Schmidt, R., Chen, C., Mok, V., de Freitas, G. R., Song, S., . . . Hankey, G. J. (2012). B vitamins and magnetic resonance imaging-detected ischemic brain lesions in patients with recent transient ischemic attack or stroke: The VITAmins TO Prevent Stroke (VITATOPS) MRI-substudy. *Stroke, 43*(12), 3266-70. doi:10.1161/STROKEAHA.112.665703

87 VITATOPS Trial Study Group, Hankey, G. J., Algra, A., Chen, C., Wong, M. C., Cheung, R., . . . Song, S. (2007). VITATOPS, the VITAmins TO prevent stroke trial: Rationale and design of a randomised trial of B-vitamin therapy in patients with recent transient ischaemic attack or stroke (NCT00097669) (ISRCTN74743444). *International Journal of Stroke, 2*(2), 144-50. doi:10.1111/j.1747-4949.2007.00111.x

88 Kaplan, E. D. (2003). Association between homocyst(e)ine levels and risk of vascular events. *Drugs of Today, 39*(3), 175-92.

89 Saposnik, G. (2011). The role of vitamin B in stroke prevention: A journey from observational studies to clinical trials and critique of the VITAmins TO Prevent Stroke (VITATOPS). *Stroke, 42*(3), 838-42.

90 Toole, J. F. (2002). Vitamin intervention for stroke prevention. *Journal of the Neurological Sciences, 203-204*, 121-24.

91 Juraschek, S. P., Guallar, E., Appel, L. J., & Miller, E. R., III. (2012). Effects of vitamin C supplementation on blood pressure: A meta-analysis of randomized controlled trials. *American Journal of Clinical Nutrition, 95*(5), 1079-88.

92 Hooper, L., Kroon, P. A., Rimm, E. B., Cohn, J. S., Harvey, I., Le Cornu, K. A., . . . Cassidy, A. (2008). Flavonoids, flavonoid-rich foods, and cardiovascular risk: A meta-analysis of randomized controlled trials. *American Journal of Clinical Nutrition, 88*(1), 38-50.

93 Moore, L. L. (2011). Functional foods and cardiovascular disease risk: Building the evidence base. *Current Opinion in Endocrinology, Diabetes and Obesity, 18*(5), 332-35.

94 McCullough, M. L., Peterson, J. J., Patel, R., Jacques, P. F., Shah, R., & Dwyer, J. T. (2012). Flavonoid intake and cardiovascular disease mortality in a prospective cohort of US adults. *American Journal of Clinical Nutrition, 95*(2), 454-64.

95 Kay, C. D. (2010). The future of flavonoid research. *British Journal of Nutrition, 104* (Suppl. 3), S91-95.

96 Lim, S. S., Vos, T., Flaxman, A. D., Danaei, G., Shibuya, K., Adair-Rohani, H., . . . Memish, Z. A. (2012). A comparative risk assessment of burden of disease and injury attributable to 67 risk factors and risk factor clusters in 21 regions, 1990-2010: A systematic analysis for the Global Burden of Disease Study 2010. *Lancet, 380*(9859), 2224-60.

97 Gardener, H., Rundek, T., Wright, C. B, Elkind, M. S, & Sacco, R. L. (2012). Dietary sodium and risk of stroke in the Northern Manhattan study. *Stroke, 43*(5), 1200-1205.

98 Chateau-Degat, M. L., Ferland, A., Dery, S., & Dewailly, E. (2012). Dietary sodium intake deleteriously affects blood pressure in a normotensive population. *European Journal of Clinical Nutrition, 66*(4), 533-35.

99 O'Donnell, M. J., Yusuf, S., Mente, A., Gao, P., Mann, J. F., Teo, K., . . . Schmeider, R. E. (2011). Urinary sodium and potassium excretion and risk of cardiovascular events. *JAMA, 306*(20), 2229-38.

100 Graudal, N. A., Hubeck-Graudal, T., & Jurgens, G. (2012). Effects of low-sodium diet vs. high-sodium diet on blood pressure, renin, aldosterone, catecholamines, cholesterol, and triglyceride (Cochrane Review). *American Journal of Hypertension, 25*(1), 1-15.

101 Alderman, M. H. (2006). Evidence relating dietary sodium to cardiovascular disease. *Journal of the American College of Nutrition, 25*(3 Suppl.), 256S-261S.

102 Alderman, M. H. (2010). Reducing dietary sodium: The case for caution. *JAMA, 303*(5), 448-49.

103 Alderman, M. H. (2011). The Cochrane review of sodium and health. *American Journal of Hypertension, 24*(8), 854-56.

104 Alderman, M. H., & Cohen, H. (2011). Dietary salt and cardiovascular disease. *Lancet, 378*(9808), 1994.

105 Alderman, M. H., & Cohen, H. W. (2002). Impact of dietary sodium on cardiovascular disease morbidity and mortality. *Current Hypertension Reports, 4*(6), 453-57.

106 Alderman, M. H., & Cohen, H. W. (2012). Dietary sodium intake and cardiovascular mortality: Controversy resolved? *Current Hypertension Reports, 14*(3), 193-201.

107 McGregor, G. A. (1988). Sodium and potassium intake and high blood pressure. *ACTA Cardiologica Supplementum, 29*, 9-19.

108 MacGregor, G. A. (1987). Sodium and potassium intake and high blood pressure. *European Heart Journal, 8* (Suppl. B), 3-8.

109 Campbell, N. R., Burgess, E., Choi, B. C., Taylor, G., Wilson, E., Cléroux, J., . . . Spence, D. (1999). Lifestyle modifications to prevent and control hypertension. 1. Methods and an overview of the Canadian recommendations. Canadian Hypertension Society, Canadian Coalition for High Blood Pressure Prevention and Control, Laboratory Centre for Disease Control at Health Canada, Heart and Stroke Foundation of Canada. *Canadian Medical Association Journal/Journal De L'association Medicale Canadienne, 160*(9 Suppl.), S1-6.

110 Umesawa, M., Iso, H., Date, C., Yananoto, A., Toyoshima, H., Watanabe, Y., . . . Tamakoshi, A.; JACC Study Group. (2008). Relations between dietary sodium and potassium intakes and mortality from cardiovascular disease: The Japan Collaborative Cohort Study for Evaluation of Cancer Risks. *American Journal of Clinical Nutrition, 88*(1), 195202.

111 Larsson, S. C., Orsini, N., & Wolk, A. (2011). Dietary potassium intake and risk of stroke: A dose-response meta-analysis of prospective studies. *Stroke, 42*(10), 2746-50.

112 O'Donnell, M. J., Yusuf, S., Mente, A., Gao, P., Mann, J. F., Teo, K., . . . Schmeider, R. E. (2011). Urinary sodium and potassium excretion and risk of cardiovascular events. *JAMA, 306*(20), 2229-38.

113 Cohn, J. N., Kowey, P. R., Whelton, P. K., & Prisant, M. (2000). New guidelines for potassium replacement in clinical practice: A contemporary review by the National Council On Potassium In Clinical Practice. *Archives of Internal Medicine, 160*(16), 2429-36.

114 Drueke, T. B. (2004). Modulation and action of the calcium-sensing receptor. *Nephrology, Dialysis, Transplantation, 19*(Suppl. 5), V20-26.

115 Torres, M. R., & Sanjuliani, A. F. (2012). Does calcium intake affect cardiovascular risk factors and/or events? *Clinics, 67*(7), 839-44.

116 Li, K., Kaaks, R., Linseisen, J., & Rohrmann S. (2012). Associations of dietary calcium intake and calcium supplementation with myocardial infarction and stroke risk and overall cardiovascular mortality in the Heidelberg cohort of the European Prospective Investigation into Cancer and Nutrition study (EPIC-Heidelberg). *Heart, 98*(12), 920-25.

117 Torres, M. R., & Sanjuliani, A. F. (2012). Does calcium intake affect cardiovascular risk factors and/or events? *Clinics, 67*(7), 839-44.

118 Bolland, M. J., Grey, A., Avenell, A., Gamble, G. D., & Reid, I. R. (2011). Calcium supplements with or without vitamin D and risk of cardiovascular events: Reanalysis of the Women's Health Initiative limited access dataset and meta-analysis. *BMJ, 342*, d2040.

119 Xiao, Q., Murphy, R. A., Houston, D. K., Harris, T. B., Chow, W. H., & Park, Y. (2013). Dietary and supplemental calcium intake and cardiovascular disease mortality: The National Institutes of Health-AARP Diet and Health Study. *JAMA Internal Medicine, 173*(8), 639-46. doi:10.1001/jamainternmed.2013.3283

120 World Health Organization (1968). *Nutritional anaemias: Report of a WHO scientific group.* World Health Organization Technical Report Series, no. 405. Geneva: World Health Organization.

121 Parikh, A., Natarajan, S., Lipsitz, S. R., & Katz, S.D. (2011). Iron deficiency in community-dwelling US adults with self-reported heart failure in the National Health and Nutrition Examination Survey III: Prevalence and associations with anemia and inflammation. *Circulation. Heart Failure, 4*(5), 599-606.

122 Van der A, D. L., Peeters, P. H. M., Grobbee, D. E., Marx, J. J. M., & van der Schouw, Y. T. (2005). Dietary haem iron and coronary heart disease in women. *European Heart Journal, 26*(3), 257-62.

123 Klipstein-Grobusch, K., Koster, J. F., & Grobbee, D. E. (1999). Serum ferritin and risk of myocardial infarction in the elderly: The Rotterdam Study. *American Journal of Clinical Nutrition, 69*(6), 1231-36.

124 Lee, D. H., Folsom, A. R., & Jacobs, D. R., Jr. (2005). Iron, zinc, and alcohol consumption and mortality from cardiovascular diseases: The Iowa Women's Health Study. *American Journal of Clinical Nutrition, 81*(4), 787-91.

125 De Oliveira Otto, M. C., Alonso, A., Lee, D. H., Delclos, G. L., Jenny, N. S., Jiang, R., . . . Nettleton, J. A. (2011). Dietary micronutrient intakes are associated with markers of inflammation but not with markers of subclinical atherosclerosis. *Journal of Nutrition, 141*(8), 1508-15. doi:10.3945/jn.111.138115

126 Zhang, W., Iso, H., Ohira, T., Date, C., Tanabe, N., Kikuchi, S., . . . JACC Study Group. (2012). Associations of dietary iron intake with mortality from cardiovascular disease: The JACC study. *Journal of Epidemiology (Japan), 22*(6), 484-493. doi:10.2188/jea.JE20120006

127 Moore, M., Folsom, A. R., Barnes, R. W., & Eckfeldt, J. (1995). No association between serum ferritin and asymptomatic carotid atherosclerosis: The Atherosclerosis Risk in Communities (ARIC) Study. *American Journal of Epidemiology, 141*(8), 719-23.

128 Moore, M., Folsom, A. R., Barnes, R. W., & Eckfeldt, J. (1995). No association between serum ferritin and asymptomatic carotid atherosclerosis: The Atherosclerosis Risk in Communities (ARIC) Study. *American Journal of Epidemiology, 141*(8), 719-23.

129 Vaskonen, T. (2003). Dietary minerals and modification of cardiovascular risk factors. *Journal of Nutritional Biochemistry, 14*(9), 492-506.

130 Naito, Y., Hirotani, S., Sawada, H., Akahori, H., Tsujino, T., & Masuyama, T. (2011). Dietary iron restriction prevents hypertensive cardiovascular remodeling in Dahl salt-sensitive rats. *Hypertension, 57*(3), 497-504.

131 Hu, F. B. (2002). Dietary pattern analysis: A new direction in nutritional epidemiology. *Current Opinion in Lipidology, 13*(1), 3-9.

132 Zarraga, I. G., & Schwarz, E. R. (2006). Impact of dietary patterns and interventions on cardiovascular health. *Circulation, 114*(9), 961-73.

133 Parikh, P., McDaniel, M. C., Ashen, M. D., Miller, J. I., Sorrentino, M., Chan, V., . . . Sperling, L. S. (2005). Diets and cardiovascular disease: An evidence-based assessment. *Journal of the American College of Cardiology, 45*(9), 1379-87.

134 Hu, F. B. (2003). The Mediterranean diet and mortality: Olive oil and beyond. *New England Journal of Medicine, 348*(26), 2595-96.

135 Ogce, F., Ceber, E., Ekti, R., & Oran, N. T. (2008). Comparison of Mediterranean, Western and Japanese diets and some recommendations. *Asian Pacific Journal of Cancer Prevention, 9*(2), 351-56.

136 Keys, A., Menotti, A., Karvonen, M. J., Aravanis, C., Blackburn, H., Buzina, R., . . . Toshima, H. (1986). The diet and 15-year death rate in the seven countries study. *American Journal of Epidemiology, 124*(6), 903-15.

137 Trichopoulou, A., & Vasilopoulou, E. (2000). Mediterranean diet and longevity. *British Journal of Nutrition, 84* (Suppl. 2), S205-9.

138 Nordmann, A. J., Suter-Zimmermann, K., Bucher, H. C., Shai, I., Tuttle, K. R., Estruch, R., . . . Briel, M. (2011). Meta-analysis comparing Mediterranean to low-fat diets for modification of cardiovascular risk factors. *American Journal of Medicine, 124*(9), 841-51.e2. doi:10.1016/j.amjmed.2011.04.024

139 Hoevenaar-Blom, M. P., Nooyens, A. C., Kromhout, D., Spijkerman, A. M. W., Beulens, J. W. J., van der Schouw, Y. T., . . . Verschuren, W. M. M. (2012). Mediterranean style diet and 12-year incidence of cardiovascular diseases: The EPIC-NL cohort study. *PLoS ONE, 7*(9), e45458. doi:10.1371/journal.pone.0045458

140 De Lorgeril, M., Renaud, S., Salen, P., Monjaud, I., Mamelle, N., Martin, J. L., . . . Delaye, J. (1994). Mediterranean alphalinolenic acid-rich diet in secondary prevention of coronary heart disease. *Lancet, 343*(8911), 1454-59. doi:10.1016/S0140-6736(94)92580-1

141 De Lorgeril, M., Salen, P., Martin, J.-L., Monjaud, I., Delaye, J., & Mamelle N. (1999). Mediterranean diet, traditional risk factors, and the rate of cardiovascular complications after myocardial infarction: Final report of the Lyon Diet Heart Study. *Circulation, 99*(6), 779-85.

142 Trichopoulou, A., Bamia, C., & Trichopoulos, D. (2005). Mediterranean diet and survival among patients with coronary heart disease in Greece. *Archives of Internal Medicine, 165*(8), 929-35. doi:10.1001/archinte.165.8.929

143 Hoevenaar-Blom, M. P., Nooyens, A. C., Kromhout, D., Spijkerman, A. M. W., Beulens, J. W. J., van der Schouw, Y. T., . . . Verschuren, W. M. M. (2012). Mediterranean style diet and 12-year incidence of cardiovascular diseases: The EPIC-NL cohort study. *PLoS ONE, 7*(9), e45458. doi:10.1371/journal.pone.0045458

144 Sofi, F., Abbate, R., Gensini, G. F., & Casini A. (2010). Accruing evidence on benefits of adherence to the Mediterranean diet on health: An updated systematic review and meta-analysis. *American Journal of Clinical Nutrition, 92*(5), 1189-96.

145 Parikh, P., McDaniel, M. C., Ashen, M. D., Miller, J. I., Sorrentino, M., Chan, V., . . . Sperling, L. S. (2005). Diets and cardiovascular disease: An evidence-based assessment. *Journal of the American College of Cardiology, 45*(9), 1379-87.

146 Appel, L. J., Moore, T. J., Obarzanek, E., Vollmer, W. M., Svetkey, L. P., Sacks, F. M., . . . Karanja, N. (1997). A clinical trial of

the effects of dietary patterns on blood pressure: DASH Collaborative Research Group. *New England Journal of Medicine, 336*(16), 1117-24.

147 Sacks, F. M., Svetkey, L. P., Vollmer, W. M., Appel, L. J., Bray, G. A., Harsha, D., . . . DASH-Sodium Collaborative Research Group. (2001). Effects on blood pressure of reduced dietary sodium and the Dietary Approaches to Stop Hypertension (DASH) diet. DASH-Sodium Collaborative Research Group. *New England Journal of Medicine, 344*(1), 3-10.

148 Parikh, P., McDaniel, M. C., Ashen, M. D., Miller, J. I., Sorrentino, M., Chan, V., . . . Sperling, L. S. (2005). Diets and cardiovascular disease: An evidence-based assessment. *Journal of the American College of Cardiology, 45*(9), 1379-87.

149 Appel, L. J., Moore, T. J., Obarzanek, E., Vollmer, W. M., Svetkey, L. P., Sacks, F. M., . . . Karanja, N. (1997). A clinical trial of the effects of dietary patterns on blood pressure: DASH Collaborative Research Group. *New England Journal of Medicine, 336*(16), 1117-24.

150 Willett, W. C. (1999). Convergence of philosophy and science: The third international congress on vegetarian nutrition. *American Journal of Clinical Nutrition, 70*(3 Suppl.), 434S-438S.

151 Gillman, M. W., Cupples, L. A., Gagnon, D., Posner, B. M., Ellison, R. C., Castelli, W. P., & Wolf, P. A. (1995). Protective effect of fruits and vegetables on development of stroke in men. *JAMA, 273*(14), 1113-17.

152 Rimm, E. B., Ascherio, A., Giovannucci, E., Spiegelman, D., Stampfer, M. J., & Willett, W. C. (1996). Vegetable, fruit, and cereal fiber intake and risk of coronary heart disease among men. *JAMA, 275*(6), 447-51.

153 Pais, P., Pogue, J., Gerstein, H., Zachariah, E., Savitha, D., Jayprakash, S., . . . Yusuf, F. (1996). Risk factors for acute myocardial infarction in Indians: A case-control study. *Lancet, 348*(9024), 358-63.

154 Crowe, F. L., Appleby, P. N., Travis, R. C., & Key, T. J. (2013). Risk of hospitalization or death from ischemic heart disease among British vegetarians and nonvegetarians: Results from the EPIC-Oxford cohort study. *American Journal of Clinical Nutrition, 97*(3), 597-603. doi:10.3945/ajcn.112.044073

155 Willett, W. C. (1999). Convergence of philosophy and science: The third international congress on vegetarian nutrition. *American Journal of Clinical Nutrition, 70*(3 Suppl.), 434S-438S.

156 Libov, C. (2012, October 1). To cook or not to cook your vegetables? *HuffingtonPost.com.* Retrieved from http://www.huffingtonpost.com/2012/09/27/cook-vegetables-health_n_1919785.html?utm_hp_ref=tw

157 Garcia, A. L., Koebnick, C., Dagnelie, P. C., Strassner, C., Elmadfa, I., Katz, N., . . . Hoffmann, I. (2008). Long-term strict raw food diet is associated with favourable plasma beta-carotene and low plasma lycopene concentrations in Germans. *British Journal of Nutrition, 99*(6), 1293-1300.

158 Dewanto, V., Wu, X., Adom, K. K., & Liu, R. H. (2002). Thermal processing enhances the nutritional value of tomatoes by increasing total antioxidant activity. *Journal of Agricultural and Food Chemistry, 50*(10), 3010-14.

159 Miglio, C., Chiavaro, E., Visconti, A., Fogliano, V., & Pellegrini, N. (2008). Effects of different cooking methods on nutritional and physicochemical characteristics of selected vegetables. *Journal of Agricultural and Food Chemistry, 56*(1), 139-47.

160 Talcott, S. T., Howard, L. R., & Brenes, C. H. (2000). Antioxidant changes and sensory properties of carrot puree processed with and without periderm tissue. *Journal of Agricultural and Food Chemistry, 48*(4), 1315-21.

161 Hu, F. B., Rimm, E. B., Stampfer, M. J., Ascherio, A., Spiegelman, D., & Willett, W. C. (2000). Prospective study of major dietary patterns and risk of coronary heart disease in men. *American Journal of Clinical Nutrition, 72*(4), 912-21.

162 Srinath Reddy, K., & Katan, M. B. (2004). Diet, nutrition and the prevention of hypertension and cardiovascular diseases. *Public Health Nutrition, 7*(1a), 167-86. doi:http://dx.doi.org/10.1079/PHN2003587

163 Shimamoto, T., Komachi, Y., Inada, H., Doi, M., Iso, H., Sato, S., . . . Nakanishi, N. (1989). Trends for coronary heart disease and stroke and their risk factors in Japan. *Circulation, 79*(3), 503-15.

164 Truswell, A. S. (1994). Review of dietary intervention studies: Effect on coronary events and on total mortality. *Australian and New Zealand Journal of Medicine, 24*(1), 98-106.

165 Srinath Reddy, K., & Katan, M. B. (2004). Diet, nutrition and the prevention of hypertension and cardiovascular diseases. *Public Health Nutrition, 7*(1a), 167-86.

166 Franco, O. H., Bonneux, L., de Laet, C., Peeters, A., Steyerberg, E. W., & Mackenbach, J. P. (2004). The Polymeal: A more natural, safer, and probably tastier (than the Polypill) strategy to reduce cardiovascular disease by more than 75%. *BMJ, 329*(7480), 1447-50.

167 Franco, O. H., Bonneux, L., de Laet, C., Peeters, A., Steyerberg, E. W., & Mackenbach, J. P. (2004). The Polymeal: A more natural, safer, and probably tastier (than the Polypill) strategy to reduce cardiovascular disease by more than 75%. *BMJ, 329*(7480), 1447-50.

168 Srinath Reddy, K., & Katan, M. B. (2004). Diet, nutrition and the prevention of hypertension and cardiovascular diseases. *Public Health Nutrition, 7*(1a), 167-86. doi: http://dx.doi.org/10.1079/PHN2003587

169 Aarsetoey, H., Grundt, H., Nygaard, O., & Nilsen, D. W. (2012). The role of long-chained marine N-3 polyunsaturated fatty acids in cardiovascular disease. *Cardiology Research and Practice, 2012*, 303456. doi:10.1155/2012/303456

170 Srinath Reddy, K., & Katan, M. B. (2004). Diet, nutrition and the prevention of hypertension and cardiovascular diseases. *Public Health Nutrition, 7*(1a), 167-86. doi:http://dx.doi.org/10.1079/PHN2003587

171 Srinath Reddy, K., & Katan, M. B. (2004). Diet, nutrition and the prevention of hypertension and cardiovascular diseases. *Public Health Nutrition, 7*(1a), 167-86. doi: http://dx.doi.org/10.1079/PHN2003587

172 American Heart Association. (2011, January 24). *Whole grains and fiber*. Retrieved from http://www.heart.org/HEARTORG /GettingHealthy/NutritionCenter/HealthyDietGoals/Whole -Grains-and-Fiber_UCM_303249_Article.jsp

173 American Heart Association. (n.d.). *Healthy diet goals*. Retrieved from http://www.heart.org/HEARTORG/GettingHealthy/Nutri tionCenter/HealthyDietGoals/Healthy-Diet-Goals_UCM _310436_SubHomePage.jsp

174 Rose, G. (1985). Sick individuals and sick populations. *International Journal of Epidemiology, 14*, 32–38.

175 Zatonski, W. A., McMichael, A. J., & Powles, J. W. (1998). Ecological study of reasons for sharp decline in mortality from ischaemic heart disease in Poland since 1991. *BMJ, 316*(7137), 1047–51.

176 Uusitalo, U., Feskens, E.J., Tuomilehto, J., Dowse, G., Haw, U., Fareed, D., . . . Zimmet, P. (1996). Fall in total cholesterol con- centration over five years in association with changes in fatty acid composition of cooking oil in Mauritius: Cross sectional survey. *BMJ, 313*(7064), 1044–46.

177 Puska, P. (2000). Nutrition and mortality: The Finnish experi- ence. *Acta Cardiologica, 55*(4), 213–20.

178 Hoevenaar-Blom, M. P., Nooyens, A. C., Kromhout, D., Spijkerman, A. M. W., Beulens, J. W. J., van der Schouw, Y. T., . . . Verschuren, W. M. M. (2012). Mediterranean style diet and 12-year incidence of cardiovascular diseases: The EPIC-NL cohort study. *PLoS ONE, 7*(9), e45458. doi:10.1371/journal .pone.0045458

179 Stafford, N. (2012). Denmark cancels "fat tax" and shelves "sugar tax" because of threat of job losses. *BMJ, 345*, e7889. doi:http://dx.doi.org/10.1136/bmj.e7889

180 MacGregor, G., Consensus Action on Salt and Health (CASH). (2008, July 2002). *CASH welcomes the news that salt intake continues to fall: 6000 lives have been saved so far*. Retrieved from http://www.actiononsalt.org.uk/news/Salt%20in%20 the%20news/2008/58266.html

181 Brownell, K. D., Farley, T., Willett, W. C, Popkin, B. M., Chaloupka, F. J., Thompson, J. W., & Ludwig, D. S. (2009). The public health and economic benefits of taxing sugar-sweetened beverages. *New England Journal of Medicine, 361*(16), 1599–1605.

182 Brownell, K. D., Farley, T., Willett, W. C, Popkin, B. M., Chaloupka, F. J., Thompson, J. W., & Ludwig, D. S. (2009). The public health and economic benefits of taxing sugar-sweetened beverages. *New England Journal of Medicine, 361*(16), 1599–1605.

183 Brownell, K. D., & Frieden, T. R. (2009). Ounces of prevention: The public policy case for taxes on sugared beverages. *New England Journal of Medicine, 360*(18), 1805–08.

184 Grynbaum, M. M. (2012, September 13). Health panel approves restriction on sale of large sugary drinks. *New York Times*. Retrieved from http://www.nytimes.com/2012/09/14/nyregion /health-board-approves-bloombergs-soda-ban.html?_r=1&

185 Brownell, K. D., & Koplan, J. P. (2011). Front-of-package nutrition labeling: An abuse of trust by the food industry? *New England Journal of Medicine, 364*(25), 2373–75.

186 Craig, P., Cooper, C., Gunnell, D., Haw, S., Lawson, K., Macintyre, S., . . . Thompson S. (2012). Using natural experiments to evalu- ate population health interventions: New Medical Research Council guidance. *Journal of Epidemiology and Public Health, 66*(12), 1182–86.

187 Gregg, E. W., Ali, M. K., Moore, B. A., Pavkov, M., Devlin, H. M., & Garfield, S. (2013). The importance of natural experiments in diabetes prevention and control and the need for better health policy research. *Preventing Chronic Disease, 10*, E14.

188 Mozaffarian, D., Appel, L. J., & Van Horn, L. (2011). Components of a cardioprotective diet: New insights. *Circulation, 123*(24), 2870–91.

189 Mozaffarian, D., Appel, L. J., & Van Horn, L. (2011). Components of a cardioprotective diet: New insights. *Circulation, 123*(24), 2870–91.

190 Bovet, P., & Paccaud, F. (2012). Cardiovascular disease and the changing face of global public health: A focus on low and mid- dle income countries. *Public Health Reviews, 33*(2), 397–415.

Chapter 20

Cardiovascular Disease: The Public Health Nutrition Impact of Hypertension in the African American Community in the Southern United States

Ralphenia D. Pace, PhD, RD, LD
Melissa Johnson, PhD, MS

"The differential nature of dietary practices is conditioned at times by the poverty and marginalization of the populace, resulting in either disadvantageous or beneficial outcomes relative to others' eating habits."–N. W. Solomons

Reproduced from Solomons, N. W. (2003). Diet and long-term health: An African Diaspora perspective. *Asia Pacific Journal of Clinical Nutrition*, *12*, 313–30.

Learning Objectives

- Put scientific principles in public health nutrition into practice to safeguard public health.
- Recognize the public health impact of diet-related chronic diseases.
- Describe disparities in hypertension risk and prevalence, with a particular emphasis on African Americans.
- Identify nutritional and public health tools and strategies for health promotion and disease prevention.
- Discuss mechanisms for mitigating hypertension risk and disparities among African Americans and other at-risk individuals.
- Examine scientific evidence regarding the success of prevention and intervention programs in reducing disease risk.
- Understand the potential for local, regional, and national programs to reduce cardiovascular disease risk.

Case Study 1: Cardiovascular Disease: Getting to the Heart of the Matter

Following an evaluation of its students' health status, the local rural school district hired Felicia, a registered dietitian and community nutritionist. Her job description is to develop a nutrition education core curriculum to improve the nutritional and health status of the children. Nearly half of the children aged 5 to 18 are overweight, and a vast majority of these are considered obese according to the Centers for Disease Control and Prevention (CDC) Growth Charts. Furthermore, 5% of the students have **hypertension**, and many are considered prehypertensive. Survey data indicate that more than 80% of the children have a family history of hypertension and **diabetes**. The median income of residents of this rural community, located in the southeastern region of the United States, is below the poverty line. Many of the students participate in the national **School Breakfast Program (SBP)** and the **National School Lunch Program (NSLP)**, and are members of households eligible for additional supplemental feeding programs.

Until now, the curriculum lacked nutrition education. Funding for the physical education program has been drastically reduced, with students participating in traditional physical education classes twice per week. Although healthier meal options are offered at lunch, many students select more popular "fast-food" options such as pizza, French fries, hamburgers, and hot dogs; fewer than half of the students select milk. Vending machines with candy, potato chips, cookies, and soda are readily accessible in the schools. The surrounding neighborhoods are characterized as poor; they have limited sidewalks and are deemed "insufficient to promote physical activity." There are various mom-and-pop stores, liquor stores, three major fast-food franchises, and only one major nearby supermarket with a limited selection of fresh fruits and vegetables. The area also has 10 churches, of which most students and their parents are active members. Parents often work at the local plant for 12-hour shifts and provide fast-food or processed meals, such as frozen dinners and sandwiches containing processed meats, to their children at least four days per week. Although many parents recognize the need to improve their children's eating and physical activity patterns, many express frustration with the school and home environments.

Discussion Questions

- What nutrition intervention program might be effective for the school district?
- What components might Felicia consider including as she designs a nutrition intervention for the school district?
- How can students and parents be included to maximize impact? How might parents be notified about their children's health status, and what guidance should they receive to help them support better nutrition for their children?
- How can the program be delivered in a culturally sensitive manner?

Case Study 2: Cardiovascular Disease and the Metabolic Syndrome

Laura, an African American, is a 45-year-old mother of three who was diagnosed with hypertension five years ago. Her blood pressure normally reads 140/90 millimeters of mercury (mm Hg). She visits her physician to discuss ways to lower her blood pressure without increasing the dose of her daily prescription medication (Diovan, 165 milligrams). Laura is five feet, four inches tall; weighs 180 pounds; and has a waist circumference of 40 inches, serum **triglycerides** of 250 milligrams per deciliter (mg/dL), normal glucose levels, and LDL cholesterol of 140 mg/dL. The physician indicates to Laura that she has three of the four symptoms of **metabolic syndrome**. He explains that metabolic syndrome is a cluster of metabolic abnormalities that increases the risk for type 2 diabetes and cardiovascular disease. Features include hyperglycemia, or fasting plasma glucose greater than 100 mg/dL, abdominal obesity, or a waist circumference for women more than 35 inches, hypertriacylglycerides greater than 150 mg/dL, low HDL cholesterol less than 50 mg/dL for women, and blood pressure greater than 130/80 mm Hg. Metabolic syndrome is diagnosed when three or more of the abnormalities are present. Its precise cause is unknown, but age and ethnic background can affect risk.

Laura's doctor tells her that certain lifestyle changes could improve her blood pressure, cholesterol, waist circumference, and weight. He recommends staying in touch with her local extension agent, a nutritionist, to discuss specific dietary changes, and joining the local gym so that she can exercise at least three days a week for 30 minutes per day.

Discussion Questions

- Why is metabolic syndrome a significant public health concern?

- Which lifestyle changes would you recommend for Laura, and why?

- If Laura is not successful with her lifestyle changes, what possible diseases could develop?

- What is the role of the public health nutritionist in this and similar cases?

- How can public health programs affect the environment to improve Laura's lifestyle decisions?

Introduction

Individual and community characteristics both affect health status and risk for certain diseases.[1,2,3,4] **Epigenetic** changes, affected by nutritional factors and passed from one generation to another, may explain in part the increased prevalence of chronic diseases, or noncommunicable diseases (NCD), among certain populations.[5] Demographic characteristics also affect nutritional status and health risk. Examples include gender, **socioeconomic status (SES)**, food availability and accessibility, access to preventive care, nutrient bioavailability and metabolism, health status, and persistent poverty across generations (**Figure 20-1**).[6,7,8,9]

> *Public Health Core Competency 4: Cultural Competency Skills 2: Recognizes the role of cultural, social, and behavioral factors in the accessibility, availability, acceptability, and delivery of public health services*
>
> Reproduced from Council on Linkages Between Academia and Public Health Practice. 2010 May. Core Competencies for Public Health Professionals. Washington, DC: Public Health Foundation. http://www.phf.org/resourcestools/Documents/Core_Competencies_for_Public_Health_Professionals_2010May.pdf. Accessed August 13, 2013. This source is used for all Public Health Core Competencies in this chapter.

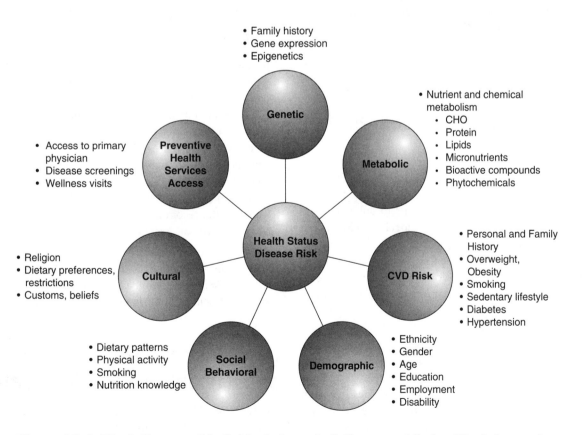

Figure 20-1 The influence of individual characteristics on public health status and disease risk

Public health programs that target these characteristics can reduce certain diseases and their risk factors. Of particular importance is the public health burden of **cardiovascular disease** (CVD), the leading cause of morbidity and mortality in the United States and globally. In particular, **hypertension**, or high blood pressure, is the most common type of CVD and a risk factor for stroke and kidney disease, as well. Hypertension is particularly prevalent among African Americans.

Healthy People 2020: HDS-5: Reduce the proportion of persons in the population with hypertension

Reproduced from the U.S. Department of Health and Human Services. Healthypeople.gov. Retrieved from http://www.healthypeople.gov/2020/default.aspx. Last updated July 30, 2013. Accessed August 13, 2013.

Public Health Core Competency 6: Basic Public Health Science Skills 1: Describes the scientific foundation of the field of public health

---

Public Health Nutrition: Principles, Practices, and Priorities

Applying the core competencies of public health, public health nutritionists help prevent diet-related diseases and mitigate nutrition-related threats to public health.[10] Strategies to improve the health of local and global communities include increasing access to safe, healthful, and nutritious foods and implementing targeted policies.[11] An extension of the basic nutritional sciences, public health nutrition includes three additional areas: (1) cultural, social, and psychological determinants of dietary behaviors; (2) fundamental principles of health education/promotion curriculums, programs, and policies; and (3) interests and contributions of stakeholders, such as institutional, government, local, national, and global health organizations.[12] This chapter examines hypertension from a public health nutrition perspective, with emphasis on nutritional relationships, disparities among African American communities, and potential community-based solutions.

Health Disparities and Public Health

Despite efforts to support the health of the general population, individuals within certain subpopulations are particularly vulnerable to adverse health outcomes. These **health disparities**, or health inequalities,[13] are often related to geography and "residential segregation."[14] Health disparities may also originate at the clinical level if doctor–patient interactions are based on preconceived perceptions and stereotypes ranging from the patient's lifestyle characteristics to symptom interpretation, particularly among minority patients.[15] In addition to reducing and eliminating health disparities, major goals of *Healthy People 2020* are to achieve health equity and improve the health of Americans in all age groups. Successful public health nutrition intervention strategies to reduce health disparities should be preventive, proactive, and dynamic, encompassing expertise from the nutritional and food sciences, biological, medical/therapeutic and biomedical sciences, and epidemiology.

Health Disparities Among African Americans

The existence of health disparities in the United States is demonstrated by evidence that African Americans have increased morbidities and mortalities related to a variety of risk factors. Poor diets may result from poverty.[16] Heart disease is one of the three major causes of death among both African American men and women, but evidence points to unique disparities among men.[17] For example, African American men have undiagnosed chronic conditions, have poorly managed chronic diseases, and eat significantly fewer than the recommended servings of fruits and vegetables than African American women.[18]

Public Health Core Competency 6: Basic Public Health Science Skills 5: Describes the scientific evidence related to a public health issue, concern, or intervention

---

Diet–Disease Relationships and Threats to Public Health

Most common NCDs and their risks result directly or indirectly from dietary imbalances (**Table 20-1**). For example, dietary factors can affect weight status, blood lipids and glucose, and blood pressure.[19] Deficiencies in **antioxidant**

Table 20-1 Relationship between diet and risk for common diet-related disease categories

		CVD	Hypertension	Diabetes	Metabolic Syndrome	Obesity	Cancer
	Excess calories	↑	↑	↑	↑	↑	↑
CHO	Monosaccharides			↑	↑	↑	
	Disaccharides						
	Polysaccharides						
	Soluble fiber	↓	↓			↓	↓
	Insoluble fiber	↓		↓			↓
Proteins	Animal protein	↑	↑	↑	↑	↑	↑
	Plant protein	↓	↓	↓	↓	↓	↓
	Amino acids						
	Arginine	↓	↓				
Fats	Trans fats, SFA	↑	↑	↑	↑	↑	↑
	Myristic, palmitic acid	↑	↑	↑	↑	↑	↑
	Cholesterol	↑					
	ω-3 fatty acids	↓	↓	↓			
	ω-6 fatty acids	↑	↑		↑	↑	↑
	ω-9 fatty acids						
	MUFAs			↓			
	PUFAs	↓	↓				
Micronutrients	Calcium						
	Folic acid	↓					
	Iron						
	Sodium	↑	↑				
	Potassium	↓	↓				
	Vitamin A						
	Vitamin D						
	Vitamin E						
	Vitamin C						
	B vitamins						
Other	Antioxidants	↓	↓	↓	↓	↓	↓
	Bioactive compounds	↓	↓	↓	↓	↓	↓
	Plant sterols	↓	↓	↓	↓	↓	↓
Dietary patterns	Green leafy vegetables	↓	↓	↓	↓	↓	
	Fruits	↓					
	Fish	↓					
	Whole grains	↓	↓	↓	↓	↓	↓
	Processed foods	↑	↑				
	Alcohol	↑					
	DASH	↓	↓	↓	↓	↓	↓
	Mediterranean	↓	↓	↓	↓	↓	↓

nutrients may decrease the body's ability to counteract oxidative stress, leading to oxidative damage, inflammation, and disease.[20]

Dietary Patterns and Health

Parental beliefs and behaviors and SES influence childhood dietary patterns, weight status, and subsequent disease risk.[21,22,23] Exploration of behavior genetics as a potential tool in explaining development of food preferences and eating habits in childhood in the presence of specific genetic and familial environment characteristics may be a useful approach.[24] Further, establishing more healthful dietary habits during childhood can help in long-term weight control and obesity prevention.[25] Public health nutritionists should identify opportunities to improve the nutrient intake, nutritional status, and physical activity levels of children to reduce the public health impacts of diet-related chronic diseases.[26]

Improved diets throughout the lifespan can reduce NCD impact.[27] The Mediterranean and more prudent dietary patterns have been associated with decreased disease risk.[28,29,30] Conversely, unhealthy habits, such as high sodium intakes and sedentary lifestyles, coupled with family history of hypertension, are risk factors for early development of hypertension.[31,32,33,34] Green, leafy, and cruciferous vegetables are particularly beneficial in promoting health and preventing disease.[35,36,37] Collard greens, purslane, and sweet potato greens are green, leafy vegetables common in the diets of African Americans, and they are sources of dietary fiber, essential fatty acids, antioxidants, and other bioactive compounds that have been demonstrated to reduce the risks associated with cancer, cardiovascular diseases, and other diseases.[38,39,40,41,42,43]

Among children, fast-food consumption is associated with higher energy intake and obesity, as well as poorer diet quality, with higher intakes of saturated fat, sodium, and soft drinks and fewer servings of cereals, milk, fruit, and dark-green and other vegetables. In addition to increased energy intake, children consuming fast food display poorer diet quality and an increased risk for obesity.[44] Similarly, associations between increased energy intake and accessibility to fast-food restaurants are seen among African Americans living in the southeastern region of the United States.[45]

Exemplifying geographic and SES disparities are children living in the Lower Mississippi Delta region of Louisiana, Arkansas, and Mississippi. Individuals living in this region and classified as food insecure have lower-quality diets and lower nutrient intake than recommended.[46] One study found lower intakes of calcium, iron, riboflavin, and vitamins A, B6, and C among these children.[47] In addition, neighborhood SES is positively associated with fruit and vegetable intake.[48]

Sodium Intake and Hypertension

The American Heart Association (AHA) recommends a daily sodium intake of less than 1,500 milligrams (mg) for the promotion of health and the prevention of disease, particularly hypertension.[49] Additionally, the United States Departments of Agriculture (USDA) and Health and Human Services (DHHS), in the *2010 Dietary Guidelines for Americans,* recommend that African Americans, individuals older than 51 years of age, and those with hypertension, chronic kidney disease, or diabetes consume less than 1,500 mg per day of sodium; all other individuals are recommended to consume no more than 2,300 mg per day of sodium.[50] Worldwide, sodium intakes exceed recommendations, increasing risk for hypertension and other CVDs.[51] Adding salt or high-sodium condiments to foods during preparation, and consuming processed foods, increases risk of elevated blood pressure, CVD, and other NCDs. The most common sources of dietary sodium worldwide are processed foods and added salt during and after food preparation.[52] Major risk factors for developing hypertension include older age, physical inactivity, smoking, dyslipidemia, and excessive intake of alcohol, energy, fat, and sodium.[53,54,55,56] High consumption of sugar-sweetened beverages may augment risk for cardiovascular, renal, and other diseases.[57,58,59,60]

Health beliefs and knowledge can influence risk behaviors related to hypertension. For example, African Americans living in rural regions were less likely to add salt at the table if they displayed knowledge regarding relationships between diet and heart disease and stroke and had personal concern for acquiring these conditions.[61] Nutrition education programs can promote dietary and lifestyle behaviors that reduce CVD risk.[62]

Public Health Core Competency 1: Analytical/Assessment Skills 2: Describes the characteristics of a population-based health problem

Assessment of Disease Risk: Emphasis on Hypertension

An estimated 60% of the American adult population is prehypertensive or hypertensive; African Americans and individuals of lower SES are particularly vulnerable.[63] The Joint National Committee on the Prevention, Detection, Evaluation, and Treatment of High Blood Pressure classifies blood pressure in four categories: normal ($\leq$ 120/80 mm Hg), prehypertensive (120–139/80–89 mm Hg), stage 1 hypertension (140–159/90–99 mm Hg), and stage 2 hypertension ($\geq$ 160/100 mm Hg).[64] In addition to genetic predisposition, dietary, lifestyle, cultural, and psychological characteristics influence hypertension risk (**Figure 20-2**).[65,66]

The prevalence of hypertension among adults worldwide is projected to increase 60% by 2025,[67] and the economic costs associated with diet-related NCDs are projected to drastically increase in developing countries with the adaptation of Westernized dietary patterns.[68] Public health professionals are critical in the surveillance, prevention, and management of hypertension to reduce its burden.[69] While many therapeutic innovations have been made in the treatment of hypertension, a large proportion of hypertensive individuals have failed to successfully control this condition.[70]

Disparities in Risk Factors for Hypertension

Although clinical and epidemiological evidence demonstrates the established relationship between dietary patterns and hypertension[71,72,73] and the importance of dietary interventions and weight management in mitigating the consequences of unmanaged hypertension,[74,75] many economically disadvantaged individuals are at an increased risk for developing hypertension. Contributing factors may include low educational attainment, limited financial resources, inadequate access to more healthful food choices, and restricted accessibility to preventive health services, as seen among rural African Americans.[76,77,78,79] Additionally, residents of neighborhoods without sidewalks and with safety concerns are less likely to engage in adequate physical activity to reduce risks associated with hypertension.[80] Low-income individuals in rural regions display exacerbated public health burden of hypertension,[81] and individuals living in rural regions of the southern United States are at higher risk for CVD and premature death due to CVD.[82,83,84]

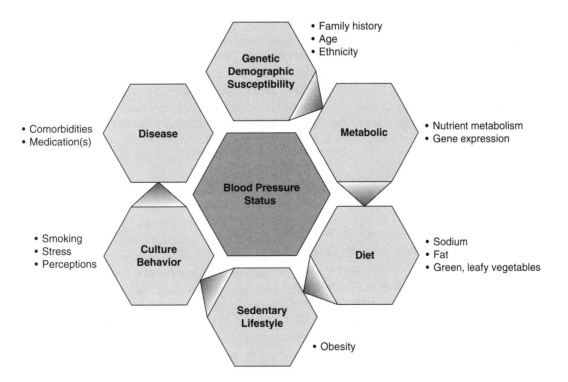

Figure 20-2 Select characteristics associated with blood pressure status

Hypertension Within the African American Community

In comparison to other subpopulations in the United States, African Americans develop hypertension at an earlier age and with greater severity.[85,86] Further, those residing in the rural south exhibit higher prevalence of hypertension and CVD mortality.[87,88] Although the prevalence of CVD is slightly greater among whites in comparison to African Americans, African Americans are 37% more likely to be hypertensive.[89] Strategies to prevent hypertension and all CVD among African Americans should be integrative and consider various components of the familial and cultural unit.[90]

Nutritional Care for Hypertension: Prevention and Treatment

Nutritional care can target general health or specific diseases such as hypertension. Hypertension (HTN) is a chronic disease starting sometimes early in life and continuing throughout the lifespan. If untreated, hypertension can cause disease conditions and comorbidities such as metabolic syndrome, diabetes, end-stage renal disease, atherosclerosis, and stroke. The best solution to this problem, prevention, entails an assessment and evaluation of lifestyle and environmental factors that can prevent hypertension and other cardiovascular diseases. Prevention should begin early in life and recognize potential racial/ethnic variations of onset and causes of the condition.

Comparison of Pre-Teen African American and White Girls

A National Heart, Lung, and Blood Institute (NHLBI) study[91] among 9- to 10-year-old African American and white girls measured frequency of breakfast consumption, dietary calcium and fiber intake, and BMI. Improving these parameters helps prevent CVD. The study found that frequency of breakfast intake declined with age, and was lower among African Americans. Eating breakfast was associated with higher calcium and dietary fiber intake and reduced BMI. These results suggest the need for nutrition education for girls, particularly high-risk African Americans, their parents, and dietetic professionals.

Food and Nutrient Intake of Teens and Young Adults

Among college students with a mean age of 20 years, participation in an eight-week dairy intake or stress management prevention/intervention using an online nutrition education program significantly increased calcium intake. The program was based on social cognitive theory and mediators that influence dietary choices. Another study, Project EAT—Eating Among Teens, found that mean daily intake of whole grains was lower than recommended among adolescents. Young people should be given opportunities to taste a variety of whole-grain foods to enhance taste preferences and self-efficacy to consume whole-grain products.[92,93] In a similar study, the diet quality and weight status of low-income urban children aged 7 to 13 years were evaluated utilizing food frequency questionnaires.[94] Food frequencies determined that more than 75% of the cross-sectional participants failed to meet recommended servings for grains, vegetables, dairy, and fruit groups, while a higher percentage of children were overweight than the national average. While the use of non-fast-food restaurants is a strong predictor of vegetable intake, fast-food and buffet restaurant use and eating while watching television were the strongest predictors of fat intake.[95]

Among urban African American children who participated in a 12-week after-school health and exercise program, increased fruit intake occurred with a significant reduction in diastolic blood pressure.[96] Systolic blood pressure improved among parents and guardians who participated in the study. Children tended to gain more diet-related benefits, while parents or guardians gained fitness-related benefits. In today's society, more parents are allowing their children to make more decisions regarding their food choices. In a study of food choices of African Americans and Latino adolescents, parents stated that their children enjoyed fast food.[97] Among African Americans, parents and children made weekday dinner decisions jointly and often allowed lunch-like alternatives with self-serve meals on the weekends. Among Latinos, parents bought their children their desired foods and had no restrictions on eating, but prepared traditional ethnic dinners without alternatives. Overall, the parents in both groups were concerned about the need to regulate their children's diets. Both groups of children are at risk for heart disease.

A workplace evaluation using the Pender's Health Promotion Model among urban and rural low-income African American women found that compared with a national sample of African American women, they had higher incidences of health risk, blood pressure, body mass index, diet and exercise behavior, and total cholesterol. Rural women had higher pre- and post-test cholesterol and fat intakes.[98] These results suggest the need for intervention among low-income pre-teen and young adult populations.

Community-Based Strategies

Intervention programs in addition to nutrition education have focused specifically on reducing plasma cholesterol, a risk factor for CVD. In a crossover trial, participants with high serum cholesterol were placed on a typical American diet, an experimental diet high in olive oil (rich in monounsaturated fats, or MUFA), or an experimental diet high in mid-oleic NuSun sunflower oil, which is high in MUFA and polyunsaturated fatty acids (PUFA). Compared to the control and olive oil diets, the NuSun sunflower diet decreased total and low-density lipoprotein cholesterol (LDL-C).[99] These results suggest the possibility that linoleic acid, abundant in sunflower oil, may reduce cholesterol levels despite controversy over the need for it over its 1–2% levels as an **essential fatty acid**. Advocates of a higher PUFA believe that higher levels have significant health benefits.[100]

Some interventions based on community involvement use focus groups to assess cardiovascular health perceptions when planning community-based interventions. Focus groups among rural women in West Virginia found that they were unaware of their personal CVD risks, did not support adopting a heart-healthy diet, and lacked skills for food selection and preparation.[101] They also preferred active learning, or hands-on experiences, coupled with group classes for learning and support. Among African Americans in the Mississippi Delta, qualitative focus group sessions preceded identification of strategies for achieving healthy energy balance. Phase I focus groups identified overeating, low self-esteem, low income, physical inactivity, unhealthy food preparation methods, and inadequate knowledge of the concept of healthy energy balance and how to achieve it. Phase 2 focus groups identified a preference for social support–based strategies for increasing physical activity levels. Current research indicates that rural regions in the deep south of the United States should emphasize social interaction at the community and family levels.[102]

Another community-oriented project[103] to refine CVD interventions found low rates of physical activity and healthy dietary patterns households in Charlotte, North Carolina. The identification of stages of readiness for change allowed

the more effective dissemination of diet and physical activity recommendations. In another community-based study[104] in North Carolina, women were evaluated for three behavioral CVD risk factors: low fruit and vegetable consumption, low physical activity, and cigarette smoking. A lay health adviser program and policy and community environment change strategies were implemented in the African American community from 2001 to 2005. All three health behaviors improved, implying the role of policy change in reducing health disparities. One study found that reading nutrition labels on food packages was more common among participants who were women, older, educated beyond high school, and obese.[105] Lay health advisers[106] or community health advisors (CHAs)[107] are becoming more useful in implementing community programs to reduce cardiovascular risk. In Uniontown, Alabama, CHAs were recruited and trained on community intervention and maintenance to increase knowledge, skills, and resources for changing behaviors that increase the risk of CVD. Additional community involvement included support from city officials, business owners, and community coalition to facilitate project activities. The unique feature of this project was that it documented that a comprehensive CHA-based intervention for CVD can facilitate side reaching in capacity to address health issues in a rural community that include improved community infrastructure that are sustained beyond the scope of the project. Researchers at the University of North Carolina in Charlotte, North Carolina, utilized an ecological perspective model that explored several levels of influences: intrapersonal, interpersonal, organization, community, and policy.[108] Fellowship among participants was identified as the primary motivator to continue positive health behaviors. Community Lay Health Advisors (LHAs) reported changes in individual health perceptions from disease- to prevention-oriented, and implementation of positive community changes like walking groups and a farmers' market. Participants reported an increase in knowledge of preventive health behaviors, the development of health-related skills, and the diffusion of knowledge to family.

Community Programs: Supplemental Feeding, Cultural Relevance, and Educational Sensitivity

Two of the largest U.S. community programs that may help improve nutritional status and prevent NCDs among low-income individuals are the **supplemental nutrition** program for **Women, Infants, and Children (WIC)** and the **Supplemental Nutrition Assistance Program (SNAP)**. Exclusive breastfeeding is considered optimal, and numerous studies link breastfeeding to lower risks for chronic diseases that include childhood-onset diabetes mellitus, obesity, and asthma.[109]

WIC and Breastfeeding

WIC participants are encouraged to breastfeed, but are also provided with baby formula if they do not exclusively breastfeed. In a cross-sectional study, 51% of participants reported breastfeeding their youngest child for a mean of 16 weeks, with higher rates among Caucasians and mothers who were breastfed as children. Most participants reported that WIC provided effective and clear education about the benefits of breastfeeding and that the information impacted their decisions to breastfeed.[110]

A mother's nutritional status affects the quality of her breast milk, and WIC helps improve dietary intake. In Los Angeles, California, low-income women in WIC received $10 per week in vouchers for the purchase of fresh fruits and vegetables. The 454 women in the program most often reported purchasing oranges, apples, bananas, peaches, grapes, tomatoes, carrots, lettuce, broccoli, and potatoes.[111]

Evidence for the Need to Reduce Disparities

Food and nutrition professionals, health club members, and WIC participants who attended the Minnesota State Fair reported that they believed the major benefit of whole-grain foods is dietary fiber, but WIC participants had fewer and more differentiated responses than the nutrition professionals.[112] In Athens, Ohio, comparisons between participants in WIC and the WIC/Farmers' Market Nutrition Program found that those in the Farmers' Market Nutrition Program reported higher education levels, higher vegetable intake, and other indicators of a healthy diet, despite the finding that these participants were not more food secure than those in the WIC comparison group.[113] A similar study in the same city found no perceived differences in food security and perceived health status, although WIC participants had greater social capital. In a Mississippi Delta study,[114] diet quality was lower among food-insecure than food-secure adults in a rural high-risk population. Overall, food insecurity was significantly inversely associated with perceived health status. Clearly, improving networking among clients and developing programs that strengthen social capital will improve health outcomes.[115]

A key component of SNAP is its nutrition education program designed to prevent disease and improve health.[116] In a "Contract for Change" of the Expanded Food and Nutrition Education/Food Stamp Nutrition Education program to increase produce consumption in low-income women below 130% of the poverty level, a four-week goal-setting exercise enhanced the effectiveness of their acceptance. Compared with the controls, the contract group significantly moved toward acceptance of vegetable consumption. This "Contract for Change" appears to be a positive workable strategy for these women. The majority of the prevention, intervention, and supplementary programs have common strategies that prevail relative to improving community outcomes (**Figure 20-3**).

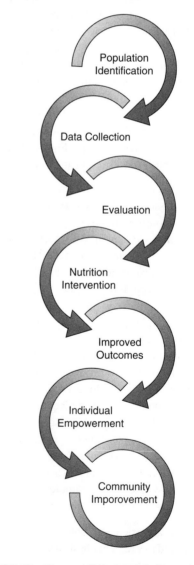

Figure 20-3 Prevention and intervention community flow chart

Local, State, and National Guidelines for Reducing Cardiovascular Disease Risk

Numerous local, state, and national guidelines aim to facilitate changes at the community level to reduce risk of CVD and other NCDs. Guidelines often result from collaborative efforts of government and nongovernment agencies.

NCEP-NHLBI Health Information Network

A sample program is the National Heart, Lung, and Blood Institute (NHLBI) of the National Institutes of Health (NIH) National Cholesterol Education Program (NCEP–NHLBI) Health Information Network. It was launched in November 1985 with the goal of reducing illness and death due to coronary heart disease (CHD) in the United States by reducing the percentage of Americans with high blood cholesterol. Since 1978, average total cholesterol levels among U.S. adults have fallen from 213 mg/dL to 203 mg/dL, and the prevalence of cholesterol levels 240 mg/dL or higher has declined from 26% to 19%.

The NCEP Coordinating Committee, with more than 40 partner organizations, promotes the implementation of NCEP's strategies and guidelines. Consisting of representatives from major medical and health professional associations, voluntary health organizations, community programs, and governmental agencies, the Coordinating Committee is the NCEP's policy-setting body and board of directors. It helps bring cholesterol information to a wide audience.

The committee also sponsors expert panels to develop guidelines for health professionals. The NCEP distributes these guidelines to physicians and other healthcare professionals and laboratories nationwide. Panel reports serve as platforms for various NCEP educational activities and materials. These panels include:

- *Expert Panel on Detection, Evaluation, and Treatment of High Blood Cholesterol in Adults (Adult Treatment Panel):* Provides guidelines for the detection, evaluation, and treatment of high blood cholesterol in adults.

- *Laboratory Standardization Panel:* Provides guidelines for standardizing laboratory measurements and reporting of blood cholesterol tests.

- *Expert Panel on Population Strategies for Blood Cholesterol Reduction (Population Panel):* Provides recommendations for reducing blood cholesterol levels through population-wide adoption of eating patterns low in saturated fat and cholesterol.

- *Expert Panel on Blood Cholesterol Levels in Children and Adolescents:* Makes recommendations for heart-healthy eating patterns for children and adolescents, and for detecting and treating high blood cholesterol in children and adolescents from high-risk families.

- *Working Group on Lipoprotein Measurement:* Develops recommendations to improve the measurement of LDL cholesterol, HDL cholesterol, and triglycerides.

The American Heart Association Scientific Statement Guide for Improving Cardiovascular Health at the Community Level

The Expert Panel on Population and Prevention Science of the American Heart Association (AHA), a nonprofit organization, provides this guide encouraging behavior change in individual patients. It is for public health practitioners, healthcare providers, and health policy makers. Improvements in facilities and resources in the places where people work and live should enhance the achievement of many goals, including cessation of tobacco use and avoidance of environmental tobacco smoke; reduction in dietary saturated fat, cholesterol, sodium, and calories; increased plant-based food intake; increased physical activity; access to preventive healthcare services; and early recognition of symptoms of heart attack and stroke.[117]

Additional Public Health Programs to Address CVD and Hypertension

The Title V Program is a federal program that applies in all states, the State Program for Children and Youth with Special Health Care Needs (CYSHCN). Under federal law every state has a program to assist children with disabilities or chronic conditions, and their families. The federal Social Security Act of 1989 requires states to provide and promote family-centered, community-based coordinated care for children with special healthcare needs and to facilitate the development of community-based systems of services. Funded with federal and state dollars, Title V programs help ensure that no child or youth with special healthcare needs goes without required services or programs.

The Department of Health and Human Services' Healthy People 2020, which lays out the health goals for the nation, states that there will be an increase in the number of states that have service systems for children with special healthcare needs and that:

1. Families of children with special healthcare needs will partner in decision making and be satisfied with services

2. All children with special healthcare needs will have coordinated and comprehensive care in a Medical Home

3. All families of children with special healthcare needs will have adequate private or public health insurance

4. All children will be screened early and continuously for special healthcare needs

5. Community-based service systems will be organized so families can use them easily

6. All youth with special healthcare needs will receive the services necessary to make transitions to all aspects of adult life, including health care, work, and independence

The four overarching goals of *Healthy People 2020* are:

- Attain high-quality, longer lives free of preventable disease, disability, injury, and premature death;

- Achieve health equity, eliminate disparities, and improve the health of all groups;

- Create social and physical environments that promote good health for all; and

- Promote quality of life, healthy development, and healthy behaviors across all life stages.

Conclusion

The leading cause of death in the United States and the world is CVD. Prevention will continue to be a priority for public health nutrition. The research presented in this chapter reveals the threat of NCDs and the significance of nutrition in their prevention. Hypertension is a major global risk factor for CVD and a financial burden on national economies. Nutritional care helps prevent and treat hypertension, and many effective community programs exist to support optimal health. Interventions must consider demographic, physical, emotional, economic, cultural, and social causes and consequences.

Hypertension affects one in three Americans and disproportionately affects African Americans, particularly those living in the southern United States. Culturally sensitive and therapeutically relevant community-based strategies are therefore required to address the needs of this vulnerable population. Managing existing conditions, evaluating potential triggers of disease initiation and progression, assessing potential protective mechanisms, and providing appropriate tools and treatment mechanisms to improve health should all be considered when designing prevention and intervention strategies, not just for cardiovascular disease but other diseases as well (**Figure 20-4**).

Advocates of public health should engage in a comprehensive, integrative team approach that addresses disease risk within the demographic, physical, emotional, economic,

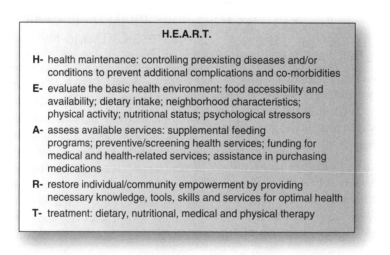

H.E.A.R.T.

H- health maintenance: controlling preexisting diseases and/or conditions to prevent additional complications and co-morbidities

E- evaluate the basic health environment: food accessibility and availability; dietary intake; neighborhood characteristics; physical activity; nutritional status; psychological stressors

A- assess available services: supplemental feeding programs; preventive/screening health services; funding for medical and health-related services; assistance in purchasing medications

R- restore individual/community empowerment by providing necessary knowledge, tools, skills and services for optimal health

T- treatment: dietary, nutritional, medical and physical therapy

Figure 20-4 A suggested integrative approach to addressing the public health impact of disease

social, and cultural paradigm. Conventional and novel factors that may be considered include: neighborhood characteristics (sidewalks, supermarkets), diet composition (traditional and novel foods), household characteristics and compositions (established meal times), eating environment (presence of television, presence of table and chairs), and psychological triggers (emotional eating, stress). Safeguarding public health, via nutrition interventions, warrants an early initiation strategy, such as promoting healthy eating during pregnancy, breastfeeding, and establishing healthful eating habits and patterns during childhood. The impact of nutrition on public health cannot be overemphasized, as nutritional requirements oscillate throughout the lifespan during stages of development and health status. Thus, prevention and intervention strategies should be revolutionized accordingly to ensure the optimal health and well-being of the public.

Acknowledgments

The contributors would like to acknowledge the College of Agriculture, Environment, and Nutritional Sciences at Tuskegee University, as well as Dr. Melissa Johnson, for her major contribution of the tables and figures.

References

1 Senauer, B., & Garcia, M. (1991). Determinants of the nutrition and health status of preschool children: an analysis with longitudinal data. *Economic Development and Cultural Change, 39,* 371-89.

2 Ene-Obong, H. N., Enugu, G. I., Uwaegbute, A. C. (2001). Determinants of health and nutritional status of rural Nigerian women. *Journal of Health, Population, and Nutrition, 19,* 320-30.

3 Gittelsohn, J., & Vastine, A. E. Sociocultural and household factors impacting on the selection, allocation and consumption of animal source foods: Current knowledge and application. *Journal of Nutrition, 133,* 4036S-4041S.

4 Bouis, H. E., Eozenou, P., & Rahman A. (2011). Food prices, household income, and resource allocation: Socioeconomic perspectives on their effects on dietary quality and nutritional status. *Food and Nutrition Bulletin, 32,* S14-23.

5 Cowley, A. W., Nadeau, J. H., Baccarelli, A., Berecek, K., Fornage, M., Gibbons, G. H., . . . Galis, Z. S. (2012). Report of the National Heart, Lung, and Blood Institute Working Group on Epigenetics and Hypertension. *Hypertension, 59,* 899-905.

6 Aranceta, J., Perez-Rodrigo, C., Ribas, L., & Serra-Majem, L. (2003). Sociodemographic and lifestyle determinants of food patterns in Spanish children and adolescents: The enKid study. *European Journal of Clinical Nutrition, 57*(Suppl. 1), S40-44.

7 Befort, C., Kaur, H., Nollen, N., Sullivan, D. K., Nazir, N., Choi, W. S., . . . Ahluwalia, J. S. (2006). Fruit, vegetable, and fat intake among non-Hispanic black and non-Hispanic white adolescents: Associations with home availability and food consumption settings. *Journal of the American Dietetic Association, 106,* 367-73.

8 Wylie, C., Copeman, J., & Kirk, S. F. L. (1999). Health and social factors affecting the food choice and nutritional intake of elderly people with restricted mobility. *Journal of Human Nutrition and Diet, 12,* 375-80.

9 Roos, E., Lahelma, E., Virtanen, M., Prattala, R., & Pietinen, P. (1998). Gender, socioeconomic status and family status as determinants of food behaviour. *Social Science and Medicine, 46,* 1519-29.

10 Hughes, R. (2003). Public health nutrition workforce composition, core functions, competencies and capacity: Perspectives of advanced-level practitioners in Australia. *Public Health Nutrition, 6,* 607-13.

11 Johnson, D. B., Eaton, D. L., Wahl, P. W., & Gleason, C. (2001). Public health nutrition practice in the United States. *Journal of the American Dietetic Association, 101,* 529-34.

12 Landman, J., Buttriss, J., & Margetts, B. Curriculum design for professional development in public health nutrition in Britain. *Public Health Nutrition, 1,* 69-74.

13 Carter-Pokras, O., & Baquet, C. (2002). What is a "health disparity"? *Public Health Reports, 117,* 426-34.

14 Osypuk, T. L., & Acevedo-Garcia, D. (2010). Beyond individual neighborhoods: A geography of opportunity perspective for understanding racial/ethnic health disparities. *Health Place, 16,* 1113-23.

15 Balsa, A. I., & McGuire, T. G. (2003). Prejudice, clinical uncertainty and stereotyping as sources of health disparities. *Journal of Health Economics, 22,* 89-116.

16 Solomons, N. W. (2003). Diet and long-term health: An African Diaspora perspective. *Asia Pacific Journal of Clinical Nutrition, 12,* 313-30.

17 Feldman, R. H., & Fulwood, R. The three leading causes of death in African Americans: barriers to reducing excess disparity and to improving health behaviors. *Journal of Health Care for the Poor and Underserved, 10,* 45-71.

18 Griffith, D. M., Metzl, J. M., & Gunter, K. (2011). Considering intersections of race and gender in interventions that address U.S. men's health disparities. *Public Health, 125,* 417-23.

19 Reddy, K. S., & Katan, M. B. (2004). Diet, nutrition and the prevention of hypertension and cardiovascular diseases. *Public Health Nutrition, 7,* 167-86.

20 Mayne, S. T. (2003). Antioxidant nutrients and chronic disease: Use of biomarkers of exposure and oxidative stress status in epidemiologic research. *Journal of Nutrition, 133*(Suppl. 3), 933S-940S.

21 Scaglioni, S., Salvioni, M., & Galimberti C. (2008). Influence of parental attitudes in the development of children's eating behaviour. *British Journal of Nutrition, 99*(Suppl. 1), S22-25.

22 Rasmussen, M., Krolner, R., Klepp, K. I., Lytle, L., Brug, J., Bere, E., & Due, P. (2006). Determinants of fruit and vegetable consumption among children and adolescents: A review of the literature. Part I: Quantitative studies. *International Journal of Behavioral Nutrition and Physical Activity, 3,* 22.

23 Tibbs, T., Haire-Joshu, D., Schechtman, K. B., Brownson, R. C., Nanney, M. S., Houston, C., & Auslander, W. (2001). The relationship between parental modeling, eating patterns, and dietary intake among African-American parents. *Journal of the American Dietetic Association, 101,* 535-41.

24 Faith, M. S. (2005). Development and modification of child food preferences and eating patterns: behavior genetics strategies. *International Journal of Obesity, 29,* 549-56.

25 Westenhoefer, J. (2002). Establishing dietary habits during childhood for long-term weight control. *Annals of Nutrition and Metabolism, 46*(Suppl. 1), 18-23.

26 Moreno, L. A., Gonzalez-Gross, M., Kersting, M., Molnar, D., de Henauw, S., Beghin, L., . . . Marcos, A., for the HELENA Study Group. (2008). Assessing, understanding and modifying nutritional status, eating habits and physical activity in European adolescents: The HELENA (Healthy Lifestyle in Europe by Nutrition in Adolescence) Study. *Public Health Nutrition, 11,* 288-99.

27 Lake, A. A., Mathers, J. C., Rugg-Gunn, A. J., & Adamson, A. J. (2006). Longitudinal change in food habits between adolescence (11-12 years) and adulthood (32-33 years): The ASH30 Study. *Journal of Public Health, 28,* 10-16.

28 Buckland, G., Gonzalez, C. A., Agudo, A., Vilardell, M., Berenguer, A., Amiano, P., . . . Moreno-Iribas, C. (2009). Adherence to the Mediterranean diet and risk of coronary heart disease in the Spanish EPIC Cohort Study. *American Journal of Epidemiology, 170,* 1518-29.

29 Sofi, F., Abbate, R., Gensini, G. F., & Casini, A. (2010). Accruing evidence on benefits of adherence to the Mediterranean diet on health: An updated systematic review and meta-analysis. *American Journal of Clinical Nutrition, 92,* 1189-96.

30 Belin, R. J., Greenland, P., Allison, M., Martin, L., Shikany, J. M., Larson, J., . . . Van Horn, L. (2011). Diet quality and the risk of cardiovascular disease: The Women's Health Initiative (WHI). *American Journal of Clinical Nutrition, 94,* 49-57.

31 Fullerton, H. J., Wu, Y. W., Zhao, S., & Johnston, S. C. (2003). Risk of stroke in children: Ethnic and gender disparities. *Neurology, 61,* 189-94.

32 Feber, J., & Ahmed, M. (2010). Hypertension in children: New trends and challenges. *Clinical Science, 119,* 151-61.

33 McCrindle, B. W. (2010). Assessment and management of hypertension in children and adolescents. *Nature Reviews Cardiology, 7,* 155-63.

34 Glover, S., Piper, C. N., Hassan, R., Preston, G., Wilkinson, L., Bowen-Seabrook, J., Meyer-Davis, B., & Williams, S. Dietary, physical activity, and lifestyle behaviors of rural African American South Carolina children. *Journal of the National Medical Association, 103,* 300-304.

35 Esposito, K., & Giugliano, D. (2011). Increased consumption of green leafy vegetables, but not fruit, vegetables or fruit and vegetables combined, is associated with reduced incidence of type 2 diabetes. *Evidence-Based Medicine, 16,* 27-28.

36 Zhang, X., Shu, X. O., Xiang, Y. B., Yang, G., Li, H., Gao, J., . . . Zheng W. (2011). Cruciferous vegetable consumption is associated with a reduced risk of total and cardiovascular disease mortality. *American Journal of Clinical Nutrition, 94,* 240-46.

37 Bosetti, C., Filomeno, M., Riso, P., Polesel, J., Levi, F., Talamini, R., . . . La Vecchia, C. (2012). Cruciferous vegetables and cancer risk in a network of case-control studies. *Annals of Oncology, 23,* 2198-2203.

38 Kahlon, T. S., Chapman, M. H., & Smith, G. E. (2007). In vitro binding of bile acids by spinach, kale, brussels sprouts, broccoli, mustard greens, green bell pepper, cabbage and collards. *Food Chemistry, 100,* 1531-36.

39 Huang, Z., Wang, B., Eaves, D. H., Shikany, J. M., & Pace, R. D. (2009). Total phenolics and antioxidant capacity of indigenous vegetables in the southeast United States: Alabama Collaboration for Cardiovascular Equality Project. *International Journal of Food Sciences and Nutrition, 60,* 100-108.

40 Kahlon, T. S., Chiu, M-C.M., & Chapman, M. H. (2008). Steam cooking significantly improves in vitro bile acid binding of collard greens, kale, mustard greens, broccoli, green bell pepper, and cabbage. *Nutrition Research, 28,* 351-57.

41 Johnson, M., & Pace, R. D. (2010). Sweet potato leaves: Properties and synergistic interactions that promote health and prevent disease. *Nutrition Reviews, 68,* 604-15.

42 Karna, P., Gundala, S. R., Gupta, M. V., Shamsi, S. A., Pace, R. D., Yates, C., . . . Aneja, R. (2011). Polyphenol-rich sweet potato greens extract inhibits proliferation and induces apoptosis in prostate cancer cells in vitro and in vivo. *Carcinogenesis, 32,* 1872-80.

43 Kris-Etherton, P. M., Hecker, K. D., Bonanome, A., Coval, S. M., Binkoski, A. E., Hilpert, K. F., . . . Etherton, T. D. (2002). Bioactive compounds in foods: Their role in the prevention of cardiovascular disease and cancer. *American Journal of Medicine, 113*(Suppl. 9B), 71S-88S.

44 Bowman, S. A., Gortmaker, S. L., Ebbeling, C. B., Pereira, M. A., & Ludwig, D. S. (2004). Effects of fast-food consumption on energy intake and diet quality among children in a national household survey. *Pediatrics, 113,* 112-18.

45 Hickson, D. A., Diez Roux, A. V., Smith, A. E., Tucker, K. L., Gore, L. D., Zhang, L., & Wyatt, S. B. (2011). Associations of fast food restaurant availability with dietary intake and weight among African Americans in the Jackson Heart Study, 2000-2004. *American Journal of Public Health, 101*(Suppl. 1), S301-9.

46 Champagne, C. M., Casey, P. H., Connell, C. L., Stuff, J. E., Gossett, J. M., Harsha, D. W., . . . Bogle, M. L.; Lower Mississippi Delta Nutrition Intervention Research Initiative. (2007).

Poverty and food intake in rural America: Diet quality is lower in food insecure adults in the Mississippi Delta. *Journal of the American Dietetic Association, 107,* 1886-94.

47 Champagne, C. M., Bogle, M. L., McGee, B. B., Yadrick, K., Allen, H. R., Kramer, T. R., . . . Weber, J. (2004). Dietary intake in the lower Mississippi delta region: Results from the Foods of our Delta Study. *Journal of the American Dietetic Association, 104,* 199-207.

48 Dubowitz, T., Heron, M., Bird, C. E., Lurie, N., Finch, B. K., Basurto-Davila, R., . . . Escarce, J. J. (2008). Neighborhood socioeconomic status and fruit and vegetable intake among whites, blacks, and Mexican Americans in the United States. *American Journal of Clinical Nutrition, 87,* 1883-91.

49 Whelton, P. K., Appel, L. J., Sacco, R. L., Anderson, C. A., Antman, E. M., Campbell, N., . . . Van Horn, L. V. (2012). Sodium, blood pressure, and cardiovascular disease: further evidence supporting the American Heart Association sodium reduction recommendations. *Circulation, 126,* 2880-89.

50 United States Department of Agriculture & United States Department of Health and Human Services. (2010). *Dietary guidelines for Americans: An overview* (7th ed.). Retrieved from http://www.nationaldairycouncil.org/Research /DairyCouncilDigestArchives/Pages/dcd82-3Page2.aspx

51 Brown, I. J., Tzoulaki, I., Candeias, V., & Elliott, P. (2009). Salt intakes around the world: Implications for public health. *International Journal of Epidemiology, 2009, 38,* 791-813.

52 Anderson, C. A., Appel, L. J., Okuda, N., Brown, I. J., Chan, Q., Zhao, L., . . . Stamler, J. (2010). Dietary sources of sodium in China, Japan, the United Kingdom, and the United States, women and men aged 40 to 59 years: The INTERMAP study. *Journal of the American Dietetic Association, 110,* 736-45.

53 Geleijnse, J. M., Kok, F. J., & Grobbee, D. E. (2004). Impact of dietary and lifestyle factors on the prevalence of hypertension in Western populations. *European Journal of Public Health, 14,* 235-39.

54 Stranges, S., Wu, T., Dorn, J. M., Freudenheim, J. L., Muti, P., Farinaro, E., . . . Trevisan, M. Relationship of alcohol drinking pattern to risk of hypertension: A population-based study. *Hypertension, 44,* 813-19.

55 Ruixing, Y., Hui, L., Jinzhen, W., Weixiong, L., Dezhai, Y., Shangling, P., . . . Xiuyan, L. (2009). Association of diet and lifestyle with blood pressure in the Guangxi Hei Yi Zhuang and Han populations. *Public Health Nutrition, 12,* 553-61.

56 Forman, J. P., Stampfer, M. J., & Curhan, G. C. (2009). Diet and lifestyle risk factors associated with incident hypertension in women. *JAMA, 302,* 401-11.

57 Johnson, R. J., Segal, M. S., Sautin, Y., Nakagawa, T., Feig, D. I., Kang, D. H., . . . Sanchez-Lozada, L. G. (2007). Potential role of sugar (fructose) in the epidemic of hypertension, obesity and the metabolic syndrome, diabetes, kidney disease, and cardio-vascular disease. *American Journal of Clinical Nutrition, 86,* 899-906.

58 Brown, I. J., Stamler, J., Van Horn, L., Robertson, C. E., Chan, Q., Dyer, A. R., . . . Elliott, P., for the International Study of Macro /Micronutrients and Blood Pressure Research Group. (2011). Sugar-sweetened beverage, sugar intake of individuals, and their blood pressure: International study of macro/micronutrients and blood pressure. *Hypertension, 57,* 695-701.

59 Douard, V., & Ferraris, R. P. (2013). The role of fructose trans-porters in diseases linked to excessive fructose intake. *Journal of Physiology, 591,* 401-14.

60 Johnson, R. J., Thomas, J., & Lanaspa, M. A. (2012). Impact of beverage content on health and the kidneys. *Nutrition Today, 47,* S22-S26.

61 Pace, R., Dawkins, N., Wang, B., Person, S., & Shikany, J. M. (2008). Rural African Americans' dietary knowledge, per-ceptions, and behavior in relation to cardiovascular disease. *Ethnicity and Disease, 18,* 6-12.

62 Qian, J., Wang, B., Dawkins, N., Gray, A., & Pace, R. D. (2007). Reduction of risk factors for cardiovascular diseases in African Americans with a 12-week nutrition education program. *Nutrition Research, 27,* 252-57.

63 Wang, Y., & Wang, Q. J. The prevalence of prehypertension and hypertension among U.S. adults according to the new joint national committee guidelines: New challenges of the old prob-lem. *Archives of Internal Medicine, 164,* 2126-34.

64 National Heart, Lung, and Blood Institute. (2003). *Seventh report of the Joint National Committee on Prevention, Detection, Evaluation, and Treatment of High Blood Pressure.* Retrieved from http://www.nhlbi.nih.gov/guidelines/hyperten sion/jnc7full.pdf

65 Djousse, L., Driver, J. A., & Gaziano, J. M. (2009). Relation between modifiable lifestyle factors and lifetime risk of heart failure. *JAMA, 302,* 394-400.

66 Gasperin, D., Netuveli, G., Dias-da-Costa, J. S., & Pattussi, M. P. (2009). Effect of psychological stress on blood pressure increase: A meta-analysis of cohort studies. *Cadernos de Saúde Pública, 25,* 715-26.

67 Kearney, P. M., Whelton, M., Reynolds, K., Muntner, P., Whelton, P. K., & He, J. (2005). Global burden of hypertension: Analysis of worldwide data. *Lancet, 365,* 217-23.

68 Popkin, B. M., Horton, S., Kim, S., Mahal, A., & Shuigao, J. (2001). Trends in diet, nutritional status, and diet-related noncommu-nicable diseases in China and India: The economic costs of the nutrition transition. *Nutrition Reviews, 59,* 379-90.

69 Campbell, N. R., Fodor, J. G., & Chockalingam, A. (2001). Hypertension recommendations: Are they relevant to public health? *Canadian Journal of Public Health, 92,* 245-47.

70 Chobanian, A. V. (2009). Shattuck Lecture. The hypertension paradox—more uncontrolled disease despite improved therapy. *New England Journal of Medicine, 361,* 878-87.

71 Bautista, L. E. (2003). Inflammation, endothelial dysfunction, and the risk of high blood pressure: Epidemiologic and biologi-cal evidence. *Journal of Human Hypertension, 17,* 223-30.

72 Vincent-Baudry, S., Defoort, C., Gerber, M., Bernard, M. C., Verger, P., Helal, O., . . . Lairon, D. (2005). The Medi-RIVAGE study: Reduction of cardiovascular disease risk factors after a 3-mo intervention with a Mediterranean-type diet or a low-fat diet. *American Journal of Clinical Nutrition, 82,* 964-71.

73 Babio, N., Bullo, M., & Salas-Salvado, J. (2009). Mediterranean diet and metabolic syndrome: The evidence. *Public Health Nutrition, 12,* 1607-17.

74 He, J., Whelton, P. K., Appel, L. J., Charleston, J., & Klag, M. J. (2000). Long-term effects of weight loss and dietary sodium reduction on incidence of hypertension. *Hypertension, 35,* 544-49.

75 Wang, L., Gaziano, J. M., Liu, S., Manson, J. E., Buring, J. E., & Sesso, H. D. (2007). Whole- and refined-grain intakes and the risk of hypertension in women. *American Journal of Clinical Nutrition, 86,* 472-79.

76 Vlismas, K., Stavrinos, V., & Panagiotakos, D. B. (2009). Socio-economic status, dietary habits and health-related outcomes in various parts of the world: A review. *Central European Journal of Public Health, 17,* 55-63.

77 Cort, N. A., & Fahs, P. S. (2001). Heart disease: The hidden killer of rural black women. *Journal of Multicultural Nursing and Health, 7,* 37-41.

78 Reschovsky, J. D., & Staiti, A. B. (2005). Access and quality: Does rural America lag behind? *Health Affairs (Millwood), 24,* 1128-39.

79 Khan, J. A., Casper, M., Asimos, A. W., Clarkson, L., Enright, D., Fehrs, L. J., . . . Greer, S. (2011). Geographic and sociodemographic disparities in drive times to Joint Commission-certified primary stroke centers in North Carolina, South Carolina, and Georgia. *Preventing Chronic Disease, 8,* A79.

80 Wilcox, S., Bopp, M., Oberrecht, L., Kammermann, S. K., & McElmurray, C. T. (2003). Psychosocial and perceived environmental correlates of physical activity in rural and older african american and white women. *Journal of Gerontolology. Series B, Psychological Sciences and Social Sciences, 58,* P329-37.

81 Appel, S. J., Harrell, J. S., & Deng, S. (2002). Racial and socioeconomic differences in risk factors for cardiovascular disease among Southern rural women. *Nursing Research, 51,* 140-47.

82 Barnett, E., Halverson, J. A., Elmes, G. A., & Braham, V. E. (2000). Metropolitan and non-metropolitan trends in coronary heart disease mortality within Appalachia, 1980-1997. *Annals of Epidemiology, 10,* 370-79.

83 Barnett, E., & Halverson, J. (2000). Disparities in premature coronary heart disease mortality by region and urbanicity among black and white adults ages 35-64, 1985-1995. *Public Health Reports, 115,* 52-64.

84 National Center for Health Statistics. (2001). Health, United States, 2001: With urban and rural health chartbook. Hyattsville, MD: National Center for Health Statistics. Retrieved from http://www.cdc.gov/nchs/data/hus/hus01.pdf

85 Brown, M. J. (2006). Hypertension and ethnic group. *BMJ, 332,* 833-36.

86 Ong, K. L., Cheung, B. M., Man, Y. B., Lau, C. P., & Lam, K.S. Prevalence, awareness, treatment, and control of hypertension among United States adults 1999-2004. *Hypertension, 49,* 69-75.

87 Hajjar, I., & Kotchen, T. (2003). Regional variations of blood pressure in the United States are associated with regional variations in dietary intakes: The NHANES-III data. *Journal of Nutrition, 133,* 211-14.

88 Danaei, G., Rimm, E. B., Oza, S., Kulkarni, S. C., Murray, C. J., & Ezzati, M. (2010). The promise of prevention: The effects of four preventable risk factors on national life expectancy and life expectancy disparities by race and county in the United States. *PLoS Medicine, 7,* e1000248.

89 Lloyd-Jones, D., Adams, R., Carnethon, M., De Simone, G., Ferguson, T. B., Flegal, K., . . . Hong, Y., for the American Heart Association Statistics Committee and Stroke Statistics Subcommittee. (2009). Heart disease and stroke statistics–2009 update: A report from the American Heart Association Statistics Committee and Stroke Statistics Subcommittee. *Circulation, 119,* e21-181.

90 Pace, R. D., Dawkins, N. L., & Johnson, M. (Eds.). (2012). *Strategies for cardiovascular disease prevention in rural southern African American communities.* Rijeka, Croatia: InTech Europe.

91 Affenito, S., Thompson, D., Barton, B., Franko, D., Daniels, S., Obarzanek, E., Schreiber, G., & Striegel-Moore, R. (2005). Breakfast consumption by African-American and White adolescent girls correlates positively with calcium and fiber intake and negatively with body mass index. *Journal of the American Dietetic Association, 105*(6), 938-45.

92 Poddar, K., Hosig, K., Anderson-Bill, E., Nickols-Richardson, S., & Duncan, S. (2012). Dairy intake and related self-regulation improved in college students using online nutrition education. *Journal of the Academy of Nutrition and Diet, 112*(12), 1976-86.

93 Larson, N., Neumark-Sztainer, D., Story, M., & Burgess-Champoux, T. (2010). Whole-grain intake correlates among adolescents and young adults: Findings from project EAT. *Journal of the American Dietetic Association, 110*(2), 230-37.

94 Langevin, D., Kwiatkowski, C., McKay, M., Mallet, J., Touger-Decker, R., Smith, J., & Perlman, A. (2007). Evaluation of diet quality and weight status of children from a low socioeconomic urban environment support "at risk" classification. *Journal of the American Dietetic Association, 107*(11), 1973-77.

95 Befort, C., Kaur, H., Nollen, N., Sullivan, D. K., Nazir, N., Choi, W. S., Hornberger, L., & Ahluwalia, J. S. (2006). Fruit, vegetable, and fat intake among non-Hispanic Black and non-Hispanic White adolescents: Associations with home availability and food consumption settings. *Journal of the American Dietetic Association, 106*(3), 367-73.

96 Engels, H., Gretebeck, R., Gretebeck, K., & Jimenez, L. (2005). Promoting healthful diets and exercise: Efficacy of a 12-week after-school program in urban African Americans. *Journal of the American Dietetic Association, 105*(3), 455-59.

97 O'Dougherty, M., Story, M., & Lytle, L. (2006). Food choices of young African-American and Latino adolescents: Where do parents fit in? *Journal of the American Dietetic Association, 106*(11), 1846-50.

98 Williams, A., Wold, J., Dunkin, J., Idleman, L., & Jackson, C. (2004). CVD prevention strategies with urban and rural African American women. *Applied Nursing Research, 17*(3), 187-94.

99 Binkoski, A., Kris-Etherton, P., Wilson, T., Mountain, M., & Nicolosi, R. (2005). Balance of unsaturated fatty acids is important to a cholesterol-lowering diet: Comparison of mid-oleic sunflower oil and olive oil of cardiovascular disease risk factors. *Journal of the American Dietetic Association*, 105(7), 1080-86.

100 Kris-Etherton, P., Fleming, J., & Harris, W. (2010). The debate about n-6 polyunsaturated fatty acids recommendations for cardiovascular health. *Journal of the American Dietetic Association, 110*(2), 201-4.

101 Krummel, D., Humphries, D., & Tessaro, I. (2002). Focus groups on cardiovascular health in rural women: implications for practice. *Journal of Nutrition Education and Behavior, 34*(1), 38-46.

102 Parham, G. P., & Scarinci, I. C. (2007. Strategies for achieving healthy energy balance among African Americans in the Mississippi Delta. *Preventing Chronic Disease, 4*(4), A97.

103 Plescia, M., & Groblewski, M. (2004). A community-oriented primary care demonstration project: refining interventions for cardiovascular disease and diabetes. *Annals of Family Medicine, 2*(2), 103-9.

104 Plescia, M., Herrick, H., & Chavis, L. (2008). Improving health behaviors in an African American community: The Charlotte Racial and Ethnic Approaches to Community Health Project. *American Journal of Public Health, 98*(9), 1678-84.

105 Satia, J. A., Galanko, J. A., & Neuhouser, M. L. (2005). Food nutrition label use is associated with demographic, behavioral, and psychosocial factors and dietary intake among African Americans in North Carolina. *Journal of the American Dietetic Association, 105*(3), 392-402.

106 Plescia, M., Herrick, H., & Chavis, L. (2008). Improving health behaviors in an African American community: The Charlotte Racial and Ethnic Approaches to Community Health Project. *American Journal of Public Health, 98*(9), 1678-84.

107 Cornell, C. E., Littleton, M. A., Greene, P. G., Pulley, L., Brownstein, J. N., Sanderson, B. K., . . . Raczynski, J. M. (2009). A community health advisor program to reduce cardiovascular risk among rural African-American women. *Health Education Research, 24*(4), 622-33.

108 DeBate, R., Plescia, M., Joyner, D., & Spann, L. (2004). A qualitative assessment of Charlotte REACH: An ecological perspective for decreasing CVD and diabetes among African Americans. *Ethnicity and Disease, 14*(3 Suppl. 1), S77-S82.

109 DiGiorgio, L., & Danoff, N. (2005). Promoting breastfeeding to mothers in the special Supplemental Nutrition Program for women, infants, and children. *Journal of the American Dietetic Association, 105*(5), 716-17.

110 Murimi, M., Dodge, C., Pope, J., & Erickson, D. (2010). Factors that influence breastfeeding decisions among special supplemental nutrition program for women, infants, and children participants from Central Louisiana. *Journal of the American Dietetic Association, 110*(4), 624-27.

111 Herman, D., Harrison, G., & Jenks, E. (2006). Choices made by low-income women provided with an economic supplement for fresh fruit and vegetable purchase. *Journal of the American Dietetic Association, 106*(5), 740-44.

112 Marquart, L., Pham, A., Lautenschlager, L., Croy, M., & Sobal, J. (2006). Beliefs about whole-grain foods by food and nutrition professionals, health club members, and special supplemental nutrition program for women, infants, and children participants /state fair attendees. *Journal of the American Dietetic Association, 106*(11), 1856-60.

113 Kropf, M., Holben, D., Holcomb, J., & Anderson, H. (2007). Food security status and produce intake and behaviors of special supplemental nutrition program for women, infants, and children and farmers' market nutrition program participants. *Journal of the American Dietetic Association, 107*(11), 1903-8.

114 Champagne, C. M., Casey, P. H., Connell, C. L., Stuff, J. E, Gossett, J. M., Harsha, D. W., . . . Bogle, M. L. (2007). Poverty and food intake in rural America: diet quality is lower in food insecure adults in the Mississippi Delta. *Journal of the American Dietetic Association, 107*(11), 1886-94.

115 Walker, J. L., Holben, D, H., Krof, M. L., Holcomb, J. P., & Anderson, H. (2007). Household food insecurity is inversely associated with social capital and health in females from special supplemental nutrition program for women, infants, and children households in Appalachian Ohio. *Journal of the American Dietetic Association, 107*(11), 1989-93.

116 Landers, P. (2007). The Food Stamp Program: History, nutrition education, and impact. *Journal of the American Dietetic Association, 107*(11), 1945-51.

117 Pearson, T. A., Blair, S. N., Daniels, S. R., Eckel, R. H., Fair, J. M., Fortmann, S. P., . . . Taubert, K. A. (2002). AHA guidelines for primary prevention of cardiovascular disease and stroke: 2002 update. *Circulation, 106*(3), 388-91.

Further Reading

Pace, R. D., Dawkins, N. L., & Johnson, M. (2011). Strategies for cardiovascular disease prevention in rural southern African American communities. In Jay Maddock (Ed.), *Public health: Social and behavioral health* (pp. 59-82). Rijeka, Croatia: InTech.

Chapter 21

Vitamin D and Bone Health: A Nutritional Perspective on a Public Health Problem

Hope Weiler, RD, PhD

"Given the growing numbers of seniors in both the developed and developing world, the issue of suboptimal vitamin D levels takes on a critical health economic significance. We must spread the urgent message that the implementation of low-cost and effective strategies to ensure optimal levels of vitamin D, particularly in high risk groups and seniors, can make a dramatic difference to health and quality of life, as well as potentially reduce a significant disease burden on healthcare systems worldwide."–Bess Dawson-Hughes, General Secretary of the International Osteoporosis Foundation (IOF) and Member of IOF Nutrition Working Group

Reproduced from Dr. Bess Dawson-Hughes and the International Osteoporosis Foundation. (2012, September 12). IOF shines spotlight on global vitamin D status with the release of interactive map. Retrieved from http://www.iofbonehealth.org/iof-shines-spotlight-global-vitamin-d-status-release-interactive-map.

Learning Objectives

- Know intake recommendations and food sources of vitamin D intake, and discuss vitamin D status in North America.

- Describe vitamin D's role in bone health and its other physiological functions.

- Understand the implications of vitamin D status on bone health and osteoporosis and link them to policy decisions.

- Identify risk factors for low vitamin D status and compromised bone health.

- Describe contributions of public health policy related to vitamin D toward meeting the Healthy People 2020 goal to reduce osteoporosis.

Case Study: Osteoporotic Fracture in Montreal, Canada

Frieda is 71 years old and Caucasian. She lives alone in Montreal, Canada, has poor eyesight, and depends on a fixed income that she stretches to meet costs of living and healthcare needs. She drinks milk only in coffee, cannot afford nutritional supplements, and receives home-delivered meals twice a week.

One snowy winter day, after going grocery shopping and picking up her salbutamol prescription for asthma, she takes public transit home. The streets are icy, and she slips near the bus stop. She arrives home without assistance, but her right arm hurts below the elbow. The next day, since her arm is fully bruised and swollen, she takes the bus to the hospital emergency department. X-rays confirm a **Colles' fracture** of the right wrist and also at the elbow, in addition to overall thinning of the **cortical** and **trabecular** bone. The diagnosis of **osteoporosis** surprised Frieda, who had always considered herself healthy, been active, maintained a healthy body mass index (BMI) of 21 kg/m², and never been told by her doctor that she was at risk for osteoporosis, or advised to take nutritional measures toward her bone health, even after the fracture.

Frieda is right handed, and her cast interferes with daily activities. Her quality of life is reduced, not only because of the cast and her fear of falling again, but also because the wrist does not heal properly, and she never regains full fine motor control of her right hand.

Discussion Questions

- Which public health strategies could have helped prevent thin bones in Frieda?
- How can public health interventions promote stronger bones in older adults?
- Which programs might prevent the initial fracture or improve recovery?

Introduction

Vitamin D is a fat-soluble vitamin best known for its roles in calcium and bone metabolism.[1] It was discovered in 1922, when a critical series of experiments demonstrated that cod liver oil, heat-treated to remove vitamin A, had antiricketic properties,[2] as seen when children with rickets are exposed to sunshine.[3] Even though vitamin D production can be **endogenous** with sufficient skin exposure to solar ultraviolet beta (UVB) radiation, recommendations now focus on **exogenous** dietary sources and are thus complementary to sun-safe practices. Vitamin D is a focus of public health nutrition strategies to achieve bone health through dietary intake, food fortification policies, and professional guidelines in the prevention and management of osteoporosis. While vitamin D is important to bone across the stages of life, this chapter will focus on adult bone health.[4]

Osteoporosis is a public health concern strongly linked to vitamin D deficiency.[5] One-third of women ages 60 to 70 and one-eighth of men over 50 years are likely to have osteoporosis or osteoporotic fractures. Global vitamin D status is not well defined, but existing data imply widespread

inadequacy,[6] especially after winter in populations living in northern climates. For example, nearly 13–48% of adults in northern China have been estimated to be deficient after winter.

Dietary Recommendations for Vitamin D

The United States and Canada jointly develop dietary recommendations for vitamin D and other nutrients for both nations. The **Institute of Medicine (IOM)** was established in 1970 by the National Academy of Sciences to oversee public health policy matters. **Health Canada** and expert scientists from both nations also help develop the **Dietary Reference Intake (DRI)** values.

The current DRI values for calcium and vitamin D are from 2011.[7] Values for adequate dietary vitamin D intake for optimal bone health were based on the assumption of minimal exposure to UVB solar radiation. For all age groups, the **Estimated Adequate Requirement (EAR)** is 10 micrograms (µg) per day (400 IU/day), whereas the **Recommended Dietary Allowance (RDA)** increases from 15 µg per day (600 IU/day) at 1 year of age to 20 µg per day (800 IU/d) for those over 70 years of age. Recommendations do not differ between males and females. At the population or public health level, the EAR value is most critical for assessing whether intakes are adequate to achieve population health. The RDA is used for setting individual-level guidelines. The **Tolerable Upper Intake Level (UL)** is of critical importance in guiding public health strategies to ensure safe intakes at all ages because monitoring is not realistic from either practical or fiscal standpoints.

Dietary Sources of Vitamin D

Cholecalciferol, or vitamin D3, is best known as the animal form. The less common form, ergocalciferol or vitamin D2, is known as the plant form. Vitamin D quantity is expressed in micrograms (μg) in the International System of Units (SI), but the common unit is the **international unit (IU):** 1 μg vitamin D is equal to 40 IU.

Natural Sources of Vitamin D

Few foods naturally contain vitamin D (**Table 21-1**). The most common natural vitamin D3 sources are fatty fish, such as salmon and tuna, and eggs. Smaller amounts of vitamin D2 are present in some irradiated mushrooms and certain bread products in Canada due to a manufacturing process with irradiated yeasts.[8] In 2013, the U.S. Food and Drug Administration (FDA) announced "that the amount of vitamin D allowed in bread and baked goods may be increased from a maximum level of 90 IU to 400 IU vitamin D per 100 g when using vitamin D baker's yeast."[9] Bioavailability and health effects of this source appear equal to vitamin D3.[10,11]

Vitamin D Fortification of Foods

In contrast to enrichment, which replaces nutrients that were removed during processing, **fortification** is the addition of a nutrient to foods. Successful fortification is

Table 21-1   Vitamin D content of foods in North America

Food	Amount (grams)	Amount (Household Measure)	Vitamin D Content (μg/IU per Amount) USDA Release 22[a]	CNF 2010[b]
Protein foods, meat, and alternatives				
Salmon, sockeye, cooked, dry heat	85	3 oz.	794	794 (USDA)
Salmon, chinook, smoked	85	3 oz.	583	439[b]
Salmon, pink canned, solids with bone and liquid	85	3 oz.	465	465 (USDA)
Tuna, light, canned in oil, drained solids	85	3 oz.	229	31[c]
Tuna, light, canned in water, drained solids	85	3 oz.	154	41[c]
Flounder and sole, cooked, dry heat	85	3 oz.	103	50[b]
Pork, shoulder, arm picnic, cooked, braised	85	3 oz.	68	68 (USDA)
Pork, cured, ham, roasted	85	3 oz.	28	28 (USDA)
Egg, whole, raw; or cooked, poached, hard boiled, or fried	46–50	1 large	25–27	28–30[d]
Turkey roast, boneless, roasted	85	3 oz.	7	7[b]
Beef, ground, 85% lean, cooked, broiled	85	3 oz.	6	6(USDA)
Chicken, breast, cooked, roasted	86	3 oz.	4	9[c]
Peanut butter, all types	16	1 tbsp.	0	0 (USDA)
Dairy, milk, and alternatives				
Milk, whole 3.25% milk fat with added vitamin D	250	1 cup	124	103[e]
Milk, reduced fat, fluid, 2% milk fat with added vitamin D	250	1 cup	120	103[e]
Milk, low fat, fluid, 1% milk fat with added vitamin D	250	1 cup	117	103[e]
Milk, non-fat (skim), fluid, with added vitamin A and vitamin D	250	1 cup	115	103[e]
Ricotta cheese, whole milk	246	1 cup	25	25 (USDA)
Rice drink, unsweetened, with added calcium, vitamins A and D	240	8 oz.	101	88[e] (250 ml)

(continues)

Table 21-1 Vitamin D content of foods in North America (continued)

Food	Amount (grams)	Amount (Household Measure)	Vitamin D Content (μg/IU per Amount) USDA Release 22[a]	CNF 2010[b]
Grains andgrain products				
Raisin Bran, General Mills, ready-to-eat (not including milk)	55	1 cup	104	0
Raisin Bran, Kellogg's, ready-to-eat (not including milk)	61	1 cup	41	0
Cheerios, General Mills, ready-to-eat (not including milk)	30	1 cup	43	0
Rice Krispies, Kellogg's, ready-to-eat (not including milk)	33	1 ¼ cup	41	0
Vegetables and fruit				
Mushrooms, shiitake, cooked	145	1 cup	45	45 (USDA)
Mushrooms, white, cooked, boiled, drained	156	1 cup	12	9-12 (USDA)
Mushrooms, Maitake, raw	72.9	1 cup	860	860 (USDA)
Orange juice with added calcium and vitamin D	250 ml	1 cup	–	100[e]

Note: One μg vitamin D3 = 40 IU vitamin D3.

Abbreviations: USDA, United States Department of Agriculture; CNF, Canadian Nutrient File.

[a] Canadian Nutrient File.

[b] Based on Canadian analytical data.

[c] Nutrient analyzed in a Canadian government lab.

[d] Nutrient analyzed in Canadian product (nongovernment lab).

[e] Nutrient levels changed to meet the Canadian regulations.

Data from USDA Agricultural Research Service. (2012). USDA National Nutrient Database for Standard Reference, Release 22 Nutrient Lists. Accessed September 10, 2013, from http://www.ars.usda.gov/SP2UserFiles/Place/12354500/Data/SR22/nutrlist/sr22w324.pdf.

affordable and safe for the general population, and it does not alter the taste of the foods. So that the majority of the population can benefit from fortification, staple foods are most commonly fortified. The FDA and Health Canada oversee food fortification policy in the United States and Canada, respectively. Vitamin D3 and D2 can both be fortificants.

Vitamin D Fortification of Foods in the United States and Canada

Fortified foods, such as fortified milk, provide the most dietary vitamin D in the United States.[12] Vitamin D was the second nutrient to be subject to voluntary food fortification in the United States in 1933, just after iodination of salt, attesting to its importance in public health. Originally added through irradiation of milk or feeding irradiated yeast to cows, vitamin D is now added to fluid milk with a target concentration of 400 IU per quart (385 IU per liter)

and allowable range of 400–600 IU per quart as per FDA regulation.[13] Even though quality control measures for vitamin D content of milk have been questioned in both Canada and the United States, data from 2007 show that U.S. manufacturers largely adhere to regulations,[14,15,16,17] with 77% of samples within the regulations, 16% below, and 7% above.[18]

Public health workers should be aware that fortification of eligible foods, including milk, is voluntary in the United States. When labeling, manufacturers may claim that milk is "fortified" only if it contains vitamin D. Therefore, public health messages should always specify "fortified milk" when referring to strategies to achieve vitamin D intake consistent with the EAR. Other dairy products made from milk, such as cheese, are often not fortified. Many ready-to-eat breakfast cereals contain added vitamin D, as do some brands of orange juice, yogurt, and margarine. The majority of the more than 600 foods whose vitamin D content has been analyzed have less than 100 IU of vitamin D per typical serving.[19]

Similarly, Canada began adding vitamin D to foods in the 1930s and 1940s. The government began regulating minimum and maximum levels in 1941 and 1949, respectively. Starting in 1950, vitamin D was added to evaporated and dried milks as a public health strategy to reduce rickets, but this was ineffective because most children consumed fluid milk. Fortification of fluid milk was permitted in the 1960s and made mandatory in 1975.[20] Under the Food and Drug Regulations at Health Canada, all fluid milk and plant-based milk alternatives[21] must contain 300 to 400 IU of vitamin D per reasonable daily intake (852 ml, or 30 fl. oz.); margarine contains 530 IU per 100 grams.

The success of vitamin D fortification policies in the United States and Canada is shown by the fact that milk is a leading source of vitamin D, and milk consumption is associated with higher vitamin D status.[22,23] However, many individuals may not be meeting the DRIs, and policy-making bodies will have to consider revision of fortification policy or education to enhance intakes of natural or fortified food sources. Some additional foods might be appropriate vehicles for fortification.[24] Furthermore, bioaddition of vitamin D is possible by incorporating vitamin D into animal feeds.

Effects of Preparation and Storage on Vitamin D Content of Foods

Food label claims must consider potential vitamin D losses during preparation and provide information based on the prepared or edible portion of a food product. In natural food sources, the specific type of food and food preparation are important considerations. Compared with raw salmon, baked salmon has 9% less vitamin D and fried salmon has 48% less. Furthermore, farmed salmon has 249 IU vitamin D in a 3.5-ounce serving, while wild salmon has 981 IU.[25] Nonetheless, farmed salmon still has a comparable content to many other fatty fish.

Vitamin D content in fortified foods can vary as well. Vitamin D is unstable with heating, sensitive to light exposure, and easily oxidized.[26] Up to 30% of vitamin D in milk may be lost in processing due to homogenization, separation, thermal treatment, and exposure to light.[27] Such losses might explain why some milk samples have vitamin D content below allowed limits.[28] Quality control in the food supply is an important public health responsibility of government agencies in the United States and Canada, especially with the dependence on fortified foods for vitamin D.

Additional Vitamin D Fortification Programs Worldwide

In Finland, vitamin D fortification of margarine began in 1950, and the program was expanded to include other fats and fluid milk to encourage adequate intake.[29] However, many individuals, such as teenage girls, young adults, or the elderly, may still have inadequate intake. Widespread vitamin D fortification was only recently allowed in the Netherlands,[30] and possibly may be allowed soon in other regions, including Europe[31] and India.[32] Population health surveys will help evaluate the success of these newer programs. The importance of selecting a food that is consumed by the majority of the population cannot be overstated.

Food Labeling

Even though Canadian and the U.S. dietary recommendations are merged through DRIs, food fortification policy varies, as does the nutritional information on food packaging. Thus, public health messages must be adjusted based on the target population. In the United States and Canada, food labels include Nutrition Facts tables. Vitamin D content of food is not required to be listed on labels, but it can be listed voluntarily. Vitamin D is expressed as a percentage of daily value (DV), which is 200 IU in Canada and 400 IU in the United States. In the United States the DV is equal to the EAR value of 400 IU for all people over the age of 1 year, and in Canada, the DV is only half of the EAR. Canadian labeling regulations are developed by Health Canada and the Food and Drugs Act and enforced by the Canadian Food Inspection Agency. U.S. guidelines are developed by the FDA. Because of the differences in DV between the two nations, a food labeled in the United States with a certain DV has a greater amount of vitamin D than a food labeled for Canadian markets. Those who purchase foods across borders must be aware of such differences, as must public health specialists who educate the public and make recommendations based on food labeling information.

Vitamin D Metabolism and Assessment of Status

Upon exposure of skin to UVB radiation, 7-dehydrocholesterol is converted to precholecalciferol that in turn is isomerized to vitamin D3. The form of vitamin D formed endogenously upon exposure to UVB radiation is cholecalciferol, or vitamin D3, which is the same form obtained from animal-based food sources, such as fish and eggs.

Risk Factors for Low Vitamin D Status

Various factors can limit endogenous synthesis and make dietary intake more relevant.

Dark Skin Tone

Melanin, a skin pigment, can reduce photosynthesis of vitamin D by 50-fold, increasing the risk for vitamin D deficiency among dark-skinned individuals.[33] Prevalence of low vitamin D status in African Americans, who compose 14% of the U.S. population, is more than twice as high as in non-Hispanic whites. Low vitamin D status in blacks may be related to higher rates of diabetes and cardiovascular disease in this group.[34]

Older Age

Age limits endogenous synthesis of vitamin D,[35] and an estimated 20.3% of the population in North America will be over 65 years of age by 2030.[36] Nearly 25% of the population is expected to be over 65 years by 2041 in Canada,[37] and by 2050, 25% of the global population will be over age 65. This increase in age is expected to contribute to an increase in hip fractures, as has been recorded in Japan, China, Sweden, and the Netherlands.[38] Expectations of aging populations are leading various nations to focus more on prevention strategies for osteoporotic fractures.

Consistent Use of Sunscreen

Sunscreen use is consistent with safe practices for skin cancer prevention, but those with a sun protection factor (SPF) of 8 or greater suppress endogenous synthesis of vitamin D.[39] These include products designed for regular outdoor activity as well as cosmetic products such as facial foundations. During the winter, endogenous synthesis is reduced because regions in the far northern latitudes of the Northern Hemisphere and far southern latitudes of the Southern Hemisphere do not receive sufficient UVB radiation to cause endogenous synthesis; furthermore, cold temperatures necessitate warm clothing, which blocks skin exposure.[40] In general, sufficient endogenous synthesis occurs only from April to October,[41] but the potential for synthesis is related to precise latitude. Populations living above the 42nd parallel north, including the United Kingdom, Scandinavia, and northern Russia, or below the 42nd parallel south, including southern New Zealand, Argentina, and Chile, are vulnerable in the winter. Individuals who are not able to be outdoors are vulnerable year-round. These situations underscore the importance of vitamin D from food or supplements.

Concealing Clothing

In addition to physiological reasons for reduced vitamin D synthesis, concealing clothing and sun-safe practices can also prevent UVB from eliciting endogenous synthesis. In fact, many women whose cultures require them to wear veils, such as the hijab in Muslim culture, have low vitamin D status.[42] The lower vitamin D status seems likely to be due to clothing, since boys[43] and men[44] have higher vitamin D status than women in these cultures. Similarly, sun-safe practices, including wearing long-sleeved shirts and pants and staying in the shade, result in lower vitamin D status in the United States.[45]

Vitamin D Metabolism

After entering circulation through endogenous synthesis or exogenous consumption, vitamin D is transported free or bound to vitamin D–binding protein. This protein, synthesized by the liver,[46] not only carries vitamin D within the blood but also extends its **half-life**. The liver removes 75% of vitamin D from circulation upon each pass for further metabolism to 25(OH)D.[47] 25(OH)D is released back into circulation, where it binds to vitamin D–binding protein, this time with stronger affinity.[48]

Serum 25(OH)D concentration is used to assess vitamin D status[49] because of its stability and long half-life of 10 to 21 days. It reflects exogenous consumption and endogenous production of vitamin D. Assays to assess vitamin D status should detect both $25(OH)D_2$ and $25(OH)D_3$, since both forms may be present. Accordingly, DRIs were set such that, with minimal sun exposure, the EAR for life-stage groups 1 to 50 years should align with a value of 40 nanomoles per liter (nmol/L) for serum 25(OH)D and the RDA with 50 nmol/L. For older adults (more than 70 years), the increased variability in the relationship between vitamin D intake and serum 25(OH)D led to an increased RDA to achieve the target concentration. Serum values of 25(OH)D below 30 nmol/L indicate deficiency.[50]

Vitamin D Intake and Status of Adults in North America

Surveillance programs can help monitor nutrient intake and status. The most common methodology for examining intakes of populations involves conducting **24-hour dietary recalls** among a random sample of the population, with correction for day-to-day variation made based on a second recall. Intake of nutrients, such as vitamin D, are then derived from a country-specific nutrient content of foods database. The **National Health and Nutrition Examination Survey (NHANES)** in the United States[51] and the 2004 Canadian Community Health Survey (CCHS) from 2004[52] suggest that in adults, vitamin D intakes from food are far below the EAR (**Table 21-2**). Fortified milk is the main source of vitamin D. Supplement use in the United States results in approximately half of men over

70 and women over 50 years of age meeting the EAR.[53] In Canada, however, the estimated contribution of supplements to total vitamin D intake is not yet available. The CCHS data indicate that 28–45% of men and 37–60% of women take vitamin/mineral supplements.[54] Similarly, national surveys in other countries, including the United Kingdom, Germany, and the Netherlands, find low vitamin D intakes.[55]

> *Public Health Core Competency 1: Analytical/ Assessment Skills 7: Identifies gaps in data sources*
>
> *Public Health Core Competency 1: Analytical/ Assessment Skills 10: Collects quantitative and qualitative community data*

Although dietary and supplemental intakes do not match the EAR, 67% of the adult population in the United States has a median serum 25(OH)D value categorized as "sufficient."[56] The risk of having vitamin D deficiency and inadequacy was higher in females than males and in adults compared with children. Canadians have similar trends.[57] Together, data showing exogenous intakes below recommended but largely sufficient serum vitamin D levels imply that the North American population likely obtains some

Table 21-2 Vitamin D intakes in adults in North America

| Age Group (years) | U.S. NHANES 2005-2006[a] | | Canada CCHS 2004[b] |
	Diet Alone µg/day	Diet + Supplements µg/day	Diet Alone µg/day
Males			
19-30	5.1 ± 0.3 (549)	6.6 ± 0.4	5.9 ± 0.2 (1804)
31-50	5.4 ± 0.3 (758)	7.9 ± 0.3	5.8 ± 0.2 (2596)
51-70	5.1 ± 0.3 (614)	8.8 ± 0.4	7.1 ± 0.5 (2550)
≥ 71	5.6 ± 0.4 (368)	10.7 ± 0.7	6.3 ± 0.4 (1520)
Females			
19-30	3.6 ± 0.3 (481)	5.8 ± 0.3	4.7 ± 0.2 (1854)
31-50	4.4 ± 0.3 (693)	7.7 ± 0.5	5.2 ± 0.3 (2686)
51-70	3.9 ± 0.4 (610)	10.1 ± 1.0	5.0 ± 0.3 (3200)
≥ 71	4.5 ± 0.2 (332)	10.0 ± 0.5	5.3 ± 0.3 (2610)

[a] Data are mean ± SE (n).

[b] Data are mean ± SE (n).

Data from: Bailey, R. L., Dodd, K. W., Goldman, J. A., Gahche, J. J., Dwyer, J. T., Moshfegh, A. J., . . . Picciano, M. F. (2010). Estimation of total usual calcium and vitamin D intakes in the United States. *Journal of Nutrition, 140*(4), 817-822. doi: jn.109.118539 [pii] 10.3945/jn.109.118539; Canadian Community Health Survey, Cycle 2.2, Nutrition (2004) - Nutrient Intakes from Food: Provincial, Regional and National Summary Data Tables, Volume 1, 2 and 3.

vitamin D from exposure to UVB. Evidence of seasonal differences of 6–14 nmol/L in randomly acquired populations in Canada support this hypothesis.[58] Milk fortification, whether voluntary or mandatory, further supports adequate vitamin D status. Canadian data associate consumption of more than one daily milk serving with 25(OH)D values at least 10 nmol/higher.[59] Efforts to maintain and enhance consumption of fortified foods are required in the public health domain to support the aging population. To allow more of the population to reach the EAR, new strategies, whether through increased food fortification or other venues, will be required.

The Canadian Food Guide recommends that adults consume two to three servings of milk and alternatives and, for adults over 50 years, a daily multivitamin supplement containing 400 IU of vitamin D.[60] The U.S. Department of Agriculture's (USDA) MyPlate guide recommends three servings.[61] Under these guidelines, dairy products alone can provide 300 IU vitamin D, with other foods providing the additional 100 IU to achieve the EAR. However, while milk provides a significant proportion of dietary vitamin D, milk consumption is well below targets. Only 26–35% of men and 16–28% of women meet recommendations in Canada;[62] in the United States, only 7.7% of adults achieve three daily servings of dairy products. Consumption is higher among higher-income individuals and non-Hispanic whites.[63] The differences in the proportions meeting the recommended servings in each nation likely reflect the differences in recommended servings. Overall, consumption of milk as a key vehicle for vitamin D fortification is below targets in North America.

Public Health Core Competency 1: Analytical/Assessment Skills 5: Identifies sources of public health data and information

Functions of Vitamin D and Physiological Roles

The best-recognized roles of vitamin D, and the focus of this chapter, are in calcium homeostasis and bone metabolism. While the best serum indicator of vitamin D status is 25(OH)D, the active form in the body is calcitriol, or 1,25-dihydroxyvitamin D ($1,25(OH)_2D$). The kidney synthesizes $1,25(OH)_2D$ from 25(OH)D for the purpose of calcium homeostasis, and other tissues synthesize the active form for other purposes.[64]

When the parathyroid glands sense a drop in serum ionized calcium concentration, parathyroid hormone (PTH) is released into the blood and reaches the kidney, resulting in conversion of 25(OH)D to $1,25(OH)_2D$. Both PTH and $1,25(OH)_2D$ work to mobilize calcium from bone, increase calcium absorption, and reduce excretion. Both 25(OH)D and PTH follow similar circannual rhythms,[65] although regardless of seasonality, PTH plateaus within the normal range when 25(OH)D concentration is over 50–80 nmol/L.[66] This plateau likely supports maintenance of bone mass.[67] Increased PTH can indicate loss of bone mineral, or bone resorption,[68] as well as low dietary intake of calcium. Elevated PTH levels and low vitamin D intake can result in the chronic conditions of **osteomalacia** and eventually osteoporosis,[69] with acute complications such as tetany and myopathy.

Osteoporosis and Public Health

Osteoporosis is "a disease characterized by low bone mass and microarchitectural deterioration of bone tissue, leading to enhanced bone fragility and a consequent increase in fracture risk."[70] The *Healthy People 2020* goals related to osteoporosis are to "prevent illness and disability related to arthritis and other rheumatic conditions, osteoporosis, and chronic back conditions."[71]

Osteoporotic fractures can occur in the vertebrae, distal forearm as a Colles' fracture, and various regions of the hip. Hip fractures are associated with the highest morbidity, mortality, and institutionalization.[72] An estimated 12 million Americans older than 50 years have osteoporosis.[73] Half of postmenopausal women will develop a fracture in their lifetime, with 25% developing a skeletal deformity and 15% suffering a hip fracture. Among women older than 50 in the United States, the prevalence of osteoporosis is lowest in non-Hispanic blacks and highest in Mexican Americans.[74] Prevalence rates for osteoporosis in adults are estimated to be 9% of the population, and for osteopenia or low bone mass, as high as 49%. In Canada, the prevalence of osteoporosis is 15.8% and 6.6% among women and men over age 50, respectively (**Figure 21-1**).[75]

The annual costs of osteoporosis and fractures in the United States are estimated to be $16 billion,[76] and fracture-related costs are as much as $137 million for women in Canada.[77] The healthcare costs for a hip fracture are $8,358 to $32,195 in U.S. dollars[78] and $21,396 to $25,306 in Canadian dollars.[79] These estimates do not include costs due to reduced

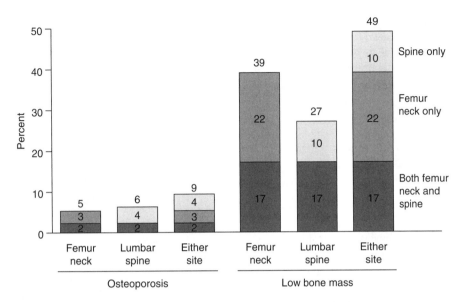

Figure 21-1 Osteoporosis or low bone mass at the femur neck only, lumbar spine only, or either site in adults aged 50 years and over

Reproduced from the Centers for Disease Control and Prevention. (2012). Osteoporosis or Low Bone Mass at the Femur Neck or Lumbar Spine in Older Adults: United States, 2005–2008. Retrieved from http://www.cdc.gov/nchs/data/data briefs/db93.htm#Fig2

quality of life. Primary prevention of osteopenia and osteoporosis and public health programs with suitable screening programs can be cost effective. Programs should reflect population needs, aging populations, and research progress.

Prevention of Osteoporosis

Clinical practice guidelines for the primary prevention and management of osteoporosis include performing weight-bearing activity and getting adequate calcium and vitamin D.[80,81] For high-risk groups, guidelines can include intakes of calcium and vitamin D that are higher than the EAR, which is for the general population. Canadian guidelines state that for adults over the age of 50 at moderate risk of deficiency, supplementation with 800–1000 IU of vitamin D is recommended, and dosages of 1000–2000 IU may be required and are safe.[82] Guidelines include assessment of vitamin D status three to four months after beginning to use vitamin D as pharmacotherapy. However, the healthcare system may not cover the test without a specific diagnosis of disease.[83] For example, vitamin D assessments based on serum 25(OH)D will be covered in Ontario, Canada, only after a diagnosis of osteoporosis, osteopenia, rickets, malabsorption syndromes, or renal disease, or with use of medications known to affect vitamin D metabolism.[84]

Public Health Core Competency 7: Financial Planning and Management Skills 13: Describes how cost-effectiveness, cost-benefit, and cost-utility analyses affect programmatic prioritization and decision making

Vitamin D nutrition has been studied most among adults over 65 years old. A National Institutes of Health review concluded that higher intakes of vitamin D are associated with better vitamin D status and increased bone mass and tooth retention, fewer falls, and improvements in physical ability.[85] The response of serum 25(OH)D to vitamin D fortification of foods seems to be better than the response from supplements,[86] although the effects of food versus supplemental vitamin D on bone health have not been as rigorously tested in aging adults. Nonetheless, achieving the EAR for vitamin D is considered beneficial to bone health.[87] Public health policy updates, task force initiatives, and communications should underscore the importance of vitamin D.

Screening for Osteoporosis

In both Canada and the United States, screening for osteoporosis is part of the public health system. The U.S. Preventive Services Task Force recommends that women of all races over 65 years of age, and those 50 to 64 years whose

Table 21-3   Indications for measuring bone mineral density in the United States

Population	Women aged ≥ 65 years without previous known fractures or secondary causes of osteoporosis	Women aged < 65 years whose 10-year fracture risk is equal to or greater than that of a 65-year-old white woman without additional risk factors	Men without previous known fractures or secondary causes of osteoporosis
Recommendation	Screen		No recommendation
	Grade: B		Grade: I (insufficient evidence)

Risk Assessment	As many as 1 in 2 postmenopausal women and 1 in 5 older men are at risk for an osteoporosis-related fracture. Osteoporosis is common in all racial groups but is most common in white persons. Rates of osteoporosis increase with age. Elderly people are particularly susceptible to fractures. According to the FRAX fracture risk assessment tool, available at www.shef.ac.uk/FRAX/, the 10-year fracture risk in a 65-year-old woman without additional risk factors is 9.3%.
Screening Tests	Current diagnostic and treatment criteria rely on dual-energy x-ray absorptiometry of the hip and lumbar spine.
Timing of Screening	Evidence is lacking about optimal intervals for repeated screening.
Interventions	In addition to adequate calcium and vitamin D intake and weight-bearing exercise, multiple U.S. Food and Drug Administration-approved therapies reduce fracture risk in women with low bone mineral density and no previous fractures, including bisphosphonates, parathyroid hormone, raloxifene, and estrogen. The choice of treatment should take into account the patient's clinical situation and the tradeoff between benefits and harms. Clinicians should provide education and how to minimize drug side effects.
Suggestions for Practice Regarding the I Statement for Men	Clinicians should consider: • Potential preventable burden: increasing because of the aging of the U.S. population • Potential harms: likely to be small, mostly opportunity costs • Current practice: routing screening of men is not widespread • Costs: additional scanners are required to screen sizable populations Men most likely to benefit from screening have a 10-year risk for osteoporotic fracture equal or greater than that of a 65-year-old white woman without risk factors. However, current evidence is insufficient to assess the balance of benefits and harms of screening for osteoporosis in men.

For a summary of the evidence systematically reviewed in making these recommendations, the full recommendation statement, and supporting documents, go to www.uspreventiveservicestaskforce.org.

Reproduced from the U.S. Preventative Services Task Force. (2011). Screening for osteoporosis: U.S. preventive services task force recommendation statement. *Annals of Internal Medicine, 154*(5), 356-64.

10-year fracture risk is as high as that of a normal 65-year-old, be screened for osteoporosis using dual-energy X-ray absorptiometry scans of the lumbar spine or hip.[88] The task force currently cites insufficient evidence to recommend such screening in men, although in 2008, the National Osteoporosis Foundation (NOF) recommended considering men and women over 50 for osteoporosis treatment.[89] The Canadian guidelines include screening women and men over 50 years of age for risk factors for osteoporosis and fracture, and assessing bone density assessment in higher-risk individuals, such as those over 65 and patients with other clinical risk factors.[90]

WHO's FRAX Prediction Tool

Launched in 2008, the World Health Organization's (WHO) fracture prediction tool called FRAX® aids in osteoporosis prevention, management, and eligibility for treatment. It is not dependent on bone density testing, and is used worldwide.[91] Assessments in the tool include age, sex, anthropometry, history of fractures in an individual and parents, lifestyle variables, such as smoking and alcohol use, and health conditions, including arthritis and medication use.[92] Healthcare providers can access the FRAX tool online to establish patients' 10-year risk of fracture risks (**Figure 21-2**).[93] For Canadians, race is not requested; for U.S.-based assessment, physicians must select the tool specific to white, black, Asian, and Hispanic ethnicities. Indicators for treatment include clinical information as well as FRAX tool results (**Table 21-4**).[94] Treatment eligibility rates are similar among Mexican American and non-Hispanic white women (32% and 32.8%) and lower among Hispanic black women (11%); in men, eligibility was 3.5% for non-Hispanic blacks, 12.6% for Mexican Americans, and 21.1% for non-Hispanic whites.[95]

Because of its biochemical nature, population-level assessment of vitamin D status can be impractical.[96] To monitor bone health and likelihood of fractures, other proposed assessment approaches include evaluating balance, dietary intake of vitamin D and other nutrients related to bone health, physical activity levels, smoking status, and vision.[97]

Vitamin D as a Treatment Measure for Osteoporosis

DRIs, food fortification guidelines, and food guides are population-level strategies to improve vitamin D status;

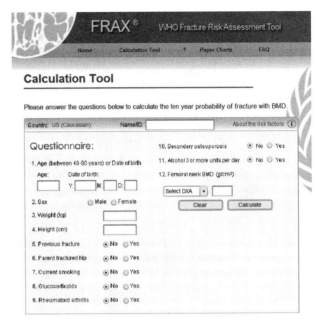

Figure 21-2 Fracture Risk Assessment Tool

Reproduced from the World Health Organization Collaborating Centre for Metabolic Bone Diseases. (2012). WHO Fracture Risk Assessment Tool. Retrieved from http://www.shef.ac.uk/FRAX/tool.jsp?country=9

clinical practice guidelines also recognize the significance of vitamin D in bone health. Public health measures should focus on adequate intake and emphasize, as appropriate, the need for daily adherence to supplementation regimens. The U.S. Preventive Services Task Force recommends vitamin D intakes consistent with the DRI values as a means to prevent falls, a primary prevention of osteoporosis measure.[98] Studies suggest that only one-quarter of adults with fractures receive therapies to prevent subsequent fractures (secondary prevention).[99,100,101] Vitamin D is an important component of treatment, but supplements are taken by less than 58% of those with fractures.[102] In the United States,

Table 21-4 Eligibility for treatment in the United States

Clinical
• Prior spine or hip fracture
• Lumbar spine or femoral neck bone mineral density (BMD) T-score ≤ −2.5
• Those with low bone mass or osteopenia (T-score −1 to −2.5) who have no prior spine or hip fracture
FRAX®
• 10-year probability ≥ 3% for a hip fracture or ≥ 20% for any major osteoporotic fracture (spine, hip, proximal humerus, or distal forearm fracture) according to FRAX

Data from National Osteoporosis Foundation. (2008). Clinician's guide to prevention and treatment of osteoporosis. Washington, DC: National Osteoporosis Foundation. http://www.nof.org/files/nof/public/content/file/344/upload/159.pdf Accessed August 28, 2013.

a study of white, black, and Hispanic adults with an average age of 79 suggests that previous fractures are directly related to adherence to vitamin D treatments.[103] Education, as simple as short video messages, was shown to triple the proportion of individuals taking vitamin D supplements three months later.[104]

Prescription-only high dosage supplements, containing as much as 50,000 IU per unit, are often covered by the respective healthcare or health insurance system. Coverage varies by region and specific policy. Based on an ambulatory setting in the United States, the most frequently prescribed medication for treatment of osteoporosis was bisphosphonates (36%) followed by calcium and vitamin D (24%).[105] Of particular importance from a public health perspective is that those with public insurance appear less likely to receive prescriptions. Whether new healthcare initiatives in the United States will change this remains to be seen. Over-the-counter vitamin D supplements are available with out-of-pocket payment.

Conclusion

Vitamin D has been the focus of many public health initiatives and policy related to bone health. Adults in North America, however, are largely underconsuming key food sources, such as vitamin D–fortified milk. Estimated population intakes are therefore below recommendations, with just over half of the population meeting recommendations. Inadequate intake is a risk factor for osteoporosis and fractures. *Healthy People 2020* goals include reduction in osteoporosis by 50%, a goal that is challenged by the limited sources of vitamin D and suboptimal dietary intake patterns. Comprehensive public health strategies are needed to enable healthier dietary intake patterns toward achievement of bone health.

References

1 Ross, A. C., Taylor, C. L., Yaktine, A. L., & Del Valle, H. B. (Eds.); Institute of Medicine. (2011). *Dietary Reference Intakes for calcium and vitamin D*. Washington, DC: National Academies Press. Retrieved from http://www.iom.edu/Reports/2010/Dietary-Reference-Intakes-for-calcium-and-vitamin-D.aspx

2 McCollum, E. V. (1967). The paths to the discovery of vitamins A and D. *Journal of Nutrition, 91*(2 Suppl. 1), 11-16.

3 Chick, H., Dalyell, E. J., Hume, M., Mackay, H. M. M., Smith, H. H., & Wimberger, H. (1922). The aetiology of rickets in infants: Prophylactic and curative observations at the Vienna University Kinderklinik. *Lancet, 2*, 7-11.

4 U.S. Department of Health and Human Services. (2012, September 26). *Arthritis, osteoporosis, and chronic back conditions*. Retrieved from HealthyPeople.gov website, http://www.healthypeople.gov/2020/topicsobjectives2020/overview.aspx?topicid=3

5 Wacker, M., & Fink, M. F. (2013). Vitamin D–Effects on skeletal and extraskeletal health and the need for supplementation. *Nutrition, 5*(1), 111-48.

6 Allen, L., Benoist, B., Dary, O., & Hurrell, R. (Eds.). (2006). *Guidelines on food fortification with micronutrients*. Geneva: World Health Organization and Food and Agricultural Organization. Retrieved from http://whqlibdoc.who.int/publications/2006/9241594012_eng.pdf

7 Ross, A. C., Taylor, C. L., Yaktine, A. L., & Del Valle, H. B. (Eds.); Institute of Medicine. (2011). *Dietary Reference Intakes for calcium and vitamin D*. Washington, DC: National Academies Press. Retrieved from http://www.iom.edu/Reports/2010/Dietary-Reference-Intakes-for-calcium-and-vitamin-D.aspx

8 Canada Gazette. (2011, February 19). *Archived–government notices*. Retrieved from http://www.gazette.gc.ca/rp-pr/p1/2011/2011-02-19/html/notice-avis-eng.html

9 Food and Drug Administration. (2013, May 28). *2012 food and color additive final rules*. Retrieved from http://www.fda.gov/Food/GuidanceRegulation/GuidanceDocumentsRegulatoryInformation/IngredientsAdditivesGRASPackaging/ucm303415.htm

10 Hohman, E. E., Martin, B. R., Lachcik, P. J., Gordon, D. T., Fleet, J. C., & Weaver, C. M. (2011). Bioavailability and efficacy of vitamin D2 from UV-irradiated yeast in growing, vitamin D-deficient rats. *Journal of Agricultural and Food Chemistry, 59*(6), 2341-46. doi:10.1021/jf104679c

11 Holick, M. F., Biancuzzo, R. M., Chen, T. C., Klein, E. K., Young, A., Bibuld, D., . . . Tannenbaum, A. D. (2008). Vitamin D2 is as effective as vitamin D3 in maintaining circulating concentrations of 25-hydroxyvitamin D. *Journal of Clinical Endocrinology and Metabolism, 93*(3), 677-81. doi:jc.2007-2308 [pii] 10.1210/jc.2007-2308

12 Drewnowski, A. (2011). The contribution of milk and milk products to micronutrient density and affordability of the U.S. diet. *Journal of the American College of Nutrition, 30*(5 Suppl. 1), 422S-428S. doi:30/5_Supplement_1/422S [pii]

13 Calvo, M. S., Whiting, S. J., & Barton, C. N. (2004). Vitamin D fortification in the United States and Canada: Current status and data needs. *American Journal of Clinical Nutrition, 80*(6 Suppl), 1710S-1716S. doi:80/6/1710S [pii]

14 Chen, T. C., Shao, A., Heath, H., III, & Holick, M. F. (1993). An update on the vitamin D content of fortified milk from the United States and Canada. *New England Journal of Medicine, 329*(20), 1507.

15 Holden, J. M., Lemar, L. E., & Exler, J. (2008). Vitamin D in foods: Development of the U.S. Department of Agriculture database. *American Journal of Clinical Nutrition, 87*(4), 1092S-96S. doi:87/4/1092S [pii]

16 Holick, M. F., Shao, Q., Liu, W. W., & Chen, T. C. (1992). The vitamin D content of fortified milk and infant formula. *New England Journal of Medicine, 326*(18), 1178-81. doi:10.1056 /NEJM199204303261802

17 Tanner, J. T., Smith, J., Defibaugh, P., Angyal, G., Villalobos, M., Bueno, M. P., et al. (1988). Survey of vitamin content of fortified milk. *Journal of the Association of Official Analytical Chemists, 71*(3), 607-10.

18 Patterson, K. Y., Phillips, K. M., Horst, R. L., Byrdwell, W. C., Exler, J., Lemar, L. E., & Holden, J. M. (2010). Vitamin D content and variability in fluid milks from a U.S. Department of Agriculture nationwide sampling to update values in the National Nutrient Database for Standard Reference. *Journal of Dairy Science, 93*(11), 5082-90. doi: S0022-0302(10)00548-5 [pii] 10.3168 /jds.2010-3359

19 Holden, J. M., Lemar, L. E., & Exler, J. (2008). Vitamin D in foods: Development of the U.S. Department of Agriculture database. *American Journal of Clinical Nutrition, 87*(4), 1092S-1096S. doi:87/4/1092S [pii]

20 Health Canada. (1999). Addition of vitamins and minerals to foods. *Proposed Policy Recommendations.* Ottawa: Bureau of Nutritional Sciences, Food Directorate, Health Protection Branch.

21 Health Canada. (1999). Addition of vitamins and minerals to foods. *Proposed Policy Recommendations.* Ottawa: Bureau of Nutritional Sciences, Food Directorate, Health Protection Branch.

22 Bailey, R. L., Dodd, K. W., Goldman, J. A., Gahche, J. J., Dwyer, J. T., Moshfegh, A. J., . . . Picciano, M. F. (2010). Estimation of total usual calcium and vitamin D intakes in the United States. *Journal of Nutrition, 140*(4), 817-22. doi:jn.109.118539 [pii] 10.3945/jn.109.118539

23 Barake, R., Weiler, H., Payette, H., & Gray-Donald, K. (2010). Vitamin D status in healthy free-living elderly men and women living in Quebec, Canada. *Journal of the American College of Nutrition, 29*(1), 25-30. doi:29/1/25 [pii]

24 Calvo, M. S., & Whiting, S. J. (2013). Survey of current vitamin D food fortification practices in the Unites States and Canada. *Journal of Steroid Biochemistry and Molecular Biology, 136*, 211-13.

25 Chen, T., Chimeh, F., Lu, Z., Mathieu, J., Person, K., Zhang, A., . . . Holick, M. (2007). Factors that influence the cutaneous synthesis and dietary sources of vitamin D. *Archives of Biochemistry and Biophysics, 460*(2), 213-17.

26 Perales, S., Alegría, A., Barberá, R., & Farré, R. (2005). Review: Determination of vitamin D in dairy products by high performance liquid chromatography. *Food Science and Technology International, 11*(6), 451-62.

27 Indyk, H., Littlejohn, V., & Woollard, D. C. (1996). Stability of vitamin D3 during spray-drying of milk. *Food Chemistry, 57*(2), 283-86.

28 Patterson, K. Y., Phillips, K. M., Horst, R. L., Byrdwell, W. C., Exler, J., Lemar, L. E., & Holden, J. M. (2010). Vitamin D content and variability in fluid milks from a U.S. Department of Agriculture nationwide sampling to update values in the National Nutrient Database for Standard Reference. *Journal of Dairy Science, 93*(11), 5082-90. doi:S0022-0302(10)00548-5 [pii] 10.3168 /jds.2010-3359

29 Pietinen, P., Mannisto, S., Valsta, L. M., & Sarlio-Lahteenkorva, S. (2010). Nutrition policy in Finland. *Public Health Nutrition, 13*(6A), 901-6.

30 Kloosterman, J., Fransen, H. P., de Stoppelaar, J., Verhagen, H., & Rompelberg, C. (2007). Safe addition of vitamins and minerals to foods: Setting maximum levels for fortification in the Netherlands. *European Journal of Nutrition, 46*(4), 220-29.

31 De Lourdes Samaniego-Vaesken, M., Alonso-Aperte, E., & Varela-Moreiras, G. (2012). Vitamin fortification today. *Food and Nutrition Research, 56*, 5459. doi:10.3402/fnr.v56i0.5459

32 Babu, U. S., & Calvo, M. S. (2010). Modern India and the vitamin D dilemma: Evidence for the need of a national food fortification program. *Molecular Nutrition and Food Research, 54*(8), 1134-47.

33 Holick, M. F. (2003). Vitamin D: A millenium perspective. *Journal of Cellular Biochemistry, 88*(2), 296-307.

34 Harris, S. S. (2006). Vitamin D and African Americans. *Journal of Nutrition, 136*(4), 1126-29.

35 Need, A. G., Morris, H. A., Horowitz, M., & Nordin, C. (1993). Effects of skin thickness, age, body fat, and sunlight on serum 25-hydroxyvitamin D. *American Journal of Clinical Nutrition, 58*(6), 882-85.

36 Centers for Disease Control and Prevention. (2003). Public health and aging: Trends in aging–United States and worldwide. *Journal of the American Medical Association, 289*(11), 1371-73.

37 Statistics Canada. (2002, July). *Profile of the Canadian population by age and sex: Canada ages.* Retrieved from www.statcan.ca

38 Marks, R. (2010). Hip fracture epidemiological trends, outcomes and risk factors, 1970-2009. *International Journal of General Medicine, 3,* 1-17.

39 Holick, M. F. (2003). Vitamin D: A millenium perspective. *Journal of Cellular Biochemistry, 88*(2), 296-307.

40 Webb, A. R., Kline, L., & Holick, M. F. (1988). Influence of season and latitude on the cutaneous synthesis of vitamin D3: Exposure to winter sunlight in Boston and Edmonton will not promote vitamin D3 synthesis in human skin. *Journal of Clinical Endocrinology and Metabolism, 67*(2), 373-78.

41 Webb, A. R., Kline, L., & Holick, M. F. (1988). Influence of season and latitude on the cutaneous synthesis of vitamin D3: Exposure to winter sunlight in Boston and Edmonton will not promote vitamin D3 synthesis in human skin. *Journal of Clinical Endocrinology and Metabolism, 67*(2), 373-78.

42 Al Attia, H. M., & Ibrahim, M. A. (2012). The high prevalence of vitamin D inadequacy and dress style of women in the sunny UAE. *Archives of Osteoporosis, 7,* 307-10,

43 Al-Ghamdi, M. A., Lanaham-New, S. A. & Kahn, J. A. (2012). Differences in vitamin D status and calcium metabolism in Saudi Arabian boys and girls aged 6 to 18 years: Effects of age, gender, extent of veiling and physical activity with concomitant implications for bone health. *Public Health Nutrition, 15*(10), 1845-53.

44 Elshafie, D. E., Al-Khashan, H. I., & Mishriky, A. M. (2012). Comparison of vitamin D deficiency in Saudi married couples. *European Journal of Clinical Nutrition, 66*(6), 742-45.

45 Linos, E., Keiser, E., Kanzler, M., Sainani, K. L., Lee, W., Vittinghoff, E., Chren, M. M., & Tang, J. Y. (2012). Sun protective behaviors and vitamin D levels in the U.S. population: NHANES 2003-2006. *Cancer Causes and Control, 23*(1), 133-40.

46 Speeckaert, M., Huang, G., Delanghe, J. R., & Taes, Y. E. (2006). Biological and clinical aspects of the vitamin D binding protein (Gc-globulin) and its polymorphism. *Clinica Chimica Acta, 372*(1-2), 33-42.

47 Miller, W. L., & Portale, A. A. (2000). Vitamin D 1 alpha-hydroxylase. *Trends in Endocrinology and Metabolism, 11*(8), 315-19.

48 Speeckaert, M., Huang, G., Delanghe, J. R., & Taes, Y. E. (2006). Biological and clinical aspects of the vitamin D binding protein (Gc-globulin) and its polymorphism. *Clinica Chimica Acta, 372*(1-2), 33-42.

49 Ross, A. C., Taylor, C. L., Yaktine, A. L., & Del Valle, H. B. (Eds.); Institute of Medicine. (2011). *Dietary Reference Intakes for calcium and vitamin D*. Washington, DC: National Academies Press. Retrieved from http://www.iom.edu/Reports/2010 /Dietary-Reference-Intakes-for-calcium-and-vitamin-D.aspx

50 Ross, A. C., Taylor, C. L., Yaktine, A. L., & Del Valle, H. B. (Eds.); Institute of Medicine. (2011). *Dietary Reference Intakes for calcium and vitamin D*. Washington, DC: National Academies Press. Retrieved from http://www.iom.edu/Reports/2010 /Dietary-Reference-Intakes-for-calcium-and-vitamin-D.aspx

51 Bailey, R. L., Dodd, K. W., Goldman, J. A., Gahche, J. J., Dwyer, J. T., Moshfegh, A. J., . . . Picciano, M. F. (2010). Estimation of total usual calcium and vitamin D intakes in the United States. *Journal of Nutrition, 140*(4), 817-22. doi:jn.109.118539 [pii] 10.3945/jn.109.118539

52 Vatanparast, H., Calvo, M. S., Green, T. J., & Whiting, S. J. (2010). Despite mandatory fortification of staple foods, vitamin D intakes of Canadian children and adults are inadequate. *Journal of Steroid Biochemistry and Molecular Biology, 121*(1-2), 301-3. doi:S0960-0760(10)00178-0 [pii] 10.1016/j.jsbmb.2010.03.079

53 Bailey, R. L., Dodd, K. W., Goldman, J. A., Gahche, J. J., Dwyer, J. T., Moshfegh, A. J., . . . Picciano, M. F. (2010). Estimation of total usual calcium and vitamin D intakes in the United States. *Journal of Nutrition, 140*(4), 817-22. doi:jn.109.118539 [pii] 10.3945/jn.109.118539

54 Vatanparast, H., Calvo, M. S., Green, T. J., & Whiting, S. J. (2010). Despite mandatory fortification of staple foods, vitamin D intakes of Canadian children and adults are inadequate. *Journal of Steroid Biochemistry and Molecular Biology, 121*(1-2), 301-3. doi:S0960-0760(10)00178-0 [pii] 10.1016/j .jsbmb.2010.03.079

55 Troesch, B., Hoeft, B., McBurney, M., Eggersdorfer, M., & Weber, P. (2012). Dietary surveys indicate vitamin intakes below recommendations are common in representative Western countries. *British Journal of Nutrition, 108*(4), 692-98. doi:S0007114512001808 [pii] 10.1017/S0007114512001808

56 Looker, A. C., Johnson, C. L., Lacher, D. A., Pfeiffer, C. M., Schleicher, R. L., & Sempos, C. T. (2011). Vitamin D status: United States, 2001-2006. *National Center for Health Statistics Data Brief*, (59), 1-8.

57 Langlois, K., Greene-Finestone, L. S., Little, J., Hidiroglou, N., & Whiting, S. (2010). Vitamin D status of Canadians as measured in the 2007 to 2009 Canadian Health Measures Survey. *Health Reports, 21*, 47-55.

58 Barake, R., Weiler, H., Payette, H., & Gray-Donald, K. (2010). Vitamin D status in healthy free-living elderly men and women living in Quebec, Canada. *Journal of the American College of Nutrition, 29*(1), 25-30. doi:29/1/25 [pii]

59 Langlois, K., Greene-Finestone, L. S., Little, J., Hidiroglou, N., & Whiting, S. (2010). *Vitamin D status of Canadians as measured in the 2007 to 2009 Canadian Health Measures Survey. Health Reports, 21*, 47-55.

60 Health Canada. (2012, September 28). *Eating well with Canada's food guide*. Retrieved from http://www.hc-sc.gc.ca /fn-an/food-guide-aliment/index-eng.php

61 United States Department of Agriculture. (2012, September 28). *ChooseMyPlate.gov*. Retrieved from http://www.choosemyplate .gov

62 Statistics Canada. (2004). *Nutrition: Findings from the Canadian Community Health Survey. Overview of Canadians' eating habits* (p. 47). Ottawa: Health Statistics Division.

63 Kirkpatrick, S. I., Dodd, K. W., Reedy, J., & Krebs-Smith, S. M. (2012). Income and race/ethnicity are associated with adherence to food-based dietary guidance among U.S. adults and children. *Journal of the Academy of Nutrition and Dietetics, 112*(5), 624-35 e626. doi:S2212-2672(11)01943-5 [pii] 10.1016 /j.jand.2011.11.012

64 Zehnder, D., Evans, K. N., Kilby, M. D., Bulmer, J. N., Innes, B. A., Stewart, P. M., & Hewison, M. (2002). The ontogeny of 25-hydroxyvitamin D(3) 1alpha-hydroxylase expression in human placenta and decidua. *American Journal of Pathology, 161*(1), 105-14.

65 Schmitt, C. P., Homme, M., & Schaefer, F. (2005). Structural organization and biological relevance of oscillatory parathyroid hormone secretion. *Pediatric Nephrology, 20*(3), 346-51.

66 Dawson-Hughes, B., Heaney, R. P., Holick, M. F., Lips, P., Meunier, P. J., & Vieth, R. (2005). Estimates of optimal vitamin D status. *Osteoporosis International, 16*(7), 713-16.

67 Bischoff-Ferrari, H. A., Willett, W. C., Wong, J. B., Giovannucci, E., Dietrich, T., & Dawson-Hughes, B. (2005). Fracture prevention with vitamin D supplementation: A meta-analysis of randomized controlled trials. *Journal of the American Medical Association, 293*(18), 2257-64.

68 Pasco, J. A., Henry, M. J., Kotowicz, M. A., Sanders, K. M., Seeman, E., Pasco, J. R., . . . Nicholson, G. C. (2004). Seasonal periodicity of serum vitamin D and parathyroid hormone, bone resorption, and fractures: The Geelong Osteoporosis Study. *Journal of Bone and Mineral Research, 19*(5), 752-58.

69 Whiting, S. J., & Calvo, M. S. (2005). Dietary recommendations for vitamin D: A critical need for functional end points to establish an estimated average requirement. *Journal of Nutrition, 135*(2), 304-9.

70 Kanis, J. A., Melton, L. J., III, Christiansen, C., Johnston, C. C., & Khaltaev, N. (1994). The diagnosis of osteoporosis. *Journal*

of Bone and Mineral Research, 9(8), 1137–41. doi:10.1002/jbmr.5650090802

71 U.S. Department of Health and Human Services. (2012, September 26). *HealthyPeople.gov Arthritis, Osteoporosis, and Chronic Back Conditions.* Retrieved from http://www.healthypeople.gov/2020/topicsobjectives2020/overview.aspx?topicId=3

72 Martinez-Reig, M., Ahmad, L., & Duque, G. (2012). The orthogeriatrics model of care: Systematic review of predictors of institutionalization and mortality in post-hip fracture patients and evidence for interventions. *Journal of the American Medical Directors Association, 13*(9), 770–77. doi:S1525-8610(12)00234-4 [pii] 10.1016/j.jamda.2012.07.011

73 U.S. Preventive Services Task Force. (2011). Screening for osteoporosis: U.S. Preventive Services Task Force recommendation statement. *Annals of Internal Medicine, 154*(5), 356–64. doi:0003-4819-154-5-201103010-00307 [pii] 10.1059/0003-4819-154-5-201103010-00307

74 Dawson-Hughes, B., Looker, A. C., Tosteson, A. N., Johansson, H., Kanis, J. A., & Melton, L. J., III. (2012). The potential impact of the National Osteoporosis Foundation guidance on treatment eligibility in the USA: An update in NHANES 2005-2008. *Osteoporosis International, 23*(3), 811–20. doi:10.1007/s00198-011-1694-y

75 Tenenhouse, A., Joseph, L., Kreiger, N., Poliquin, S., Murray, T. M., Blondeau, L., . . . Prior, J. C. (2000). Estimation of the prevalence of low bone density in Canadian women and men using a population-specific DXA reference standard: The Canadian Multicentre Osteoporosis Study (CaMos). *Osteoporosis International, 11*(10), 897–904.

76 Blume, S. W., & Curtis, J. R. (2011). Medical costs of osteoporosis in the elderly Medicare population. *Osteoporosis International, 22*(6), 1835–44.

77 Leslie, W. D., Lix, L. M., Finlayson, G. S., Metge, C. J., Morin, S. N., & Majumdar, S. R. (2013). Direct healthcare costs for 5 years post-fracture in Canada: A long-term population-based assessment. *Osteoporosis International, 24,* 1697–1705.

78 Budhia, S., Mikyas, Y., Tang, M., & Badamgarav, E. (2012). Osteoporotic fractures: A systematic review of U.S. healthcare costs and resource utilization. *Pharamacoeconomics, 30*(2), 147–70.

79 Leslie, W. D., Lix, L. M., Finlayson, G. S., Metge, C. J., Morin, S. N., & Majumdar, S. R. (2013). Direct healthcare costs for 5 years post-fracture in Canada: A long-term population-based assessment. *Osteoporosis International, 24,* 1697–1705.

80 Papaioannou, A., Morin, S., Cheung, A. M., Atkinson, S., Brown, J. P., Feldman, S., . . . Leslie, W. D. (2010). 2010 clinical practice guidelines for the diagnosis and management of osteoporosis in Canada: summary. *Canadian Medical Association Journal, 182*(17), 1864–73. doi:cmaj.100771 [pii] 10.1503/cmaj.100771

81 U.S. Preventive Services Task Force. (2011). Screening for osteoporosis: U.S. Preventive Services Task Force recommendation statement. *Annals of Internal Medicine, 154*(5), 356–64. doi: 0003-4819-154-5-201103010-00307 [pii] 10.1059/0003-4819-154-5-201103010-00307

82 Papaioannou, A., Morin, S., Cheung, A. M., Atkinson, S., Brown, J. P., Feldman, S., . . . Leslie, W. D. (2010). 2010 clinical practice guidelines for the diagnosis and management of osteoporosis in Canada: Summary. *Canadian Medical Association Journal, 182*(17), 1864–73. doi: cmaj.100771 [pii] 10.1503/cmaj.100771

83 Vieth, R. (2012). Implications for 25-hydroxyvitamin D testing of public health policies about the benefits and risks of vitamin D fortification and supplementation. *Scandinavian Journal of Clinical and Laboratory Investigation Supplement, 243,* 144–53. doi:10.3109/00365513.2012.682893

84 Ontario Ministry of Health and Long-Term Care. (2012, September 26). *Ontario Health Insurance Plan vitamin D testing.* Retrieved from http://www.health.gov.on.ca/en/public/programs/ohip/changes/vitamin_d.aspx

85 Cranney, A., Horsley, T., O'Donnell, S., Weiler, H., Puil, L., Ooi, D., . . . Mamaladze, V. (2007). Effectiveness and safety of vitamin D in relation to bone health. *Evidence Report/Technology Assessment,* (158), 1–235.

86 Cranney, A., Horsley, T., O'Donnell, S., Weiler, H., Puil, L., Ooi, D., . . . Mamaladze, V. (2007). Effectiveness and safety of vitamin D in relation to bone health. *Evidence Report/Technology Assessment,* (158), 1–235.

87 Ross, A. C., Taylor, C. L., Yaktine, A. L., & Del Valle, H. B. (Eds.), for the Institute of Medicine. (2011). *Dietary Reference Intakes for calcium and vitamin D.* Washington, DC: National Academies Press. Retrieved from http://www.iom.edu/Reports/2010/Dietary-Reference-Intakes-for-calcium-and-vitamin-D.aspx

88 U.S. Preventive Services Task Force. (2011). Screening for osteoporosis: U.S. Preventive Services Task Force recommendation statement. *Annals of Internal Medicine, 154*(5), 356–64. doi: 0003-4819-154-5-201103010-00307 [pii]10.1059/0003-4819-154-5-201103010-00307

89 National Osteoporosis Foundation. (2008). *Clinician's guide to prevention and treatment of osteoporosis.* Washington, DC: National Osteoporosis Foundation.

90 Papaioannou, A., Morin, S., Cheung, A. M., Atkinson, S., Brown, J. P., Feldman, S., . . . Leslie, W. D. (2010). 2010 clinical practice guidelines for the diagnosis and management of osteoporosis in Canada: Summary. *Canadian Medical Association Journal, 182*(17), 1864–73. doi:cmaj.100771 [pii] 10.1503/cmaj.100771

91 McCloskey, E., & Kanis, J. A. (2012). FRAX updates 2012. *Current Opinion in Rheumatology, 24*(5), 554–60. doi:10.1097/BOR.0b013e328356d2f5

92 Kanis, J. A., Johnell, O., Oden, A., Johansson, H., & McCloskey, E. (2008). FRAX and the assessment of fracture probability in men and women from the UK. *Osteoporosis International, 19*(4), 385–97. doi:10.1007/s00198-007-0543-5

93 World Health Organization Collaborating Centre for Metabolic Bone Diseases. (2012, September 26). *WHO fracture risk assessment tool.* Retrieved from http://www.shef.ac.uk/FRAX/

94 Papaioannou, A., Morin, S., Cheung, A. M., Atkinson, S., Brown, J. P., Feldman, S., . . . Leslie, W. D. (2010). 2010 clinical practice guidelines for the diagnosis and management of osteoporosis in Canada: Summary. *Canadian Medical Association Journal, 182*(17), 1864–73. doi:cmaj.100771 [pii] 10.1503/cmaj.100771

95 Dawson-Hughes, B., Looker, A. C., Tosteson, A. N., Johansson, H., Kanis, J. A., & Melton, L. J., III. (2012). The potential impact of the National Osteoporosis Foundation guidance on treatment eligibility in the USA: An update in NHANES 2005–2008. *Osteoporosis International, 23*(3), 811–20. doi:10.1007/s00198-011-1694-y

96 Allen, L., Benoist, B., Dary, O., & Hurrell, R. (Eds.). (2006). Guidelines on food fortification with micronutrients. *World Health Organization and Food and Agricultural Organization.* Retrieved from http://whqlibdoc.who.int/publications/2006/9241594012_eng.pdf

97 Marks, R. (2010). Hip fracture epidemiological trends, outcomes and risk factors, 1970–2009. *International Journal of General Medicine, 3,* 1–17.

98 Moyer, V. A. (2012). Prevention of falls in community-dwelling older adults: U.S. Preventive Services Task Force Recommendation Statement. *Annals of Internal Medicine, 157*(3), 197–204. doi:1305528 [pii] 10.7326/0003-4819-157-3-201208070-00462

99 Bessette, L., Ste-Marie, L. G., Jean, S., Davison, K. S., Beaulieu, M., Baranci, M., . . . Brown, J. P. (2008). The care gap in diagnosis and treatment of women with a fragility fracture. *Osteoporosis International, 19*(1), 79–86. doi:10.1007/s00198-007-0426-9

100 Fraser, L. A., Ioannidis, G., Adachi, J. D., Pickard, L., Kaiser, S. M., Prior, J., . . . Papaioannou, A. (2011). Fragility fractures and the osteoporosis care gap in women: The Canadian Multicentre Osteoporosis Study. *Osteoporosis International, 22*(3), 789–96. doi:10.1007/s00198-010-1359-2

101 Papaioannou, A., Giangregorio, L., Kvern, B., Boulos, P., Ioannidis, G., & Adachi, J. D. (2004). The osteoporosis care gap in Canada. *BMC Musculoskeletal Disorders, 5,* 11.

102 Bessette, L., Ste-Marie, L. G., Jean, S., Davison, K. S., Beaulieu, M., Baranci, M., . . . Brown, J. P. (2008). The care gap in diagnosis and treatment of women with a fragility fracture. *Osteoporosis International, 19*(1), 79–86. doi:10.1007/s00198-007-0426-9

103 Unson, C. G., Litt, M., Reisine, S., Mahoney-Trella, P., Sheperd, T., & Prestwood, K. (2006). Adherence to calcium/vitamin D and estrogen protocols among diverse older participants enrolled in a clinical trial. *Contemporary Clinical Trials, 27*(3), 215–26. doi:S1551-7144(06)00007-3 [pii] 10.1016/j.cct.2006.02.006

104 Kulp, J. L., Rane, S., & Bachmann, G. (2004). Impact of preventive osteoporosis education on patient behavior: Immediate and 3-month follow-up. *Menopause, 11*(1), 116–19. doi:10.1097/01.GME.0000079221.19081.11 00042192-200411010-00019 [pii]

105 Teschemaker, A., Lee, E., Xue, Z., & Wutoh, A. K. (2008). Osteoporosis pharmacotherapy and counseling services in U.S. ambulatory care clinics: Opportunities for multidisciplinary interventions. *American Journal of Geriatric Pharmacotherapy, 6*(5), 240–48. doi:S1543-5946(08)00073-1 [pii] 10.1016/j.amjopharm.2008.12.002

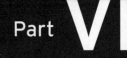

Community and Global Public Health Nutrition in a Changing World

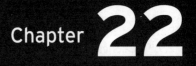
Global Changes in Diet and Physical Activity: The Nutrition Transition

Hala Madanat, PhD
Iyas Masannat, RPh, MS

"It's an urgent question. It's one we have to ask, and we have to start answering. We know we are what we eat. We need to realize that the world is also what we eat. But if we take that idea, we can use food as a really powerful tool to shape the world better."–Carolyn Steele, Architect, in a Ted Talk

Reproduced from: C Steele. (July 2009). How food shapes our cities. (Ted Talk). http://www.ted.com/talks/carolyn_steel_how_food_shapes_our_cities.html Accessed. August 28, 2013.

Learning Objectives

- Define the nutrition transition and place it in the context of economic and demographic transitions.

- Describe the dietary patterns associated with the nutrition transition.

- Identify the driving forces of the nutrition transition.

- Describe the effects of the nutrition transition on nutritional status, health outcomes, and healthcare systems.

- Discuss some of the ongoing research and the documented examples of the nutrition transition globally.

- Consider strategies that can reduce negative consequences of the nutrition transition and the dual burden of malnutrition.

Case Study: Jordan

Jordan is a small Middle Eastern country with limited resources. Its population of over 6.5 million has a very young demographic, with median age 22.4 years.[1] Like many developing nations, Jordan has been rapidly undergoing significant economic and social transition. Jordan's location, bordering Iraq, Syria, Saudi Arabia, Palestine, and Israel, puts it amid much of the political unrest in the region and makes it a destination for refugees. In 2012,

Jordan had 1,979,580 Palestinian, 173,680 Syrian, and 29,286 Iraqi refugees.[2] These population changes, combined with high rates of urbanization (79%)[3] and changes in economic conditions, have affected food systems, food supply, agriculture, and physical activity levels and have resulted in a rapid nutrition transition.[4]

Changes in Diet Intake

As in many other developing countries, Jordan's dietary energy supply (DES) has increased in recent decades.[5]

Data from 2005 to 2007 indicate that the DES had reached 2,979 kcalories per person per day (kcal/capita/day), exceeding estimated requirements of 2,056 kcal/capita/day.[6] Over the past four decades, fruit, vegetable, and cereal consumption has decreased, and consumption of meat and other animal products has increased.[7] Self-reported data suggest that in 2007, only 17% of survey adults ate three or more cups of fruits and vegetables per day.[8] The proportion of calories from fat has increased to 30% of total calories.[9]

Consequences of the Nutrition Transition in Jordan

Effects of the nutrition transition are evident in increases in nutrition-related noncommunicable diseases (NCDs), which are now the leading cause of morbidity and mortality within the country.[10] In 2003, cardiovascular disease accounted for 38.2% of all deaths in Jordan, while cancer accounted for 14.3%.[11] In 2004, NCD prevalence among adults included 19.5% for obesity, 7.5% for diabetes, 30.2% for high blood pressure, and 23.1% for hyperlipidemia.[12] By 2007, obesity prevalence was 36%.[13]

Research on the Nutrition Transition

Since 2006, researchers have used the Hawks et al. model[14] described later in the chapter to describe the nutrition transition among Jordanian women, collecting data such as body mass index (BMI), eating styles, and body size preferences. Researchers determined that the nutrition transition was occurring rapidly, and they found high levels of overweight and obesity, as well as disordered eating attitudes and behaviors, such as emotional and restrained eating.[15] However, level of body esteem was higher than expected, and these women reported desire to have a healthy body size. In contrast, the replicated study among young, urban college women found that most were normal weight, but wanted to lose weight, and indicated high levels of body dissatisfaction. These young women also had high levels of external and restrained eating, and disordered eating attitudes and behaviors.[16] Further research in Jordan needs to address the healthcare costs of this transition and the potential for high rates of eating disorders in this population, and assess whether these changes are occurring among males and at what rate.

Discussion Questions

- Which factors are contributing to the nutrition transition in Jordan?
- How does Jordan's large refugee population affect average dietary intake and food availability?
- Which dietary and physical activity patterns have changed as Jordan experiences the nutrition transition, and how do they affect health?
- Which elements of the nutrition transition still need to be explored in Jordan, and how can they be studied? How can this information help guide public health nutrition interventions?
- How can the government develop policies to improve nutrition in Jordan?

Introduction

The **nutrition transition** refers to a global phenomenon characterized by changes in dietary patterns and physical activity levels in populations. It leads to increases in obesity and other NCDs, such as diabetes, hypertension, and stroke.[17] Diets shift from traditional diets, high in grains, fibers, vegetables, and fruits,[18] toward "Westernized diets," higher in fat, sugar, animal proteins, and sodium.[19] Concurrently, physical activity is replaced by sedentary behaviors, and reliance on technology is increased. This chapter discusses various models explaining the nutrition transition, public health implications of the transition, and case studies from a variety of countries at different stages of this transition.

Popkin's Models

Barry Popkin, known for his groundbreaking research on the nutrition transition, proposes that the nutrition transition accompanies **demographic** and **epidemiologic transitions** (**Figure 22-1**). The **demographic transition** is the shift from high to low fertility and mortality rates,[20] and the **epidemiologic transition** is the shift from high prevalence of infectious diseases to high rates of chronic and degenerative diseases.[21]

> *Public Health Core Competency 8: Leadership and Systems Thinking Skills 2: Describes how public health operates within a larger system*
>
> Reproduced from Council on Linkages Between Academia and Public Health Practice. 2010 May. Core Competencies for Public Health Professionals. Washington, DC: Public Health Foundation. http://www.phf.org/resourcestools/Documents/Core_Competencies_for_Public_Health_Professionals_2010May.pdf. Accessed August 13, 2013. This source is used for all Public Health Core Competencies in this chapter.

Popkin has proposed a five-pattern model of the nutrition transition.[22] In Pattern 1, undernutrition, high levels of

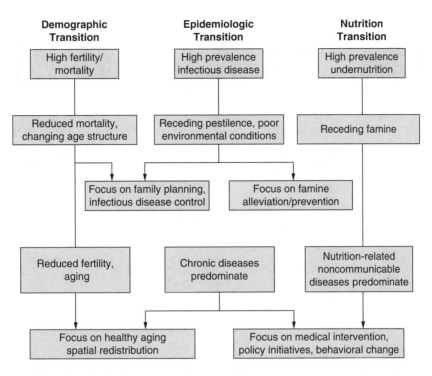

Figure 22-1 Stages of health, nutrition and demographic change

Data from Popkin, B. M. (2002). An overview on the nutrition transition and its health implications: The Bellagio meeting. *Public Health Nutrition, 5*(1A), 93-103.

fertility and mortality, and infectious diseases, are evident. In Pattern 2, famine is receding, environmental conditions, such as access to clean water, are improving, and infectious diseases are less burdensome. As mortality decreases and life expectancy increases, the population ages. Pattern 3 includes minimizing famine, reducing fertility, and decreasing mortality from infectious diseases. The result is Pattern 4, with more NCDs, lower fertility, and an aging population. Pattern 5 is marked by dietary change associated with promoting health. The behavior changes seen in Pattern 5 often result from multilevel interventions aimed at the policy level of the **socioecological model**. However, these changes may be driven by individuals or governments. Currently occurring in only a few nations, this stage is expected to improve length and quality of life by delaying degenerative and chronic diseases. Consistent with the literature, this chapter uses the term "nutrition transition" to refer specifically to the shift from receding famine (Pattern 3) to the increase in nutrition-related noncommunicable diseases (Pattern 4).[23]

In Popkin's five-stage model, physical activity changes accompany the nutrition transition (**Table 22-1**). Patterns 1, 2, and 3 are labor intensive, Pattern 4 is characterized by sedentary lifestyles, and Pattern 5 includes "purposeful activity," or planned physical activity, such as exercise, distinct from necessary physical activity, such as that required in labor-intensive occupations.

The Nutrition Transition Model: Looking at Individuals

A model to explain the mechanism of the nutrition transition[24] indicates that prior to the nutrition transition, people are intuitive/physical eaters; they do not overeat, and regulate their food intake based on appeal and satisfy hunger. At this stage, people are generally thin, although the prevailing culture may perceive a larger body size as more beautiful and a sign of wealth.

In this model, economic and demographic transitions cause a shift not only in dietary intake, but also in eating styles. Increased **social eating** and **environmental eating** increases obesity levels.[25] "**Emotional eating**" due to anxiety, depression, loneliness, boredom, or anger also contributes. During the transition, preference for body thinness over plumpness increases, leading to restrictive dieting and emotional eating in the population. Replacement of social and environmental eating styles by restrictive dieting and emotional eating has been shown to lead to negative physical and psychological consequences.[26] The Western media may also contribute to these effects.

Table 22-1 Stages of the nutrition transition

Stage	Diet Patterns	Activity Patterns	Main Nutritional Health Concern	Result
Stage 1	Wild plants and animals, water	Labor intensive	High disease rate	Low fertility and life expectancy
Stage 2	Grains, water	Labor intensive	Nutritional deficiencies	High maternal and child mortality, low life expectancy
Stage 3	Starches: low-fat, high-fiber, water	Labor intensive	Maternal and child health deficiencies	Slow mortality decline
Stage 4	Fat, sugar, processed foods, caloric beverages	Sedentary	Obesity, noncommunicable disease	Increased obesity and noncommunicable disease
Stage 5	Increased fruit/ vegetable/fiber consumption, lower fat diets, decreased intake of caloric beverages	Purposeful activity	Reduced health concerns	Reduced noncommunicable disease, extended aging

Data from Popkin, B. M. (2002). An overview on the nutrition transition and its health implications: The Bellagio meeting. *Public Health Nutrition*, 5(1A), 93-103.

Constant restrictive dieting lowers metabolic rates and energy expenditure.[27] These changes contribute to future weight gains characterized by increased storage of visceral fat that increases the risk of chronic diseases. Psychologically, restrictive eating tends to stimulate binge eating through a sense of food deprivation, which later leads to a negative relationship with food and potentially to eating disorders (**Figure 22-2**).[28]

Factors Influencing the Nutrition Transition

Several causal mechanisms, primarily demographic and economic changes, have been linked to the nutrition transition.[29] Nations that are more urbanized, Westernized, and developed are further in the nutrition transition. Within

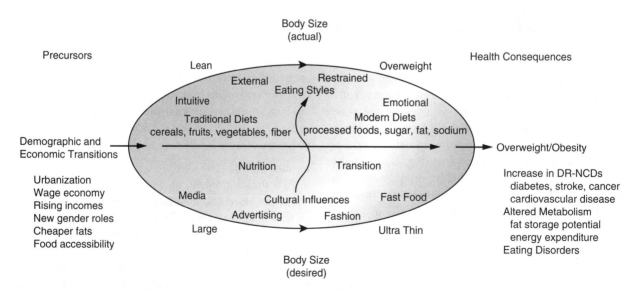

Figure 22-2 The nutrition transition, eating styles and public health consequences

Data from: Hawkes, S. R., Merrill, R. M., Madanat, H. N., Takeo, M., Suwanteerangkul, J., Guarin, C. M., & Shaofang, C. (2004). Intuitive eating and the nutrition transition in Asia. Asia Pacific *Journal of Clinical Nutrition*, 13(2): 194-203.

nations, differences are evident between **socioeconomic status (SES)** and rural and urban areas. In China, for example, more traditional low-fat diets are associated with poverty. Fat consumption decreases as economic development surges,[30] likely due to corporate food advertising, exposure to mass media, greater availability of food, increased incomes, decreased prices of unhealthy foods such as fats and sugars, and the resulting changes in the population's food preferences.[31]

Modernization and urbanization also influence the nutrition transition as developing nations have increased exposure to Western lifestyles. Levels of physical activity have dropped significantly as the job market has shifted from rural agricultural occupations that required more physical labor to more sedentary urban occupations that utilize high-level technologies in the manufacturing of their products.[32]

Socioeconomic Status

Changes in socioeconomic status can influence the nutrition transition through higher incomes and increased affordability and consumption of fat, sugar, and animal-source foods (ASF). These foods replace vegetables and grains, whose consumption declines.[33,34] Higher SES also affects the nutrition transition through modern conveniences and changes in the food preparation process. In low-SES households without refrigerators to preserve perishable foods, meals must be prepared daily and typically include more fresh fruits and vegetables. Thus, an increase in SES contributes to the nutrition transition by facilitating access to modern conveniences, which reduce diet quality and require less physical activity, since food need not be purchased daily. Furthermore, higher SES allows for eating out.

Urbanization

To improve SES, individuals often move to urban settings, where industrialization offers more employment opportunities.[35,36,37,38] **Urbanization** influences the nutrition transition in several ways. First, food is cheaper and available in larger quantities and more varieties. This typically leads to increased calorie intake, even if income does not change.[39] Second, urbanization is associated with gender role changes. Women tend to participate more in the labor force, and have less time for household chores, such as food selection and preparation.[40] The result is a decrease in the quality of diets eaten by families, since the more convenient meal options tend to be more processed; higher in fat, sodium, and sugar; and lower in vitamins and minerals.

Third, urbanization can also lead to reduced physical activity,[41] with one-stop shops for groceries, mass transportation, and, usually, less physically demanding jobs.

Western Influences and Modernization

Globalization promotes progression through the nutrition transition as a country further encourages foreign investments.[42] Western influences affect the nutrition transition through several mechanisms.[43] Fast food becomes available, and there is an increased investment in advertising it and making it appealing to the public. Second, changes are evident in eating patterns and the way people, especially women, view their bodies. Also, cultural attitudes toward female gender roles in the home and the society change.[44] Individuals are exposed to modern conveniences, such as washers and dryers, microwaves, and televisions, which reduce physical activity or affect diet quality. Increased influence of Western advertising and media can occur through exposure to foreign news sources and to movies and music.[45] This can facilitate shifts in eating styles.[46,47]

Food Advertising

Food advertisements often promote unhealthy foods. The 1996 Consumers International study indicated that half of all foods advertised in Norway, Australia, the United States, and 10 European Union nations were of low nutritional value, with high levels of sugar and sodium.[48] In the United States, fast-food restaurants account for one-third of the money spent on food advertising.[49] McDonald's has an annual advertising budget of $1.4 billion,[50] and Coca-Cola's budget was $2.9 billion in 2010.[51] Humans' innate preferences for high-fat, high-sugar foods not only promote obesity during the nutrition transition,[52] but also make the market for these energy-dense foods more profitable.[53] Additionally, processed foods have higher profit margins than individual ingredients.[54]

Controversy over Reduced Energy Expenditure

Technological advances promote the nutrition transition through reductions in physical activity. For example, using personal motorized vehicles instead of walking to commute may increase the risk of becoming obese.[55] However, while most current research indicates an association between technology and reduced energy expenditure, conflicting data remain. In one study,[56] the **doubly-labeled water** method was used to measure and compare total daily energy expenditure in Hadza hunter-gatherers of Tanzania and their Western counterparts. Hadza foragers had higher levels of physical activity than Westerners, but not higher total daily energy expenditure after controlling for body size. The study concludes that "the similarity in metabolic rates across a broad range of cultures challenges current models of obesity suggesting that Western lifestyles lead to decreased energy expenditure."

Consequences of the Nutrition Transition

Obesity rates in the United States began to increase sharply in the 1980s.[57] Initially thought to be a country's isolated experience, the trend was attributed to changes in school policies, and increased consumption of foods away from home, fast food, and prepared meals. However, by the 1990s, similar patterns of obesity emerged in other industrialized and developing countries.[58] Public health professionals were concerned by the rapid pace of this transition. The United States and some European countries had taken more than 70 years to transition from Pattern 3 to Pattern 4, but many of the countries were undergoing this transition in less than 50 years, and some in as little as 20. This rapid pace has significant consequences, such as the double burden of malnutrition and a negative impact on healthcare systems.

Obesity and NR-NCDs

Increased prevalence of obesity is a significant consequence of the nutrition transition. Worldwide, over 2 billion adults are overweight and obese; by 2030, 2.2 billion adults may be overweight, with an additional 1.1 billion obese.[59] Obesity has negative implications for health and healthcare costs, as well as quality of life. Adding to the burden is that while standard **body mass index (BMI)** indicators are used to compare obesity rates across countries, available data suggest that unhealthy changes in body composition and cardiometabolic effects occur at lower BMI levels for individuals in these developing countries.[60,61] Consequently, screening for NCD may be indicated in these populations even when BMI is not a risk factor according to standard cutoff values.

Double (Dual) Burden of Malnutrition

With the rapid transition comes the presence of high rates of undernutrition and overnutrition simultaneously within nations and even households, where parents may be overweight or obese while children are undernourished.[62,63] The "**double (or dual) burden of malnutrition**" is most common in middle-income countries where the transition has been occurring fastest. Dual-burden households present a challenge for public health interventions, since efforts to reduce undernutrition may contradict efforts to reduce overweight and obesity.[64] For example, supplementary feeding programs for acute malnutrition may need to be monitored to ensure that these programs do not lead to increased obesity.[65] When possible, interventions should avoid harming nontarget populations within the same household as the target population.[66]

> *Millennium Development Goal 1: Eradicate Extreme Poverty and Hunger. Target 1.C: Halve, between 1990 and 2015, the proportion of people who suffer from hunger*
>
> Reproduced from the United Nations. (n.d.). 2015 Millennium Development Goals. Retrieved from http://www.un.org/millenniumgoals/. Accessed August 13, 2013. This source is used for all Millennium Development Goals in this chapter.

Healthcare Systems

The nutrition transition also affects healthcare spending and healthcare systems. During the transition, nations shift to higher rates of obesity and NCDs after building a healthcare system based on high rates of infectious diseases, such as diarrheal diseases, that are relatively inexpensive to treat. Exponential increases in spending costs can result from a lagging healthcare system and the need for more expensive equipment and drugs to diagnose and treat chronic conditions. One estimate predicts that the indirect cost of the nutrition transition for China between 2000 and 2025 may increase from 3.58% to 8.7% of gross national product (GNP), or an increase of $6.3 billion.[67] During this time, the cost attributable to overweight and obesity in China is estimated to increase from $49 billion to $112 billion.[68] These are important costs to consider, especially in low- and middle-income countries, where resources may not be available to support these large increases in healthcare spending.[69] Thus, addressing underlying causes of the nutrition transition and preventing its consequences is warranted.

Global Recognition and Surveys to Investigate the Nutrition Transition

The following section addresses some of the projects related to the nutrition transition, including the 2001

Bellagio Conference in Bellagio, Italy; the China Health and Nutrition Survey (CHNS); and the Russia Longitudinal Monitoring Survey of the Higher School of Economics (RLMS-HSE). Case studies from China and Brazil follow.

Bellagio Conference

In 2001, the International Union of Nutrition Sciences Committee organized the Bellagio Conference to address the rapid shifts toward the nutrition transition observed in many countries. This was the first worldwide recognition of the importance of addressing the transition, and research on the nutrition transition has expanded since then. Conference presentations are available on the conference's website.[70] Participants signed the Bellagio declaration, which included two important points:

1. "Four out of five deaths from nutrition-related chronic diseases occur in middle- and low-income countries. The burden of cardiovascular disease alone is now far greater in India, and also in China, than in all economically developed countries in the world added together."

2. "Immediate action to control and prevent nutrition-related chronic diseases is not only a public health imperative but also a political, economic, social necessity."[71]

The China Health and Nutrition Survey

The CHNS, a collaborative effort of researchers in China and the United States, is an ongoing open cohort. It aims to understand the effects of health, nutrition, and family planning policies and programs implemented in China. It also documents the nation's social and economic transformations and their impacts on the health and nutritional status of the Chinese population. These impacts are measured by changes at the community and policy levels as well as by changes in economic, demographic, and social factors at the individual and household levels. Community data include measures in food markets and health facilities, and surveys of key informants, such as family planning public health professionals, social services workers, and community leaders. A random survey of 19,000 individuals in nine provinces of China provides information at the household and individual levels.[72] Data from the CHNS are valuable for understanding the nutrition transition.

Russia Longitudinal Monitoring Survey of the Higher School of Economics

The RLMS-HSE is a series of nationally representative surveys to improve understanding of the effects of national reforms on the health and economic welfare of its population.[73] This project, initiated in 1992, has so far collected 16 serial surveys. As with the CHNS, the RLMS-HSE includes measures at the community, household, and individual levels. The individual and household measures include health status and dietary intake, household expenditures, and healthcare service utilization. This longitudinal approach is crucial for understanding the dynamics of the nutrition transition.

Case Studies on the Nutrition Transition in Various Nations

China

China's rapid social and economic transitions significantly influenced its nutrition transition and effects. Urbanization is a major force. Between 1949 and 1957, rural–urban migration increased significantly, and the urban population rose at a rate of 7% per year while the rural population was increasing by only 1.4% annually. By the early 1960s, 20% of China's population, or 130 million people, lived in urban settings.[74] By 2011, more than half of the population was urban, with the proportion continuing to increase. By 2025, 65.4% are expected to live in urban settings, and the number will reach 77.3% by 2050.[75] Although the proportion remains lower than in industrialized nations, the number of urban dwellers in China exceeds the total population of any country in the world besides India.[76]

Due to changes in China's taxation system and its economic development policies, China is one of the most rapidly developing countries in the world. This rapid industrialization has had significant impact on both dietary habits and physical activity. China's economy is shifting away from traditional sectors, such as farming and mining, to service-oriented jobs. Furthermore, due to technological advancement, the amount of energy expended within a given occupation has declined. The result is lower occupational energy expenditure and a decrease in physical activity. Adding to the positive energy balance is that "China is experiencing the world's fastest growth in supermarkets with sales growing by as much as 40% annually."[77]

Changes in Diet Intake

Due in part to urbanization, the agricultural sector decreased from 41% to 29% of GDP between 1970 and 1992.

Simultaneously, agriculture shifted from producing grains, oil, cotton, and other cash crops, to raising livestock, maintaining fisheries, and producing other commodities. The decrease in grain production and fear of scarcity caused a hike in grain prices in autumn of 1993 that lasted for years.[78] The price spike led to increased consumption of fats. Between 1952 and 1992, the individual daily fat intake increased from 28.3 grams to 58.3 grams and contributed from 11% to 22% of total calories, as the proportion of energy from carbohydrates decreased from 77% to 66%. The proportion of energy from ASF increased from 4.9% to 9.3%,[79] and national use of soybean oil increased from almost no use to 14 million metric tons annually in 2006.[80] These changes help describe the "Westernization" of the Chinese diet.

The use of meat and oil has recently expanded beyond home-cooked meals into Western restaurants, which are relatively new to China.[81] In 1985, Beijing had no restaurants selling Western fast foods, but by 2010 had more than 100 McDonald's or Kentucky Fried Chicken restaurants. More than 3,700 KFC establishments exist in the entire country. These American restaurants are increasingly fashionable[82] and, though not yet universally affordable, are accessible to a large portion of the population. This, combined with the high caloric content of the foods sold in these restaurants, has resulted in dietary changes. These changes in nutrition in turn affect the health of the Chinese people. Between 1989 and 2000, the rates of overweight had tripled among adult males and females and were almost 25% by 2004. The proportion of overweight or obese adults was 25% in 2002 and 38.5% in 2010, and projected to be 50–57% by 2015.[83] The corresponding result is a significant increase in NCDs, including cancer and coronary heart disease. From 1985 to 1995, NCDs went from accounting for 48% to 61.8% of deaths in urban areas, and 34.5% to 45.9% of deaths in rural areas.

Without interventions to improve China's food systems and physical activity environments, dietary habits, physical activity levels, rates of overweight/obesity, and NCDs will continue to worsen in response to the rapid social and economic transitions.

Brazil

Brazil, a middle-income country, has been undergoing the nutrition transition for years, and it faces the double burden of malnutrition. In 1975, the ratio of underweight to obesity was 2:1; the ratio was to 1:2 by 1997.[84] As in other transitioning countries, low-income Brazilian women are at higher risk for both underweight and obesity than higher-income women. "In Brazil, from 1974–1975 to 2008–2009, the prevalence rates of obesity increased more than fourfold among men (2.8% to 12.4%) and more than twofold among women (from 8.0% to 16.9%)."[85] The nutrition transition is also evident when studying Brazilian children. Between 1982 and 2004, stunting among 4-year-olds declined from 10.9% to 3.6%, while overweight increased from 7.6% to 12.3%.[86] The increase in overweight must be addressed to minimize long-term consequences. To understand the nutrition transition among indigenous populations, the first national survey of these groups was conducted in 2008–2009. Data are still being analyzed.[87]

Brazil provides an example not only of the nutrition transition's causes and progression, but also of government responses to these changes. Since the late 1990s, Brazil's government has been working at the national and local levels to develop policies aimed at addressing the double burden of malnutrition in the country. Brazil developed a national food and nutrition policy with three specific areas: legislation, information/communication, and capacity building. Understanding these policies and their effects can help Brazil and other nations continue to prepare for and minimize negative effects of the nutrition transition.[88]

Legislative Progress

Legislative progress includes nutrition labeling and serving guidelines. All packaged foods in Brazil are required to list their contents of calories, protein, carbohydrates, total fats, saturated fats, cholesterol, calcium, iron, sodium, and dietary fiber in a standardized manner designed to enable all consumers to understand it. Also, "nutritionally adequate serving sizes" were developed for mandatory use to prevent consumers from being misled.

Additionally, Brazil was among the first countries to recognize the importance of school settings in the promotion of healthy eating. The federal government financed a national school meal program with standards for meal quality. Purchase of fresh vegetables, fruits, and minimally processed foods should compose 70% of the budget, and foods should be purchased locally when possible. This legislation addresses previous concern from schools regarding the lack of available staff to prepare these foods by providing resources to local farmers to prepare the fresh foods prior to school delivery. More recently, taxation of sugar-sweetened beverages (SSBs) has been discussed. Data support an inverse relationship between increased price and reduced consumption of SSBs, with greater effects among low-income individuals.[89,90]

> *Public Health Core Competency 5: Community Dimensions of Practice Skills 5: Maintains partnerships with key stakeholders*

Information and Communication

The Brazilian government established a "step-by-step route to healthy eating" that encouraged individuals to select 1 of 10 possible goals to achieve either individually or as a family. Additionally, the goals were presented in a manner intended to encourage individuals to pick the first goal, reanalyze, and then move to the next goal. This proposal also included two physical activity steps focused on the importance of achieving 30 minutes of daily physical activity, and the ability to exercise anywhere. Also, a "shop smart" software program was developed to help consumers make better decisions regarding what should be purchased on their food budget. This was a point-of-sale tool that also integrated price, sales, and seasonality in providing consumers with suggestions on what to purchase. The program relies on businesses to integrate it into their stores.[91]

> *Public Health Core Competency 5: Communication Skills 2: Communicates in writing and orally, in person, and through electronic means, with linguistic and cultural proficiency*

Capacity-Building Activities

The government developed a special television channel aimed at teachers to educate them about a broad array of issues, including healthy eating. For healthy eating, the network repeated the screening of four 10-minute videos every two months that could be recorded by the teachers for use in classrooms and were accompanied by additional materials to help teachers develop class-related activities. Videos focused on obesity, malnutrition, physical activity, health, food and culture, and food safety.

Guidelines and manuals from the government increased the capacity of health workers to provide advice on healthy diets and physical activity for individuals in all stages of their lives. For example, the government studied more than 100 Brazilian indigenous plants whose use in food preparation had declined significantly. In one such manual, it provides the micronutrient analysis of these plants to show Brazilians how nutritious they are and to encourage their reintroduction into the Brazilian diet. It also launched national screening campaigns, such as screening for diabetes in adults over age 40. Protocols for hypertensive and diabetic patients were added to the standard practice.

Innovative local programs supplemented these large federal-level programs. For example, the Healthy Streets program was established in the most impoverished parts of Rio de Janeiro, where safe physical activity opportunities are scarce. To allow individuals to exercise safely in the city's streets, traffic is restricted and sometimes banned during certain hours of the day and night. Each municipality determines the streets to be affected, the hours, and days during which the traffic restriction or ban occurs. Another program developed in Rio de Janeiro is the assurance of healthy cooking in the city's first-class restaurants.[92] These two programs are promising because they can easily be extended to additional cities.

Conclusion

The nutrition transition is under way in many countries worldwide, especially middle-income countries. However, addressing the nutrition transition and the associated obesity and NCD rates requires a broad approach that considers the multiple levels of the socioecological model and recognizes that physical activity and nutrition go hand in hand. Countries that are rapidly transitioning often do not have the time or means to respond to the changes to prepare their healthcare systems. Much remains to be done to mitigate the negative effects of the nutrition transition.

References

1 Central Intelligence Agency. (2013, April 10). *The world fact book: Jordan*. Retrieved from https://www.cia.gov/library/publications/the-world-factbook/geos/jo.html

2 Central Intelligence Agency. (2013, April 10). *The world fact book: Jordan*. Retrieved from https://www.cia.gov/library/publications/the-world-factbook/geos/jo.html

3 Central Intelligence Agency. (2013, April 10). *The world fact book: Jordan*. Retrieved from https://www.cia.gov/library/publications/the-world-factbook/geos/jo.html

4 Madanat, H. N., Troutman, K. P., & Al-Madi, B. (2008). The nutrition transition in Jordan: The political, economic and food consumption contexts. *Promotion and Education, 15*, 6-10.

5   Hourani, H. A. (2011). *Food nutrition profile: Jordan*. Nutrition and Consumer Protection Division, Food and Agriculture Organization. Retrieved from http://www.fao.org/ag/agn/nutrition/jor_en.stm

6   Food and Agriculture Organization. (2004). *Calculating population energy requirements and food needs* [software program]. FAO Food and Nutrition Technical Report Series No. 1. Rome: Food and Agriculture Organization of the United Nations.

7   Hourani, H. A. (2011). *Food nutrition profile: Jordan*. Nutrition and Consumer Protection Division, Food and Agriculture Organization. Retrieved from http://www.fao.org/ag/agn/nutrition/jor_en.stm

8   Al-Nsour, M., Zindah, M., Belbeisi, A., Hadaddin, R., Brown, D. W., & Walke, H. (2012). Prevalence of selected chronic, noncommunicable disease factors in Jordan: Results of the 2007 Jordan behavioral risk factor surveillance survey. *Preventing Chronic Disease: Public Health Research, Practice, and Policy, 9*, 1-9.

9   Hourani, H. A. (2011). *Food nutrition profile: Jordan*. Nutrition and Consumer Protection Division, Food and Agriculture Organization. Retrieved from http://www.fao.org/ag/agn/nutrition/jor_en.stm

10 Zindah, M., Belbeisi, A., Walke, H., & Mokdad, A. H. (2008). Obesity and diabetes in Jordan: Findings from the behavioral risk factor surveillance system, 2004. *Preventing Chronic Disease: Public Health Research, Practice, and Policy, 5*, 1-8.

11 Zindah, M., Belbeisi, A., Walke, H., & Mokdad, A. H. (2008). Obesity and diabetes in Jordan: Findings from the behavioral risk factor surveillance system, 2004. *Preventing Chronic Disease: Public Health Research, Practice, and Policy, 5*, 1-8.

12 Zindah, M., Belbeisi, A., Walke, H., & Mokdad, A. H. (2008). Obesity and diabetes in Jordan: Findings from the behavioral risk factor surveillance system, 2004. *Preventing Chronic Disease: Public Health Research, Practice, and Policy, 5*, 1-8.

13 Al-Nsour, M., Zindah, M., Belbeisi, A., Hadaddin, R., Brown, D. W., & Walke, H. (2012). Prevalence of selected chronic, noncommunicable disease factors in Jordan: Results of the 2007 Jordan behavioral risk factor surveillance survey. *Preventing Chronic Disease: Public Health Research, Practice, and Policy, 9*, 1-9.

14 Hawks, S. R., Merrill, R. M., Madanat, H. N., Miyagawa, T., Suwanteerangkul, J., Guarin, C. M., & Shaofang, C. (2004). Intuitive eating and the nutrition transition in Asia. *Asia Pacific Journal of Clinical Nutrition, 13*, 194-203.

15 Madanat, H. N., Brown, R. B., & Hawks, S. R., (2007). The impact of body mass index and Western advertising and media on eating style, body image, and nutrition transition among Jordanian women. *Public Health Nutrition, 10*, 1039-46.

16 Madanat, H. N., Lindsay, R., & Campbell, T., (2010). Young urban women and the nutrition transition in Jordan. *Public Health Nutrition, 14*, 599-604.

17 Popkin, B. M. (2002). An overview of the nutrition transition and its health implications: The Bellagio meeting. *Public Health Nutrition, 5*, 93-103.

18 Gordon-Larsen, P., Adair, L. S., Nelson, M. C., & Popkin, B. M., (2004). Five-year obesity incidence in the transition period between adolescence and adulthood: The National Longitudinal Study of Adolescent Health. *American Journal of Clinical Nutrition, 80*, 69-575.

19 Popkin, B. M. (2002). An overview of the nutrition transition and its health implications: The Bellagio meeting. *Public Health Nutrition, 5*, 93-103.

20 Caldwell, J. (2006). *Demographic transition theory* (p. 426). Dordrecht: Springer.

21 Omran, A. R. (2005), The epidemiological transition: A theory of the epidemiology of population change. *Milbank Quarterly, 83*(4), 731-57.

22 Popkin, B. M. (2002). An overview of the nutrition transition and its health implications: The Bellagio meeting. *Public Health Nutrition, 5*, 93-103.

23 Popkin, B. M. (2001). Nutrition in transition: The changing global nutrition challenge. *Asia Pacific Journal of Clinical Nutrition, 10*(Suppl.), S13-S18.

24 Hawks, S. R., Merrill, R. M., Madanat, H. N., Miyagawa, T., Suwanteerangkul, J., Guarin, C. M., & Shaofang, C. (2004). Intuitive eating and the nutrition transition in Asia. *Asia Pacific Journal of Clinical Nutrition, 13*, 194-203.

25 Hawks, S. R., Merrill, R. M., Madanat, H. N., Miyagawa, T., Suwanteerangkul, J., Guarin, C. M., & Shaofang, C. (2004). Intuitive eating and the nutrition transition in Asia. *Asia Pacific Journal of Clinical Nutrition, 13*, 194-203.

26 Hawks, S. R., Merrill, R. M., Madanat, H. N., Miyagawa, T., Suwanteerangkul, J., Guarin, C. M., & Shaofang, C. (2004). Intuitive eating and the nutrition transition in Asia. *Asia Pacific Journal of Clinical Nutrition, 13*, 194-203.

27 Hawks, S. R., Madanat, H. N., & Christley, H. (2008). Behavioral and biological associations of dietary restraint: A review of the literature. *Ecology of Food and Nutrition, 47*(5), 415-49.

28 Hawks, S. R., Madanat, H. N., & Christley, H. (2008). Psychosocial associations of dietary restraint: Implications for healthy weight promotion. *Ecology of Food and Nutrition, 47*(5), 450-83.

29 Hawks, S. R., Merrill, R. M., Madanat, H. N., Miyagawa, T., Suwanteerangkul, J., Guarin, C. M., & Shaofang, C. (2004). Intuitive eating and the nutrition transition in Asia. *Asia Pacific Journal of Clinical Nutrition, 13*, 194-203.

30 Popkin, B. M., Horton, S., Kim, S., Mahal, A., & Shuigo, J. (2001). Trends in diet, nutritional stats, and diet-related noncommunicable diseases in China and India: The economic costs of the nutrition transition. *Nutritional Reviews, 59*, 379-90.

31 Drewnowski, A., & Popkin, B. M. (1997). The nutrition transition: New trends in the global diet. *Nutrition Reviews, 55*, 31-43.

32 Drewnowski, A., & Popkin, B. M. (1997). The nutrition transition: New trends in the global diet. *Nutrition Reviews, 55*, 31-43.

33 Haddad, L. (2003). Redirecting the diet transition: What can food policy do? *Developmental Policy Review, 21*, 599-615.

34 Popkin, B. M. (2003). The nutrition transition in the developing world. *Developmental Policy Review, 21*, 581-97.

35 Gunewardene, A., Huon, G. F., & Zheng, R. (2001). Exposure to westernization and dieting: A cross-cultural study. *International Journal of Eating Disorders, 29*, 289-93.

36 Hawks, S. R., Merrill, R. M., Madanat, H. N., Miyagawa, T., Suwanteerangkul, J., Guarin, C. M., & Shaofang, C. (2004). Intuitive eating and the nutrition transition in Asia. *Asia Pacific Journal of Clinical Nutrition, 13*, 194-203.

37 Popkin, B. M., Horton, S., Kim, S., Mahal, A., & Shuigo, J. (2001). Trends in diet, nutritional stats, and diet-related noncommunicable diseases in China and India: The economic costs of the nutrition transition. *Nutritional Reviews, 59*, 379-90.

38 Popkin, B. M. (2002). An overview of the nutrition transition and its health implications: The Bellagio meeting. *Public Health Nutrition, 5*, 93-103.

39 Ruel, M. T., & Garret, J. (1999). *Urban challenges to food and nutrition security in the developing world.* Washington, DC: International Food Policy Research Institute.

40 Popkin, B. M., Horton, S., Kim, S., Mahal, A., & Shuigo, J. (2001). Trends in diet, nutritional stats, and diet-related noncommunicable diseases in China and India: The economic costs of the nutrition transition. *Nutritional Reviews, 59*, 379-90.

41 Popkin, B. M. (2002). An overview of the nutrition transition and its health implications: The Bellagio meeting. *Public Health Nutrition, 5*, 93-103.

42 Popkin, B. M., Horton, S., Kim, S., Mahal, A., & Shuigo, J. (2001). Trends in diet, nutritional stats, and diet-related noncommunicable diseases in China and India: The economic costs of the nutrition transition. *Nutritional Reviews, 59*, 379-90.

43 Popkin, B. M. (2001). Nutrition in transition: The changing global nutrition challenge. *Asia Pacific Journal of Clinical Nutrition, 10*(Suppl.), S13-S18.

44 Popkin, B. M. (2001). Nutrition in transition: The changing global nutrition challenge. *Asia Pacific Journal of Clinical Nutrition, 10*(Suppl.), S13-S18.

45 Popkin, B. M. (2001). Nutrition in transition: The changing global nutrition challenge. *Asia Pacific Journal of Clinical Nutrition, 10*(Suppl.), S13-S18.

46 Drewnowski, A., & Popkin, B. M. (1997). The nutrition transition: New trends in the global diet. *Nutrition Reviews, 55*, 31-43.

47 Nestle, M., Wing, R., Birch, L., DiSogra, L., Drewnowski, A., Middleton, S., . . . Economos, C. (1998). Behavioral and social influences on food choice. *Nutrition Reviews, 56*, S50-S64; discussion S64-S74.

48 Dibb, S., & Harris, L. (1996). *A spoonful of sugar: Television food advertising aimed at children: An international comparative study.* London, UK: Consumers International.

49 Gallo, A. E. (1998). *Food advertising in the United States.* Retrieved from the U.S. Department of Agriculture website, http://www.ers.usda.gov/media/91050/aib750i_1_.pdf

50 Austin, C. (2012). The billionaires' club: Only 36 companies have $1,000 million plus budgets. *Business Insider.* Retrieved from http://www.businessinsider.com/the-35-companies-that-spent-1-billion-on-ads-in-2011-2012-11?op=1

51 McWilliams, J. (2011). Coca-Cola spent more than $2.9 billion on advertising in 2010. Retrieved from http://www.ajc.com/news/business/coca-cola-spent-more-than-29-billion-on-advertisin/nQq6X

52 Popkin, B. M., Adair, L. S., & Ng, S. W. (2011). Global nutrition transition and the pandemic of obesity in developing countries. *Nutrition Reviews, 70*(1), 3-21.

53 Gardner, G., & Halweil, B. (2000). *Overfed and underfed: The global epidemic of malnutrition.* Washington, DC: Worldwatch Institute.

54 Gardner, G., & Halweil, B. (2000). *Overfed and underfed: The global epidemic of malnutrition.* Washington, DC: Worldwatch Institute.

55 Popkin, B. M. (2006). Technology, transport, globalization and the nutrition transition food policy. *Food Policy, 31*(6), 554-69.

56 Pontzer, H., Raichlen, D. A., Wood, B. M., Mabulla, A. Z. P., Racette, S. B., & Marlowe, F. W. (2012). Hunter-gatherer energetics and human obesity. *PLoS One, 7*(7), e40503.

57 Popkin, B. M., Adair, L. S., & Ng, S. W. (2011). Global nutrition transition and the pandemic of obesity in developing countries. *Nutrition Reviews, 70*(1), 3-21.

58 Popkin, B. M., Adair, L. S., & Ng, S. W. (2011). Global nutrition transition and the pandemic of obesity in developing countries. *Nutrition Reviews, 70*(1), 3-21.

59 Popkin, B. M., Adair, L. S., & Ng, S. W. (2011). Global nutrition transition and the pandemic of obesity in developing countries. *Nutrition Reviews, 70*(1), 3-21.

60 Nguyen, T. T., Adair, L. S., Suchindran, C. M., He, K., & Popkin, B. M. (2009). The association between body mass index and hypertension is different between East and Southeast Asians. *American Journal of Clinical Nutrition, 89*, 1905-12.

61 WHO Expert Consultation. (2004). Appropriate body-mass index for Asian populations and its implications for policy and intervention strategies. *Lancet, 363*, 157-63.

62 Caballero, B. (2005). A nutrition paradox-underweight and obesity in developing countries. *New England Journal of Medicine, 325*, 15.

63 Doak, C. M., Adair, L. S., Monteiro, C., & Popkin, B. M. (2000). Overweight and underweight coexist within households in Brazil, China, and Russia. *Journal of Nutrition, 130*, 2965-71.

64 Doak, C. M., Adair, L. S., Bentley, M., Monteiro, C., & Popkin, B. M. (2005). The dual burden household and the nutrition transition paradox. *International Journal of Obesity, 29*, 129-36.

65 Uauy, R., & Kain, J. (2002). The epidemiological transition: Need to incorporate obesity prevention into nutrition programmes. *Public Health Nutrition, 5*, 223-29.

66 Doak, C. M., Adair, L. S., Bentley, M., Monteiro, C., & Popkin, B. M. (2005). The dual burden household and the nutrition transition paradox. *International Journal of Obesity, 29*, 129-36.

67 Popkin, B. M. (2008). Will China's nutrition transition overwhelm its health care system and slow economic growth? *Disease and Demography, 27*(4), 1064-76.

68 Popkin, B. M. (2008). Will China's nutrition transition overwhelm its health care system and slow economic growth? *Disease and Demography, 27*(4), 1064-76.

69 Popkin, B. M. (2008). Will China's nutrition transition overwhelm its health care system and slow economic growth? *Disease and Demography, 27*(4), 1064-76.

70 *Bellagio conference papers.* (2001). Retrieved from the Nutrition Transition website, http://www.cpc.unc.edu/projects/nutrans/research/bellagio/papers

71 Popkin, B. M., et al. (2002). Bellagio declaration: Nutrition and health nutrition in the developing world: The time to act. *Public Health Nutrition, 5*(1a), 279-80.

72 *The China Health and Nutrition Survey.* (2012). Retrieved from http://www.cpc.unc.edu/projects/nutrans/research/chns

73 *Russian Longitudinal Monitoring Survey of HSE.* (2012). Retrieved from http://www.cpc.unc.edu/projects/nutrans/research/rlms

74 Sidel, R., & Sidel, V. W. (1982). Problems of daily life. In *The health of China* (pp. 101-24). Boston, MA: Beacon Press.

75 United Nations, Department of Economic and Social Affairs. (2012). *Population division urban and rural areas, 2011.* Retrieved from http://esa.un.org/unup/Wallcharts/urban-rural-areas.pdf.

76 Federal Research Division, Library of Congress. (1998). *A country study: China.* Retrieved from the Library of Congress website, http://lcweb2.loc.gov/frd/cs/cntoc.html.

77 Popkin, B. M. (2008). Will China's nutrition transition overwhelm its health care system and slow economic growth? *Disease and Demography, 27*(4), 1064-76.

78 Lin, J. Y., Huang, J., & Rozelle, S. (1996). China's food economy: Past performance and future trends. In Organisation for Economic Co-operation and Development, *China in the 21st century: Long-term global implications* (pp. 71-93). Paris, France: Organisation for Economic Co-operation and Development.

79 Du, S., Lu, B., Zing, F., & Popkin, B. M. (2002). The nutrition transition in China: A new stage of the Chinese diet. In B. Caballero & B. M. Popkin (Eds.), *The nutrition transition: Diet and disease in the developing world* (pp. 205-21). San Diego, CA: Academic Press.

80 Drewnoswski, A. (1987). Sweetness and obesity. In J. Dobbing (Ed.), *Sweetness* (pp. 177-92). Berlin, Germany: Springer-Verlag.

81 Watson, J. L. (Ed.). (1997). *Golden arches east: McDonald's in East Asia.* Stanford, CA: Stanford University Press.

82 Federal Research Division, Library of Congress. (1998). *A country study: China.* Retrieved from the Library of Congress website, http://lcweb2.loc.gov/frd/cs/cntoc.html

83 Bruno, D. (2012, December 31). In China, obesity becomes a problem that's foreign to survivors of its great famine. *Washington Post.* Retrieved from http://articles.washingtonpost.com/2012-12-31/national/36103804_1_chinese-waistlines-chinese-center-obesity.

84 Monteiro, C. A, Conde, W. L., & Popkin, B. M. (2004). The burden of disease from undernutrition and overnutrition in countries undergoing rapid nutrition transition: A view from Brazil. *American Journal of Public Health, 94*(3), 433-34.

85 Madeira, F. B., Silva, A. A., Veloso, H. F., Goldani, M. Z., Kac, G., Cardoso, V. C., Bettiol, H., & Barbieri, M. A. (2013). Normal weight obesity is associated with metabolic syndrome and insulin resistance in young adults from a middle-income country. *PLoS One, 8*(3), e60673.

86 Matijasevich, A., Santos, I. S., Menezes, A. M., Barros, A. J., Gigante, D. P., Horta, B. L., . . . Victora, C. G. (2012). Trends in socioeconomic inequalities in anthropometric status in a population undergoing the nutritional transition: Data from 1982, 1993, and 2004 Pelotas birth cohort studies. *BMC Public Health, 12,* 511.

87 Coimbra, C. E., Santos, R. V., Welch, J. R., Cardoso, A. M., de Souza, M. C., Garnelo, L., . . . Horta, B. L. (2012). The first national survey of indigenous people's health and nutrition in Brazil: Rationale, methodology, and overview of results. *BMC Public Health, 13,* 52.

88 Coitinho, D., Monteiro, C. A., & Popkin, B. M. (2001). What Brazil is doing to promote healthy diets and active lifestyles. *Public Health Nutrition, 5*(1A), 263-67.

89 Claro, R. M., Levy, R. B., Popkin, B. M., & Monteiro, C. A. (2012). Sugar-sweetened beverage taxes in Brazil. *American Journal of Public Health, 102*(1), 178-83.

90 Coitinho, D., Monteiro, C. A., & Popkin, B. M. (2001). What Brazil is doing to promote healthy diets and active lifestyles. *Public Health Nutrition, 5*(1A), 263-67.

91 Coitinho, D., Monteiro, C. A., & Popkin, B. M. (2001). What Brazil is doing to promote healthy diets and active lifestyles. *Public Health Nutrition, 5*(1A), 263-67.

92 Coitinho, D., Monteiro, C. A., & Popkin, B. M. (2001). What Brazil is doing to promote healthy diets and active lifestyles. *Public Health Nutrition, 5*(1A), 263-67.

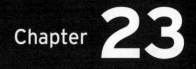
Food Policies in a Changing Nutrition Landscape: Assessing Child Nutrition in Pastoralist Communities in Africa

Emily Mitchard Turano, MS, MPH
Elizabeth Stites, PhD

"Most of them [the children] now are malnourished. They are missing milk. The older children are now in school, healthy, playful. The [young] kids now eat greens. They are used to never having milk. They are sickly, tired. . . . They eat green vegetables and they are stricken with diarrhea. The infants survive on breast milk but the mothers are eating only greens, salt and sim sim [sesame]."–Women in the Lobalangit subcounty, Kaabong

Interview with women, Lobalangit sub-county, Kaabong, February 12, 2011

Learning Objectives

- Recognize how socioeconomic, political, and environmental factors can affect the nutrition status of a population, particularly in complex environments.

- Understand the evolution, role, and variety of tools used in a nutrition assessment.

- Recognize the role and appropriate use of participatory approaches and methods of investigation.

- Understand how to make evidence-based recommendations in a complex environment.

Case Study: Milk Matters in Karamoja

Basic Factors Affecting Malnutrition

Various factors, many beyond an individual's control, affect health and nutrition status. Chronic or acute illness changes the body's basic nutrient requirements, routine or seasonal availability of and physical and economic access to nutritious foods affect the ability to satisfy nutrient needs, and nutrition knowledge, beliefs, and cultural practices permeate an individual's behaviors related to food consumption. Further removed from an individual's control, but still of critical importance, are the basic, or "upstream," factors that compose the socioeconomic, political, and environmental context. The United Nations Children's Fund's (UNICEF's) conceptual framework for **malnutrition**, the most widely agreed upon framework for assessing the causal factors of malnutrition, differentiates these upstream factors from immediate and underlying factors.[1]

Background: (Agro-)Pastoralists in a Changing World

Pastoralist and **agro-pastoralist** populations exist in regions around the world, including the Andes of South America, the steppes of Mongolia, the deserts of Africa, and the icy frontiers of Siberia. Characteristics of these populations include historic lack of sedentary agriculture due to climatically variable environments, mobile herding lifestyles that maximize scarce natural resources of pasture and water, and household economies and diets that rely extensively on livestock and livestock products, such as milk, blood, and less frequently, meat.[2,3]

Milk in particular is a universally valued product for pastoralist and agro-pastoralist households (**Figure 23-1**). Economically, the sale of milk and milk products generates income for those groups with access to markets. Socially, the exchange and gifting of milk and use in ceremonies strengthens relationships, a critical component of a broader risk management strategy. Nutritionally, milk and milk products are highly renewable sources of energy and essential nutrients, including protein, fat, and many **micronutrients.**[4,5,6,7,8] Indeed, the considerable consumption of milk and milk products by (agro-)pastoralists has been linked to tall and lean statures and historically high levels of nutritional **resiliency.**[9]

However, many pastoralists and agro-pastoralists around the globe are **vulnerable** to threats to the resiliency of their livelihood **strategies** and in turn their nutrition status. Their dependence on animals makes them particularly vulnerable to factors that interfere with the ability to maintain large, healthy herds. Long histories of social, economic, and political marginalization, as well as progressive encroachment of agriculture into traditional grazing lands in many areas, have greatly increased (agro-)pastoralists' vulnerability to poverty and malnutrition around the world.[10,11,12]

(Agro-)pastoralists in the Karamoja region of northeastern Uganda have been negatively affected by the dearth of basic infrastructure and services, such as transportation networks, markets, and veterinary services, and the loss of land to agriculture, national gaming parks, and nature preserves (**Figure 23-2**). Additional concerns are a semi-arid environment becoming harsher with a climate change, widespread violence and insecurity from cattle-raiding and an influx of weapons, regional military presence resulting from flawed disarmament policy and implementation, and policy restrictions on movement of herds and the establishment of government-protected mobile cattle camps (*kraals*).[13,14,15,16,17,18]

These complex factors restrict mobility of animals and humans, leading to increased livestock morbidity and mortality, reduced availability of and access to animal products, especially milk, and major disruption of household

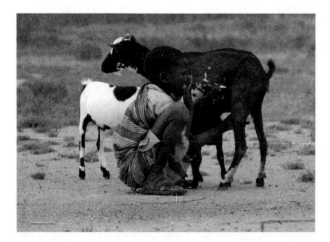

Figure 23-1 Child drinking milk

Courtesy of Khristopher Carlson.

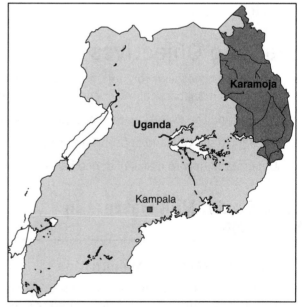

Figure 23-2 Map of Karamoja, Uganda

livelihoods and ability to cope with change. The Africa Pastoral Regional Initiative, launched by the Save the Children Alliance in 2007, aimed to generate new knowledge and understanding of pastoral systems that would contribute to an evidence base from which to improve programming and advocate for better policies and practices in pastoral settings. A key component of the Regional Initiative was the Pastoral Health and Nutrition Initiative (PHNI), which prompted investigation of factors underscoring child health and nutrition in pastoral areas.

The Origins of the Milk Matters Project

The Milk Matters project emerged as a regional research agenda under the realization that while substantial information over the decades has been generated around pastoral livelihoods, diets, and vulnerabilities, large gaps remained in the understanding of linkages and reciprocal impacts among these broad contextual changes, shifts in livelihoods, household **food security**, and child malnutrition. The research study was conducted by the Feinstein International Center (FIC) of Tufts University, in partnership with the **international nongovernmental organization** (INGO) Save the Children in Uganda (SCiUG) and funded by UNICEF Kampala.

Feinstein International Center and Save the Children (SC) conducted Milk Matters in the Somali region of Ethiopia beginning in 2007 and progressing in several stages over the next five years. A key finding of Milk Matters Ethiopia was that when *milk is absent in the pastoral diet, there are no adequate nutritional substitutes and child nutrition status deteriorates significantly.* Milk Matters Karamoja developed from collaborative discussions with the FIC-SC Milk Matters Ethiopia team. Responding to the unique characteristics and constraints of operating within a complex environment, Milk Matters Karamoja was designed to use a qualitative participatory approach to explore the stated linkages of interest.

Discussion Questions

- Describe the traditional significance of milk among pastoral communities, both for dietary and other purposes.
- Which upstream factors have forced shifts in livelihoods among pastoral and agro-pastoral communities? What are the social, nutritional, and economic consequences?

- Which local considerations were necessary when modifying the original Milk Matters in Ethiopia as a base for Milk Matters in Karamoja?
- What is the role of exploratory studies in improving population health? How can governments, research institutions, and aid organizations collaborate?

Introduction

Achieving the first Millennium Development Goal (MDG) will require attention to pastoralist and agro-pastoralist regions. Uganda is not on track for achieving MDG 1, as **undernourishment** actually increased from 26.6% in 1990 to 34.6% in 2012.[19] Rates of malnutrition are higher in Karamoja than in the rest of the country. In 2012, rates of **underweight, wasting,** and **stunting** in Karamoja were 26%, 12%, and 32%, respectively, compared with respective averages in Uganda of 16%, 6%, and 38%.[20] Nutrition surveillance demonstrates that these indicators have changed little since 2009.[21]

Millennium Development Goal 1: Eradicate Extreme Poverty and Hunger. Target 1.A: Halve, between 1990 and 2015, the proportion of people whose income is less than $1 a day

Millennium Development Goal 1: Eradicate Extreme Poverty and Hunger. Target 1.C: Halve, between 1990 and 2015, the proportion of people who suffer from hunger

Reproduced from the United Nations. (n.d.). 2015 Millennium Development Goals. Retrieved from http://www.un.org/millenniumgoals/. Accessed August 13, 2013. This source is used for all Millennium Development Goals in this chapter.

This chapter, using Milk Matters Karamoja as an example, examines population-level nutrition assessment and determinants in complex environments. The first section provides a background on pastoralist livelihoods; the role of milk in livelihoods, diets, and nutrition; and the influence of upstream factors on persistent nutritional vulnerability. The second section introduces selected quantitative and qualitative methods for evaluating the nutritional status of a population. Such assessments help identify the nutritionally vulnerable and assess causal factors of malnutrition, and qualitative participatory methods, as used in Milk Matters Karamoja, can investigate more deeply relationships between upstream factors and malnutrition. The third section, again using Karamoja as an example, describes challenges in making and implementing recommendations.

Background

Pastoralist Livelihoods and Diets

Mobility is central to pastoralist and agro-pastoralist livelihood strategies. In environments with seasonal availability of water and pasture, movement is necessary for herders to maintain herd health and conserve scarce resources. Pastoralism can vary from highly **nomadic** to **transhumant**,[22] while agro-pastoralists, in contrast, incorporate opportunistic agricultural production, displaying partial settlement while retaining some mobility. Agro-pastoralism is dominant in the Karamoja region of Uganda. Households historically split their time between a permanent settlement site, or *manyatta,* located near good sites for cultivation, and multiple *kraals,* in close proximity to key sites for pasture and water.[23,24]

Pastoralists and agro-pastoralists pursue various livelihood strategies. For example, nomadic pastoralists, whose diets are heavily reliant on animal products, maintain large and diversified herds that provide milk year-round for their own consumption and for sale and exchange for other food items, such as cereals, vegetables, and oils.[25,26] Few if any (agro-)pastoralist populations rely solely on livestock products for their food. In particular, in regions with monomodal rainfall patterns or low annual rainfall and where livestock rely on natural forage without added supplementation, milk supply tends to be more seasonal and food items from hunting and gathering feature more prominently in the diet.[27,28] For agro-pastoralists, the incorporation of agriculture supplements the animal-based food supply, while additional food items are still obtained

through sale or exchange of livestock products. Seasonally available foraged and hunted products may further supplement the diets of pastoralists and agro-pastoralists.[29,30,31,32]

Groups' movement patterns affect diets. They are traditionally determined by seasonality and rainfall but increasingly dictated by extreme weather, such as drought, conflict, and political and economic restrictions. Historically in Karamoja, herders, mostly men and boys, moved herds during the dry season between strategic *kraals,* with access to these sites maintained through political and social alliances with neighboring groups. Women, young children, and the elderly remained at the *manyatta,* cultivating small plots and tending to a few small livestock that provided limited milk. Communities often sent their most nutritionally vulnerable members, including young children and pregnant or lactating mothers, to the *kraals* to ensure regular access to the main supply of milk.[33,34] Food scarcity characterized the dry season, but the food supply improved quickly with the return of the rains and rapid resumption of milk production, particularly in comparison to the prolonged gap between rains and the crop harvest.[35] Past research on pastoral nutrition found that outside of drought years, pastoralist livelihoods exhibited a high degree of resiliency to seasonal malnutrition, as milk yields resume much more quickly than food productions with the return of the rains.[36]

Today, however, an insecure environment, loss of land, policies limiting movement, and recurrent drought have restricted animal and human movement and disrupted the balance between human and animal needs and scarce natural resources. Results include deteriorating animal health and reduced availability of and access to animal milk.

Role of Milk in Pastoralist Child Nutrition

Milk and milk products, such as sour milk, yogurt, butter, and ghee, are among the "most nutritionally complete foods in the world," providing energy and essential nutrients, and are central to the pastoralist diet.[37] Milk is a highly renewable food source, but household supply is extremely variable. Biological factors, such as the animal's reproductive cycle and health status, affect the quantity of milk produced. Physical factors, such as proximity of livestock to the household, are critical in the dry season, when herders must often take animals far to find pasture and water. Traditional (agro-)pastoralist strategies for maintaining a stable milk supply include keeping a diversified herd with different milk production patterns, closely managing animals' reproductive cycles, and protecting animal health and nutritional status, in part through maintaining access to food and water. However, many uncontrollable factors affect access to milk. For example, as rainfall increases, pastures and water sources improve, animal nutrition improves, and milk production increases; the opposite is true during drought.[38] In addition, different animal species have different pregnancy and lactation periods. Thus, a herd composed of a variety of types of animals, when healthy and managed appropriately, can allow for year-round milk supply. In Karamoja, people typically supplement cattle herds with goats, sheep, and sometimes camels.

Children require energy- and nutrient-dense foods to support growth and development. The main source of protein, fat, and micronutrients for pastoralist children is milk, either alone or mixed with grain dishes in fresh, sour, or processed forms.[39,40] Due to its significance, milk is typically prioritized for consumption by children during periods of scarcity, such as during droughts.[41,42,43] High milk consumption among pastoralist children leads to a protein-rich, calorie-poor diet based in animal products, while children in poor agricultural populations, with heavily cereal-based diets, are more likely to obtain sufficient energy while struggling to get adequate protein and fat.[44,45,46] While calories may be low, children in (agro-)pastoralist populations tend to be thin but healthy.[47]

Assessment and Investigation

In any discipline, planning field-based research involves considering various methods and approaches, such as quantitative versus qualitative or participatory versus extractive. Both internal and external factors influence these decisions. Internal factors include specific research goals and objectives, nature of the research questions, needs and interests of the stakeholders, and partnerships between researchers, development agencies, and the community. External factors include the security environment and logistics, such as time allotted, field access, and finances.

Quantitative and qualitative approaches can complement each other to assess a public health nutrition context in depth. **Nutrition assessment**, a predominantly quantitative approach, is used for identifying and monitoring nutritionally vulnerable populations and investigating causal determinants of malnutrition at national, regional, and project levels. Qualitative methods in nutrition research permit situation-specific exploration of nuances in causal linkages, culture- and gender-sensitive aspects, and community

perceptions that would not otherwise be captured through quantitative methods. Milk Matters Karamoja provides an example of qualitative research that includes participatory approaches and methods.

Nutrition Assessment

Assessment is the first core function of public health. In public health nutrition, valid, timely, and reliable assessment is crucial for informed decision making, including for humanitarian response planning, intervention and program design, monitoring and program evaluation, and policy development. While various guidelines for nutrition assessments have emerged, the choice of tools employed has remained flexible to allow for differing needs, objectives, resources, and situational constraints. Nutrition assessments can be predominantly quantitative, but may also include qualitative strategies, with focus group discussions, key informant interviews, and observation.

> *Public Health Core Competency 1: Analytical/ Assessment Skills 1: Identifies the health status of populations and their related determinants of health and illness*
>
> *Public Health Core Competency 2: Policy Development/ Program Planning Skills 1: Gathers information relevant to specific public health policy issues*

History and Evolution of Nutrition Assessments

"Nutrition assessments," a term coined by the League of Nations in 1932 as disparities in hunger and malnutrition around the world came into the limelight, refers to the medical set of tools used to measure the nutritional status of a population.[48] In 1949, the newly established United Nations (UN) called for a Joint Expert Committee on Nutrition that would advise two of its specialized agencies, the Food and Agriculture Organization (FAO) and the World Health Organization (WHO), on collaborative approaches to improving malnutrition and hunger around the world.[49] Over the next few decades, the Joint Committee sought to establish guidelines for evaluating, measuring, and monitoring the nutrition status of a population.[50,51] Although no definitive guidelines were set, a widely recognized set of direct and indirect tools was established for use in nutrition assessments (**Table 23-1**).

In following years, numerous countries undertook large-scale national nutrition surveys, often with aid from

Table 23-1 Direct and indirect tools for nutrition assessment

Direct	Anthropometric measurements	Weight, height/length, age, and sex
		Indices: weight-for-age, height-for-age, weight-for-height, BMI
	Biochemical (lab) measurements	Hemoglobin, stool and urine tests, analysis of hair and nails
	Clinical signs	Signs associated with micronutrient deficiencies
	Dietary intake measurements	24-hour dietary recall, food frequency questionnaire, dietary histories, observation
Indirect	Ecological variables	Socioeconomic factors, food production, food consumption, cultural influences, infrastructure, and facilities
	Economic variables	Population density, income
	Vital health statistics	Mortality, morbidity, fertility

Data from Jelliffe, D. B. (1966). The assessment of the nutritional status of the community (with special reference to field surveys in developing regions of the world). *Monograph Series. World Health Organization, 53*, 3-271.

international organizations, but outcomes were variable. In 1988, WHO responded to the lack of standardization for nutrition surveillance and assessment by publishing guidelines for national, regional, and project levels.[52] By the mid-1990s, the U.S. Agency for International Development (USAID) and UNICEF had, respectively, initiated the Demographic Health Survey (DHS) and Multiple Indicator Cluster Survey (MICS), two major national-level surveys with clearly defined public health and nutrition-related modules and structured guidelines and standards for data collection. These surveys improved the availability of reliable and internationally comparable data.[53,54]

The **Sphere Project** was a voluntary initiative within the global movement to "improve the quality of humanitarian assistance and the accountability of humanitarian actors to their constituents."[55] Established in 1997, the Sphere Project generated an invaluable resource for humanitarian assistance in the form of a handbook of internationally accepted guidelines and standards, including guidance on conducting food security and nutrition assessments in emergencies.[56]

A nutrition assessment can include numerous modules, such as those investigating mortality and morbidity, food consumption, micronutrient deficiencies, supplementation and vaccination coverage, water and sanitation, breastfeeding, and infant and young child feeding practices. Nutrition assessments continue to evolve with the emergence of new, more rapid, accessible, and noninvasive "bedside" tools, such as the finger-prick blood sample.[57] Assessments may

vary in size and scale from large national-level or regional-level assessments to local, program-oriented efforts.

Nutritional Assessments in Karamoja, Uganda

Since 2000, nutritional assessments in pastoralist areas, particularly in the Horn of Africa, indicate increasing malnutrition among pastoralist children during the dry season, indicating susceptibility, or loss of traditional resiliency to traditional fluctuations in milk supply.[58,59,60] Nutritional assessments conducted in Karamoja before Milk Matters Karamoja included the DHS in 2006, the World Food Programme's Emergency Food Security Assessment (EFSA) of the Karamoja region in 2007, the Comprehensive Food Security and Vulnerability Analysis (CFSVA) in 2009, and the nutrition surveillance system for the region implemented jointly by the District Health Offices and the INGO Action Against Hunger (ACF) between 2009 and 2012. The surveys revealed ongoing prevalence of malnutrition in the region, with average **severe acute malnutrition (SAM)** rates exceeding WHO's critical threshold of 2.0% in May 2012, and average **global acute malnutrition (GAM)** levels of 8.1–12.8%, with district-specific levels occasionally exceeding WHO standard thresholds for emergency levels. Because these extensive quantitative surveillance data had already clearly established vulnerable populations, Milk Matters Karamoja focused on qualitative methods for further investigating factors related to the high rates of child malnutrition.

Participatory Approach and Methods: An Example of Qualitative Nutrition Research

Qualitative research methods aim to objectively explore complex social phenomena and interactions in a specific context. Participatory approaches recognize the significance of including individuals and communities in research, assessment, and program planning.

> *Public Health Core Competency 3: Communication Skills 3: Solicits community-based input from individuals and organizations*
>
> *Public Health Core Competency 4: Cultural Competency Skills 1: Incorporates strategies for interacting with persons from diverse backgrounds*

History and Evolution of Participatory Methods

In traditional field research, outside researchers would assess and analyze poor communities with little or no inclusion of the studied populations in the research design and analysis phase. Participatory strategies gained momentum in the early 1990s with the growing popularity of a **Participatory Rural Appraisal (PRA)** promoting a fundamental shift in thinking toward the involvement of local people in the analysis, planning, and enacting of change.[61] It was influenced by various approaches, including the **Rapid Rural Appraisal (RRA)**. Since the 1970s, RRA had been exploring quicker and more cost-effective techniques for assessing and understanding rural life, emphasizing the use of local people's knowledge and information. RRA recognized the value of local input, but was still extractive in nature, seeking information from community members for analysis by outside experts. PRA, however, began to emphasize the roles of local people throughout the entire process, not just in providing data.[62]

Robert Chambers, a principal developer and proponent of PRA, realized that participatory approaches would continue to evolve as the result of innovation and sharing, and therefore the core principles of PRA were most important.[63] These principles focused on placing the needs and interests of the community members first, being prepared to listen and adapt to a more flexible learning process and pace, engaging first and foremost as a facilitator rather than a leader and accepting that the community has

a greater capacity to understand the concerns and realities of their lives than an outsider.[64]

Since the 1990s, participatory methods have been incorporated into a wide range of applications beyond PRAs, including but not limited to topical research, monitoring assessments, and impact assessment. The choice of tools may depend on the nature of the research questions, but generally fall into five categories (**Table 23-2**). The list is by no means exhaustive.

Methodology of Milk Matters Karamoja

Three overarching questions informed the conceptual framework, study design, and data collection and analysis of Milk Matters Karamoja:

- How have the amount and sources of household milk changed?
- How has what households do with available milk changed?
- What are the impacts of these changes on child nutrition and household livelihoods?

Table 23-2 Participatory tools and examples

Type of Participatory Approach	Example of Tools
Spatial data	Transects
	Village walk
	Village resource map
Temporal data	Daily activity clocks
	Timelines
	Seasonal calendars
Social/ institutional information	Flow diagram
	Social network map
	Wealth ranking
	Venn diagram
Discrete data	Farming systems diagram
	Pairwise/preference ranking
	Livelihood profiles
Indigenous or local data	Cultural histories
	Myths and legends
	Indigenous ways of expressing realities

Data from Food and Agriculture Organization (n.d.) Field tools. Acces' September 3, 2013, from http://www.fao.org/Participation/tools/PRA '

The depth of these inquiries makes them well suited to qualitative methods that allow for extended and open-ended discussions using participatory approaches (**Figure 23-3**).

Participatory methods in Milk Matters Karamoja included gender- and age-specific **focus group discussions (FGDs)** and **semistructured key informant interviews** with open-ended questioning, **community timelines**, **proportional piling**, and **pairwise ranking**. The interviews began by asking male and female community members of varying ages to create a timeline illustrating periods of recent change. This exercise led to two important outcomes. First, community members were introduced to the project and became engaged in the process. Second, the timelines established two clear time periods, one referred to as the *before* period, with traditional livelihoods and conditions, and one referred to as the *now* period, characterized by worsening security environment and intensifying drought conditions. The timeline and establishment of two distinct time periods were then used as reference points in the participatory exercises and questions related to shifts in milk supply, diets, and livelihood activities. Community members also participated in discussion of which solutions they felt would best address the factors and trends revealed through the interview.

Sample size, sampling method, and site selection are critical elements of research, whether quantitative or qualitative. Decisions are influenced by such factors as study design, availability of financial and human resources, accessibility, time, and sociopolitical and security environments. In the qualitative Milk Matters Karamoja, the emphasis was on depth rather than breadth, and applicability of the findings to a broader population was not a priority. Study sites were selected strategically, not randomly, to satisfy predetermined criteria: (1) representation across the three government-classified different livelihood zones in the region, or pastoral, agro-pastoral, and agricultural; (2) varying distances to trading centers in order to understand the impact of market access; and (3) in proximity to neighboring, potentially hostile, groups in order to understand the impact of conflict.

Two subcounties were chosen from each of the three livelihood zones, and two settlements were visited in each subcounty, for a total of 12 study sites. The team conducted at least nine focus group discussions (FGDs) and on average 12 individual interviews per subcounty. All interviews and FGDs were conducted in the *manyattas* and targeted men and women who were parents to children under 5 years of age. Men and women participated in separate FGDs. The team intentionally oversampled women, at a frequency twice as high as men, because women are considered more reliable informants on household diets.

Implementation and Making Recommendations

Constraints and Challenges in Implementation

Balance Context and Speed

Complex environments pose multiple constraints and challenges when conducting research. For example, gathering context-specific information must be balanced with the speed of response. This challenge threatens nutritional and emergency assessments in **complex humanitarian emergencies** (CHEs), as practitioners must collect situation-specific information but work quickly to save lives and livelihoods. Available guidelines and other resources include the aforementioned Sphere Project handbook, *Emergency Nutrition Assessment: Guidelines for Field Workers*,[65] produced by Save the Children UK, and *Emergency Food Security Assessment (EFSA): Guidelines* established by the World Food Programme (WFP).[66] Both recommend first carefully evaluating all available secondary data on the population before making decisions about data needs. Sufficient data may already be available, making further collection redundant. It is best to identify the primary information gaps and, if needed, select the appropriate methodology for data collection.

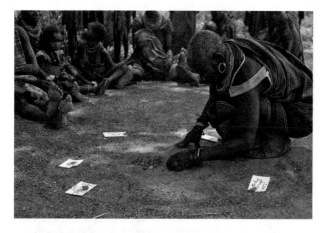

Figure 23-3 Participatory methods

Courtesy of Khristopher Carlson.

Milk Matters Karamoja, while occurring in a complex environment, was not implementing an assessment nor responding to an emergency, but rather was seeking to understand and inform responses to a long-term, gradual change in the context of a protracted crisis. More time was available for designing and testing an appropriate study methodology. In addition, various team members had years of experience in Karamoja or with pastoralist populations in the greater region, providing advantages of familiarity with the context, underlying situation, local culture, institutional history, and conflict dynamics.

Representativeness

Study site and population sample selection in all studies are critical to the logistics of collecting data, and directly influence data quality analysis. The manner in which sites and the study sample are selected determines the level of representativeness that the study can achieve. Other factors affecting sampling include budget, relationship between community and researcher, and accessibility, which can be affected by seasonality, conflict, and political atmosphere.

Reports and analyses of assessments that do not aim for representativeness of a given population or area must clearly state this fact. In qualitative research, for example, the focus is depth rather than breadth. In Milk Matters Karamoja, where representativeness was not the priority, the study findings can be taken as reflections of experiences and reality *only* of the *exact* population involved. They do not represent an entire national population.

Insecurity

Security can be a major constraint to any assessment or research in conflict- or violence-prone areas. Team security and physical safety must be paramount, as well as any possible protection threats that the presence of a research team may bring to local communities. At times the emphasis on team security can introduce an important bias into the research or assessment data. In the case of the Karamoja region, for instance, studies that seek to understand the impact and effects of violence and conflict on livelihoods and nutrition are often unable to gather data in the most insecure areas, thereby potentially underestimating the impacts for the population. In addition, insecurity in study areas often poses logistical problems, causing delays in fieldwork, inaccessibility of sites, limited periods of fieldwork, additional costs and ethical considerations of hiring security escorts, and difficulties in hiring qualified personnel willing to work in such areas.

Respondents' experiences with insecurity can also pose challenges to the accuracy of the data. Respondents may be distrustful of outsiders, hesitant to disclose information on assets that may be targeted for theft (including livestock, savings, remittances, regular forms of cash inflow, personal possessions, and so on), and wary of interventions that may appear to be linked to state actors in situations where state forces are a party to a conflict.

Experiences with Humanitarian Relief

Nutritional assessments are often conducted in areas with recurring or protracted food insecurity or nutritional crises. Long experiences with assessments and humanitarian operations can lead to bias in the data. In Karamoja, for example, food relief has been part of the region's economy for over 40 years. Respondents in such contexts have often integrated humanitarian assistance into their livelihoods in the forms of household nutritional support, extensive markets for the resale and exchange of relief items, and labor markets for the support services, such as offloading, protection, and community liaisons, that accompany relief operations. Respondents are often aware of the answers most likely to ensure the continuation of relief aid, and are motivated to provide them.

This phenomenon occurred in Milk Matters. Although the team always stressed the independence of their academic project from relief agencies, and lack of any direct link between the research and the provision of assistance, respondents often overemphasized the extent of poverty or loss of assets. The team sought to counter this bias by conducting multiple interviews in each location and including perspectives of key informants, but the bias likely persisted given the region's history of relief assistance.

Recall

Many nutritional assessments and research studies rely partly on respondents' memories of diets, conditions, or experiences. Women may be asked, for instance, to list all the foods they fed to their children over the past day or week, or even over the past few years, for the purpose of establishing a retroactive baseline for longitudinal purposes or defining a "now" and "before" comparison, as in Karamoja. While less concerning in humanitarian nutrition assessments, sources of error in dietary recall can include faulty memory and inaccurate depictions of diet that may occur when participants attempt to tell interviewers what they think are "better" answers, such as reporting higher intake of nutrient-dense foods. Methods to limit bias in dietary recalls include standardized interview protocols, training of interviewers and coders, "probing" methods in the interview, and an increase in the number of observations to reduce the effects of poor recall.[67]

In Milk Matters Karamoja, problems with recall were apparent upon analysis of data from separate field visits in September, during the rainy, prosperous season, and in February, during the drier season with more food insecurity. In both visits, participants were asked to compare conditions in the previous rainy season with current conditions at the time of data collection. In general, respondents described a less prosperous and productive previous rainy season when asked in February than when asked in September. This reflects the impact on perceptions of the passage of time as well as of current experiences, given that February falls during the depths of the dry season and is generally marked by greater food insecurity and hardship. This clear example illustrates the shortcomings of recall combined with the bias resulting from a long history of humanitarian intervention.

Biases of Data Collectors

Individual biases of each member of research or assessment teams affect data collection, transcription, analysis, and reporting. Demographic and ideological background, such as gender, age, nationality, culture, religion and political ideology, past experience, and expertise can all lead to bias. Some of these biases can be countered by hiring team members from the region, but these individuals will have their own biases.

In the case of Milk Matters Karamoja, biases displayed by external researchers resulted from their tendency to be expatriate and well educated. Local biases were also evident. For example, one problem was hiring literate team members who did not have preestablished negative opinions of the rural population and way of life. The team sought to avoid this bias through the interview process, but was still forced to dismiss two team members who made disparaging comments about the attire and cleanliness of the respondents.

Team Composition

The ideal composition of a research or assessment team balances experience, expertise, and likely biases. Milk Matters Karamoja sought to have more local team members than outsiders to limit the expatriate presence to one person at any one time, and to seek a gender balance. A critical team

member was a former large-animal veterinarian with over 30 years of experience in the region. His presence in the project allowed better access to remote communities who either remembered him specifically or would welcome any veterinarian.

Translation

Translators are the direct communicators with interviewees. They must clearly understand not only the day-to-day aspects of the work but also the larger picture and objectives in order to help guide the researcher during the interview. Careful training of translators can enable them to contribute as observers during the interview. They may be able to recognize key behaviors that might otherwise be missed by an outsider, such as body language and tone of voice. Translators must understand the importance of translating responses in as much detail as possible, instead of providing broad interpretations, to ensure detection of small nuances that may trigger additional follow-up questions or discussion. It is also important to remember that translation is incredibly tiring, and translators need frequent breaks. Ideally, postinterview debriefings should occur to ask translators about any observations, thoughts, and reactions they may have had during the interview. Such feedback can be useful in adjusting work for the next day or site.

Findings from Milk Matters Karamoja

The findings of the study reflect community perceptions of changes over time from the *before* period to the *now* period, as established through community timelines, in four interrelated areas: (1) sources of milk within the households; (2) uses of milk by the household; (3) milk in the diets of children; and (4) livelihood adaptations. These findings also demonstrate the depth of information that can be obtained through appropriate implementation of participatory qualitative methods.

Sources of Milk

Shift in Source of Milk and Sharp Decline in Total Milk

Households in the three livelihood zones reported declines in milk production from their own animals, from 76% to 88% in the *before* period to 23%, 48%, and 67% in the agricultural, pastoral, and agro-pastoral zones, respectively, in the *now* period. They also noted a sharp increase in purchased milk. Overall, the data indicate that purchased milk has replaced households' own production as the primary source of milk in the *now* period in all livelihood zones, with women in particular noting this change.

Households need cash to purchase milk. They often acquire cash through the sale of natural resources and by engaging in casual labor for pay or in-kind exchanges, either milk or other goods that can then be traded or sold for milk. However, milk often sells out quickly in all locations, and women who live farther from markets or *kraals* report that there is often no milk left to buy by the time they reach the seller. Because of the cost and availability constraints, households can rarely obtain enough milk via purchasing to fully replace what they previously had through their own production. Indeed, the most profound overall change from *before* to *now* is the decrease in overall household milk supply.

Underlying Factors

Households were accustomed to normal seasonality of milk production in the *before* period. However, decreased availability of and access to milk in the *now* period exceeded seasonal fluctuations in the *before* period. This decrease is due primarily to a household's loss of its own production due to the following interlinking factors:

Loss of livestock: Many animals died or were sold.

Distance from herds: Milk herds, once kept near the household, became largely kept in government *kraals* or near military barracks, which limits household access.

Animal health: Animal morbidity increased due to overcrowding in government *kraals*, decreasing access to pasture, and the spread of animal disease.

Involvement of the military in animal husbandry: Military personnel limit access to livestock to specific times of the day, thereby constraining both milk off-take and the management of herds for optimal milk production.

Shifts in livelihood strategies: With widespread insecurity, mobility was decreased and herders were often unable to access traditional sites for grazing.

Furthermore, means of procuring milk through other avenues, except for purchasing, also decreased. These alternative sources in the *before* time period included sharing among households, exchange with migrating pastoralists from other areas, and gifts. These systems of exchange were the means of building social reciprocity and allegiances between groups, and the erosion of these sources has not only reduced the amount of milk coming into households, but has also heightened vulnerability by eliminating potential sources of assistance that were maintained through these regular exchanges and interactions.

Uses of Milk

Household use of milk has shifted with the decrease in milk supply at the household level. The primary shift is an increase in the portion of available milk allocated to young children, with a decrease in all other uses of milk.

Narrowed Range of Uses

In the *before* time period, milk was an important part of household diets, social exchange, gifting, ceremonies and rituals, and commerce. In the *now* period, by contrast, respondents reported little use of milk outside of consumption by household members, although women reported less than 4% of milk being sold, while men reported almost 29% of milk being sold, used in rituals or ceremonies, and given to visitors. Cash generated from the sale can be used for the purchase of essential commodities and other food items. The appearance of multiple locations outside of town for selling milk in the *now* period reflects the declining overall supply, as such sites did not exist in the *before* period because "everyone in the village had enough milk."[68]

Fewer Social Uses

The amount of milk used in ceremonies, given as gifts, and offered to visitors declined from *before* to *now*. As one group of women said, "How can we have ceremonies? Milk is necessary to perform ceremonies."[69] Milk is traditionally important in weddings, initiations, and the naming of babies. A decrease in the regularity of ceremonies is paralleled by a decrease in political and social cohesion within and between communities. The decline in sharing of milk through gifts or with visitors indicates both the overall loss of milk across the population and the erosion of social exchanges that previously helped to mitigate vulnerability. Gifts most often went to those who had newborn babies, did not have milk animals of their own, or had animals that had not yet reproduced. A group of men in the Regnen sub-county stated that "a household with milking cows supported those households without."[70] While some of these gifts were expected to be reciprocated, gifts of milk made to households in hardship were acts of kindness or charity.[71] Superstition may have also played a role, as one focus group of men reported that "it is a belief that such poor household could [cast] bad omens onto the family if they were denied milk."[72]

Milk in the Diets of Young Children

Prioritization of Milk for Children

Young children receive top priority for milk consumption. Women reduce the amount of milk used for other purposes, including for consumption by other household members. In the *before* time period, women reported that 57% of total household milk consumed was by young children, and other members received 47%; in the *now* time period, women reported that other household members, including the very old, received only 19% of total milk consumed. While the responses of men differed slightly from those of the women, responses from both groups showed clear trends in increasing the portion given to children from the *before* to the *now* time period at the expense of consumption by other household members.

It is important to remember that even though young children are receiving a greater percentage of the total milk supply than they were previously, the precipitous drop in total available milk means that children are receiving significantly less milk than in the previous time period.

Less Nutritious Replacements for Milk in the Diet

Milk went from being the primary food item in all livelihood zones to one of the least represented foods in children's diets. Other forms of animal protein also dropped markedly in all areas, from an average of 20% to only 8% of total calories. Children's consumption of wild fruits and vegetables jumped from 11–15% in the *before* period to 40–50% in the *now* period. Purchased and self-produced cereals contributed 20–25% of calories in the *before* period, and a greater proportion in the *now* time period.

In Karamoja, families struggled to provide adequate substitutes for milk in children's diets. Mothers most commonly reported wild greens in their children's diets in the *now* period, but also used tamarind, sesame paste, and oil pressed from sunflower seeds in place of milk when possible. These substitute foods lack the nutrient density of milk

and fail on their own to meet growing children's requirements for nutrients such as protein and calcium.

Concern for Health and Nutrition of Children

Men and women in the study population were well aware of the health benefits of milk for young children. Respondents reported that milk is "good for growth," that children who consume a lot of milk are "strong and healthy," and that butter "keeps coughs and colds away." Furthermore, "those who have access to milk are brighter, smarter children. Those who have access to milk can develop into healthy, growing children and are more suited to become strong shepherd boys."[73]

Respondents ascribe many negative health outcomes to the relative lack of milk in children's diets and the decrease in dietary diversity in recent years. The most common complaints regarding children's health were emaciation, diarrhea, malaria, scabies, "hair that is yellowish, silky and scant," and general "fevers" and "cough." Children were said to be weak and lethargic and to have dry skin, "puffy eyes and swollen faces," and big bellies "from eating porridge without milk." Various respondents said that children without regular milk were stunted or did not grow quickly.

Livelihood Adaptations

Households across Karamoja are seeking ways to adapt to changes in livelihoods due to loss of livestock, repeated drought, insecurity, and external pressures on animal-based production systems. Livelihood strategies at the household level are usually quite diverse and involve multiple activities by different household members. The patterns of livelihood change apparent in the study population and aimed at improving food security fall into one of the following broad categories: (1) adaptations to acquire cash or equivalents to replace items that have been lost within the diet, (2) adaptations to decrease reliance on these same items in the diet, and (3) adoption of new or different livelihood strategies in an effort to prevent increased food insecurity.

Specific strategies and adaptations at the household level vary in their duration and reversibility. Some strategies can increase household vulnerability, while others may bring greater resilience over time. Many of these adaptations are related to household decisions regarding specific members of the household, such as whether a young person should be in school, should migrate to another area, or should engage in a given activity. The tension between the needs of the individual and those of the household or community remains a primary challenge in changing landscapes.

> *Public Health Core Competency 4: Cultural Competency Skills 3: Responds to diverse needs that are the result of cultural differences*

Participants in the study categorically expressed despair about their current situations and anxiety about the future for themselves and their children. While additional research would be needed to investigate the impact of specific livelihood adaptations on overall well-being, the data from this study indicate that people's efforts to improve their situations have not yet been successful.

Making Recommendations in Complex Environments

Public health nutrition problems with a complex web of upstream factors invariably require complicated solutions. Too often there is a tendency in such situations to react by simply treating a symptom, such as malnutrition, with a one-dimensional response, such as relief aid, rather than addressing the underlying complex problems and systems, such as poverty. Such direct symptomatic responses can be important components of immediate humanitarian responses, but they should not overshadow long-term, multifaceted approaches. Producing changes through holistic approaches in complex environments can be challenging. They can require, for example, an overhaul of national, regional, or local policy, a change in long-standing perceptions and attitudes, a substantial investment in infrastructure, or broad intersectoral cooperation. Such solutions can be controversial and face difficulty in gaining traction among political and local actors. Addressing such challenges requires careful consideration of the context and appropriateness of recommendations, consulting the local residents and including their ideas of solutions to the problems, and setting goals for immediate, short-term, and long-term recommendations.

Considering the Context

Karamoja provides an example of a problem that on the surface may appear as straightforward as the loss of milk leading to declining nutrition, but in reality there are diverse factors, including historical patterns, policy decisions, and animal epidemics. Viable solutions must consider these realities. Interventions may draw from comparable situations among similar populations, but must also reflect the unique characteristics of the region. In the case of Milk Matters, the parent project, Milk Matters Ethiopia, had compiled and reviewed a list of interventions that could help to tackle the problem of seasonal decline in milk availability and accessibility to households in pastoralist regions of Africa.[74] These interventions included:

- Increasing the number of milking animals to households with few animals;
- Improving the nutrition of lactating animals in the seasons when the forage is insufficient or of low quality;
- Improving livestock health so as to increase milk supply;
- Introducing or promoting different livestock breeds so as to prolong the seasonal availability of milk; and
- Introducing methods of preserving or selling milk in less perishable forms.

Some of these practices could have potential in Karamoja, but should not be applied in Karamoja without careful consideration of any differences in the original setting from that of Karamoja. Milk Matters Karamoja, using data from local perceptions and input as well as long experience in the region, critically assessed the opportunities with an eye for unintended consequences, anticipating that:

- Restocking (or introducing new breeds) would be a potentially major liability for households in Karamoja due to the chronic insecurity caused by cattle thefts and raids;
- Increasing milk yields by boosting animal nutrition with supplementary feeding would likely be challenged by politicians and donors on the premise that human malnutrition, at astonishing high levels throughout the region, and not animals, should be the primary target of limited resources, such as cost of relief assistance. In addition, an approach such as this would likely require a national policy context that values and promotes pastoralism, which is not currently the case in Uganda; and
- Introducing new methods for preserving or selling milk might be viable in Karamoja in the future, as data demonstrate a strong demand for milk. However, this sort of intervention would be cost effective only *after* the livestock milk supply had been increased.

Supporting Local Priorities

Local community members often have a better understanding of the situation than external researchers, and should be engaged in discussions of possible solutions. In Milk Matters Karamoja, participants were asked which factors they believed were causing the loss of milk, and which solutions were best. Responses indicated the belief that the absence of milk represented a broader erosion of the traditional way of life and uncertainty about the future. Regarding solutions, participants identified the need to address the pervasive situation of insecurity through complete and uniform disarmament and improved protection. However, based on history, the complete and uniform removal of all weapons is not straightforward.[75] While the policy of disarmament intended to improve security through the removal of guns, its uncoordinated and uneven implementation, lack of adequate security for disarmed households, ongoing loss of household assets (for example, livestock), and reports of human rights abuses have been problematic. Additional suggestions from the community focused on improving the health and security of the livestock and increasing education for children to improve opportunities and combat the pull of cattle raiding.

Setting Short- and Long-Term Goals

In complex situations, the best solutions often take considerable time and effort from various stakeholders. Such goals in Karamoja include advocating for propastoral policies, improved security and better protection for local populations, and a holistic approach requiring intersectoral collaboration. Even while pursuing these long-term objectives, areas for immediate attention should be identified and short-term recommendations should be required. Recommendations in Milk Matters Karamoja were for immediate and short-term action that supported and incorporated local priorities.

- Support and expand programs focused on improving animal health (for example, expand training and facilitation of Community Animal Health Workers–CAHWs).

- Support and expand programs aimed at greater well-being for children (for example, school feeding).

- Support initiatives to improve and diversify markets and increase access (for example, encouraging small traders in marketing of animal products).

Conclusion

Nutrition assessments and participatory methods have a significant role in investigating the nutrition status and the linkages between upstream factors, livelihoods, and nutrition. In addition, researchers face many key challenges and constraints, including difficulties in making recommendations, in complex environments. A major goal of such research is to fill gaps in knowledge and provide evidence-based resources to policy makers for improved decision making.

Milk Matters Karamoja established that milk does indeed matter, and people know it. By working at multiple levels to address upstream factors such as improving the policy, economic, and security environment in the region, stakeholders should be able to improve both child nutrition and livelihood sustainability of local populations. On a broader scale, Milk Matters Karamoja is part of a large and ongoing discussion about the future of pastoralism and an attempt to redress past inappropriate polices for pastoral development. Participatory and investigative research in such ever-changing situations can help to ensure that the voices of affected communities, including the (agro-)pastoralists of Karamoja, are heard.

References

1 United Nations Children's Fund (UNICEF). (1990). *Strategy for improved nutrition of children and women in developing countries.* Policy Review Paper E/ICEF/1990/1.6. New York, NY: UNICEF.

2 Blench, R. (2001). *Pastoralism in the new millennium.* FAO Animal Production and Health Paper 150. Rome, Italy: Food and Agriculture Organization.

3 Sadler, K., Kerven, C., Calo, M., Manske, M., & Catley, A. (2010). The fat and the lean: Review of the production and use of milk by pastoralists. *Pastoralism, 1*(2), 34.

4 Kerven, C. (1987). *The role of milk in a pastoral diet and economy: The case of South Darfur, Sudan.* International Livestock Centre for Africa (ILCA) Bulletin No. 27. Addis Ababa: ILCA.

5 Sikana, P. M., Kerven, C., & Behnke, R. H. (1993). *From subsistence to specialized commodity production: Commercialization and pastoral dairying in Africa.* Pastoral Development Network Set 35. London, UK: Overseas Development Institute.

6 Gray, S. (2000). A memory of loss: Ecological politics, local history, and the evolution of Karimojong violence. *Human Organizations, 59*(4), 18.

7 Rugadya, M. (2006). *Pastoralism and conservation studies: Uganda country report.* Kampala, Uganda: IUCN.

8 Sadler, K., Kerven, C., Calo, M., Manske, M., & Catley, A. (2010). The fat and the lean: Review of the production and use of milk by pastoralists. *Pastoralism, 1*(2), 34.

9 Sadler, K., Kerven, C., Calo, M., Manske, M., & Catley, A. (2009). *Milk matters: A literature review of pastoral nutrition and programming responses*. Medford, MA: Feinstein International Center, Tufts University.

10 Markakis, J. (2004). *Pastoralism on the margin*. Minority Rights Group International. Retrieved from http://dev135.buchwald.ca/docs/MRG-Pastorialists-Markakis%202004.pdf.

11 Rass, N. (2006). *Policies and strategies to address the vulnerability of pastoralists in sub-Saharan Africa*. PPLPI Working Paper 37. Rome, Italy: Food and Agriculture Organization.

12 Pavanello, S. (2009). *Pastoralist vulnerability in the Horn of Africa: Exploring political marginalization, donors' policies and cross-border issues–literature review*. London, UK: Humanitarian Policy Group, Overseas Development Institute.

13 Ocan, C. E. (1992). *Pastoral crisis in northeastern Uganda: The changing significance of cattle raids*. Center for Basic Research, Working paper 21.

14 Mirzeler, M., & Young, C. (2000). Pastoral politics in the northeast periphery in Uganda: AK-47 as a change agent. *Journal of Modern African Studies, 38*(3), 407-29.

15 Gray, S. (2000). A memory of loss: Ecological politics, local history, and the evolution of Karimojong violence. *Human Organizations, 59*(4), 18.

16 Gray, S., Sundal, M., Wiebusch, B., Little, M., et al. (2003). Cattle raiding, cultural survival, and adaptability of east African pastoralists. *Current Anthropology, 44*, S3.

17 Stites, E., & Akabwai, D. (2009). *Changing roles, shifting risks: Livelihood impacts of disarmament in Karamoja, Uganda*. Medford, MA: Feinstein International Center, Tufts University.

18 Stites, E., & Akabwai, D. (2010). "We are now reduced to women": Impacts of forced disarmament in Karamoja, Uganda. *Nomadic Peoples, 14*(2), 24-43.

19 Food and Agriculture Organization. (2012.) *The state of food insecurity in the world 2012*. Rome, Italy: FAO.

20 United Nations Children's Fund. (2012). *Country statistics: Uganda*. Retrieved from http://www.unicef.org/infobycountry/uganda_statistics.html

21 District Health Offices, Action Against Hunger, & United Nations Children's Fund. (2012, May). *Nutrition surveillance, Karamoja Region, Uganda, Round 8, May 2012*. Retrieved from http://www.actionagainsthunger.org/sites/default/files/publications/DHO-ACF_Karamoja_Nutrition_Surveillance_Round_8_-_Final_Report_2012.05.pd

22 Blench, R. (2001). *Pastoralism in the new millennium*. FAO Animal Production and Health Paper 150. Rome, Italy: Food and Agriculture Organization.

23 Dyson-Hudson, N. (1969). Subsistence herding in Uganda. *Scientific American, 220*(2), 76-89.

24 Stites, E., & Akabwai, D. (2009). *Changing roles, shifting risks: Livelihood impacts of disarmament in Karamoja, Uganda*. Medford, MA: Feinstein International Center, Tufts University.

25 Nicholson, M. J. L. (1984). Pastoralism and milk production. In A. J. Smith (Ed.), *International Conference on Milk Production in Developing Countries*. Edinburgh, Scotland: University of Edinburgh.

26 Sadler, K., Kerven, C., Calo, M., Manske, M., & Catley, A. (2010). The fat and the lean: Review of the production and use of milk by pastoralists. *Pastoralism, 1(2)*, 34.

27 Nicholson, M. J. L. (1984). Pastoralism and milk production. In A. J. Smith (Ed.), *International Conference on Milk Production in Developing Countries*. Edinburgh, Scotland: University of Edinburgh.

28 Sadler, K., Kerven, C., Calo, M., Manske, M., & Catley, A. (2010). The fat and the lean: Review of the production and use of milk by pastoralists. *Pastoralism, 1(2)*, 34.

29 Galvin, K. A. (1992). Nutritional ecology of pastoralists in dry tropical Africa. *American Journal of Human Biology, 4*, 13.

30 Shell-Duncan, B. (1995). Impact of seasonal variation in food availability and disease stress on the health status of nomadic Turkana children: A longitudinal analysis of morbidity, immunity, and nutritional status. *American Journal of Human Biology, 7*(3), 17.

31 Nathan, M. A., Fratkin, E. M., & Roth, E. A. (1996). Sedentism and child health among Rendille pastoralists of northern Kenya. *Social Science and Medicine, 43*(4), 13.

32 World Food Programme (WFP). (2007). *Emergency food security assessment of Karamoja Region, March-April 2007*. Kamapala, Uganda: WFP.

33 Dyson-Hudson, N. (1969). Subsistence herding in Uganda. *Scientific American, 220*(2), 76-89.

34 Stites, E., Akabwai, D., Mazurana, D., & Ateyo, P. (2007). *Angering Akuju: Survival and suffering in Karamoja*. Medford, MA: Feinstein International Center, Tufts University.

35 Sadler, K., Kerven, C., Calo, M., Manske, M., & Catley, A. (2009). *Milk Matters: A literature review of pastoral nutrition and programming responses*. Medford, MA: Feinstein International Center, Tufts University.

36 Sadler, K., Kerven, C., Calo, M., Manske, M., & Catley, A. (2009). *Milk Matters: A literature review of pastoral nutrition and programming responses*. Medford, MA: Feinstein International Center, Tufts University.

37 Sadler, K., Kerven, C., Calo, M., Manske, M., & Catley, A. (2010). The fat and the lean: Review of the production and use of milk by pastoralists. *Pastoralism, 1(2)*, 34.

38 Sadler, K., Kerven, C., Calo, M., Manske, M., & Catley, A. (2010). The fat and the lean: Review of the production and use of milk by pastoralists. *Pastoralism, 1(2)*, 34.

39 Catley, A., Leyland, T., & Bishop, S. (2008). Policies, practice and participation in protracted crises: The case of livestock interventions in south Sudan. In L. Alinovi, G. Hemrich, & L. Russo (Eds.), *Beyond relief: Food security in protracted crises*. Warwickshire, UK: Practical Action Publishing.

40 Sadler, K., Kerven, C., Calo, M.,Manske, M., & Catley, A. (2010). The fat and the lean: Review of the production and use of milk by pastoralists. *Pastoralism, 1(2)*, 34.

41 Catley, A., Abebe, D., Admassu, B., Bekele, G., Abera, B., Eshete, T., Rufael, T., & Haile, T. (2009). Impact of drought-related

vaccination on livestock mortality in pastoralist areas of Ethiopia. *Disasters, 32*(2): 167-68.

42 Stites, E., & Mitchard, E. (2011). *Milk Matters in Karamoja: Milk in the children's diets and household livelihoods.* Medford, MA: Feinstein International Center, Tufts University.

43 Sadler, K., Mitchard, E., Abdi, A., Shiferaw, Y., Bekele, G., & Catley, A. (2012). *Milk Matters: The impact of dry season livestock support on milk supply and child nutrition in Somali region, Ethiopia.* Medford, MA: Feinstein International Center, Tufts University.

44 Galvin, K. A. (1985). *Food procurement, diet, activities and nutrition of Ngisonyoko, Turkana: Pastoralists in an ecological and social context.* Binghamton, NY: Department of Anthropology, SUNY, Binghamton.

45 Galvin, K. A. (1992). Nutritional ecology of pastoralists in dry tropical Africa. *American Journal of Human Biology, 4,* 13.

46 Fratkin, E., Nathan, M. A., & Roth, E. A. (2006). *Is settling good for pastoralists? The effects of pastoral sedentarization on children's nutrition, growth, and health among Rendille and Ariaal of Marsabit District, Northern Kenya.* Paper presented at Pastoralism and Poverty Reduction in East Africa, A Policy Research Conference, International Livestock Research Institute (ILRI), Nairobi.

47 Rutishauser, I. H. E., & Whitehead, R.G. (1969). Field evaluation of two biochemical tests which may reflect nutritional status in three areas of Uganda. *British Journal of Nutrition, 23,* 13.

48 Gibson, R. (2005). *Principles of nutrition assessment* (2nd ed.). Oxford, UK: Oxford University Press.

49 World Health Organization & Food and Agriculture Organization. (1949). *Joint FAO/WHO Expert Committee on Nutrition, Report on the First Session.* World Health Organization Technical Report Series No. 16. Geneva: World Health Organization.

50 Jeliffe, D. B. (1966). *The assessment of the nutritional status of the community.* World Health Organization Monograph Series No. 53. Geneva: World Health Organization.

51 Gibson, R. (2005). *Principles of nutrition assessment* (2nd ed.). Oxford, UK: Oxford University Press.

52 Beghin, I., Cap, M., & Dujardin, B. (1988). *A guide to nutritional assessment.* Geneva: World Health Organization.

53 UNICEF. Multiple INdicator Cluster Survey (MICS). Updated May 25, 2012. Retrieved from http://www.unicef.org/statistics /index_24302.html

54 USAID. Measure DHS. Retrieved from http://www.measuredhs .com/

55 The Sphere Project. http://www.sphereproject.org/

56 Sphere Project. (2010), *The Humanitarian Charter and minimum standards in Humanitarian Response.* Retrieved from www.spherehandbook.org.

57 Gibson, R. (2005). *Principles of nutrition assessment* (2nd ed.). Oxford, UK: Oxford University Press.

58 Mason, J. B., Chotard, S., et al. (2008). *Fluctuations in wasting in vulnerable child populations in the Greater Horn of Africa.* Working Papers in International Health and Development, No. 08-02. New Orleans, LA: Department of International Health and Development, Tulane University.

59 Ethiopian Health and Nutrition Research Institute, UNICEF, et al. (2009). *Final report from nutrition and mortality surveys conducted in seven mega livelihood zones in Somali Regional State, Ethiopia.* Addis Ababa, Ethiopia: Ethiopian Health and Nutrition Research Institute.

60 United Nations Children's Fund (UNICEF). (2009). *Humanitarian action report: Uganda in 2009.* Kampala, Uganda: UNICEF.

61 Chambers, R. (1994). The origins and practice of Participatory Rural Appraisal. *World Development, 22*(7), 953.

62 Chambers, R. (1994). The origins and practice of Participatory Rural Appraisal. *World Development, 22*(7), 953.

63 Chambers, R. (1994). *Paradigm shifts and the practice of participatory research and development.* Institute of Development Studies Working Paper 2.

64 Food and Agriculture Organization. (n.d.). *Overview of Participatory Rural Appraisal.* Retrieved from http://www.fao .org/Participation/tools/PRA.html.

65 Save the Children UK. (2004). *Emergency nutrition assessment guidelines for field workers.* Retrieved from United Nations System, Standing Committee on Nutrition website, http://www.unscn.org /en/resource_portal/index.php?&themes=211&resource=181.

66 World Food Programme. (2009). *Emergency food security assessment handbook.* Retrieved from http://www.wfp.org /content/emergency-food-security-assessment-handbook.

67 Gibson, R. (2005). *Principles of nutrition assessment* (2nd ed.). Oxford, UK: Oxford University Press.

68 Stites, E., & Mitchard, E. (2011). *Milk Matters in Karamoja: Milk in the children's diets and household livelihoods.* Medford, MA: Feinstein International Center, Tufts University.

69 Stites, E., & Mitchard, E. (2011). *Milk Matters in Karamoja: Milk in the children's diets and household livelihoods.* Medford, MA: Feinstein International Center, Tufts University.

70 Stites, E., & Mitchard, E. (2011). *Milk Matters in Karamoja: Milk in the children's diets and household livelihoods.* Medford, MA: Feinstein International Center, Tufts University.

71 Stites, E., & Mitchard, E. (2011). *Milk Matters in Karamoja: Milk in the children's diets and household livelihoods.* Medford, MA: Feinstein International Center, Tufts University.

72 Stites, E., & Mitchard, E. (2011). *Milk Matters in Karamoja: Milk in the children's diets and household livelihoods.* Medford, MA: Feinstein International Center, Tufts University.

73 Stites, E., & Mitchard, E. (2011). *Milk Matters in Karamoja: Milk in the children's diets and household livelihoods.* Medford, MA: Feinstein International Center, Tufts University.

74 Sadler, K., Kerven, C., Calo, M., Manske, M. & Catley, A. (2010). The fat and the lean: Review of the production and use of milk by pastoralists. *Pastoralism, 1*(2), 34.

75 Stites, E., & Akabwai, D. (2010). "We are now reduced to women": Impacts of forced disarmament in Karamoja, Uganda. *Nomadic Peoples, 14*(2), 24-43.

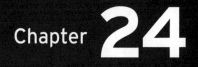
Telehealth, Telemedicine, eHealth, and mHealth in Nutrition Programs

P. Greg Gulick, JD, MHA, MBA

"The average person looks at their smartphone 150 times a day, so all of a sudden they're able to diagnose if their blood pressure's adequately controlled and what are the circumstances when it's not."
—Cardiologist Eric Topol

Cardiologist Eric Topol (quoted on http://www.npr.org/blogs/health/2013/06/18/192777704/patients-lead-the-way-as-medicine-grapples-with-apps)

Learning Objectives

- Distinguish between telehealth, telemedicine, eHealth, and mHealth in nutrition.

- Be familiar with the history of telehealth and factors that are leading to the adoption of telemedicine in public health nutrition programs.

- Know current domestic and international applications of telemedicine, eHealth, and mHealth to improve population nutrition status.

- Recognize the importance of assessing the impact of cost, quality, access, and satisfaction of telemedicine, eHealth, and mHealth programs.

Case Study: Type 2 Diabetes in Rural South Carolina, United States

Stella is a 10-year-old girl in rural South Carolina who was recently diagnosed with type 2 diabetes. She does not have access to nutritious food or to medical specialists trained in dealing with pediatric diabetes in her small town. Stella attends the local elementary school, which does not have the finances to keep a nurse on staff, and she has trouble remembering how and when to take her insulin.

Stella's mother, Maya, is a single parent. Maya's nutrition-related conditions include obesity, hypertension, and pre-diabetes, and she also has undiagnosed depression. Her full-time factory job does not leave her time to make dinner each night, to get Stella to all of her doctor's appointments, or to manage her own chronic conditions. Maya and Stella have health insurance through Maya's employer, but Maya is unable to take time off of work to see a physician. Furthermore, the specialist healthcare providers that she and Stella need are located in the nearest big city, 50 miles away.

Discussion Questions

- Which risk factors do Stella and Maya have that impede their access to care?

- How might access to a computer impact the ability of Stella and Maya to receive the specialized care and counseling they need?

- Which innovations in eHealth might help Stella and Maya manage their conditions and improve their dietary habits?

- How might Stella and Maya be able to regularly receive counseling from a nutritionist?

- How is the situation of Stella and Maya analogous to situations in developing nations where individuals and communities might lack nearby nutritional services and health care, but benefit from telehealth?

Introduction

Challenges such as an increasing population, an aging population,[1] and increasing prevalence of obesity and other chronic conditions are straining the U.S. healthcare system. The shortage of primary care and specialist physicians is further straining the system.[2] Residents of rural areas are particularly likely to have inadequate access to health care.

A substantial portion of the healthcare system's resources is used for treating chronic conditions. Only 3% of all healthcare expenditures in 2007 were for public health programs. To reduce costs and improve health, more focus should be placed on relatively inexpensive public health programs. Increasing funding for nutrition programs can be a cost-effective approach to meeting modern healthcare needs in the United States and the rest of the world. Technology to reduce costs, improve quality of care, and increase accessibility should be integral to public health systems' preparations for the future. Factors that facilitate the adoption of telemedicine, eHealth, and mHealth programs include:

- The development of easy-to-use, inexpensive computers, including tablet personal computers, smartphones, cellphones, and other related technologies;

- The widespread accessibility of the Internet through wireless, satellite, and other means;

- The digitization of healthcare information through the adoption of electronic medical records (EMRs) and electronic health records (EHRs);

- Physician, healthcare professional, and patient demand for better access to health care; and

- Shortages of healthcare professionals.

This chapter examines the differences between telehealth, telemedicine, eHealth, and mHealth and how these programs are improving health care, with a special focus on nutrition programs. The chapter also discusses implementation and evaluation of telemedicine/eHealth/mHealth programs.

Telemedicine, eHealth, and mHealth Defined

Telehealth

The term **telehealth** can "describe electronic information and telecommunications technology used to support and improve clinical health services, health administration, patient information, public health, and professional education and supervision."[3] However, people have engaged in medical practices similar to telehealth for centuries. Since telehealth is the application of communication technologies to health care, any communications designed to transmit healthcare information can be considered to be telehealth. By this definition, during the bubonic plague, villagers who lit fires, which both notified others that the plague had spread to the village and also disposed of the infected dead, were essentially engaging in telehealth.[4]

Health-related radio programs broadcast in the United States in the 1920s are another example of telehealth. Some programs shared general health information, while others focused on a particular condition. Telehealth progressed with the invention of television, and with the Internet, health information can be rapidly disseminated with the click of a button. Countless television programs and websites, such as Yahoo! Health and WebMD, provide health information.[5] Seventy-two percent of Internet users reported using the Internet to search for some type of health information within the past year.[6] With 35% of people using the Internet to identify a medical condition and only half of them following up with a medical professional, the Internet is a powerful means of delivering health-related information.[7]

Hundreds of sites are dedicated to nutrition-related topics such as proper diet, managing chronic conditions such as obesity and diabetes, and losing weight.[8] Many, such as those hosted by health systems and universities, provide trustworthy information, but many others provide misinformation or promote "snake-oil" cures or false science. Verification of the legitimacy of any health information found online before applying it is critical.

Telemedicine

Telemedicine is a more specific form of telehealth, defined by the World Health Organization (WHO) as "the delivery of healthcare services, where distance is a critical factor, by all health care professionals using information and communications technologies for the exchange of valid information for diagnosis, treatment and prevention of disease and injuries, research and evaluation, and for the continuing education of health care providers."[9] Furthermore, WHO notes that the purpose is to promote the health of individuals and communities.

In healthcare settings, "telemedicine" can refer to the use of telecommunications technologies to facilitate interactions between physicians and patients. As with telehealth, telemedicine has been used for many years. For example, primary care physicians (PCPs) could seek consultations from specialists by letter, and later by telephone.[10] Computers and the Internet have greatly improved the ability of healthcare professionals to collaborate and share information.

Synchronous and Asynchronous Telemedicine

Synchronous telemedicine occurs in real time, using a streaming data connection, as in the case of a telephone call or videoconference. **Asynchronous** telemedicine, also known as "store and forward" telemedicine, involves uploading of medical information to a central repository, such as an Internet site, and retrieval of the information by another party. One example of asynchronous telemedicine is when patients email physicians about their medical issues, and physicians review the email and respond with a diagnosis or a suggested course of treatment. Or, a patient might send a text message containing a photo of a rash to a dermatologist, who can review it and send back a recommendation. Synchronous telemedicine generally requires a high-speed Internet connection, while asynchronous telemedicine requires only an Internet connection, making it especially useful in low-resource areas such as rural areas or developing nations.

> *Healthy People 2020: AHS-6.2: Reduce the proportion of persons who are unable to obtain or delay in obtaining necessary medical care*

The Swinfen Charitable Trust and Asynchronous Telemedicine

Asynchronous telemedicine is extremely useful in areas with low bandwidth Internet connections. The Swinfen Charitable Trust established a telemedicine program in 1998.[11] To accomplish its aim of "assisting poor, sick and disabled people in the developing world," the trust "establish[es] telemedicine links between medical practitioners in the developing world and expert medical and surgical specialists who generously give free advice via the Internet." Since many clients live in developing countries with poor telecommunication infrastructures, asynchronous telemedicine can be necessary. The program allows this by sending technicians out into the field with computers connected to the Internet via a solar-powered satellite dish. A technician or nurse in the field then meets with the local doctors or caregivers and writes up the case, including pictures and anything else that can help with diagnosis or developing treatment plans. This write-up is then uploaded to a database for a Swinfen Charitable Trust volunteer to access. The volunteer triages the case and sends it to an appropriate specialist who has agreed to donate his or her time. The specialist can respond with questions, or, if the write-up is sufficient, with a diagnosis or treatment plan, which is then administered by the local physician or caregiver. In regions with poor telecommunication technologies and limited access to the Internet, this asynchronous telemedicine program delivers a much-needed connection to specialist care that would otherwise not be available.

The Hub and Spoke and Project ECHO Models

The **hub and spoke model** and the **Project ECHO model** are commonly used to describe telemedicine. These models are often referenced in grant applications, so it is useful to understand them.

Hub and Spoke Model

The hub and spoke model is so named because it resembles a wagon wheel with multiple spokes connected to a single hub. The hub can be a tertiary care center, or a single specialty provider, and the spokes are the rural or underserved clinics that may not otherwise have access to the specialist (**Figure 24-1**). The hub and spoke model can also be reversed, with the patient placed at the hub, as the center of care, and various specialty care options placed at the spokes.

In most cases, the patient and the patient's PCP are at the hub, and various specialty care providers, such as cardiologists, dermatologists, and infectious disease and other specialist physicians, as well as social workers, nutritionists, and even family members who may be located at a distance, can be placed at the spokes, all connected by telemedicine (**Figure 24-2**).

> *Healthy People 2020: HC/HIT-7: Increase the proportion of adults who report having friends and family members with whom they talk about their health*

As the U.S. population ages, patients increasingly need multifaceted care to manage chronic conditions. Family and friends have increasing roles in assisting in the coordination of this care. This social network of health will utilize various health information technologies to assist families in coordinating care for family members (typically elderly parents or grandparents). By engaging the patient's social network of health, the patient benefits by having multiple people working together to ensure that appointments are made, medicine is taken, and exercise or eating programs are realized.

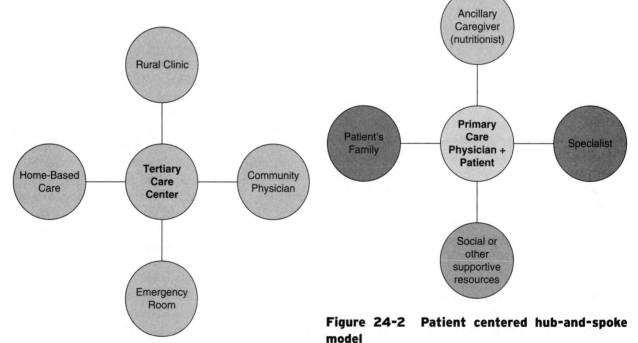

Figure 24-1 Traditional hub-and-spoke model

Data from Tan, J. (2005). *E-Health Care Information Systems: An Introduction for Students and Professionals*. San Francisco, CA: Jossey-Bass.

Figure 24-2 Patient centered hub-and-spoke model

Data from Roh, C-Y. (2008). Telemedicine: What it is, Where it Came From, and Where it Will Go, *Comparative Technology Transfer and Society*, 6(1), 35–57. Data also from Christensen, C et al. (2009). *The Innovator's Prescription: A Disruptive Solution for Health Care*. New York, NY: McGraw Hill.

Project ECHO

The Extension for Community Health Outcomes (ECHO) is a program established by the University of New Mexico to "develop the capacity to safely and effectively treat chronic, common and complex diseases in rural and underserved areas, and to monitor outcomes of this treatment."[12] Project ECHO established community outreach programs to improve the health of rural and underserved communities in New Mexico and incorporated telemedicine to connect physicians and other providers in these communities to specialty care in the urban settings. The program focuses on training PCPs in rural and underserved settings to diagnose, treat, and manage chronic conditions. This occurs through videoconferencing technology to connect providers in rural and underserved areas with specialists in tertiary care centers and academic medical centers. Project ECHO is an effective model to manage chronic conditions such as hepatitis C, asthma, diabetes, HIV/AIDS, pediatric obesity, chronic pain, substance abuse disorders, rheumatoid arthritis, cardiovascular conditions, and mental illness suffered by people in underserved areas.[13]

The basic Project ECHO model consists of regular weekly, biweekly, or monthly teleconferences with providers in rural and underserved communities. Prior to the teleconference, the rural/underserved providers submit questions regarding their patient populations. For example, the University of New Mexico implemented an ECHO program focused on hepatitis C in which rural/underserved providers could submit questions specific to their patients that had been diagnosed with hepatitis C.[14] During the teleconference, the rural/underserved providers connect with the academic medical center and the appropriate specialist panel, or, in the case of the hepatitis C program, hepatologists or infectious disease physicians. The specialists present information and also respond to the patient-specific case studies and/or questions that were submitted prior to the teleconference. By reviewing actual case studies, the rural/underserved providers receive guidance for their own patients and are able to learn from other cases. This program was found to be an effective way to treat hepatitis C in rural and underserved areas.[15]

Telemedicine Programs

Radiology was among the first fields to use telemedicine. In this medical specialty, radiologists examine and interpret X-rays, computed tomography (CT), and magnetic resonance imaging (MRI) scans and other types of images. Since images need not be read on-site, the only obstacle to teleradiology had been image quality to allow accurate readings on a high-resolution monitor. Modern computer monitors, especially high-definition ones, are suitable. This allows radiologists to do their jobs from anywhere with access to a computer or even a smartphone.

Telemedicine can also facilitate treatment of stroke patients. The expression "time is brain" refers to the fact that more time passing after a stroke before initiation of treatment leads to more brain damage. Telemedicine has reduced the response time by connecting the patient with a neurologist, who can diagnose the stroke by observing or talking to the patient and also by reviewing the diagnostic results. Once the neurologist confirms that the patient is suffering from a stroke, medication can be administered to quickly treat the stroke.

Telepathology is effective and especially useful in developing countries that lack adequate pathologists.[16] In one program, technicians in Zambia prepared pathology slides and then transmitted pictures of specimens to pathologists located in Italy.[17] This program greatly reduced the time to interpret a specimen and initiate treatment, and increased the accuracy of the interpretations of the specimens. In addition, the telepathology interpretations were found to be as accurate as interpretations done using traditional methods.

Telemedicine has also been shown to be effective in cardiology (telecardiology), dermatology (teledermatology), ophthalmology (teleophthalmology), and many other types of specialty care. In addition, studies have shown that the care delivered via telemedicine is generally as good as the care provided by traditional means in diabetes management,[18] in psychology,[19] and in general.[20]

> *Public Health Core Competency 1: Analytical/ Assessment Skills 11: Uses information technology to collect, store, and retrieve data*

eHealth

Telehealth and telemedicine primarily involve the application of telecommunication technologies to the provision of health care, the sharing of health information, and health education. Electronic health, or **eHealth**, is broader, and can be defined as "an emerging field of medical informatics referring to the organization and delivery of health services and information using the Internet and related technologies."[21]

eHealth also includes "a new way of working, an attitude, and a commitment for networked, global thinking, to improve healthcare locally, regionally, and worldwide by using information and communication technologies."[22] The term also describes commercial applications of telehealth or telemedicine, using the Internet as a platform to connect healthcare professionals and patients.

> *Healthy People 2020: HC/HIT-10: Increase the proportion of medical practices that use electronic health records*

Adoption of **electronic health records (EHRs)** and **electronic medical records (EMRs)** allows greater coordination of patient care (**Box 24-1**). Traditional paper records can lead to fragmented care if patients' various providers, including PCPs, specialists, and dietitians, are not all able to access patients' full records. This can lead to wasteful practices, such as the duplication of tests, or conflicting care. Consider patients being treated for multiple obesity-related conditions. With EHRs, care management plans from various providers can be updated in real time, allowing PCPs to be aware of visits to endocrinologists, cardiologists, dietitians, and rehabilitation specialists. When patients meet with PCPs, PCPs can initiate telemedicine consultations with one or more specialists, such as a nutritionist, to provide joint counseling to patients.

As eHealth connections among providers, payers, and patients develop, greater coordination and collaboration can potentially increase efficiency and improve patient health outcomes. This connectivity also supports objectives of patient-centered medical homes (PCMHs). The U.S. Department of Health and Human Services (DHHS) established these centers as a way of financially motivating providers to focus on overall patient health rather than individual symptoms, which often led to fragmented care as the patient sought care from multiple specialists. The fee-for-service system that is currently dominant in the United States encourages physicians to treat health conditions, and not necessarily cure or prevent them, since physicians receive payment for seeing and treating patients.[23] PCMHs reduce the emphasis on fee-for-service compensation and increase incentives based on patient outcomes. eHealth can facilitate communication among providers and promote preventive care.

mHealth

The proliferation of cellphones, especially smartphones, makes **mHealth**, or mobile health, a rapidly growing area

---

Box 24-1 EMRs versus EHRs

Electronic Medical Record (EMR): "The legal record of what happened to the patient during their encounter" at the provider or healthcare facility. This record is owned by the provider or healthcare facility.

Electronic Health Record (EHR): The EHR is broader in scope than an EMR and contains more patient history and previous/current medical treatment. This record "spans episodes of care across" many different types of providers and caregivers. The EHR is owned by the patient and is typically linked to a National or State Health Information Network.

If Stella, as described in this chapter's opening case study, seeks care from a particular hospital, this care is documented in that hospital's EMR system. If she then seeks care from a second provider not affiliated with the first hospital, this care may be recorded in a different EMR system. Not all EMR systems are compatible with each other, and many cannot share information. This is where the EHR comes in. If Stella lives in a state in which a Health Information Network (HIN) has been developed, all of Stella's care information, including information obtained by health insurers, public health agencies, and any other source of health or medical data connected to the HIN, would be accessible to Stella in her EHR. Since this information is now in digital format, Stella can take her EHR and share it with a new caregiver, review it with her family, or even email it to another, possibly remote, provider for a second opinion. EMRs are useful for patients whose care is provided in one location or in a health system connected to a single EMR, but EHRs are even more useful because patients can take them with them. The federal HITECH (Health Information Technology for Economic and Clinical Health) Act provides financial incentives for physician practices and hospitals that can demonstrate the "meaningful use" of electronic health records.

of telehealth. mHealth is a promising method for delivering healthcare and health-related information and managing chronic conditions because so many people use mobile phones and almost always keep their phones with them. By harnessing something that people use every day, healthcare providers are able to better manage their patients. Cellphones can make phone calls, send and receive text messages, and take and send digital photographs. Smartphones have additional capabilities, such as running applications that can perform various functions and deliver various services, accessing the Internet, and supporting peripheral devices that convert the smartphone into a medical device. Because smartphones can perform so many functions from nearly anywhere and because they are so easy to use, they are potential vehicles for the delivery of healthcare services and information to people. mHealth is especially prevalent in developing countries such as African countries and India.

Smartphones can deliver care through a variety of software programs known as "apps," which can assist patients in self-managing chronic conditions, including complying with medication schedules. Apps can also help physicians provide direct patient care. Another use of smartphones for mHealth is to convert them into medical tools by attaching them to peripheral devices. These uses are described in more detail below.

Managing Chronic Conditions

Mobile phone users are rarely far from their phones, making smartphones ideal for chronic condition management. Early management tools included simple apps that utilized the phone's ringer to remind people to take their medications. Text messages are more effective, and further, patients prefer a customizable approach, with phone reminders, text message reminders, phone call reminders, and emailed reminders.[24]

Some mHealth management programs are web-based and designed for patients to take regular readings of various health factors, such as blood pressure and blood glucose, and input them into the website through the smartphone's web browser. The patient regularly inputs the various vital signs that need to be monitored, and this information is overseen by a nurse, physician, or even a family member. No intervention is taken when measurements are within a specified range. Predetermined interventions will take place when the information falls outside of the patient's normal range. Possible interventions include a text message providing the patient with education or a friendly warning, a phone call to the patient to determine the cause of the

abnormal readings, and even the summoning of an ambulance or other immediate care, using the smartphone's geographic positioning system to find the patient's location.

More advanced mHealth programs allow health information to be input directly into an app that is installed on the phone. These data are uploaded from the smartphone to a destination website, such as a physician's office, when the smartphone is connected to the Internet. This method eliminates the need for the patient to have to open the phone's browser and input data on the small screen. Certain medical equipment with Bluetooth technology also allows physicians to receive data from users' cellphones. Patients use the device, such as a blood pressure cuff, a glucometer, or a scale, and data are automatically uploaded to the phone and then to the website. Bluetooth-enabled devices are easy, but remain relatively expensive.

In a **body area network (BAN)**, a smartphone can also be used as a "data collector" for various body-worn sensors that monitor such physiological functions as heart rate, temperature, and skin alkalinity. Again, data are automatically uploaded to the smartphone and then to a website. BANs are low cost and versatile in the types of information they can gather. A challenge, as is the case with other mHealth programs, is maximizing this method without creating more work for caregivers. Computer programs can use algorithms to process the data and can be assigned tasks of gathering, analyzing, and reacting to the data received. Providers can then review reports and adjust the treatment protocol during their next visit with the patient.

The programs described above are used in more formal programs with a care manager or some other type of supervisor overseeing the patient's health. iTunes and other app sites offer hundreds of nonformal applications that allow patients to self-manage their conditions.

In addition to being used to simply collect and analyze data, the smartphone can also be transformed into a medical device by attaching a peripheral device. For example, a smartphone can be transformed into an electrocardiogram device (EKG or ECG) by clipping an attachment onto the smartphone. The user can then hold the smartphone to his or her chest (or someone else's chest) to obtain an EKG. This signal can then be sent to a medical professional to interpret, and the appropriate care can then be coordinated.

A smartphone can also be turned into a stethoscope and ultrasound device by attaching a specially designed stethoscope or ultrasound to the smartphone. These devices require U.S. Food and Drug Administration (FDA) approval as a medical device, so they remain relatively expensive and are not widely available. There are also restrictions on how they can be used. For example, the EKG attachment can transmit an EKG only to a medical professional, so it is not currently designed for personal use.[25]

Costs of these peripheral devices are expensive, but expected to eventually decrease, making these devices more accessible. A technician or a nurse could be deployed to a rural or underserved area with a smartphone and a bag of peripheral devices and would be able to give physical examinations to patients with a physician readily available to interpret the data from the devices. The physician could then direct the nurse in providing care or treatment, or could recommend follow-up care that is needed (and could be provided via telemedicine in some cases).

mHealth is in its infancy in terms of development and deployment in the healthcare industry. The potential for bringing chronic condition management, diagnosis, treatment, information, and education to patients and communities through their smartphones is nearly limitless. There are also many opportunities for public health agencies to utilize mHealth to collect data and conduct community health assessments and other evaluations of community health. Some eHealth programs focused on nutrition will be discussed later in this chapter.

Barriers to Telemedicine/ eHealth/mHealth

Telemedicine/eHealth/mHealth can be useful in improving access to care, reducing costs associated with care, maintaining and improving the quality of care delivered to patients, and improving patient and healthcare provider satisfaction. However, the following barriers to the adoption of telemedicine in the United States remain.[26]

Reimbursement

Providers are less likely to use telemedicine if they will not get paid for it. **Medicare** reimburses for telemedicine only under limited circumstances. **Medicaid** programs in some states reimburse for telemedicine consultations if the only available specialist is a certain distance from the patient, typically 50 miles.[27] Those without transportation to a provider within 50 miles remain uncovered for telemedicine. Private insurance companies have traditionally not reimbursed for telemedicine, but laws in 16 states now require private insurers to reimburse for telemedicine consultations as they would traditional consultations.[28] Many more

states were taking up proposed bills in the 2013 legislative session. Most reimbursement laws require that the telemedicine be synchronous in order to be reimbursable.

Licensure

Physicians must be licensed by each state in which they practice medicine. Most state laws clarify that for telemedicine consultations, a physician must be licensed in the patient's state. Thus, if a patient is located in Indiana and is consulting with a physician in Michigan, that physician must be licensed in Indiana.

Technology and Security

Telemedicine can be inexpensive, but is commonly believed to require expensive equipment. In reality, only Internet access and a computer, preferably with a web camera, are needed. Any videoconferencing tool used for synchronous telemedicine consultations must be compliant with the Health Insurance Portability and Accountability Act (HIPAA) standards for privacy and security. Both the videoconferencing itself and any data transmitted between the patient and provider should be compliant. Although videoconferencing is a good tool for telemedicine consultations, providers will also need to document each encounter with patients for legal and billing purposes, so using a dedicated telemedicine platform rather than just a standalone videoconferencing tool may be efficacious.

Lack of Common Standards

Since many EMR systems consist of proprietary software, creating the ability to share data across different platforms is difficult. Without a common platform, the likelihood of interoperable systems is decreased, and the potential utility of such a system is reduced.

Medical Liability and Malpractice Issues

So far, physicians have not been sued for a misdiagnosis or other form of malpractice during a telemedicine consultation. However, as telemedicine becomes increasingly common, lawsuits are inevitable. The same standards of regular office visits should apply to telemedicine consultations. Providers must use their professional judgment to decide whether a telemedical consult is appropriate or whether the patient should be seen in person. Providers should also check with their professional liability carriers to ensure that they are covered for telemedical consultations.

Personnel Concerns

Telemedicine disrupts the traditional methods of health-care delivery.[29] As such, there will be people who resist adopting or implementing telemedicine programs for a variety of reasons, from "it's never been done that way" to "it's too much like science fiction." In addition, some people are not comfortable with technology. Education and training are strategies for resolving these issues and demonstrating the effectiveness of telemedicine compared with traditional health care.

> *Healthy People 2020: HC/HIT 5: Increase the proportion of persons who use electronic personal health management tools*
>
> *Healthy People 2020: HC/HIT 5.1: Increase the proportion of persons who use the Internet to keep track of personal health information, such as care received, test results, or upcoming medical appointments*
>
> *Healthy People 2020: HC/HIT 5.2: Increase the proportion of persons who use the Internet to communicate with their health provider*

Telemedicine, eHealth, and mHealth as Applied to Nutrition Programs

As noted, telemedicine/eHealth/mHealth is convenient for keeping patients engaged in their health care and in eliminating obstacles, such as distance, to care. Examples of telemedicine in nutrition programs are videoconferencing and phone calls to link dietitians to patients. Patients receive more immediate support and direct feedback on their programs, and they are also more likely to utilize the services of dietitians if it is convenient for them.

Telemedicine and Obesity: Program in Greece

A telemedicine program in Greece examined the efficacy of telemedicine in treating overweight and obese patients.[30] This program utilized electronic blood pressure cuffs and electronic weight scales to allow patients to input data, and also had participants respond daily to certain lifestyle questions ("Did you follow your diet plan during the past two days?" and "Did you follow your exercise plan during

the past two days?"). Participants could utilize one of three methods to respond to the questions:

1. Automated call center through a regular phone
2. Wireless application protocol server through a cellular phone
3. Internet server through a personal computer

Participants also participated in monthly in-person meetings with a physician and a dietitian. Participants who utilized telemedicine had greater decreases in body weight than patients who participated in the standard program without.[31] This study focused on short-term weight loss, but found convincing evidence for the use of telemedicine as an intervention in treating overweight and obese patients.

Application of Telemedicine to Improve Rural Nutrition

Telemedicine has also been used for nutrition counseling sessions with dietitians for patients in rural areas.[32] In one study, patients located in a rural area, who were more likely to forgo counseling because of the distance they would have to travel, were given the option of meeting with a dietitian by way of videoconferencing.[33] The dietitians reported that the counseling sessions were adequate, but could not replace in-person sessions.[34] Patients reported greater satisfaction with the videoconferencing sessions, and one reported that in-person sessions were not necessary.[35]

Telemedicine and the U.S. Military

The U.S. military has deployed telemedicine to deliver nutrition services to its soldiers worldwide.[36] Nutritionists at the Tripler Army Medical Center in Hawaii successfully counseled military members and families in the Marshall Islands on weight loss and proper nutrition.[37] The videoconferencing system was also useful in educating PCPs on the importance of nutrition counseling.[38] Each telemedicine intervention that prevented a specialist provider from needing to travel from Hawaii to the Marshall Islands, or a patient from the Marshall Islands to Hawaii, saved $2,000.[39]

eHealth has also provided nutritional information to scientists, nutritionists, and dietitians for a variety of epidemiological research, clinical practice, health promotion, policy, and food manufacturing purposes.[40] Many eHealth programs provide information on food composition data.[41] The online availability of this information facilitates online, research, and clinical efforts.

Telemedicine and Diabetes Programs

Telemedicine has been effective in diabetes education, treatment, and management. In one randomized trial, patients with diabetes were assigned either to travel to a health center in a larger city for meetings with a diabetes nurse educator and dietitian in person, or to stay in their local communities and meet with a diabetes nurse educator and dietitian via videoconferencing.[42] This study concluded that "telemedicine is an effective means of providing diabetes education to patients."[43]

In another randomized trial, diabetes patients received medical nutrition therapy via standard carbohydrate counting education using a paper diary or via a smartphone application called a Diabetes Interactive Diary or DID.[44] The DID is a carbohydrate/bolus calculator, an information technology device, and a telemedicine system in which the healthcare professional (physician or dietitian) can communicate with the patient via text message.[45] This study concluded that the "system is safe, easy to use, and well accepted by the vast majority of patients."[46] The DID also halved the amount of educational time needed for learning to count carbohydrates and insulin dose adjustment; resulted in lower weight gain, likely due to lower dosages of long-acting insulin required; and was associated with a significant improvement in several mental and physical components of the SF-36 Health Survey (as compared with the control group).[47]

Telemedicine has also been deployed in Diabetes Case Management (DCM) programs.[48] Patients might receive a home telemedicine unit allowing them to upload blood glucose and blood pressure readings, connect with a nurse case manager and dietitian, and access educational materials.[49] In a study involving elderly diabetes patients, DCM using telemedicine resulted in "significantly improved diabetes self-efficacy . . . but not improved depression or diabetes distress."[50] DCM has the potential to enhance the care of patients with diabetes, especially when access to care is reduced because of mobility or another age-related factor. BAN programs can also assist diabetic patients in monitoring blood glucose. The diabetic patient wears sensors that automatically measure blood glucose concentrations, which can then automatically trigger an insulin pump to deliver the appropriate amount of insulin.[51]

Telemedicine has also been deployed by the Project ECHO program in New Mexico and other programs to screen patients at risk for diabetes retinopathy in rural and underserved areas.[52] Technicians are sent to rural and underserved areas with a retinoscope connected to a computer (which is connected to the Internet). The technician performs the screenings, and the image is sent back to the ophthalmologist to interpret the image and direct care. By using lesser resources (technicians and others with college degrees), costs can be contained and higher-level resources, such as nurses and physicians, can be better utilized.

mHealth Nutrition Programs

mHealth is particularly well suited to support nutrition programs because it is convenient for patients, and is a powerful and portable tool.

Digital photography can help in dietary assessment and help patients understand their dietary intake. In one study, patients in Bolivia were instructed to take photographs of their meals to assist dietitians in conducting dietary assessments. Digital photographs were found to be more useful than other methods of dietary assessment, such as a weighted food diary, because individuals in developing countries are often illiterate or busy working on farms with less spare time for other types of dietary assessments or self-reporting.[53] Since cellphones and even smartphones are extremely prevalent in developing countries, programs whereby the participant sends photographs of their meals to a dietitian via cellphone to assist in dietary assessments make sense. Teledietetics incorporates the Internet in allowing for the sharing of digital photographs of food with dietitians and nutritionists along with direct feedback to patients via email and videoconferencing.[54]

Other types of mHealth nutrition programs have also been used. Barcode recognition apps for smartphones allow users to photograph a barcode and almost instantaneously access food composition data for that barcode.[55] Text messages have also been studied as a strategy to change eating habits and behaviors among teenagers and young adults, and appear promising.[56]

International Telemedicine and mHealth Programs

Telemedicine programs are especially useful in bringing specialty care to patients who may not otherwise have access to it, such as in developing countries where access to basic and specialty care is limited. The tremendous resource of telemedicine must be provided in a culturally competent way.[57] Development of telehealth interventions should include input from target populations, including healthcare providers and patients who are representative of their communities. Beyond using appropriate language, messages must be designed for the likely level of literacy of users, and treatment plans should fit within cultural norms, beliefs, and social structures.[58]

> *Public Health Core Competency 4A: Cultural Competency Skills 1: Incorporates strategies for interacting with persons from diverse backgrounds*

One such program, the Cambodia Teleconsultation Programme or Village Leap Program, uses email to connect U.S. physicians with people in Cambodia.[59] The Village Leap Program involves a nurse who works a clinic in Cambodia and intakes patients by completing a template that collects various types of health information. This information is then emailed to U.S. physicians, at Massachusetts General Hospital, Brigham and Women's Hospital, and the Dana Farber Cancer Center, who review each case and email back a diagnosis and/or recommended treatment protocol. The nurse then delivers the care to the patients. Using this program, both the patients, as well as the nurse, benefit: the patients are receiving top-notch medical advice, and the nurse is also enriched by the education he or she receives.[60] The local nurse, who delivers the care, can ensure that the treatment is culturally appropriate.

Another telemedicine program, in Zambia, is designed to provide primary care to people located in rural, underserved areas. This program, known as the Virtual Doctor Project, uses mobile clinics (vans outfitted with clinical equipment and satellite telecommunication) to travel the countryside to see patients and then upload case studies (including images and case notes) to the Internet (another example of store and forward, or asynchronous telemedicine), where they are then reviewed by a physician.[61] In 1999, South Africa rolled out a national telemedicine program that implemented teleradiology, tele-ultrasound, telepathology, and teleophthalmology.[62] Telemedicine has also been deployed in Tanzania, where it has been deployed to support pediatric care in small hospitals.[63] The Tanzanian Telemedicine Network delivers teleconsultations in pediatrics, obstetrics and gynecology, surgery, anesthesiology, radiology, dermatology, internal medicine, infectious diseases, and ophthalmology with the support of physicians in Tanzania, Britain, Germany, Switzerland, Finland, Norway, the United States, India, Australia, and New Zealand.[64] This telemedicine program is an asynchronous and low-cost solution to bringing specialty care to rural Tanzania.

Telemedicine can also be useful in industrialized nations. In Finland, for example, a teledentistry program intended to reduce the disparity in the number of specialist dentists in Finland.[65] The program involved synchronous lectures that were offered to students twice a week, and also involved case studies (including pictures of actual patients that were transmitted along with the lecture). Taking into account the travel that would have been involved to attend these lectures in person, it is estimated that this teledentistry program saved about 40,000 euros (approximately $50,500) per student, even taking into account the cost of the equipment.[66]

In developing countries, mHealth is even more prevalent and has even more potential to deliver care to individuals. The reason for this is that cellphones are especially prevalent in developing countries such as India and many African nations. Cellphones are readily available in developing countries because a telecommunications infrastructure built around landlines was not developed, but a cellular network was implemented. An mHealth program in Kenya was shown to be effective in improving and maintaining health workers' adherence to treatment guidelines for managing outpatient pediatric malaria.[67] Text message reminders were sent to the health workers in Kenya, reminding them of the appropriate treatment/management protocols for their case management patients. This text-message reminder approach was found to be successful in increasing adherence to the treatment/management protocols.[68] The findings in Kenya also support similar mHealth programs that focus on the patient's adherence to treatment protocols (for HIV/AIDS medications).[69]

Telemedicine programs are still in their early stages, so as telecommunication infrastructures in developing countries continue to improve, telemedicine will continue to emerge as a cost-effective way of delivering care to the underserved. Perhaps more than telemedicine, mHealth will emerge in developing countries to allow access to care, and also to assist patients and health providers in managing various conditions. mHealth can also be used for public health purposes by collecting and sharing data among clinics to combat the spread of disease. In developing countries, mHealth can also be deployed to educate patients on better nutrition and the importance of purifying water before consuming it. The possible uses of mHealth and telemedicine are limitless in these resource-constrained countries.

> *Public Health Core Competency 2: Policy Development/ Program Planning Skills 7: Identifies mechanisms to monitor and evaluate programs for their effectiveness and quality*

Assessing and Implementing Telemedicine, eHealth, and mHealth Programs

Telemedicine, eHealth, and mHealth are simply ways to enhance and supplement the care of the patient; they are not in any way intended to replace traditional methods of care or eliminate the face-to-face relationship altogether. Telemedicine, eHealth, and mHealth programs can be designed to fit within an existing process or practice, but can also be deployed as standalone programs. This may be the case in areas in which health care simply is not available, such as rural or underserved areas. In this case, care delivered via telemedicine, or even text message, can be better than no care at all.

Implementation of Telemedicine Programs

Sustainability is a significant challenge for telemedicine programs. Frequently, telemedicine programs are established with grant funding or some other type of limited time investment, and the program disappears with the funding. In cases where proper planning and due diligence are not conducted, telemedicine programs are used and put away in the closet, never to be used again. Many studies have demonstrated the various success factors inherent in successful telemedicine programs (studies have also demonstrated factors inherent in unsuccessful telemedicine programs as well). These factors are discussed below.

Telemedicine Coordinator or Telemedicine Director Role

A telemedicine coordinator/director is someone who is responsible for overseeing the telemedicine program, including establishing protocols (and ensuring that the protocols are followed), troubleshooting technical issues, and overseeing the telemedicine program.[70] A telemedicine coordinator/director will generally have a background in (or training in) the delivery of care as well as technology. Successful telemedicine programs generally have someone who is dedicated to serving in this role, regardless of whether this person has the formal title or not. In the Tanzanian Telemedicine Network, for example, a telemedicine coordinator sends emailed reminders to specialists if they do not respond to a request for consult within a certain amount of time depending on the urgency of the request.[71]

Telemedicine Program Champion

As with any new program, leadership is important. Successful telemedicine programs generally have someone in a leadership role (typically a physician or other caregiver) who provides leadership and support in implementing and adopting a telemedicine program.[72]

Protocols

As with many other medical processes, a protocol allows all users of a telemedicine platform to understand the steps to be taken when using the system. Protocols should be developed for both the initiating site (the site that initiates the telemedicine connection; this is generally where the patient is located) as well as the receiving site (the site that connects to the telemedicine connection). The protocol for the initiating site should include steps such as patient registration, the taking of vital signs or other information necessary for the consult, and initiating the computer/videoconferencing connection. The protocol for the receiving site should include steps such as detailing the information that must be collected at the initiating site, connecting to the computer/videoconferencing site, and putting together a record of the visit (a record of the visit is a requirement for reimbursement, as well as a required practice for physicians).

Long-Term Planning and Budgeting

In order for a telemedicine program to be sustainable, it must be incorporated into the long-term planning of the physician office, hospital, or other provider site.[73] In addition, proper funding is necessary for successful telemedicine programs (especially beyond the initial investment). Fortunately, as more and more states enact laws requiring reimbursement for telemedicine consultations, telemedicine can become self-sustaining (and can allow the organization to also realize efficiencies).

User-Friendly Technology

If a telemedicine platform is difficult or cumbersome to use, users will not use it.[74] Telemedicine programs need to be incorporated into current processes and should not be disruptive or difficult to use.

Evaluation and Measurement

In order to demonstrate success, telemedicine programs must be evaluated and assessed. This should be a continuous process so that corrective action can be taken if certain goals are not met.

Assessing Telemedicine Programs

In order for telemedicine programs to be adopted and sustained, it is important to measure and assess these programs. The Institute of Medicine emphasizes four areas of focus for telemedicine programs to be evaluated to demonstrate the value of telemedicine: outcomes/quality, costs, access, and patient/provider satisfaction.

Outcomes/Quality

Telemedicine programs must deliver the same quality of care and produce the same outcomes as traditional methods of delivering care. Outcome evaluations of telemedicine programs should be conducted and compared with existing outcome results for traditional methods of care.

Costs

Telemedicine programs should be designed to reduce costs (for both the provider and the patient). For example, costs associated with travel and gained efficiencies should be taken into account.

Access

Telemedicine programs should increase access to care, including primary care, and (in more cases) specialty care. Increased access to care should be easy to measure and can be an important success factor for telemedicine programs.

Patient/Provider Satisfaction

Providers and patients need to be comfortable and satisfied using telemedicine for the provision of care. Satisfaction surveys are the easiest way to collect feedback on user satisfaction with the program.[75] Evaluating and assessing telemedicine programs is crucial to demonstrating the utility and effectiveness of these programs.

Conclusion

Stella and her mother, Maya, introduced in the opening case study, could benefit greatly from a telemedicine and an mHealth program. Telemedicine can be deployed to bring care directly to Stella and Maya without requiring them to travel or take much time off of work or school. mHealth can also be deployed, using a device that Stella already uses, to train her in managing her condition.

Telemedicine, eHealth, and mHealth have the potential to change the way in which care is delivered by allowing for specialty care to be readily available to rural and underserved areas, allowing health information to be readily available to all caregivers, and allowing for patient information to be collected and shared with a caregiver from wherever the patient may be using a device that he or she regularly uses anyway. There are limitless possibilities for implementing telemedicine and mHealth programs, both domestic and international. As technology and telecommunications continue to improve, telemedicine and mHealth have the potential to change people's lives for the better by educating them, giving them access to treatment, care management, or even data that they otherwise would not have had access to, and bringing down the cost of health care. People who otherwise would not have access to a specialist, a nutritionist, a dietitian, a case manager, or even a support group will be able to access these resources from the comfort of their own living room. Technology and telecommunications will also allow patients like Stella or Maya to engage their social network of health and gain support from family, friends, other patients, and different types of providers to stay on track and manage their conditions. If Stella fails to take her medications, Maya or Stella's friends or family could get an email or a text message notifying them that they need to keep Stella on track.

Telemedicine, eHealth, and mHealth will not soon replace traditional doctor's visits, but they can enhance the traditional visit. Telemedicine increases patient access to providers by preventing the need to travel long distances. As eHealth continues to connect providers, a patient's information will be readily available and patients can receive more coordinated, likely higher quality, care.

References

1 Howden, L. M., & Mayer, J. A. (2001, May). *Age and sex composition.* 2010 U.S. Census Briefs. Retrieved from U.S. Census Bureau website, http://www.census.gov/prod/cen2010/briefs/c2010br-03.pdf

2 Kirch, D. G., Henderson, M. K., & Dill, M. J. (2012). Physician workforce projections in an era of health care reform. *Annual Review of Medicine, 63,* 435.

3   Baker, D. C., & Bufka, L. F. (2011). Preparing for the telehealth world: Navigating legal, regulatory, reimbursement, and ethical issues in an electronic age. *Professional Psychology: Research and Practice, 42*(6), 405-11.

4   Bashshur, R., & Shannon, G. (2009*). The history of telemedicine: Evolution, context, and transformation.* New Rochelle, NY: Mary Ann Liebert.

5   *Top 15 most popular health websites.* (2013, April). Retrieved from eBiz MBA website, www.ebizmba.com/articles/health-websites

6   Fox, S., & Duggan, M. (2013). *Health online 2013 report.* Retrieved from Pew Research Center website, http://pewinternet.org/reports/2013/health-online.aspx

7   Fox, S., & Duggan, M. (2013). *Health online 2013 report.* Retrieved from Pew Research Center website, http://pewinternet.org/reports/2013/health-online.aspx

8   Bodkin, C., & Miaoulis, G. (2007). eHealth information quality and ethics issues: An exploratory study of consumer perceptions. *International Journal of Pharmaceutical and Health Marketing, 1*(1), 27-42.

9   World Health Organization. (2010). *Telemedicine: Opportunities and developments in member states, report on the Second Global Survey on eHealth.* Geneva: World Health Organization.

10 Bashshur, R., & Shannon, G. (2009*). The history of telemedicine: Evolution, context, and transformation.* New Rochelle, NY: Mary Ann Liebert.

11 Swinfen Charitable Trust. (n.d.). *Have you got a Swinfen Telemedical Link?* Retrieved from http://www.swinfencharitabletrust.org

12 University of New Mexico, Project ECHO website, http://echo.unm.edu

13 Arora, S., Kalishman, S., Dion, D., Som, D., Thornton, K., Bankhurst, A., . . . Yutzy, S. (2011). Partnering urban academic medical centers and rural primary care clinicians to provide complex chronic disease care. *Health Affairs, 30*(6), 1176.

14 Arora, S., Thornton, K., Murata, G., Deming, P., Kalishman, S., Dion, D., . . . Qualls, C. (2011). Outcomes of treatment for hepatitis C virus infection by primary care providers. *New England Journal of Medicine, 364*(23), 2199-207.

15 Arora, S., Thornton, K., Murata, G., Deming, P., Kalishman, S., Dion, D., . . . Qualls, C. (2011). Outcomes of treatment for hepatitis C virus infection by primary care providers. *New England Journal of Medicine, 364*(23), 2199-207.

16 Pagni, F., Bono, F., Di Bella, C., Faravelli, A., & Cappellini, A. (2011). Virtual surgical pathology in underdeveloped countries: The Zambia Project. *Archives of Pathology and Laboratory Medicine, 135,* 215-19.

17 Pagni, F., Bono, F., Di Bella, C., Faravelli, A., & Cappellini, A. (2011). Virtual surgical pathology in underdeveloped countries: The Zambia Project. *Archives of Pathology and Laboratory Medicine, 135,* 215-19.

18 Johnson, A., Gorman, M., Coulehan, N., Lewis, C., Baker, F., & Rader, J. (2011). Interactive videoconferencing improves nutrition intervention in a rural population. *Journal of the American Diabetic Association, 101*(2), 173.

19 Slone, N. C., Reese, R. J., & McClellan, M. J. (2012). Telepsychology outcome research with children and adolescents: A review of the literature. *Psychological Services,* 9(3), 272-92.

20 Horner, K., Wagner, E., & Tufano, J. *Electronic consultations between primary and specialty care clinicians: Early insights.* Commonwealth Fund, Publication 1554, Vol. 23. Retrieved from http://www.commonwealthfund.org/~/media/Files/Publications/Issue%20Brief/2011/Oct/1554_Horner_econsultations_primary_specialty_care_clinicians_ib.pdf

21 Pagliari, C., Sloan, D., Gregor, P., Sullivan, F., Detmer, D., Kahan, J. P., . . . MacGillivray, S. (2005). What is eHealth (4)? A scoping exercise to map the field. *Journal of Medical Internet Research,* 7(1), e9.

22 Pagliari, C., Sloan, D., Gregor, P., Sullivan, F., Detmer, D., Kahan, J. P., . . . MacGillivray, S. (2005). What is eHealth (4)? A scoping exercise to map the field. *Journal of Medical Internet Research,* 7(1), e9.

23 Christensen, C. M., Grossman, J. H., & Hwang, J. (2009). *The innovator's prescription: A disruptive solution for health care.* New York, NY: McGraw-Hill.

24 Harris, L. T., Lehavot, K., Huh, D., Yard, S., Andrasik, M. P., Dunbar, P. J., & Simoni, J. M. (2010). Two-way text messaging for health behavior change among human immunodeficiency virus-positive individuals. *Telemedicine and eHealth, 16*(10), 1024-29.

25 Dolan, B. (2012, December 3). *FDA clears AliveCor heart monitor, doctors can pre-order.* Retrieved from MobileHealthNews website, http://mobihealthnews.com/19306/fda-clears-alivecor-heart-monitor-doctors-can-pre-order

26 Gulick, P. G. (2002). E-health and the future of medicine: The economic, legal, regulatory, cultural and organizational obstacles facing telemedicine and cybermedicine programs. *Albany Law Journal of Science and Technology, 12,* 351.

27 Center for Telehealth and eHealth Law. (2011, February). *50 state Medicaid statute survey* [Webinar].

28 American Telemedicine Association. (2013, April 2). *State telemedicine policy matrix.* Retrieved from http://www.americantelemed.org/get-involved/public-policy-advocacy/state-telemedicine-policy

29 Christensen, C. M., Grossman, J. H., & Hwang, J. (2009). *The innovator's prescription: A disruptive solution for health care.* New York: McGraw-Hill.

30 Goulis, D. G., Giaglis, G. D., Boren, S. A., Lekka, I., Bontis, E., Balas, E. A., . . . Avramides, A. (2004). Effectiveness of home-centered care through telemedicine applications for overweight and obese patients: A randomized controlled trial. *International Journal of Obesity, 28,* 1391-98.

31 Goulis, D. G., Giaglis, G. D., Boren, S. A., Lekka, I., Bontis, E., Balas, E. A., . . . Avramides, A. (2004). Effectiveness of home-centered care through telemedicine applications for overweight and obese patients: A randomized controlled trial. *International Journal of Obesity, 28,* 1391-98.

32 Johnson, A., Gorman, M., Coulehan, N., Lewis, C., Baker, F., & Rader, J. (2001). Interactive videoconferencing improves

nutrition intervention in a rural population. *Journal of the American Diabetic Association, 101*(2), 173.

33 Johnson, A., Gorman, M., Coulehan, N., Lewis, C., Baker, F., & Rader, J. (2001). Interactive videoconferencing improves nutrition intervention in a rural population. *Journal of the American Diabetic Association, 101*(2), 173.

34 Johnson, A., Gorman, M., Coulehan, N., Lewis, C., Baker, F., & Rader, J. (2001). Interactive videoconferencing improves nutrition intervention in a rural population. *Journal of the American Diabetic Association, 101*(2), 173.

35 Johnson, A., Gorman, M., Coulehan, N., Lewis, C., Baker, F., & Rader, J. (2001). Interactive videoconferencing improves nutrition intervention in a rural population. *Journal of the American Diabetic Association, 101*(2), 173.

36 Cline, A. D., & Wong, M. (1999). New frontiers in using telemedicine for nutrition intervention. *Journal of the American Diabetes Association, 99*(11), 1442.

37 Cline, A. D., & Wong, M. (1999). New frontiers in using telemedicine for nutrition intervention. *Journal of the American Diabetes Association, 99*(11), 1442.

38 Cline, A. D., & Wong, M. (1999). New frontiers in using telemedicine for nutrition intervention. *Journal of the American Diabetes Association, 99*(11), 1442.

39 Cline, A. D., & Wong, M. (1999). New frontiers in using telemedicine for nutrition intervention. *Journal of the American Diabetes Association, 99*(11), 1442.

40 Koroušić Seljak, B. (2010). Web-based eHealth applications with reference to food composition data. *European Journal of Clinical Nutrition, 64*, S121–S127.

41 Koroušić Seljak, B. (2010). Web-based eHealth applications with reference to food composition data. *European Journal of Clinical Nutrition, 64*, S121–S127.

42 Izquierdo, R. E., Knudson, P. E., Meyer, S., Kearns, J., Ploutz-Snyder, R., & Weinstock, R. S., A comparison of diabetes education administered through telemedicine versus in person. *Diabetes Care, 26*(4), 1002.

43 Izquierdo, R. E., Knudson, P. E., Meyer, S., Kearns, J., Ploutz-Snyder, R., & Weinstock, R. S., A comparison of diabetes education administered through telemedicine versus in person. *Diabetes Care, 26*(4), 1002.

44 Rossi, M. C. E., Nicolucci, A., Di Bartolo, P., Bruttomesso, D., Girelli, A., Amputia, F. J., . . . Vespasiani, G. (2010). Diabetes Interactive Diary: A new telemedicine system enabling flexible diet and insulin therapy while improving quality of life. *Diabetes Care, 33*(1), 109.

45 Rossi, M. C. E., Nicolucci, A., Di Bartolo, P., Bruttomesso, D., Girelli, A., Amputia, F. J., . . . Vespasiani, G. (2010). Diabetes Interactive Diary: A new telemedicine system enabling flexible diet and insulin therapy while improving quality of life. *Diabetes Care, 33*(1), 109.

46 Rossi, M. C. E., Nicolucci, A., Di Bartolo, P., Bruttomesso, D., Girelli, A., Amputia, F. J., . . . Vespasiani, G. (2010). Diabetes Interactive Diary: A new telemedicine system enabling flexible diet and insulin therapy while improving quality of life. *Diabetes Care, 33*(1), 109.

47 Rossi, M. C. E., Nicolucci, A., Di Bartolo, P., Bruttomesso, D., Girelli, A., Amputia, F. J., . . . Vespasiani, G. (2010). Diabetes Interactive Diary: A new telemedicine system enabling flexible diet and insulin therapy while improving quality of life. *Diabetes Care, 33*(1), 109.

48 Trief, P. M., Teresi, J. A., Izquierdo, R., Morin, P. C., Goland, R., Field, L., . . . Ruth, S. (2007). *Psychosocial outcomes of telemedicine case management for elderly patients with diabetes, 30*(5), 1266.

49 Trief, P. M., Teresi, J. A., Izquierdo, R., Morin, P. C., Goland, R., Field, L., . . . Ruth, S. (2007). *Psychosocial outcomes of telemedicine case management for elderly patients with diabetes, 30*(5), 1266.

50 Trief, P. M., Teresi, J. A., Izquierdo, R., Morin, P. C., Goland, R., Field, L., . . . Ruth, S. (2007). *Psychosocial outcomes of telemedicine case management for elderly patients with diabetes, 30*(5), 1266.

51 Koroušić Seljak, B. (2010). Web-based eHealth applications with reference to food composition data. *European Journal of Clinical Nutrition, 64*, S121–S127.

52 University of New Mexico, Project ECHO website, http://echo.unm.edu.

53 Lazarte, C., Encinas, M. E., Alegre, C., & Granfeldt, Y. (2012). Validation of digital photographs, as a tool in 24-h recall, for the improvement of dietary assessment among rural populations in developing countries. *Nutrition Journal, 11*, 61.

54 Chung, L. M., & Chung, J. W. (2010). Tele-dietetics with food images as dietary intake record in nutrition assessment. *Telemedicine and e-Health, 16*(6), 691–98.

55 Koroušić Seljak, B. (2010). Web-based eHealth applications with reference to food composition data. *European Journal of Clinical Nutrition, 64*, S121–S127.

56 Kerr, D. A., Pollard, C. M., Howat, P., Delp, E. J., Pickering, M., Kerr, K. R., . . . Boushey, C. J. (2012). Connecting Health and Technology (CHAT): Protocol of a randomized controlled trial to improve nutrition behaviours using mobile devices and tailored text messages in young adults. *Nutrition Journal, 12*, 477.

57 Edworthy, S. M. (2001). Telemedicine in developing countries. *British Medical Journal, 323*, 7312, 524.

58 Nimmon, L., Poureslami, I., & Fitzgerald, J. M. (2012). What counts as cultural competency in telehealth interventions? A call for new directions. *Journal of Telemedicine and Telecare, 18*, 425–26.

59 Lugh, N. E. (2006). Global health care—bridging the gap. *Journal of Telemedicine and Telecare, 12*(3), 109.

60 Lugh, N. E. (2006). Global health care—bridging the gap. *Journal of Telemedicine and Telecare, 12*(3), 109.

61 Mupela, E. N., Mustarde, P., & Jones, H. L. (2011). Telemedicine in primary health: The virtual doctor project Zambia. *Philosophy, Ethics, and Humanities in Medicine, 6*, 9.

62 Mupela, E. N., Mustarde, P., & Jones, H. L. (2011). Telemedicine in primary health: The virtual doctor project Zambia. *Philosophy, Ethics, and Humanities in Medicine, 6*, 9.

63 Kruger, C., & Niemi, M. (2012). A telemedicine network to support paediatric care in small hospitals in rural Tanzania. *Journal of Telemedicine and Telecare, 18*, 59-62.

64 Kruger, C., & Niemi, M. (2012). A telemedicine network to support paediatric care in small hospitals in rural Tanzania. *Journal of Telemedicine and Telecare, 18*, 59-62.

65 Ignatius, E., Makela, K., Happonen, R-P., & Perala, S. (2006). Teledentistry in dental specialist education in Finland. *Journal of Telemedicine and Telecare, 12*(Suppl. 3), S3:46-49.

66 Ignatius, E., Makela, K., Happonen, R-P., & Perala, S. (2006). Teledentistry in dental specialist education in Finland. *Journal of Telemedicine and Telecare, 12*(Suppl. 3), S3:46-49.

67 Zurovac, D., Sudoi, R. K., Akhwale, W. S., Ndiritu, M., Hamer, D. H., Rowe, A. K., & Snow, R. W. (2011). The effect of mobile phone text-message reminders on Kenyan health workers' adherence to malaria treatment guidelines: A cluster randomised trial. *Lancet, 378*, 795-803.

68 Zurovac, D., Sudoi, R. K., Akhwale, W. S., Ndiritu, M., Hamer, D. H., Rowe, A. K., & Snow, R. W. (2011). The effect of mobile phone text-message reminders on Kenyan health workers' adherence to malaria treatment guidelines: A cluster randomised trial. *Lancet, 378*, 795-803.

69 Zurovac, D., Sudoi, R. K., Akhwale, W. S., Ndiritu, M., Hamer, D. H., Rowe, A. K., & Snow, R. W. (2011). The effect of mobile phone text-message reminders on Kenyan health workers' adherence to malaria treatment guidelines: A cluster randomised trial. *Lancet, 378*, 795-803.

70 Whitten, P., Holtz, B., & Nguyen, L. (2010). Keys to a successful and sustainable telemedicine program. *International Journal of Technology Assessment in Health Care, 26*(2), 211-16.

71 Kruger, C., & Niemi, M. (2012). A telemedicine network to support paediatric care in small hospitals in rural Tanzania. *Journal of Telemedicine and Telecare, 18*, 59-62.

72 Yellowlees, P. M. (2005). Successfully developing a telemedicine system. *Journal of Telemedicine and Telecare, 11*, 331-35.

73 Whittaker, S. L., Adkins, S., Phillips, R., Jones, J., Horsley, M. A., & Kelley, G. (2004). Success factors in the long-term sustainability of a telediabetes programme. *Journal of Telemedicine and Telecare, 10*(2), 84.

74 Yellowlees, P. M. (2005). Successfully developing a telemedicine system. *Journal of Telemedicine and Telecare, 11*, 331-35.

75 Institute of Medicine. (1996). *Telemedicine: A guide to assessing telecommunications in health care*. Washington, DC: National Academy Press.

Millennium Development Goals and Targets

In 2000, members of the United Nations (UN) established the eight Millennium Development Goals (MDGs) at the Millennium Summit of the United Nations (UN). They were designed to guide nations and aid organizations to reduce disparities in the world by the year 2015. Each goal is divided into more specific targets with benchmarks for progress. Following are the MDGs and their targets.

Goal 1: Eradicate Extreme Poverty and Hunger

Target 1.A: Halve, between 1990 and 2015, the proportion of people whose income is less than $1.25 a day

- The target of reducing extreme poverty rates by half was met five years ahead of the 2015 deadline.
- The global poverty rate at $1.25 a day fell in 2010 to less than half the 1990 rate. 700 million fewer people lived in conditions of extreme poverty in 2010 than in 1990. However, at the global level 1.2 billion people are still living in extreme poverty.

Target 1.B: Achieve full and productive employment and decent work for all, including women and young people

- Globally, 384 million workers lived below the $1.25 a day poverty line in 2011—a reduction of 294 million since 2001.

- The gender gap in employment persists, with a 24.8 percentage point difference between men and women in the employment-to-population ratio in 2012.

Target 1.C: Halve, between 1990 and 2015, the proportion of people who suffer from hunger

- The hunger reduction target is within reach by 2015.
- Globally, about 870 million people are estimated to be undernourished.
- More than 100 million children under age 5 are still undernourished and underweight.

Goal 2: Achieve Universal Primary Education

Target 2.A: Ensure that, by 2015, children everywhere, boys and girls alike, will be able to complete a full course of primary schooling

- Enrollment in primary education in developing regions reached 90% in 2010, up from 82% in 1999, which means more kids than ever are attending primary school.
- In 2011, 57 million children of primary school age were out of school.
- Even as countries with the toughest challenges have made large strides, progress on primary school enrolment has

slowed. Between 2008 and 2011, the number of out-of-school children of primary age fell by only 3 million.

- Globally, 123 million youth (aged 15 to 24) lack basic reading and writing skills. 61% of them are young women.

- Gender gaps in youth literacy rates are also narrowing. Globally, there were 95 literate young women for every 100 young men in 2010, compared with 90 women in 1990.

Goal 3: Promote Gender Equality and Empower Women

Target 3.A: Eliminate gender disparity in primary and secondary education, preferably by 2005, and in all levels of education no later than 2015

- The world has achieved equality in primary education between girls and boys, but only 2 out of 130 countries have achieved that target at all levels of education.

- Globally, 40 out of every 100 wage-earning jobs in the non-agricultural sector were held by women in 2011. This is a significant improvement since 1990.

- In many countries, gender inequality persists and women continue to face discrimination in access to education, work and economic assets, and participation in government. For example, in every developing region, women tend to hold less secure jobs than men, with fewer social benefits.

- Violence against women continues to undermine efforts to reach all goals.

- Poverty is a major barrier to secondary education, especially among older girls.

- Women are largely relegated to more vulnerable forms of employment.

Goal 4: Reduce Child Mortality

Target 4.A: Reduce by two-thirds, between 1990 and 2015, the under-five mortality rate

- Despite population growth, the number of deaths in children under five worldwide declined from 12.4 million in 1990 to 6.9 million in 2011, which translates into about 14,000 fewer children dying each day.

- Since 2000, measles vaccines have averted over 10 million deaths.

- Despite determined global progress in reducing child deaths, an increasing proportion of child deaths are in sub-Saharan Africa where 1 in nine children die before the age of five and in Southern Asia where 1 in 16 die before age five.

- As the rate of under-five deaths overall declines, the proportion that occurs during the first month after birth is increasing.

- Children born into poverty are almost twice as likely to die before the age of five as those from wealthier families.

- Children of educated mothers—even mothers with only primary schooling—are more likely to survive than children of mothers with no education.

Goal 5: Improve Maternal Health

Target 5.A: Reduce by three-quarters the maternal mortality ratio

- Maternal mortality has nearly halved since 1990. An estimated 287,000 maternal deaths occurred in 2010 worldwide, a decline of 47% from 1990. All regions have made progress but accelerated interventions are required in order to meet the target.

- In Eastern Asia, Northern Africa, and Southern Asia, maternal mortality has declined by around two-thirds.

- Nearly 50 million babies worldwide are delivered without skilled care.

- The maternal mortality ratio in developing regions is still 15 times higher than in the developed regions.

- The rural–urban gap in skilled care during childbirth has narrowed.

Target 5.B: Achieve universal access to reproductive health

- More women are receiving antenatal care. In developing regions, antenatal care increased from 63% in 1990 to 81% in 2011.

- Only half of women in developing regions receive the recommended amount of health care they need.

- Fewer teens are having children in most developing regions, but progress has slowed.
- The large increase in contraceptive use in the 1990s was not matched in the 2000s.
- The need for family planning is slowly being met for more women, but demand is increasing at a rapid pace.
- Official Development Assistance for reproductive health care and family planning remains low.

Goal 6: Combat HIV/AIDS, Malaria, and Other Diseases

Target 6.A: Have halted by 2015 and begun to reverse the spread of HIV/AIDS

- New HIV infections continue to decline in most regions.
- More people than ever are living with HIV due to fewer AIDS-related deaths and the continued large number of new infections with 2.5 million people newly infected each year.
- Comprehensive knowledge of HIV transmission remains low among young people, along with condom use.
- More orphaned children are now in school due to expanded efforts to mitigate the impact of AIDS.

Target 6.B: Achieve, by 2010, universal access to treatment for HIV/AIDS for all those who need it

- While the target was missed by 2011, access to treatment for people living with HIV increased in all regions.
- At the end of 2011, 8 million people were receiving antiretroviral therapy for HIV. This total constitutes an increase of over 1.4 million people from December 2010.
- By the end of 2011, 11 countries had achieved universal access to antiretroviral therapy.

Target 6.C: Have halted by 2015 and begun to reverse the incidence of malaria and other major diseases

- The global estimated incidence of malaria has decreased by 17% since 2000, and malaria-specific mortality rates by 25%.

- In the decade since 2000, 1.1 million deaths from malaria were averted.
- Countries with improved access to malaria control interventions saw child mortality rates fall by about 20%.
- Thanks to increased funding, more children are sleeping under insecticide-treated bed nets in sub-Saharan Africa.
- Treatment for tuberculosis saved some 20 million lives between 1995 and 2011.

Goal 7: Ensure Environmental Sustainability

Target 7.A: Integrate the principles of sustainable development into country policies and programmes and reverse the loss of environmental resources

- Forests are a safety net for the poor, but they continue to disappear at an alarming rate.
- Of all developing regions, South America and Africa saw the largest net losses of forest areas between 2000 and 2010.
- Global emissions of carbon dioxide (CO_2) have increased by more than 46% since 1990.
- In the 25 years since the adoption of the Montreal Protocol on Substances that Deplete the Ozone Layer, there has been a reduction of over 98% in the consumption of ozone-depleting substances.
- At Rio+20, the United Nations Conference on Sustainable Development, world leaders approved an agreement entitled "The Future We Want," and more than $513 billion was pledged toward sustainable development initiatives.

Target 7.B: Reduce biodiversity loss, achieving, by 2010, a significant reduction in the rate of loss

- More areas of the earth's surface are protected. Since 1990, protected areas have increased in number by 58%.
- Growth in protected areas varies across countries and territories and not all protected areas cover key biodiversity sites.
- By 2010, protected areas covered 12.7% of the world's land area but only 1.6% of total ocean area.

Target 7.C: Halve, by 2015, the proportion of the population without sustainable access to safe drinking water and basic sanitation

- The world has met the target of halving the proportion of people without access to improved sources of water, five years ahead of schedule.

- Between 1990 and 2010, more than two billion people gained access to improved drinking water sources.

- The proportion of people using an improved water source rose from 76% in 1990 to 89% in 2010.

- Over 40% of all people without improved drinking water live in sub-Saharan Africa.

- In 2011, 768 million people remained without access to an improved source of drinking water.

- Over 240,000 people a day gained access to improved sanitation facilities from 1990 to 2011.

- Despite progress, 2.5 billion in developing countries still lack access to improved sanitation facilities.

Target 7.D: Achieve, by 2020, a significant improvement in the lives of at least 100 million slum dwellers

- The target was met well in advance of the 2020 deadline.

- The share of urban slum residents in the developing world declined from 39% in 2000 to 33% in 2012. More than 200 million of these people gained access to improved water sources, improved sanitation facilities, or durable or less crowded housing, thereby exceeding the MDG target.

- 863 million people are estimated to be living in slums in 2012 compared to 650 million in 1990 and 760 million in 2000.

Goal 8: Develop a Global Partnership for Development

Target 8.A: Develop further an open, rule-based, predictable, non-discriminatory trading and financial system

- Despite the pledges by G20 (Group of 20 Finance Ministers and Central Bank Governors) members to resist protectionist measures initiated as a result of the global financial crisis, only a small percentage of trade restrictions introduced since the end of 2008 have been eliminated. The protectionist measures taken so far have affected almost 3% of global trade.

Target 8.B: Address the special needs of least developed countries

- Tariffs imposed by developed countries on products from developing countries have remained largely unchanged since 2004, except for agricultural products.

- Bilateral aid to sub-Saharan Africa fell by almost 1% in 2011.

- There has been some success of debt relief initiatives reducing the external debt of heavily indebted poor countries (HIPCs), but 20 developing countries remain at high risk of debt distress.

Target 8.C: Address the special needs of landlocked developing countries and small island developing States

- Aid to landlocked developing countries fell in 2010 for the first time in a decade, while aid to small island developing States increased substantially.

Target 8.D: Deal comprehensively with the debt problems of developing countries

- At this time, it appears developing countries weathered the 2009 economic downtown and in 2011 the debt to GDP ratio decreased for many developing countries. Vulnerabilities remain. Expected slower growth in 2012 and 2013 may weaken debt ratios.

Target 8.E: In cooperation with pharmaceutical companies, provide access to affordable essential drugs in developing countries

- Resources available for providing essential medicines through some disease-specific global health funds increased in 2011, despite the global economic downturn.

- There has been little improvement in recent years in improving availability and affordability of essential medicines in developing countries.

Target 8.F: In cooperation with the private sector, make available benefits of new technologies, especially information and communications

- 74% of inhabitants of developed countries are Internet users, compared with only 26% of inhabitants in developing countries.

- The number of mobile cellular subscriptions worldwide by the end of 2011 reached 6 billion.

Selected *Healthy People 2020* Objectives

The U.S. Department of Health and Human Services publishes the Healthy People (HP) objectives decennially based on the most pressing health problems in the United States. The four overarching categories are general health status, health-related quality of life and well-being, determinants of health, and disparities. *Healthy People 2020* topics include Nutrition and Weight Status (NWS), Physical Activity (PA), Early and Middle Childhood (EMC), and Heart Disease and Stroke (HDS); each topic includes multiple objectives to be reached by 2020. The Healthy People objectives also include consumer information, clinical strategies, and evidence-based resources for public health policy interventions. The following objectives are some of the ones addressed and identified in this book. The complete set of objectives, along with baseline and target figures, target-setting methods, data sources, and further resources, is available at the Healthy People website.

Nutrition and Weight Status Objectives

Healthier Food Access

NWS-1   Increase the number of States with nutrition standards for foods and beverages provided to preschool-aged children in child care

NWS-2   Increase the proportion of schools that offer nutritious foods and beverages outside of school meals

NWS-2.1   Increase the proportion of schools that do not sell or offer calorically sweetened beverages to students

NWS-2.2   Increase the proportion of school districts that require schools to make fruits or vegetables available whenever other food is offered or sold

NWS-3   Increase the number of States that have State-level policies that incentivize food retail outlets to provide foods that are encouraged by the Dietary Guidelines for Americans

NWS-4   (Developmental) Increase the proportion of Americans who have access to a food retail outlet that sells a variety of foods that are encouraged by the Dietary Guidelines for Americans

Health Care and Worksite Settings

NWS-5   Increase the proportion of primary care physicians who regularly measure the body mass index of their patients

NWS-5.1   Increase the proportion of primary care physicians who regularly assess body mass index (BMI) in their adult patients

NWS-5.2   Increase the proportion of primary care physicians who regularly assess body mass index (BMI) for age and sex in their child or adolescent patients

NWS-6   Increase the proportion of physician office visits that include counseling or education related to nutrition or weight

NWS-6.1   Increase the proportion of physician office visits made by patients with a diagnosis of cardiovascular disease, diabetes, or hyperlipidemia that include counseling or education related to diet or nutrition

NWS-6.2   Increase the proportion of physician office visits made by adult patients who are obese that include counseling or education related to weight reduction, nutrition, or physical activity

NWS-6.3   Increase the proportion of physician visits made by all child or adult patients that include counseling about nutrition or diet

NWS-7   (Developmental) Increase the proportion of worksites that offer nutrition or weight management classes or counseling

Weight Status

NWS-8   Increase the proportion of adults who are at a healthy weight

NWS-9   Reduce the proportion of adults who are obese

NWS-10   Reduce the proportion of children and adolescents who are considered obese

NWS-10.1   Reduce the proportion of children aged 2 to 5 years who are considered obese

NWS-10.2   Reduce the proportion of children aged 6 to 11 years who are considered obese

NWS-10.3   Reduce the proportion of adolescents aged 12 to 19 years who are considered obese

NWS-10.4   Reduce the proportion of children and adolescents aged 2 to 19 years who are considered obese

NWS-11   (Developmental)   Prevent   inappropriate weight gain in youth and adults

NWS-11.1   (Developmental) Prevent inappropriate weight gain in children aged 2 to 5 years

NWS-11.2   (Developmental) Prevent inappropriate weight gain in children aged 6 to 11 years

NWS-11.3   (Developmental) Prevent inappropriate weight gain in adolescents aged 12 to 19 years

NWS-11.4   (Developmental) Prevent inappropriate weight gain in children and adolescents aged 2 to 19 years

NWS-11.5   (Developmental) Prevent inappropriate weight gain in adults aged 20 years and older

Food Insecurity

NWS-12   Eliminate very low food security among children

NWS-13   Reduce household food insecurity and in doing so reduce hunger

Food and Nutrient Consumption

NWS-14   Increase the contribution of fruits to the diets of the population aged 2 years and older

NWS-15   Increase the variety and contribution of vegetables to the diets of the population aged 2 years and older

NWS-15.1   Increase the contribution of total vegetables to the diets of the population aged 2 years and older

NWS-15.2   Increase the contribution of dark green vegetables, orange vegetables, and legumes to the diets of the population aged 2 years and older

NWS-16   Increase the contribution of whole grains to the diets of the population aged 2 years and older

NWS-17   Reduce consumption of calories from solid fats and added sugars in the population aged 2 years and older

NWS-17.1   Reduce consumption of calories from solid fats

NWS-17.2   Reduce consumption of calories from added sugars

NWS-17.3   Reduce consumption of calories from solid fats and added sugars

NWS-18   Reduce consumption of saturated fat in the population aged 2 years and older

NWS-19   Reduce consumption of sodium in the population aged 2 years and older

NWS-20   Increase consumption of calcium in the population aged 2 years and older

Iron Deficiency

NWS-21   Reduce iron deficiency among young children and females of childbearing age

NWS-21.1   Reduce iron deficiency among children aged 1 to 2 years

NWS-21.2   Reduce iron deficiency among children aged 3 to 4 years

NWS-21.3   Reduce iron deficiency among females aged 12 to 49 years

NWS-22   Reduce iron deficiency among pregnant females

Heart Disease and Stroke

HDS-1   (Developmental) Increase overall cardiovascular health in the U.S. population

HDS-2   Reduce coronary heart disease deaths

HDS-3   Reduce stroke deaths

HDS-4   Increase the proportion of adults who have had their blood pressure measured within the preceding 2 years and can state whether their blood pressure was normal or high

HDS-5   Reduce the proportion of persons in the population with hypertension

HDS-5.1   Reduce the proportion of adults with hypertension

HDS-5.2   Reduce the proportion of children and adolescents with hypertension

HDS-6   Increase the proportion of adults who have had their blood cholesterol checked within the preceding 5 years

HDS-7   Reduce the proportion of adults with high total blood cholesterol levels

HDS-8   Reduce the mean total blood cholesterol levels among adults

HDS-20   (Developmental) Increase the proportion of adults with coronary heart disease or stroke who have their low-density lipoprotein (LDL) cholesterol level at or below recommended levels

HDS-20.1   (Developmental) Increase the proportion of adults with coronary heart disease who have their low-density lipoprotein (LDL) cholesterol at or below recommended levels

HDS-20.2   (Developmental) Increase the proportion of adults who have had a stroke who have their low-density lipoprotein (LDL) cholesterol at or below recommended levels

Physical Activity

PA-1   Reduce the proportion of adults who engage in no leisure-time physical activity

PA-2   Increase the proportion of adults who meet current Federal physical activity guidelines for aerobic physical activity and for muscle-strengthening activity

PA-2.1   Increase the proportion of adults who engage in aerobic physical activity of at least moderate intensity for at least 150 minutes/week, or 75 minutes/week of vigorous intensity, or an equivalent combination

PA-2.2   Increase the proportion of adults who engage in aerobic physical activity of at least moderate intensity for more than 300 minutes/week, or more than 150 minutes/week of vigorous intensity, or an equivalent combination

PA-2.3   Increase the proportion of adults who perform muscle-strengthening activities on 2 or more days of the week

PA-2.4   Increase the proportion of adults who meet the objectives for aerobic physical activity and for muscle-strengthening activity

PA-4   Increase the proportion of the Nation's public and private schools that require daily physical education for all students

PA-4.1   Increase the proportion of the Nation's public and private elementary schools that require daily physical education for all students

PA-4.2   Increase the proportion of the Nation's public and private middle and junior high schools that require daily physical education for all students

PA-4.3   Increase the proportion of the Nation's public and private senior high schools that require daily physical education for all students

PA-5   Increase the proportion of adolescents who participate in daily school physical education

PA-6   Increase regularly scheduled elementary school recess in the United States

PA-6.1   Increase the number of States that require regularly scheduled elementary school recess

PA-6.2 Increase the proportion of school districts that require regularly scheduled elementary school recess

PA-8 Increase the proportion of children and adolescents who do not exceed recommended limits for screen time

PA-8.1 Increase the proportion of children aged 0 to 2 years who view no television or videos on an average weekday

PA-8.2 Increase the proportion of children and adolescents aged 2 years through 12th grade who view television, videos, or play video games for no more than 2 hours a day

PA-8.2.1 Increase the proportion of children aged 2 to 5 years who view television, videos, or play video games for no more than 2 hours a day

PA-8.2.2 Increase the proportion of children and adolescents aged 6 to 14 years who view television, videos, or play video games for no more than 2 hours a day

PA-8.2.3 Increase the proportion of adolescents in grades 9 through 12 who view television, videos, or play video games for no more than 2 hours a day

PA-8.3 Increase the proportion of children and adolescents aged 2 years to 12th grade who use a computer or play computer games outside of school (for nonschool work) for no more than 2 hours a day

PA-8.3.1 Increase the proportion of children aged 2 to 5 years who use a computer or play computer games outside of school (for nonschool work) for no more than 2 hours a day

PA-8.3.2 Increase the proportion of children and adolescents aged 6 to 14 years who use a computer or play computer games outside of school (for nonschool work) for no more than 2 hours a day

PA-8.3.3 Increase the proportion of adolescents in grades 9 through 12 who use a computer or play computer games outside of school (for nonschool work) for no more than 2 hours a day

PA-13 (Developmental) Increase the proportion of trips made by walking

PA-13.1 (Developmental) Increase the proportion of trips of 1 mile or less made by walking by adults aged 18 years and older

PA-13.2 (Developmental) Increase the proportion of trips of 1 mile or less made to school by walking by children and adolescents aged 5 to 15 years

Early and Middle Childhood

EMC-4 Increase the proportion of elementary, middle, and senior high schools that require school health education

EMC-4.1 Increase the proportion of schools that require newly hired staff who teach required health education to have undergraduate or graduate training in health education

EMC-4.1.1 Increase the proportion of elementary schools that require newly hired staff who teach required health education to have undergraduate or graduate training in health education

EMC-4.1.2 Increase the proportion of middle schools that require newly hired staff who teach required health education to have undergraduate or graduate training in health education

EMC-4.1.3 Increase the proportion of high schools that require newly hired staff who teach required health education to have undergraduate or graduate training in health education

EMC-4.2 Increase the proportion of schools that require newly hired staff who teach required health instruction to be certified, licensed, or endorsed by the State in health education

EMC-4.2.1 Increase the proportion of elementary schools that require newly hired staff who teach required health instruction to be certified, licensed, or endorsed by the State in health education

EMC-4.2.2 Increase the proportion of middle schools that require newly hired staff who teach required health instruction to be certified, licensed, or endorsed by the State in health education

EMC-4.2.3 Increase the proportion of high schools that require newly hired staff who teach required health instruction to be certified, licensed, or endorsed by the State in health education

EMC-4.3 Increase the proportion of schools that require cumulative instruction in health education that meet the U.S. National Health Education Standards for elementary, middle, and senior high schools

EMC-4.3.1 Increase the proportion of elementary schools that require cumulative instruction in health education that meet the U.S. National Health Education Standards for elementary, middle, and senior high schools

EMC-4.3.2   Increase the proportion of middle schools that require cumulative instruction in health education that meet the U.S. National Health Education Standards for elementary, middle, and senior high schools

EMC-4.3.3   Increase the proportion of high schools that require cumulative instruction in health education that meet the U.S. National Health Education Standards for elementary, middle, and senior high schools

EMC-4.4   Increase the proportion of required health education classes or courses with a teacher who has had professional development related to teaching personal and social skills for behavior change within the past 2 years

Maternal, Infant, and Child Health

MICH-1   Reduce the rate of fetal and infant deaths

MICH-1.1   Reduce the rate of fetal deaths at 20 or more weeks of gestation

MICH-1.2   Reduce the rate of fetal and infant deaths during perinatal period (28 weeks of gestation to 7 days after birth)

MICH-1.3   Reduce the rate of all infant deaths (within 1 year)

MICH-1.4   Reduce the rate of neonatal deaths (within the first 28 days of life)

MICH-1.5   Reduce the rate of postneonatal deaths (between 28 days and 1 year)

MICH-1.6   Reduce the rate of infant deaths related to birth defects (all birth defects)

MICH-1.7   Reduce the rate of infant deaths related to birth defects (congenital heart defects)

MICH-1.8   Reduce the rate of infant deaths from sudden infant death syndrome (SIDS)

MICH-1.9   Reduce the rate of infant deaths from sudden unexpected infant deaths (includes SIDS, Unknown Cause, Accidental Suffocation, and Strangulation in Bed)

Pregnancy Health and Behaviors

MICH-10   Increase the proportion of pregnant women who receive early and adequate prenatal care

MICH-10.1   Increase the proportion of pregnant women who receive prenatal care beginning in first trimester

MICH-10.2   Increase the proportion of pregnant women who receive early and adequate prenatal care

Preconception Health and Behaviors

MICH-14   Increase the proportion of women of child-bearing potential with intake of at least 400 µg of folic acid from fortified foods or dietary supplements

MICH-15   Reduce the proportion of women of child-bearing potential who have low red blood cell folate concentrations

Infant Care

MICH-21   Increase the proportion of infants who are breastfed

MICH-21.1   Increase the proportion of infants who are ever breastfed

MICH-21.2   Increase the proportion of infants who are breastfed at 6 months

MICH-21.3   Increase the proportion of infants who are breastfed at 1 year

MICH-21.4   Increase the proportion of infants who are breastfed exclusively through 3 months

MICH-21.5   Increase the proportion of infants who are breastfed exclusively through 6 months

MICH-22   Increase the proportion of employers that have worksite lactation support programs

MICH-23   Reduce the proportion of breastfed newborns who receive formula supplementation within the first 2 days of life

MICH-24   Increase the proportion of live births that occur in facilities that provide recommended care for lactating mothers and their babies

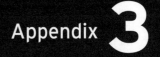

Core Competencies of Public Health Professionals

This book integrates the core competencies of public health. These competencies were revised in 2010 by the Council on Linkages between Academia and Public Health Practice, which represents universities, government agencies, and professional organizations relating to public health. The competencies are multidisciplinary skills that are referenced in this book to assist users in developing their confidence in public health settings. The core competencies "were designed for public health professionals at three different levels: Tier 1 (entry level), Tier 2 (supervisors and managers), and Tier 3 (senior managers and CEOs)." This book presents Tier 1 competencies. The full set and examples are available from the Public Health Foundation.

1. **Analytical/Assessment Skills:**

   Competency in this area is defined as possessing the ability to identify and utilize appropriate data resources to define, assess and understand the health status of populations, determinants of health and illness, factors contributing to health promotion and disease prevention, and factors influencing the use and success of health services.

   Necessary skills include:

   1. Identifies the health status of populations and their related determinants of health and illness
   2. Describes the characteristics of a population-based health problem

   3. Uses variables that measure public health conditions
   4. Uses methods and instruments for collecting valid and reliable quantitative and qualitative data
   5. Identifies sources of public health data and information
   6. Recognizes the integrity and comparability of data
   7. Identifies gaps in data sources
   8. Adheres to ethical principles in the collection, maintenance, use, and dissemination of data and information
   9. Describes the public health applications of quantitative and qualitative data
   10. Collects quantitative and qualitative community data
   11. Uses information technology to collect, store, and retrieve data
   12. Describes how data are used to address scientific, political, ethical, and social public health issues

2. **Policy Development/Program Planning Skills:**

   Competency in this area is defined as possessing the ability to identify and articulate the health, fiscal, administrative, legal, social and political implications of public health policies and regulations and translates such policies into public health organizational structure and programs.

Necessary skills include:

1. Gathers information relevant to specific public health policy issues
2. Describes how policy options can influence public health programs
3. Explains the expected outcomes of policy options
4. Gathers information that will inform policy decisions
5. Describes the public health laws and regulations governing public health programs
6. Participates in program planning processes
7. Identifies mechanisms to monitor and evaluate programs for their effectiveness and quality
8. Demonstrates the use of public health informatics practices and procedures
9. Applies strategies for continuous quality improvement
10. Incorporates policies and procedures into program plans and structures

3. **Communication Skills:**

Competency in this area is defined as possessing the ability to utilize multiple approaches to communicate with individuals and organizations to present accurate statistical, programmatic, and scientific information, facilitate community partnerships, and to promote the expression of diverse opinions and perspectives.

Necessary skills include:

1. Identifies the health literacy of populations served
2. Communicates in writing and orally, in person, and through electronic means, with linguistic and cultural proficiency
3. Solicits community-based input from individuals and organizations
4. Conveys public health information using a variety of approaches
5. Participates in the development of demographic, statistical, programmatic and scientific presentations
6. Applies communication and group dynamic strategies in interactions with individuals and groups

4. **Cultural Competency Skills:**

Competency in this area is defined as possessing the ability to understand the importance of diversity and the role of cultural, social and behavioral factors in the effective delivery of public health services and utilizes appropriate methods for adapting approaches to work with persons from diverse cultural, socioeconomic, educational, racial, ethnic and professional backgrounds and persons of all ages and lifestyles.

Necessary skills include:

1. Incorporates strategies for interacting with persons from diverse backgrounds
2. Recognizes the role of cultural, social, and behavioral factors in the accessibility, availability, acceptability, and delivery of public health services
3. Responds to diverse needs that are the result of cultural differences
4. Describes the dynamic forces that contribute to cultural diversity
5. Describes the need for a diverse public health workforce
6. Participates in the assessment of the cultural competence of the public health organization

5. **Community Dimension of Practice Skills:**

Competency in this area is defined as possessing the ability to understand the role of public and private organizations in the delivery of community health services and establishes and facilitates linkages with key stakeholder groups to promote the health of the population.

Necessary skills include:

1. Recognizes community linkages and relationships among multiple factors (or determinants) affecting health
2. Demonstrates the capacity to work in community-based participatory research efforts
3. Identifies stakeholders
4. Collaborates with community partners to promote the health of the population
5. Maintains partnerships with key stakeholders
6. Uses group processes to advance community involvement
7. Describes the role of governmental and non-governmental organizations in the delivery of community health services

8. Identifies community assets and resources

9. Gathers input from the community to inform the development of public health policy and programs

10. Informs the public about policies, programs, and resources

6. Basic Public Health Science Skills:

Competency in this area is defined as possessing the ability to understand the interaction of individuals, public health and healthcare systems within the context of the Essential Public Health Services, applies the basic public health sciences appropriately and in accordance with current relevant scientific evidence.

Necessary skills include:

1. Describes the scientific foundation of the field of public health

2. Identifies prominent events in the history of the public health profession

3. Relates public health science skills to the Core Public Health Functions and Ten Essential Services of Public Health

4. Identifies the basic public health sciences (all fields)

5. Describes the scientific evidence related to a public health issue, concern, or intervention

6. Retrieves scientific evidence from a variety of text and electronic sources

7. Discusses the limitations of research findings

8. Describes the laws, regulations, policies, and procedures for the ethical conduct of research

9. Partners with other public health professionals in building the scientific base of public health

7. Financial Planning and Management Skills:

Competency in this area is defined as possessing the ability to develop, manage, and evaluate public health programs, services, and budgets through the application of human relations strategies.

Necessary skills include:

1. Describes the local, state, and federal public health and healthcare systems

2. Describes the organizational structures, functions, and authorities of local, state, and federal public health agencies

3. Adheres to the organization's policies and procedures

4. Participates in the development of a programmatic budget

5. Operates programs within current and forecasted budget constraints

6. Identifies strategies for determining budget priorities based on federal, state, and local financial contributions

7. Reports program performance

8. Translates evaluation report information into program performance improvement action steps

9. Contributes to the preparation of proposals for funding from external sources

10. Applies basic human relations skills to internal collaborations, motivation of colleagues, and resolution of conflicts

11. Demonstrates public health informatics skills to improve program and business operations

12. Participates in the development of contracts and other agreements for the provision of services

13. Describes how cost-effectiveness, cost-benefit, and cost-utility analyses affect programmatic prioritization and decision making

8. Leadership and Systems Thinking Skills:

Competency in this area is defined as possessing the ability to create and promote an organizational culture of shared learning, values and vision based on ethical standards of professional practice.

Necessary skills include:

1. Incorporates ethical standards of practice as the basis of all interactions with organizations, communities, and individuals

2. Describes how public health operates within a larger system

3. Participates with stakeholders in identifying key public health values and a shared public health vision as guiding principles for community action

4. Identifies internal and external problems that may affect the delivery of Essential Public Health Services

5. Uses individual, team, and organizational learning opportunities for personal and professional development

6. Participates in mentoring and peer review or coaching opportunities

7. Participates in the measuring, reporting, and continuous improvement of organizational performance

8. Describes the impact of changes in the public health system, and larger social, political, economic environment on organizational practices

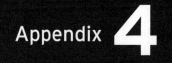

Resources

Academy of Nutrition and Dietetics	www.eatright.org
American Heart Association	www.heart.org
American Obesity Treatment Association	www.americanobesity.org
American Public Health Association	www.apha.org
Association of Schools and Programs of Public Health	www.aspph.org
Bellagio Conference Papers: The Nutrition Transition	www.cpc.unc.edu/projects/nutrans/research/bellagio/papers
Best Bones Forever	www.bestbonesforever.gov
Bill & Melinda Gates Foundation	www.gatesfoundation.org
Body Mass Index (BMI) Calculator	www.cdc.gov/healthyweight/assessing/bmi/adult_bmi/english_bmi_calculator/bmi_calculator.html
California Baby Behavior Campaign	www.cdph.ca.gov/programs/wicworks/Pages/WICCaliforniaBabyBehaviorCampaign.aspx
Centers for Disease Control and Prevention (CDC)	www.cdc.gov
CDC National Health and Nutrition Examination Survey (NHANES)	www.cdc.gov/NCHS/nhanes.htm
CDC Evaluation Steps (for public health efforts)	www.cdc.gov/eval/steps/index.htm
Centers for Medicare and Medicaid Services	http://cms.gov/
Chamber Maps	http://chambermaps.com/
Clinton Foundation	www.clintonfoundation.org
Commodity Supplemental Food Program	http://www.fns.usda.gov/csfp/commodity-supplemental-food-program-csfp
Feed the Future	www.feedthefuture.gov/about
Food and Agriculture Organization (FAO)	www.fao.org
Food and Nutrition Technical Assistance III Project	www.fantaproject.org
Hormone Health Network	www.hormone.org
International Confederation of Dietetic Associations	www.internationaldietetics.org
International Diabetes Federation	www.idf.org
International Food Policy Research Institute	www.ifpri.org
International Life Sciences Institute (ILSI)	www.ilsi.org

International Nutrition Foundation	www.inffoundation.org
International Union of Nutritional Sciences (IUNS)	www.iuns.org
Let's Move!	www.letsmove.gov
Johns Hopkins Bloomberg School of Public Health Center for a Livable Future	http://www.jhsph.edu/research/centers-and-institutes/johns-hopkins-center-for-a-livable-future
Millennium Development Goals	www.un.org/millenniumgoals/
National Center for Health Statistics (NCHS)	www.cdc.gov/nchs/
National Heart, Lung, and Blood Institute (NHLBI)	www.nhlbi.nih.gov
National Institutes of Health (NIH)	http://nih.gov/
National School Lunch Program (NSLP)	www.fns.usda.gov/slp
Pan American Health Organization (PAHO)	www.paho.org
Planning Guide for National Implementation of the Global Strategy for Infant and Young Child Feeding	www.who.int/maternal_child_adolescent/documents/9789241595193/en/
Public Health Foundation	www.phf.org
Robert Wood Johnson Foundation Center to Prevent Childhood Obesity	www.rwjf.org
Supplemental Nutrition Assistance Program (SNAP)	www.fns.usda.gov/snap/
Ten Steps to Breastfeeding Friendly Child Care Centers: Resource Kit	www.dhs.wisconsin.gov/publications/P0/P00022.pdf
The World Bank	www.worldbank.org
United Nations Children's Fund (UNICEF)	www.unicef.org
United Nations Standing Committee on Nutrition	www.unscn.org
U.S. Agency for International Development (USAID)	www.usaid.gov
U.S. Census Bureau: Maps & Data	www.census.gov/geo/maps-data/index.html
U.S. Department of Agriculture	http://usda.gov/wps/portal/usda/usdahome
U.S. Department of Health and Human Services	www.hhs.gov
U.S. Department of Health and Human Services, Office on Women's Health	www.womenshealth.gov
U.S. Peace Corps	www.peacecorps.gov
U.S. Geological Survey: Maps, Imagery, and Publications	www.usgs.gov/pubprod/maps.html
WHO. Vitamin and Mineral Nutrition Information System (VMNIS)	www.who.int/vmnis/en/index.html
Weight-control Information Network	www.win.niddk.nih.gov
World Food Programme	www.wfp.org
Women, Infants, and Children (WIC)	www.fns.usda.gov/wic/
World Health Organization (WHO)	www.who.int/en/
World Health Organization: Nutrition	www.who.int/nutrition/
World Health Organization: Global Strategy on Diet, Physical Activity and Health	www.who.int/dietphysicalactivity/en
World Vision International	www.wvi.org/wvi/wviweb.nsf
Yale Rudd Center for Food Policy and Obesity	http://yaleruddcenter.org/

Index